NUTRITIONAL ASSESSMENT

Seventh Edition

David C. Nieman, DrPH, FACSM
Appalachian State University,
North Carolina Research Campus

NUTRITIONAL ASSESSMENT, SEVENTH EDITION

3 4 5 6 7 8 9 BRP 21 20 19

ISBN 978-1-260-08448-1
MHID 1-260-08448-5

Cover Image: ©*liquidlibrary/PictureQuest;* ©*David C. Nieman*

To my loving wife, Cathy, who has supported me and shared her insights as a practicing dietitian throughout the writing process.

BRIEF CONTENTS

CONTENTS

CHAPTER 10

CLINICAL ASSESSMENT OF NUTRITIONAL STATUS   *319*

CHAPTER 11

COUNSELING THEORY AND TECHNIQUE   *336*

PREFACE

The leading causes of death are chronic, non-communicable diseases, including heart disease, stroke, cancer, and diabetes, which are and most often linked to dietary patterns. The continuing presence of nutrition-related disease makes it essential for health professionals to have the ability to determine the nutritional status of individuals. As defined by the Academy of Nutrition and Dietetics, nutritional assessment is "a systematic method for obtaining, verifying, and interpreting data needed to identify nutrition-related problems, their causes, and significance." In other words, nutritional assessment is critical to determine whether a person is at nutritional risk, the nutritional problem, and best strategy to monitor responses to nutrition- and lifestyle-based treatment. Nutritional assessment methods can be divided into anthropometric, biochemical, clinical, and dietary categories, and each is fully described in this textbook.

The Seventh Edition of *Nutritional Assessment* addresses these and many other topics, including computerized dietary analysis systems, national surveys of dietary intake and nutritional status, assessment techniques and standards for the hospitalized patient, nutritional assessment for the prevention of diseases such as coronary heart disease, osteoporosis, and diabetes. Proper counseling and clinical assessment techinques are also featured.

This extensively revised edition builds on the strengths of the previous six editions. Nearly all photos and graphs in this textbook have been updated, and the reference list for each chapter has been refreshed with essential, topical references. The appendices have been reorganized, with numerous tables added to provide current reference data important to the field of nutritional assessment.

This textbook was written for students of dietetics and public health nutrition, but is also intended to be a valuable reference for health professionals who work with patients who have diet-related medical problems.

CHANGES IN THE SEVENTH EDITION

Numerous revisions and additions to the Seventh Edition of *Nutritional Assessment* make it the most comprehensive and up-to-date textbook available on the subject. Included in this edition are extensive updates to nutrient intake recommendations, guidelines, and indices including the 2015–2020 Dietary Guidelines for Americans, Healthy Eating Index, American Heart Association's Cardiovascular Disease Metrics, Evidence-Based Guidelines for the Management of High Blood Pressure in Adults, and American College of Cardiology/American Heart Association practice guidelines on the treatment of blood cholesterol to reduce atherosclerotic cardiovascular risk in adults. Updated methods and standards for a wide variety of anthropometric, body composition, and malnutrition assessment procedures have also been added. Photos, graphs, tables, and references are updated throughout the entire textbook, while the appendices have been thoroughly reorganized and updated to provide the most current nutritional assessment standards and reference data.

Chapter 1 Introduction to Nutritional Assessment (Provides thorough introduction to Nutritional Assessment and Nutrition Care Process; explores definitions and concepts)

- Updated section on opportunities in nutrition assessment with current information provided on monitoring the incidence and prevalence of conditions such as diabetes, obesity, heart disease, cancer, and osteoporosis.

Chapter 2 Standards for Nutrient Intake (Reviews standards for nutrient intake)

- Detailed description of the five guidelines and 13 key recommendations of the 2015–2020 Dietary Guidelines for Americans.

- Updated information on the Healthy Eating Index, a review of the new Nutrition Facts label and most current standards for Daily Values, and a description of the "Choose Your Foods" system.

Chapter 3 Measuring Diet (Explores methods for measuring diet)

- New assessment activity on dietary screeners, and summary of nutrients and food components analyzed by the Diet History Questionnaire II.

Chapter 4 National Dietary and Nutrition Surveys (Reviews statistics on the trends in food availability)

- Revised data and graphs on food security and insecurity from the USDA.
- Updated tables summarize the major components of the continuous NHANES and the Total Diet Study.
- New graphs summarize nutrient intake information from food availability estimates and the NHANES What We Eat in America surveys, and current Behavioral Risk Factor Surveillance System Questionnaire (Appendix F).

Chapter 5 Computerized Dietary Analysis Systems (Reviews the use of computerized dietary analysis systems and provides guidelines for evaluation)

- Updated tables and information from the USDA Nutrient Database for Standard Reference and the USDA Food and Nutrient Database for Dietary Studies (FNDDS).
- A revised summary of databases maintained by the USDA, Nutrient Data Laboratory (NDL), and Agricultural Research Service (ARS).

Chapter 6 Anthropometry (Describes anthropometric techniques)

- This chapter has been extensively revised with the inclusion of new photos, current prevalence data for overweight and obesity in adults, children, and adolescents.
- Added information on the sagittal abdominal diameter measurement as an anthropometric index of visceral adiposity and a description of the American Body Composition Calculator (ABCC) (with a new, related assessment activity).
- Updated sections on segmental multi-frequency bioelectrical impedance (BIA) and dual-energy X-ray absorptiometry (DXA) testing for body composition and osteoporosis.
- Many new tables on body composition, bone mineral density, and anthropometric reference data in Appendices H through L.

Chapter 7 Assessment of the Hospitalized Patient (Provides a thorough description of methods to assess malnutrition)

- This chapter has also been completely revised, with a focus on current recommendations for the assessment of malnutrition using the Mini Nutritional Assessment Short Form (MNA-SF), Malnutrition University Screening Tool (MUST), Subjective Global Assessment (SGA), Nutritional Risk Screening (NRS), and the Simplified Nutritional Appetite Questionnaire (SNAQ).
- New sections have been added on the use of hand-grip strength testing to determine weakness and sarcopenia, arm anthropometry, the use of the Pediatric Nutrition Screening Tool (PNST), mental health and quality of life (QOL) testing, functional status assessment using activities of daily living (ADLs) and instrumental activities of daily living (IADLs), and guidelines for measuring energy expenditure using indirect calorimetry.

Chapter 8 Nutritional Assessment in Prevention and Treatment of Cardiovascular Disease (Relates nutrition to the prevention of disease)

- This chapter has also been completed revised, with emphasis placed on the American Heart Association's (AHA) cardiovascular disease metrics system for tracking key health factors and behaviors in children, adolescents, and adults. Current AHA diet and lifestyle recommendations are described in detail, with information provided for six tools to assess and monitor dietary patterns.
- Prevalence data on risk factors for heart disease and stroke have been updated with numerous new graphs and tables (also see new reference and trend tables in Appendix M).
- A detailed description of the American College of Cardiology (ACC) and AHA guidelines for the treatment of high blood cholesterol is provided, with a new related assessment activity. Screening guidelines for dyslipidemia in children and adolescents are detailed.
- Updated information is given for hypertension, with a focus on the current Evidence-Based Guideline for the Management of High Blood Pressure in Adults from the Eight Joint National Committee Panel (JNC8).
- The section on diabetes mellitus has been completely updated, with emphasis on risk factors and screening guidelines for diabetes mellitus in children, adolescents, and adults, and related medical nutrition therapy (MNT) recommendations.

Chapter 9 Biochemical Assessment of Nutritional Status (Interprets laboratory tests and reviews methods for assessing nutrient status)

- A new section has been added on using the complete blood count (CBC) to assess nutritional status and updated guidelines and graphs for assessment of vitamin D status.

Chapter 10 Clinical Assessment of Nutritional Status (Provides overview of clinical assessment of nutrition status)

- This chapter now includes the World Health Organization (WHO) clinical staging criteria for HIV/AIDS for adults and adolescents.
- Updated information on diagnostic criteria, signs and symptoms, and potential medical consequences for anorexia nervosa and bulimia nervosa.

Appendices

- Updated anthropometric, skinfold, body composition, and bone density reference and trend data are presented in Appendices H through L.
- Appendix M provides current reference and trend data for serum lipid and lipoprotein levels in adults.

NUTRITIONAL ASSESSMENT WEBSITE (www.mhhe.com/nieman7)

This website provides instructors with a convenient and authoritative online source for additional information and resources on nutritional assessment. It serves to update readers about new information and developments in the field of nutritional assessment as they become available. A password-protected test bank and PPT lecture outlines are also available.

FEATURES

Chapter Outline and Student Learning Outcomes

Each chapter begins with an outline of the chapter contents and set of student learning outcomes. Reading these before beginning the chapter gives the student an idea of the material to be covered and key concepts contained in the chapter, while serving as useful review tools when the student studies for exams.

Figures and Tables

There are more than 100 tables in the text, supplemented with over 150 graphs, illustrations, photographs, and nearly 70 text boxes. Figures in Chapter 4, for example, illustrate trends in food and nutrient intake based on data from the National Health and Nutrition Examination Survey and U.S. Department of Agriculture's monitoring of food available for consumption from the U.S. food supply. Chapters 6 and 7 contain numerous photographs illustrating the exact procedures involved in skinfold measurement and other anthropometric techniques used to assess nutritional status.

Summaries

A summary at the end of each chapter highlights all important chapter information and will be especially helpful when the student reviews for exams.

References

A complete list of up-to-date references is included at the end of each chapter. This list provides the student and instructor with extensive sources for continued study.

Assessment Activities

Most of the chapters end with two or three practical assessment activities to help the student better understand concepts presented in the chapter. For example, some activities involve the analysis of diet records using software on a personal computer, obtaining information on food composition from online databases, accessing nutritional monitoring data from government websites, practicing anthropometry, one-on-one dietary counseling, and interpreting serum lipid and lipoprotein results.

Appendices

Appendices A through F provide numerous recording forms and questionnaires used to measure diet intake at the individual and population level. Appendix G provides the CDC clinical growth charts for children and adolescents, including charts for infants and children from birth to two years of age. Anthropometric, skinfold, body composition, and bone density reference and trend data are presented in Appendices H through L. Appendix M gives reference and trend data for serum lipid and lipoprotein levels in adults. Appendix N contains a form for self-monitoring dietary intake, and Appendix O has a checklist for counseling competencies.

Glossary

Throughout the text, important terms are shown in bold-face type. Concise definitions for more than 360 terms can be found in the glossary.

McGraw-Hill Create™

Craft your teaching resources to match the way you teach! With McGraw-Hill Create, you can easily rearrange chapters, combine material from other content sources, and quickly upload content you have written like your course syllabus or teaching notes. Arrange your book to fit your teaching style. Experience how McGraw-Hill Create empowers you to teach *your* students *your* way.

ACKNOWLEDGMENTS

I would like to express my sincere gratitude to the editorial and production teams at McGraw-Hill Education—they have been highly professional and supportive throughout the entire writing process. I am particularly indebted to my wife, Cathy, for her encouragement, support, and patience.

INTRODUCTION TO NUTRITIONAL ASSESSMENT

STUDENT LEARNING OUTCOMES

After studying this chapter, the student will be able to:

1. Describe the factors that contributed to a change in the leading causes of death during the 20th century.
2. Name the leading causes of death in the United States in which diet plays a role.
3. Distinguish between nutritional screening and nutritional assessment.
4. Name the four methods used to collect nutritional assessment data.
5. Explain the Nutrition Care Process Model.
6. Discuss the role of nutritional assessment in the Nutrition Care Process.
7. Discuss the role of nutritional assessment in the prevention and treatment of disease.

INTRODUCTION

Throughout most of human history, agriculture has been a labor-intensive process with relatively small yields of a limited number of crops. Hunger, nutrient deficiency, and starvation were common, and infectious diseases were the leading causes of death. Beginning in the late 19th century and early 20th century, improvements in plant breeding, the mechanization of agriculture, and the widespread use of fertilizers and pesticides resulted in dramatic increases in crop yields per unit of land. Food became much more available and less expensive, and by the middle of the 20th century developed nations went from a dismal era of food scarcity to one of food excess. Nutrient deficiency diseases have become much less common and chronic diseases related to excess consumption of food, tobacco and alcohol use, and a lack of physical activity are now the leading causes of death and disability throughout the world. During the same time, improvements in sanitation, convenient access to safe drinking water, vaccine and antibiotic development, and improvements in health care have dramatically reduced the **incidence** and **prevalence** of infectious diseases and dramatically increased **life expectancy** in developed countries. However, many developing countries experience a double burden of death from chronic diseases and infectious diseases.[1,2]

These changes have resulted in an **epidemic** of chronic diseases, many of which are directly linked to excess consumption of high-fat foods and alcoholic beverages, inadequate consumption of foods high in complex carbohydrates and fiber, and a sedentary lifestyle. This situation, along with heightened public and professional interest in the role of nutrition in health and disease, has created an increased need for health professionals proficient in nutritional assessment. The ability to identify persons at nutritional risk, describe and label an existing nutrition problem, and then plan and implement a nutrition intervention addressing the nutrition problem has made nutritional assessment an essential element of health care and a necessary skill for health professionals concerned about making health care more cost-effective.

GOOD NUTRITION ESSENTIAL FOR HEALTH

Good nutrition is critical for the well-being of any society and to each individual within that society. The variety, quality, quantity, cost, and accessibility of food and the patterns of food consumption can profoundly affect health.

Scurvy, for example, was among the first diseases recognized as being caused by a nutritional deficiency. One of the earliest descriptions of scurvy was made in 1250 by French writer Joinville, who observed it among the troops of Louis IX at the siege of Cairo. When Vasco da Gama sailed to the East Indies around the Cape of Good Hope in 1497, more than 60% of his crew died of scurvy.[3] In 1747, James Lind, a British naval surgeon, conducted the first controlled human dietary experiment showing that consumption of citrus fruits cures scurvy.[4]

Deficiency Diseases Once Common

Up until the middle of the 20th century, scurvy and other **deficiency diseases,** such as **rickets, pellagra, beriberi, xerophthalmia,** and iodine-deficiency diseases such as **goiter** and **cretinism** (caused by inadequate dietary vitamin D, niacin, thiamin, vitamin A, and iodine, respectively), were commonly seen in the United States and throughout the world and posed a significant threat to human health.[3,4]

Infectious disease and malnutrition remain serious problems in developing nations. According to the World Health Organization, infectious diseases are responsible for 52% of deaths in children less than 5 years of age, and improved breast-feeding practices and nutrition interventions are needed to reduce deaths from infections and improve child survival.[5] Sanitation measures, improved health care, vaccine development, and mass immunization programs have dramatically reduced the incidence of infectious disease in developed nations. An abundant food supply, **fortification** of some foods with important nutrients, **enrichment** to replace certain nutrients lost in food processing, and better methods of determining the nutrient content of foods have made nutrient-deficiency diseases relatively uncommon in developed nations. Despite these gains, 5% of American households experience very low food security, meaning that the food intake of one or more household members was reduced and their eating patterns were disrupted at times during the year because the household lacked money.[6]

Chronic Diseases Now Epidemic

Despite the many advances of nutritional science, nutrition-related diseases not only continue to exist but also result in a heavy toll of disease and death. In recent decades, however, they have taken a form different from the nutrient-deficiency diseases common in the early 1900s. Diseases of dietary excess and imbalance now rank among the leading causes of illness and death in North America and play a prominent role in the epidemic of chronic disease that all nations are currently experiencing.[5] Table 1.1 ranks the 10 leading causes of death in the United States. Four of these are related directly to diet, including heart disease, cancer, stroke, and diabetes.[7]

Overweight and obesity prevalence has risen to high levels and contributes to risk for heart disease, certain types of cancer, and type 2 diabetes. In the United States, 71% of adults are overweight or obese (body mass index, or BMI, of 25 kg/m^2 and higher), and 38% are obese (BMI of 30 and higher). About one in five children (ages 6–11 years) and adolescents (ages 12–19 years) is considered obese, according to the National Center for Health Statistics.[8]

The continuing presence of nutrition-related disease makes it essential that health professionals be able to determine the nutritional status of individuals. Nutritional assessment is critical in determining whether a person is at nutritional risk, what the nutritional problem is, and

TABLE 1.1	**Leading Causes of Death, United States**	
Rank	**Cause of Death**	**% of all Deaths**
1*	**Heart Disease**	23.5
2*	**Cancer**	22.5
3	**COPD**	5.7
4	**Injuries**	5
5*	**Stroke**	5
6	**Alzheimer's disease**	3.3
7*	**Diabetes**	2.9
8	**Pneumonia/influenza**	2.2
9	**Kidney disease**	1.8
10	**Suicide**	1.6

Source: National Center for Health Statistics.

*Causes of death in which diet plays a role.

how best to treat it and to monitor the person's response to the treatment. Nutritional assessment is the first of the four steps in the Nutrition Care Process.[9–12]

NUTRITIONAL SCREENING AND ASSESSMENT

Nutritional screening can be defined as "a process to identify an individual who is malnourished or who is at risk for malnutrition to determine if a detailed nutrition assessment is indicated."[13] If nutritional screening identifies a person at nutritional risk, a more thorough assessment of the individual's nutritional status can be performed. Nutritional screening can be done by any member of the health-care team such as a dietitian, dietetic technician, dietary manager, nurse, or physician. Nutritional screening and how it fits into the nutritional care process are discussed in greater detail in Chapter 7, and examples of screening instruments are shown there.

Nutritional assessment is defined by the American Society for Parenteral and Enteral Nutrition as "a comprehensive approach to diagnosing nutrition problems that uses a combination of the following: medical, nutrition, and medication histories; physical examination; anthropometric measurement; and laboratory data."[13] The Academy of Nutrition and Dietetics defines nutritional assessment as "a systematic method for obtaining, verifying, and interpreting data needed to identify nutrition-related problems, their causes, and their significance."[9] It involves initial data collection and continuous reassessment and analysis of data, which are compared to certain criteria such as the Dietary Reference Intakes or other nutrient intake recommendations.[9]

Nutritional Assessment Methods

Four different methods are used to collect data used in assessing a person's nutritional status: anthropometric, biochemical or laboratory, clinical, and dietary. The reader may find the mnemonic "ABCD" helpful in remembering these four different methods.

Anthropometric Methods

Anthropometry is the measurement of the physical dimensions and gross composition of the body. Examples of anthropometry include measurements of height, weight, and head circumference and the use of measurements of **skinfold thickness, body density** (underwater weighing), **air-displacement plethysmography, magnetic resonance imaging,** and **bioelectrical impedance** to estimate the percentage of fat and lean tissue in the body. These results often are compared with standard values obtained from measurements of large numbers of subjects. Anthropometry will be covered in Chapters 6 and 7. At the end of most chapters are suggested exercises,

called assessment activities, that allow you to apply the concepts covered. In the assessment activities of Chapter 6, you will try your hand at skinfold measurements to estimate percent body fat and compare several methods of determining body composition.

Biochemical Methods

In nutritional assessment, biochemical or laboratory methods include measuring a nutrient or its metabolite in blood, feces, or urine or measuring a variety of other components in blood and other tissues that have a relationship to nutritional status. The quantity of **albumin** and other **serum proteins** frequently is regarded as an indicator of the body's protein status, and **hemoglobin** and serum ferritin levels reflect iron status. Serum lipid and lipoprotein levels, which are influenced by diet and other lifestyle factors, reflect coronary heart disease risk.

Biochemical methods are covered in Chapters 7 through 9. An assessment activity in Chapter 8 suggests that you have your blood drawn and tested at a clinical laboratory and compare your results with recommended values. Assessment activities in Chapters 7 and 9 guide you through the application of key concepts as you evaluate biochemical and other data from patient records.

Clinical Methods

The patient's personal and family history, medical and health history, and physical examination are clinical methods used to detect **signs** and **symptoms** of **malnutrition.** Symptoms are disease manifestations that the patient is usually aware of and often complains about. Signs are observations made by a qualified examiner during physical examination. Enlargement of the salivary glands and loss of tooth enamel are clinical signs of frequent vomiting sometimes seen in patients with bulimia nervosa. Examining a patient for loss of subcutaneous fat and muscle in the neck, shoulders, and upper arms, a clinical sign of inadequate calorie intake, is included in **Subjective Global Assessment,** a clinical approach for assessing nutritional status that relies on information collected by the clinician through observation and interviews at the patient's bedside. Clinical signs and symptoms in nutritional assessment will be discussed in Chapter 10.

Dietary Methods

Dietary methods generally involve surveys measuring the quantity of the individual foods and beverages consumed during the course of one to several days or assessing the pattern of food use during the previous several months. These can provide data on intake of nutrients or specific classes of foods. Chapters 2 through 4 cover dietary methods. One of the assessment activities in Chapter 3 involves collecting a 24-hour dietary recall from a classmate and analyzing his or her nutrient intake using food composition tables.

Included among dietary methods is the use of computers to analyze dietary intake. A number of online dietary and physical activity assessment tools are available, as are numerous software programs for computers that allow nutritionists and dietitians to quickly analyze the nutrient composition of dietary intake. These online systems and software programs vary widely in price and certain features, such as the number and types of different foods and nutrients that each contains. Chapter 5 covers selection and use of nutritional analysis software and online systems. The assessment activity in Chapter 5 involves computerized analysis of the 24-hour recall and 3-day food record collected as part of the assessment activities in Chapter 3.

Importance of Nutritional Assessment

The use of nutritional assessment to identify diet-related disease has increased in importance in recent years because of our greater knowledge of the relationship between nutrition and health and our expanded ability to alter the nutritional state.

Evidence related to the role of diet in maternal and child health indicates that well-nourished mothers produce healthier children.[15,16] Sufficient intake of energy and nutrients, including appropriate body weight before pregnancy and adequate weight gain during pregnancy, improves infant birth weight and reduces infant **morbidity** and **mortality.** Consequently, nutritional assessment has become an integral part of maternity care at the beginning of pregnancy and periodically throughout pregnancy and lactation.[15,17] Nutrition also can have a profound influence on health, affecting growth and development of infants, children, and adolescents; immunity against disease; morbidity and mortality from illness or surgery; and risk of such diseases as cancer, coronary heart disease, and diabetes.[17–19]

Interventions to alter a person's nutritional state can take many forms. In certain situations, nutrient mixes can be delivered into the stomach or small intestine through feeding tubes **(enteral nutrition)** or administered directly into veins **(parenteral nutrition)** to improve nutritional status. Thus, nutritional assessment is important in identifying persons at nutritional risk, in determining what type of nutrition intervention, if any, may be appropriate to alter nutritional status, and in monitoring the effects of nutrition intervention.

THE NUTRITION CARE PROCESS

The Nutrition Care Process (NCP) is "a systematic problem-solving method" in which dietetic practitioners use critical-thinking skills to make evidence-based decisions addressing the nutrition-related problems of those they serve, whether it be patients, clients, groups, or communities of any age or health condition (collectively referred to as "patients/clients").[9–12] Developed by the Academy of Nutrition and Dietetics (formerly known as the American Dietetic Association), the NCP establishes a consistent, *standardized process* for the delivery of nutrition-related care to patients/clients that is safe, effective, and of high quality. In addition, the Academy of Nutrition and Dietetics has created a set of standardized phrases or "terms" that are organized into categories or "domains," with each phrase having its own unique alphanumeric code for identification and documentation purposes. These phrases or terms were developed to allow dietetic practitioners to clearly describe, document, and evaluate the nutrition-related care they provide to their patients/clients. The terms facilitate clear and specific communication among practitioners and with other members of the health-care team.[9,12] This standardized terminology is described in greater detail later in this chapter.

It is important to note that while the NCP is intended to help standardize the process of delivering nutrition-related care, is not intended to standardize the actual nutrition care that different patients/clients receive.[9,10] The nutrition-related problems experienced by different patients/clients are highly variable, depending on numerous individual characteristics and circumstances that are unique to each patient/client and that will require an intervention that is uniquely suited to the condition of each individual patient/client. The NCP is designed to improve the consistency and quality of nutrition-related care that patients/clients receive and to ensure that the outcomes or results of that care are more predictable.[9,10]

There are four steps in the NCP: nutritional assessment, nutrition diagnosis, nutrition intervention, and nutritional monitoring and evaluation, as depicted in Figure 1.1.[9,10] Nutritional assessment, the first step, involves collecting, verifying, recording, and interpreting a variety of data that are relevant to the nutritional status of the patient or client. These data, also referred to as **nutrition care indicators,** allow the practitioner to determine whether a nutrition problem exists and to make informed decisions about the nature, cause, and significance of nutrition-related problems that do exist.[10] Thus, nutritional assessment is essential to and an initial step in the delivery of cost-effective and high-quality nutrition care.

The Nutrition Care Process Model

At the very center of the NCP is the relationship between the dietetic professional and the patient/client, illustrating that the nutrition care provided is to be patient/client-centered. The practitioner should interact with the patient/client in a respectful, empathetic, nonjudgmental, and culturally sensitive manner and demonstrate good listening skills. This will help ensure that the patient/client is actively involved in setting the goals and outcomes of any intervention and that these are patient-focused, reasonable, achievable, incremental, and measurable.

Nutritional assessment is the initial step in the NCP, and its purpose is to establish a foundation for progressing

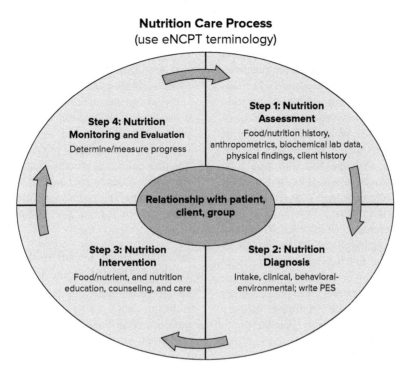

Nutrition Care Process
(use eNCPT terminology)

Step 1: Nutrition Assessment
Food/nutrition history, anthropometrics, biochemical lab data, physical findings, client history

Step 2: Nutrition Diagnosis
Intake, clinical, behavioral-environmental; write PES

Step 3: Nutrition Intervention
Food/nutrient, and nutrition education, counseling, and care

Step 4: Nutrition Monitoring and Evaluation
Determine/measure progress

Relationship with patient, client, group

Figure 1.1 The four distinct but interrelated and connected steps of the Nutrition Care Process and model.

through the remaining three steps. The strengths and abilities that the practitioner brings to the process include unique dietetics knowledge, skills and competencies, critical-thinking skills, collaboration, communication, evidence-based practice, and a code of ethics. Evidence-based practice involves incorporating the most current available scientific information in the nutrition-related care provided. Adherence to a professional code of ethics ensures that patients/clients are cared for in a manner conforming to strict social, professional, and moral standards of conduct.[9,10]

Environmental factors that can impact the patient/client's ability to receive and benefit from the NCP include practice settings, health-care systems, social systems, and economics. For example, the patient/client's income and health insurance coverage will significantly impact the type and extent of nutrition care that is provided. The patient/client's living arrangements, access to food, and social-support system can impact the ability to adopt and maintain healthful changes in diet, physical activity, etc. These environmental factors can have either a positive or a negative effect on the outcome of the nutrition care provided and must be assessed and considered in providing care.

Two supporting systems that play important roles in providing nutrition care include a screening and referral system and an outcomes management system. Nutritional screening can be defined as "a process to identify an individual who is malnourished or who is at risk for malnutrition to determine if a detailed nutritional assessment is indicated."[13] Because nutritional screening may be done by

someone other than a dietetics professional, such as a registered dietitian or dietetic technician, this is considered an external supportive system and not a step within the NCP.[10] If nutritional screening identifies a person at nutritional risk, a more thorough assessment of the individual's nutritional status should be performed. Nutritional screening is discussed in greater detail in Chapter 7, and examples of screening instruments are shown there. The outcomes management system evaluates the effectiveness and efficiency of the process by collecting and analyzing relevant data in a timely manner in order to adjust and improve the performance of the process.[10]

Nutritional Assessment in the Nutrition Care Process

Nutrition assessment is the first step in the Nutrition Care Process and involves obtaining, verifying, and interpreting data that are needed to identify a particular nutrition-related problem. Nutritional assessment is organized into five domains: food/nutrition-related history, anthropometric measurements, biochemical data (with medical tests and procedures), and client history. Nutritional assessment begins once the nutritional screening indicates that the patient/client is at risk of malnutrition or may benefit from nutrition-related care. This in-depth assessment involves collecting a variety of relevant data, reviewing the data for factors affecting nutritional and health status, clustering or grouping various data points in order to establish a nutrition diagnosis, and then identifying nutrition care criteria against which the data will be compared for purposes of analysis. The NCP groups these nutrition care criteria into two categories: (1) a nutrition prescription or goal established by the nutrition practitioner in consultation with the medical team and (2) reference standards for food and nutrient intake. A nutrition prescription or goal for a patient whose nutrition diagnosis is inadequate energy intake would include a level of energy intake that is considered appropriate for the patient's height, activity, and age and that would be expected to return the patient to a healthy body weight over time. Examples of reference standards for food and nutrient intake include the Dietary Reference Intakes (DRIs), the Dietary Reference Values for Food and Energy for the United Kingdom, the Dietary Guidelines for Americans, and clinical practice guidelines for specific conditions established by organizations such as the American Diabetes Association, the Canadian Diabetes Association, Diabetes UK, the National Kidney Foundation, or the Kidney Foundation of Canada.

When evaluating biochemical measures such as lipid and lipoprotein values, standards established by the American Heart Association, the Canadian Heart and Stroke Foundation, the British Heart Foundation, or the National Heart, Lung, and Blood Institute can be used. Individual health-care facilities generally have their own criteria for evaluating anthropometric, biochemical, and clinical indicators of nutritional status. Anthropometric measurements can be compared against what are considered normal values or ranges typically seen in healthy populations, such as the pediatric growth charts issued by the U.S. Centers for Disease Control and Prevention. Because laboratory values may vary depending on the laboratory performing the assay, as discussed in Chapter 8, normal ranges provided by the individual laboratory should be consulted.[9,10]

When assessing food and nutrient intake using information provided by the patient/client, it is important to remember that such assessments are only *estimates* of actual consumption because they are based on subjective information provided by the patient or a member of the patient's family. One exception to this is when the patient's sole source of nutrition is enteral and/or parenteral nutrition support, which can be objectively and accurately measured. Data on food and nutrient intake can then be compared to the patient/client's nutrition prescription or goal or to some reference standard such as the DRIs. When using the DRIs, it is important to note that they are intended for healthy populations and that clinical judgment is necessary when applying them to those who are ill or injured. In addition, an intake less than the Recommended Dietary Allowance or Adequate Intake does not necessarily mean that a nutrient deficiency exists. Finally, a thorough assessment of nutritional status must also include evaluation of anthropometric, biochemical, and clinical data, consideration of the patient's

history, and relevant information collected by other members of the health-care team.[9–12]

If a nutrition problem exists, the data collected during the nutritional assessment and its analysis serve as the foundation for establishing the nutrition diagnosis, which is the second step in the NCP. Nutritional assessment is not a one-time, isolated event occurring at the beginning of a patient's nutrition-related care. It is more than simply the initial step of the NCP. It is a continuous, ongoing, nonlinear, data collection process spanning the entire duration of the patient/client's care and serving as the basis for the reassessment and reanalysis of relevant data in the fourth step of the NCP, nutritional monitoring and evaluation.[9,10]

Standardized Terminology in the Nutrition Care Process

In the NCP, numerous types of data or nutrition care indicators are used to assess, describe, and document a patient's nutritional status and to monitor and evaluate the outcomes of the nutritional intervention. The Nutrition Care Process Terminology, or NCPT, contains more than 1000 terms categorized to describe the four steps of the Nutrition Care Process: nutrition assessment, nutrition diagnosis, nutrition intervention, and nutrition monitoring and evaluation. The electronic Nutrition Care Process Terminology (eNCPT) is the online publication that provides access to the most up-to-date terminology and requires a modest subscription. Also included are reference sheets that provide clear definitions and explanation of all terms, including indicators, criteria for evaluation, etiologies, and signs and symptoms. Go to this website for more information: https://ncpt.webauthor.com/. The standardized language ensures that individuals in the dietetic profession will clearly articulate the exact nature of the nutrition problem, the intervention, and goals and approaches. When the nutritional assessment identifies a nutrition problem in a patient (that is, the patient's nutrition care indicator deviates in a clinically significant way from what would be expected or considered normal), a standardized term is used so that the problem can be specifically identified, clearly described, and easily documented. Because nutritional assessment and nutritional monitoring and evaluation share common elements (as discussed in greater detail below), most of the terms used in nutritional assessment are also used in monitoring, evaluating, and documenting the patient's response to any nutrition intervention he or she is receiving.[9] Similar sets of standardized terms have been developed for use when making nutrition diagnoses and planning and implementing any nutrition intervention.

Because of the large amount of data that could potentially be considered for analysis, critical-thinking skills are necessary to enable the practitioner to limit the selection of data for analysis to only the data that are clinically relevant to the unique circumstances of the patient/client. Likewise, critical-thinking skills are necessary in the appropriate interpretation of the collected data. The set of data that is considered relevant and how those data are interpreted will vary from one patient to another, depending on the patient's status.[9]

Nutrition Diagnosis in the Nutrition Care Process

Nutrition diagnosis is a critical bridge in the Nutrition Care Process between nutrition assessment and nutrition intervention. The purpose of the second step in the NCP is to establish a nutrition diagnosis that specifically identifies and describes a nutrition problem that a dietetic practitioner is responsible for independently treating.[9] The eNCPT provides standardized nutrition diagnosis language so that the information is clear within and outside the profession. Nutrition diagnosis is organized into three domains, including food/nutrient intake, clinical conditions, and behavioral-environmental factors. It is important to note that a nutrition diagnosis is different from a medical diagnosis. The medical diagnosis refers to the process of determining the existence of a disease and identifying or classifying the disease based on various criteria, such as the patient's **signs** and **symptoms,** the results of diagnostic tests, and relevant data from the nutritional assessment. The medical diagnosis then allows the medical practitioner (e.g., physician, physician assistant, nurse practitioner) to make medical decisions about treating the disease and predicting the likely outcome of the disease. In contrast, the nutrition diagnosis is the "identification and labeling of a specific nutrition problem that food and nutrition professionals are responsible for treating independently."[9] The nutrition diagnosis and subsequent intervention focus on specific nutrition and dietary issues and food-related behaviors that may cause a disease or be a consequence of a disease. In other words, the dietetic practitioner establishes the nutrition diagnosis by identifying and labeling a nutrition problem which he or she is legally and professionally responsible for treating by working collaboratively with the patient and with other members of the health-care team to improve the patient's nutritional status.[9,11] Data from the nutritional assessment are the basis for establishing the nutrition diagnosis and for setting reasonable and measurable outcomes that can be expected from any subsequent intervention in the third step of the NCP.

During documentation, the nutrition diagnosis is summarized in a single, structured sentence or nutrition diagnosis statement having three distinct components: the problem (P), the etiology (E), and the signs and symptoms (S). Also known as a PES statement, it identifies the problem using the appropriate diagnostic term, addresses the etiology or root cause or contributing risk factors of the problem, and lists signs and symptoms and other data from the nutritional assessment that provide evidence to support the nutrition diagnosis.

The problem or diagnostic term describes the alteration in the patient's nutritional status that the dietetic practitioner is responsible for independently treating. It allows the practitioner to identify reasonable and measurable outcomes for an intervention and to monitor and evaluate changes in the patient's nutritional status. The etiology is the factors that are causally related to the problem or contribute to it. Clearly identifying the etiology will allow the practitioner to design a nutrition intervention intended to resolve the underlying cause of the nutrition problem, if possible. Evidence substantiating the nutrition diagnosis is relevant data from the nutritional assessment, the signs (objective data) reported by a physician or other qualified member of the health-care team, and the symptoms (subjective data) reported by the patient.

The PES statement is to be written following a specific format beginning with the nutrition diagnostic label, followed by the etiology, and ending with the signs and symptoms. These three components of the PES statement are linked together with the words "related to" and "as evidenced by." The format is (the nutrition diagnostic label) related to (the etiology) as evidenced by (the signs and symptoms). For example, consider a 61-year-old male who has had a poor appetite and an unintentional weight loss of 15% during the past three months since he had a medical diagnosis of colon cancer, underwent a partial resection of his colon, and began receiving chemotherapy. The weight loss is based on the patient's weight history as documented in the medical record. The patient complains that since beginning chemotherapy, "food has tasted funny" and consequently he doesn't eat as much as usual. Dysgeusia, a distorted sense of taste, is a common drug–nutrient interaction associated with the chemotherapy agents he is receiving, and this often leads to inadequate oral intake. An assessment of the patient's usual diet for the past three months shows that his usual energy intake is approximately 60% of his estimated needs, clearly indicating inadequate oral intake (eNCPT provides the appropriate terminology). An example of a PES statement for this patient would be "Inadequate oral intake related to chemotherapy-associated dysgeusia as evidenced by oral intake at 60% of estimated needs." In this instance, the nutrition diagnostic label is inadequate oral intake, the etiology is the chemotherapy-associated dysgeusia, and the signs and symptoms are an oral intake at 60% of the patient's estimated needs.

Nutrition Intervention in the Nutrition Care Process

The purpose of nutrition intervention is to resolve or improve the patient/client's nutrition problem by planning and implementing appropriate strategies that will change nutritional intake, nutrition-related knowledge and behavior, environmental conditions impacting diet, or access to supportive care and services.[9] The dietetics professional works in conjunction with patients, other health-care providers, and agencies during the nutrition intervention phase. The selection of the intervention is driven by the nutrition diagnosis and its etiology. The objectives and goals of the intervention serve as the basis for measuring the outcome of the intervention and monitoring the patient/client's progress.[9,11]

Nutrition intervention has two basic components: planning and implementation. During planning, multiple nutrition diagnoses must be prioritized based on the severity of the nutrition problem, the intervention's potential impact on the problem, and the patient's needs and perceptions. Ideally, the intervention should target the etiology or root cause of the nutrition problem, although in some instances it may not be possible for the dietetic practitioner to change the etiology, in which case the signs and symptoms may have to be targeted. When determining the patient's recommended intake of energy, nutrients, and foods, the most current and appropriate reference standards and dietary guidelines should be used and modified, if necessary, based on the patient's nutrition diagnosis and health condition. These intake recommendations, along with a brief description of the patient's health condition and the nutrition diagnosis, are concisely summarized in a statement known as the nutrition prescription. Once the nutrition prescription is written, the specific strategies and goals of the intervention can be established. The intervention strategies should be based on the best available evidence and consistent with institutional policies and procedures. The goals of the intervention should be patient-focused, reasonable, achievable, measurable, and incremental, and, whenever possible, established in collaboration with the patient. During implementation, the dietetic practitioner communicates the plan to all relevant parties and carries it out. Relevant data on the patient's nutritional status are collected and used to monitor and evaluate the intervention's effectiveness and the patient's progress and, when warranted, to change the intervention to improve its safety and effectiveness.[9,11]

Nutritional Monitoring and Evaluation in the Nutrition Care Process

The purpose of the fourth step in the NCP, nutritional monitoring and evaluation, is to determine whether and to what extent the goals and objectives of the intervention are being met. In the NCP, nutritional monitoring and evaluation begins by identifying specific and measurable nutrition care indicators of the patient's behavior and/or nutritional status that are the desired results of the patient's nutrition care. These nutrition care indicators should be carefully selected so that they are relevant to the nutrition diagnosis, the etiology of the nutrition problem, the patient's signs and symptoms, and the goals and objectives of the intervention. In many instances the nutrition care indicators selected for monitoring and

evaluation will be the same as those used in the initial assessment of the patient's nutritional status. The practitioner then monitors, measures, and evaluates changes in these nutrition care indicators to determine whether the patient's behavior and/or nutritional status are improved in response to the intervention.[9] The practitioner monitors the patient's knowledge, beliefs, and behaviors for evidence indicating whether the nutrition intervention is meeting its intended goals and objectives. Measurements of specific nutrition care indicators provide objective data on whether intervention outcomes are being met. The practitioner then evaluates the intervention's overall impact on the patient's behavior or status by comparing the current findings to those obtained earlier—for example, during the initial assessment of the patient's nutritional status.[9]

The definition of nutritional monitoring used in the NCP is somewhat different from that used when discussing national surveys of diet and health, which are covered in Chapter 4. When discussing these surveys of population groups, the term *nutritional monitoring* is defined as "an ongoing description of nutrition conditions in the population, with particular attention to subgroups defined in socioeconomic terms, for purposes of planning, analyzing the effects of policies and programs on nutrition problems, and predicting future trends."[14]

OPPORTUNITIES IN NUTRITIONAL ASSESSMENT

Numerous opportunities currently exist for applying nutritional assessment skills. As our understanding of the relationships between nutrition and health increases, these opportunities will only increase. Following are some examples of areas in which nutritional assessment is making a significant contribution to health care.

Meeting the *Healthy People 2020* Objectives

The *Healthy People 2020* objectives outline a comprehensive, nationwide health promotion and disease prevention agenda designed to improve the health of all people in the United States during the second decade of the 21st century.[20] Like the preceding *Healthy People 2010* initiative, *Healthy People 2020* is committed to a single, fundamental purpose: promoting health and preventing illness, disability, and premature death.[21] The 2020 objectives focus on four overarching goals: attain high-quality, longer lives free of preventable disease, disability, injury, and premature death; achieve health equity, eliminate disparities, and improve the health of all groups; create social and physical environments that promote good health for all; and promote quality of life, healthy development, and healthy behaviors across all life stages.[21] There are approximately 1200 objectives organized into 42 topic areas, with each topic area representing

Box 1.1   *Healthy People 2020* Topic Areas

1. Access to health services
2. Adolescent health
3. Arthritis, osteoporosis, and chronic back pain
4. Blood disorders and blood safety
5. Cancer
6. Chronic kidney disease
7. Dementias, including Alzheimer's disease
8. Diabetes
9. Disability and health
10. Early and middle childhood
11. Educational and community-based programs
12. Environmental health
13. Family planning
14. Genomics
15. Global health
16. Health communication and information technology
17. Healthcare-associated infections
18. Health-related quality of life and well-being
19. Hearing, sensory, and communication disorders
20. Heart disease and stroke

21. HIV
22. Immunization and infectious disease
23. Injury and violence prevention
24. Lesbian, gay, bisexual, and transgender health
25. Maternal, infant, and child health
26. Medical product safety
27. Mental health and mental disorders
28. Nutrition and weight status
29. Occupational safety and health
30. Older adults
31. Oral health
32. Physical activity
33. Preparedness
34. Public health infrastructure
35. Respiratory diseases
36. Sexually transmitted diseases
37. Sleep health
38. Social determinants of health
39. Substance abuse
40. Tobacco use
41. Vision

Source: U.S. Department of Health and Human Services. 2010. *Healthy People 2020.* Office of Disease Prevention and Health Promotion. www.healthypeople.gov.

an important public health concern. The 42 topic areas are shown in Box 1.1. Of the approximately 1200 objectives, 22 are listed in the nutrition and weight status topic area, as shown in Box 1.2. Numerous other nutrition-related objectives are listed under other topic areas, such as cancer, diabetes, food safety, heart disease and stroke, physical activity, and maternal, infant, and child health.

For example, meeting objective NWS-10 (Reduce the proportion of children and adolescents who are considered obese) requires health professionals skillful in anthropometry and able to intelligently use the CDC growth charts or other appropriate methods for assessing body mass index or body composition. The ability to evaluate dietary intake and interpret laboratory data and physical signs and symptoms reflecting iron status would be important in evaluating progress on objectives NWS-21 and NWS-22. Objective NWS-18 (Reduce consumption of saturated fat in the population aged 2 years and older) requires a working knowledge of dietary survey methods to initially assess fat intake and to monitor long-term adherence to the objective.

Health-Care Organizations

Health-care organizations such as physicians' offices, urgent-care clinics, emergency rooms, acute-care hospitals, and long-term care facilities offer many opportunities for health professionals trained in nutritional assessment. Inadequate food and nutrient intake are commonly seen in chronically ill patients, and one manifestation of this is **protein-energy malnutrition (PEM),** which is a loss of lean body mass resulting from inadequate consumption of energy and/or protein or resulting from the increased energy and nutrient requirements of certain diseases.[23]

Although the relationship between malnutrition and treatment outcome often is obscured by other factors that can affect the outcome of a patient's hospital stay (for example, the nature and severity of the disease process), several researchers have reported that patients with PEM tend to have a longer hospital stay, a higher incidence of complications, and a higher mortality rate.[22–26]

Identifying patients at nutritional risk is a major activity necessary for providing cost-effective medical treatment and helping contain health-care costs. Good medical practice and economic considerations make it imperative that hospital patients be nutritionally assessed and that steps be taken, if necessary, to improve their nutritional status. Evaluation of a patient's weight, height, midarm muscle area, and triceps skinfold thickness and values from various laboratory tests can be valuable aids in assessing protein and energy nutriture. Some researchers believe that rapid, nonpurposeful weight loss is the single best predictor of malnutrition currently available. These and other assessment techniques for hospitalized patients will be discussed in detail in Chapter 8.

Box 1.2

Healthy People 2020 Objectives for the Nutrition and Weight Status (NWS) Topic Area*

NWS–1: Increase the number of States with nutrition standards for foods and beverages provided to preschool-aged children in child care.

NWS–2: Increase the proportion of schools that offer nutritious foods and beverages outside of school meals.

NWS–3: Increase the number of States that have State-level policies that incentivize food retail outlets to provide foods that are encouraged by the Dietary Guidelines for Americans.

NWS–4: Increase the proportion of Americans who have access to a food retail outlet that sells a variety of foods that are encouraged by the Dietary Guidelines for Americans.

NWS–5: Increase the proportion of primary care physicians who regularly measure the body mass index of their patients.

NWS–6: Increase the proportion of physician office visits that include counseling or education related to nutrition or weight.

NWS–7: Increase the proportion of work sites that offer nutrition or weight management classes or counseling.

NWS–8: Increase the proportion of adults who are at a healthy weight.

NWS–9: Reduce the proportion of adults who are obese.

NWS–10: Reduce the proportion of children and adolescents who are considered obese.

NWS–11: Prevent inappropriate weight gain in youth and adults.

NWS–12: Eliminate very low food security among children.

NWS–13: Reduce household food insecurity and in so doing reduce hunger.

NWS–14: Increase the contribution of fruits to the diets of the population aged 2 years and older.

NWS–15: Increase the variety and contribution of vegetables to the diets of the population aged 2 years and older.

NWS–16: Increase the contribution of whole grains to the diets of the population aged 2 years and older.

NWS–17: Reduce consumption of calories from solid fats and added sugars in the population aged 2 years and older.

NWS–18: Reduce consumption of saturated fat in the population aged 2 years and older.

NWS–19: Reduce consumption of sodium in the population aged 2 years and older.

NWS–20: Increase consumption of calcium in the population aged 2 years and older.

NWS–21: Reduce iron deficiency among young children and females of childbearing age.

NWS–22: Reduce iron deficiency among pregnant females.

*NWS = nutrition and weight status

Source: U.S. Department of Health and Human Services. 2010. *Healthy People 2020.* Office of Disease Prevention and Health Promotion. www.healthypeople.gov.

Diabetes Mellitus

Diabetes is an increasingly common chronic disease in both developed and developing countries.[1,2] According to data from the National Center for Health Statistics, the prevalence of diabetes has increased in the United States in recent decades and among all U.S. adults is estimated to be 12%. As shown in Figure 1.2, there are marked differences in the prevalence of diabetes, depending on one's age or gender. Nutritional assessment has been an important component in diagnosing and managing diabetes in recent decades and plays a major role in the American Diabetes Association's nutrition recommendations and principles for people with diabetes.[27] Goals for the person with diabetes are based on dietary history, nutrient intake, and clinical data. A thorough knowledge of the patient gained through nutritional assessment will assist the dietitian—the primary provider of nutrition therapy—in guiding the patient to a successful treatment outcome. The role of nutritional assessment in managing diabetes is discussed further in Chapter 8.

Weight Management

The *Dietary Guidelines for Americans*[7] defines a "healthy weight" range for most adults as a body mass index, or BMI (weight in kilograms divided by height in meters squared), of 18.5 kg/m^2 to 24.9 kg/m^2. **Overweight** is defined as a BMI range of 25.0 kg/m^2 to 29.9 kg/m^2, while **obesity** is defined as a BMI ≥ 30.0 kg/m^2. Based on these definitions, 73.0% of U.S. adult males and 66.2% of U.S. adult females are considered either overweight or obese (i.e., they have a BMI > 25.0 kg/m^2), while 34.5% of U.S. adult males and 38.1% of U.S. adult females are considered obese (i.e., they have a BMI ≥ 30.0 kg/m^2). Figure 1.3 shows how the prevalence of U.S. adults who are either overweight or obese (i.e., a BMI ≥ 25.0 kg/m^2) has increased since the early 1960s. Figure 1.4 shows the prevalence of obesity among adults based on gender and ethnicity. Since the early 1960s the prevalence of obesity has also increased among U.S. children and adolescents, as shown in Figure 1.5. In persons 2 to 20 years of age, obesity is now defined as a BMI greater than or equal to the 95th percentile of BMI for sex and age using the pediatric growth charts developed by the U.S. Centers for Disease Control and Prevention, which are discussed in detail in Chapter 6.

National surveys conducted in Canada during the past three decades have shown a steady increase in the prevalence of overweight and obesity.[28–31] Between 1985 and 2011, the prevalence of adult obesity in Canada increased from 6.1% to 18.3%, and will reach a prevalence of 21.2% in the year 2019.[31]

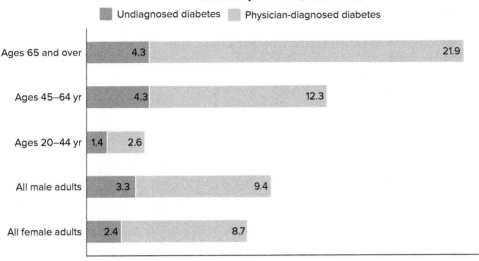

Figure 1.2 **Percent of U.S. adults with diagnosed and undiagnosed diabetes by age and gender.**
The values represent both physician-diagnosed diabetes and undiagnosed diabetes. Undiagnosed
diabetes is defined as a fasting blood glucose $\geq$ 126 mg/dL or a hemoglobin A1c $\geq$ 6.5% and no
reported physician diagnosis.
Source: National Center for Health Statistics.

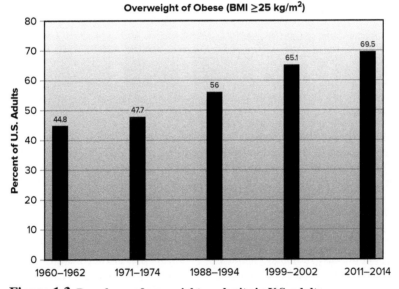

Figure 1.3 **Prevalence of overweight or obesity in U.S. adults.**
Nearly 7 in 10 adults are now overweight or obese (BMI equal to or greater
than 25 kg/m^2).
Source: National Center for Health Statistics.

The increasing prevalence of overweight and obesity
is not limited to the people of developed nations such as
the United States, Canada, and the European Union. The
urban populations of many developing nations are experiencing a marked increase in the prevalence of overweight,
obesity, and diet-related diseases such as cardiovascular
disease and type 2 diabetes, paradoxically, while

malnutrition, hunger, and starvation continue to plague
the rural populations of these countries.[1] The term
globesity has been coined to identify what many epidemiologists consider to be a global epidemic of obesity. While
the term *epidemic* is typically used to describe a marked
increase in the number of cases of an infectious or communicable disease over a certain period of time, the term

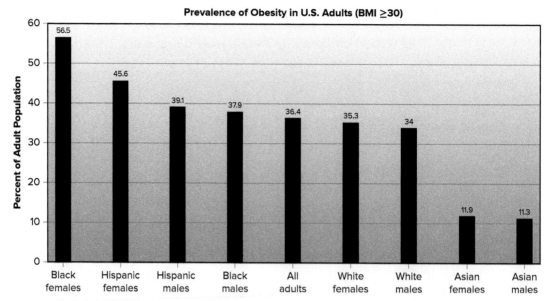

Figure 1.4 **Prevalence of obesity among U.S. adults.**
The prevalence of obesity (BMI equal to or greater than 30 kg/m²) varies widely across gender and ethnic groups.
Source: National Center for Health Statistics.

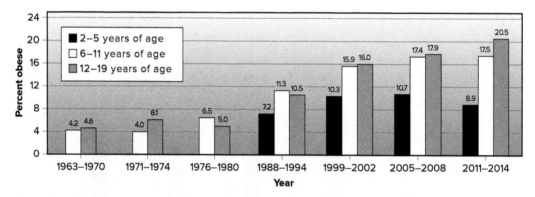

Figure 1.5 **Prevalence of obesity among U.S. children and adolescents.**
In the past several decades, the prevalence of obesity has increased among U.S. children and adolescents. In persons 2 to 20 years of age, obesity is defined as a BMI greater than or equal to the 95th percentile of BMI for sex and age using the pediatric growth charts developed by the U.S. Centers for Disease Control and Prevention, or a BMI of 30 kg/m², whichever is smaller. Obesity prevalence data for persons 2–5 years old are not available prior to the 1988–1994 survey period.
Source: National Center for Health Statistics.

can appropriately be used in the case of noncommunicable diseases or other adverse health conditions such as overweight and obesity, motor vehicle crashes, domestic violence, and firearm deaths. The World Health Organization estimates that by 2020 two-thirds of the global burden of disease will be due to noncommunicable diseases—such as cardiovascular diseases, type 2 diabetes, and obesity—that are linked to such dietary factors as increased consumption of fats, refined and processed foods, and foods of animal origin, and lifestyle factors such as tobacco smoking and physical inactivity.[1,32,33]

One of the *Healthy People 2020* objectives is to increase the proportion of U.S. adults who are at a healthy weight from the current proportion of approximately 30.8% who are at a healthy weight to the target of 33.9%, which is a 10% improvement.

National surveys provide important nutritional assessment data, such as prevalence of overweight and obesity in a particular population. Dietary methods can be valuable in initially assessing the quantity and quality of caloric intake and in monitoring dietary intake throughout treatment for obesity. Anthropometry is important in monitoring changes in percent body fat to help ensure that decrements in weight primarily come from body fat stores and that losses of lean body mass (mostly viscera and skeletal muscle) are minimized. Techniques for monitoring changes in percent body fat will be discussed in Chapter 6.

Box 1.3	**Risk Factors for Heart Disease According to the American Heart Association**
	(www.heart.org; www.cdc.gov)

MAJOR RISK FACTORS THAT *CAN* BE CHANGED	**% U.S. ADULTS WITH RISK FACTOR**
1. Cigarette/tobacco smoke	17%
2. High blood pressure	29% ($\geq$ 140/90 mm Hg)
3. High blood cholesterol	13% ($\geq$ 240 mg/dl)
4. Physical inactivity	32%
5. Obesity and overweight	70% (BMI $\geq$ 25 kg/m^2)
6. Diabetes	12%
MAJOR RISK FACTORS THAT *CAN'T* BE CHANGED	**% ADULTS WITH RISK FACTOR**
1. Heredity	—
2. Male	—
3. Increasing age	14% (over age 65)
CONTRIBUTING FACTOR	
1. Individual response to stress	—
2. Excessive alcohol intake	5%
3. Poor diet quality	—

Heart Disease and Cancer

Heart disease and cancer are the first and second leading causes of death in the United States, respectively. Together they account for 46% of all deaths in a given year. Dietary factors playing a major role in heart disease are consumption of saturated and trans fats, low intake of fruits, vegetables, nuts, seeds, and whole grains, and an imbalance between energy intake and energy expenditure leading to obesity.

Coronary heart disease (CHD) risk factors are shown in Box 1.3. The "major risk factors that can be changed" are the major causal risk factors for CHD. When these are modified, CHD risk is reduced.[34,35] CHD incidence and death rates are markedly lower in individuals who avoid smoking, high blood pressure, high blood cholesterol, obesity, diabetes, and physical inactivity. Keeping stress under control, avoiding high alcohol intake, and ingesting a heart-healthy diet are contributing factors for lowering CHD risk.

Since 1950, the death rate for heart disease decreased 70%. This is one of the greatest health success stories of the past half-century and is due to improvements in American health habits and medical care. Heart disease still accounts for 23.5% of all deaths, and much work yet remains to be accomplished in improving the lifestyles of adults and children. Because dietary therapy is the cornerstone of lowering serum low-density lipoprotein cholesterol, nutritional assessment skills are vitally important in its management. Proficiency in measuring diet, for example, would enable a dietitian to assess a client's consumption of saturated fat, *trans* fatty acids, dietary fiber, and antioxidant nutrients and

suggest appropriate dietary changes. Chapter 3 includes a discussion of a questionnaire for assessing adherence to a heart-healthy diet. Chapter 8 covers nutritional assessment in preventing heart disease.

Cancer is largely a preventable disease that results in more than a half-million deaths annually, which is more than 22.5% of all deaths in the United States.[36] Among Americans less than 85 years of age, cancer is the leading cause of death, although heart disease remains the leading cause of death when all Americans are grouped together.[36] Roughly two-thirds of all cancer deaths in the United States are linked to tobacco use, obesity, physical inactivity, and certain dietary choices, all of which can be modified by both individual and societal action. The percentage of cancer deaths attributable to dietary factors is estimated to be one-third.

The American Cancer Society guidelines on nutrition and physical activity for cancer prevention are shown in Box 1.4.[37] Methods for assessing dietary levels of fruits, vegetables, cereals, legumes, meats and other animal products, and alcoholic beverages will be necessary in applying these guidelines, as will anthropometric skills.

Nutrition Monitoring

When discussing national surveys of diet and health, which are covered in Chapter 4, nutrition monitoring is defined as "those activities necessary to provide timely information about the contributions of food and nutrient consumption and nutritional status to the health of the U.S. population."[14] As previously discussed, this definition of the term *nutrition monitoring* is different from when it is used within the

Box 1.4   **American Cancer Society Guidelines on Nutrition and Physical Activity for Cancer Prevention**

ACS Recommendations for Individual Choices

Achieve and maintain a healthy weight throughout life.

- Be as lean as possible throughout life without being underweight.
- Avoid excess weight gain at all ages. For those who are currently overweight or obese, losing even a small amount of weight has health benefits and is a good place to start.
- Engage in regular physical activity and limit consumption of high-calorie foods and beverages as key strategies for maintaining a healthy weight.

Adopt a physically active lifestyle.

- Adults should engage in at least 150 minutes of moderate intensity or 75 minutes of vigorous intensity activity each week, or an equivalent combination, preferably spread throughout the week.
- Children and adolescents should engage in at least 1 hour of moderate or vigorous intensity activity each day, with vigorous intensity activity occurring at least 3 days each week.
- Limit sedentary behavior such as sitting, lying down, watching television, or other forms of screen-based entertainment.
- Doing some physical activity above usual activities, no matter what one's level of activity, can have many health benefits.

- Consume a healthy diet, with an emphasis on plant foods.
- Choose foods and beverages in amounts that help achieve and maintain a healthy weight.
- Limit consumption of processed meat and red meat.
- Eat at least 2.5 cups of vegetables and fruits each day.
- Choose whole grains instead of refined grain products.

If you drink alcoholic beverages, limit consumption.

- Drink no more than 1 drink per day for women or 2 per day for men.

ACS Recommendations for Community Action

Public, private, and community organizations should work collaboratively at national, state, and local levels to implement policy and environmental changes that:

- Increase access to affordable, healthy foods in communities, worksites, and schools, and decrease access to and marketing of foods and beverages of low nutritional value, particularly to youth.
- Provide safe, enjoyable, and accessible environments for physical activity in schools and worksites, and for transportation and recreation in communities.

Source: Kushi LH, Doyle C, McCullough M, Rock CL, Demark-Wahnefried W, Bandera EV, Gapstur S, Patel AV, Andrews K, Gansler T, American Cancer Society 2010 Nutrition and Physical Activity Guidelines Advisory Committee. 2012. American Cancer Society Guidelines on Nutrition and Physical Activity for Cancer Prevention. *CA: A Cancer Journal for Clinicians* 62:30–67.

context of the Nutrition Care Process. A milestone in nutrition monitoring in the United States was passage of the National Nutrition Monitoring and Related Research Act of 1990. Key provisions of the act were development of a 10-year comprehensive plan for coordinating the activities of more than 20 different federal agencies involved in nutrition monitoring and assurance of the collaboration and coordination of nutrition monitoring at federal, state, and local levels.[14] This included all data collection and analysis activities associated with health and nutrition status measurements, food composition measurements, dietary knowledge, attitude assessment, and surveillance of the food supply. Considerable nutritional assessment expertise is required for conducting such surveys as the National Health and Nutrition Examination Survey and the Behavioral Risk Factor Surveillance System. These will be discussed in Chapter 4.

Nutritional Epidemiology

Practically all nutrition research undertaken by universities, private industry, and government involves some aspect of nutritional assessment. An understanding of the theory behind assessment techniques, an awareness of the

strengths and weaknesses of assessment methods, and proficiency in their use are essential skills for anyone currently involved in or contemplating a career in **nutritional epidemiology.**

For example, to arrive at valid conclusions about the relationships between the intake of antioxidant nutrients, such as β-carotene, and risk of cancer or heart disease, nutritional epidemiologists need to know which methods best assess β-carotene nutriture and how to appropriately use those methods. Failing to do so, they would likely arrive at erroneous conclusions and disseminate inaccurate information about diet-health relationships. Methods for measuring diet are discussed in Chapter 3, and measurement of vitamin A status is presented in Chapter 9.

Epidemiologists examining the prevention and treatment of **osteoporosis** must understand, among other things, the strengths and weaknesses of various techniques to assess changes in bone mineralization. Such techniques will be discussed in Chapter 8. Researchers investigating the influence of diet and/or exercise on weight loss and changes in percent body fat use a variety of dietary and anthropometric methods to monitor caloric intake and changes in weight and body composition.

Studying the relationship between diet and disease risk is complicated by the difficulty of measuring the diet of humans, the considerable variety of foods people consume, the many nutrients and food components found in food, incomplete data on the nutrient composition of food, and the many other factors besides diet that influence disease risk. Consequently, there is considerable need for improved methods of measuring diet and assessing the body's vitamin and mineral status, as well as a need for better data on the nutrient composition of foods.

SUMMARY

1. The relationship between nutrition and health has long been recognized. Scientific evidence confirming this relationship began accumulating as early as the mid-18th century, when James Lind showed that consumption of citrus fruits cured scurvy.

2. Before the middle of the 20th century, infectious disease was the leading cause of death worldwide, and nutrient deficiency diseases and starvation were common. Because of advances in public health, medicine, and agriculture, chronic diseases such as coronary heart disease, cancer, and stroke now surpass infectious diseases as the leading causes of death throughout the world and hunger and nutrient deficiencies remain problematic but are less common.

3. Although many factors contribute to the high incidence of chronic disease, diet plays an important role in 4 of the 10 leading causes of death in the United States. The increasing prevalence of overweight and obesity is a particularly troubling global trend, even in developing nations where malnutrition, hunger, and starvation are, paradoxically, also common. Epidemiologists have coined the term *globesity* to identify what many regard as a global epidemic of obesity.

4. The continuing presence of nutrition-related disease makes it important that health professionals be able to assess nutritional status to identify who might benefit from nutrition intervention and which interventions would be appropriate.

5. Nutritional screening allows persons who are at nutritional risk to be identified, so that a more thorough evaluation of the individual's nutritional status can be performed. Nutritional assessment is an attempt to evaluate the nutritional status of individuals or populations through measurements of food and nutrient intake and nutrition-related health.

   Nutritional assessment techniques can be classified according to four types: anthropometric, biochemical or laboratory, clinical, and dietary. Use of the mnemonic "ABCD" can help in remembering these four types.

6. Our expanded ability to alter the nutritional state of a patient and our increased knowledge of the relationship between nutrition and health have made nutritional assessment an important tool in health care.

7. The Nutrition Care Process is a standardized problem-solving approach in which practitioners use critical-thinking skills to make evidence-based decisions addressing the nutrition-related problems of their clients/patients.

8. Nutritional assessment is the first step in the Nutrition Care Process and is critical to providing cost-effective and high-quality nutrition care in any health-care organization.

9. Objectives related to nutrition and health have a prominent place in the *Healthy People 2020* objectives. Skill in applying nutritional assessment techniques will play a major part in the health professional's efforts to help achieve those objectives.

10. Nutritional assessment is a major component of the American Diabetes Association's nutrition recommendations and principles for people with diabetes.

11. Nutritional assessment also plays a significant role in identifying diet-related risk factors for heart disease and cancer and in monitoring efforts to reduce risk.

12. Nutritional assessment is central to current government efforts to monitor and improve the nutritional status of its citizens. It is also a skill essential for nutritional epidemiologists and other nutrition researchers investigating links between diet and health.

REFERENCES

1. World Health Organization. 2014. Global Status Report on Noncommunicable Diseases. http://www.who.int/nmh/publications/ncd-status-report-2014/en/.

2. Stein AD, Martorell R. 2006. The emergence of diet-related chronic diseases in developing countries. In Bowman BA, Russell RM (eds.), *Present knowledge in nutrition,* 9th ed., 891–905. Washington, DC: International Life Science Institute.

3. Todhunter EN. 1976. Chronology of some events in the development and application of the science of nutrition. *Nutrition Reviews* 34:353–365.

4. Todhunter EN. 1962. Development of knowledge in nutrition. *Journal of the American Dietetic Association* 41:335–340.

5. Liu L, Oza S, Hogan D, Perin J, Rudan I, Lawn JE, Cousens S, Mathers C, Black RE. 2015. Global, regional, and national causes of child mortality in 2000-13, with projections to inform post-2015 priorities: An updated systematic analysis. *Lancet* 385(9966):430–440.

6. Coleman-Jensen A, Rabbitt MP, Gregory CA, Singh A. 2016. *Household Food Security in the United States in 2015, ERR-215,* U.S. Department of Agriculture, Economic Research Service.

7. U.S. Department of Health and Human Services and U.S. Department of Agriculture. 2015. *2015–2020 Dietary Guidelines for Americans,* 8th ed. Available at http://health.gov/dietaryguidelines/2015/guidelines/.

8. National Center for Health Statistics. 2016. *Health, United States, 2015: With Special Feature on Racial and Ethnic Health Disparities.* Hyattsville, MD: NCHS.

9. Academy of Nutrition and Dietetics. 2016. *eNCPT. Nutrition Terminology Reference Manual. Dietetics Language for Nutrition Care.* https://ncpt.webauthor.com/.

10. Lacey K, Pritchett E. 2003. Nutrition care process and model: ADA adopts road map to quality care and outcomes management. *Journal of the American Dietetic Association* 103:1061–1072.

11. Writing Group of the Nutrition Care Process/Standardized Language Committee. 2008. Nutrition Care Process and model part I: The 2008 update. *Journal of the American Dietetic Association* 108:1113–1117.

12. Writing Group of the Nutrition Care Process/Standardized Language Committee. 2008. Nutrition Care Process part II: Using the International Dietetics and Nutrition Terminology to document the nutrition care process. *Journal of the American Dietetic Association* 108:1287–1293.

13. Mueller C, Compher C, Druyan ME. 2011. ASPEN clinical guidelines: Nutrition screening, assessment, and intervention in adults. *Journal of Parenteral and Enteral Nutrition* 35:16–24.

14. Briefel RR. 2006. Nutrition monitoring in the United States. In Bowman BA, Russell RM (eds.), *Present knowledge in nutrition,* 9th ed., 838–858. Washington, DC: International Life Science Institute.

15. Turner RE. 2006. Nutrition during pregnancy. In Shils ME, Shike M, Ross AC, Cabellero B, Cousins RJ (eds.), *Modern nutrition in health and disease,* 10th ed., 771–783. Philadelphia: Lippincott Williams & Wilkins.

16. Institute of Medicine. 2009. *Weight Gain During Pregnancy: Reexamining the Guidelines.* Washington, DC: National Academies Press.

17. Picciano MF, McDonald SS. 2006. Lactation. In Shils ME, Shike M, Ross AC, Cabellero B, Cousins RJ (eds.), *Modern nutrition in health and disease,* 10th ed., 784–796. Philadelphia: Lippincott Williams & Wilkins.

18. Heird WC, Cooper A. 2006. Infancy and childhood. In Shils ME, Shike M, Ross AC, Cabellero B, Cousins RJ (eds.), *Modern nutrition in health and disease,* 10th ed., 797–817. Philadelphia: Lippincott Williams & Wilkins.

19. Treuth MS, Griffin IJ. 2006. Adolescence. In Shils ME, Shike M, Ross AC, Cabellero B, Cousins RJ (eds.), *Modern nutrition in health and disease,* 10th ed., 818–829. Philadelphia: Lippincott Williams & Wilkins.

20. U.S. Department of Health and Human Services. 2010. *Healthy People 2020.* Office of Disease Prevention and Health Promotion. www.healthypeople.gov.

21. Koh HK. 2010. A 2020 vision for healthy people. *New England Journal of Medicine* 362:1653–1656.

22. Torun B. 2006. Protein-energy malnutrition. In Shils ME, Shike M, Ross AC, Cabellero B, Cousins RJ (eds.), *Modern nutrition in health and disease,* 10th ed., 881–908. Philadelphia: Lippincott Williams & Wilkins.

23. Hensrud DD. 1999. Nutrition screening and assessment. *Medical Clinics of North America* 83:1526–1546.

24. Jeejeebhoy KN. 1998. Nutritional assessment. *Gastroenterology Clinics of North America* 27:347–369.

25. Pirlich M, Schutz T, Kemps M, Luhman N, Burmester GR, Baumann G. 2003. Prevalence of malnutrition in hospitalized medical patients: Impact of underlying disease. *Digestive Diseases* 21:245–251.

26. Donini LM, De Bernardini L, De Felice MR, Savina C, Coletti C, Cannella C. 2004. Effect of nutritional status on clinical outcome in a population of geriatric rehabilitation patients. *Aging Clinical and Experimental Research* 16:132–138.

27. Evert AB, Boucher JL, Cypress M, Dunbar SA, Franz MJ, Mayer-Davis EJ, Neumiller JJ, Nwankwo R, Verdi CL, Urbanski P, Yancy WS Jr. 2014. Nutrition therapy recommendations for the management of adults with diabetes. *Diabetes Care* 37 Suppl 1:S120–143.

28. Katzmarzyk PT. 2002. The Canadian obesity epidemic, 1985–1998. *Canadian Medical Association Journal* 166:1039–1040.

29. Sanmartin C, Ng E, Blackwell D, Gentleman J, Martinez M, Simile C. 2004. *Joint Canada/United States Survey of Health, 2002–03.* Ottawa: Statistics Canada.

30. Katzmarzyk PT, Mason C. 2006. Prevalence of class I, II and III obesity in Canada. *Canadian Medical Association Journal* 174:156–157.

31. Twells LK, Gregory DM, Reddigan J, Midodzi WK. 2014. Current and predicted prevalence of obesity in Canada: A trend analysis. *CMAJ Open* 2(1):E18–26.

32. World Health Organization. 2016. *World Health Statistics.* http://www.who.int/gho/publications/world_health_statistics/en/.

33. World Health Organization. 2013. *Global Action Plan for the Prevention and Control of Noncommunicable Diseases 2013–2020.* http://www.who.int/nmh/publications/ncd-status-report-2014/en/.

34. Mozaffarian D, Benjamin EJ, Go AS, et al. 2015. Heart disease and stroke statistics—2015 update: A report from the American Heart Association. *Circulation* 131(4):e29–322.

35. Stone NJ, Robinson JG, Lichtenstein AH, et al. 2014. ACC/AHA guideline on the treatment of blood cholesterol to reduce atherosclerotic cardiovascular risk in adults: A report of the American College of Cardiology/American Heart Association Task Force on Practice Guidelines. *Circulation* 129(25 Suppl 2):S1–45.

36. American Cancer Society. 2016. *Cancer Facts & Figures 2016.* Atlanta: American Cancer Society. www.cancer.org.

37. Kushi LH, Doyle C, McCullough M, Rock CL, Demark-Wahnefried W, Bandera EV, Gapstur S, Patel AV, Andrews K, Gansler T, American Cancer Society 2010 Nutrition and Physical Activity Guidelines Advisory Committee. 2012. American Cancer Society guidelines on nutrition and physical activity for cancer prevention. *CA: A Cancer Journal for Clinicians* 62:30–67.

2 STANDARDS FOR NUTRIENT INTAKE

STUDENT LEARNING OUTCOMES

After studying this chapter, the student will be able to:

1. Compare and contrast the factors that influenced the development of early and more recent dietary standards.

2. Differentiate between observational and scientifically based dietary standards.

3. Discuss the development of the Dietary Reference Intakes.

4. Name the characteristics of nutrient-dense foods.

5. Describe how the Healthy Eating Index-2005 is used to score dietary intake.

6. Discuss the key differences between the latest edition of the *Dietary Guidelines for Americans* and earlier editions.

7. Identify the purposes of the Nutrition Labeling and Education Act of 1990.

8. Demonstrate an understanding of the key aspects of the Nutrition Facts label.

9. Explain the Institute of Medicine's recent recommendations for the design of front-of-package labels.

INTRODUCTION

This chapter discusses a variety of recommendations and standards that can be used for evaluating the food and nutrient intake of groups and individuals. Prominent among these are the Dietary Reference Intakes, the *Dietary Guidelines for Americans,* regulations governing the nutrition labeling of food, the USDA's MyPlate graphic, and various other graphics developed to pictorially communicate recommendations for food intake and principles of good nutrition. Although most of these standards originally were designed to serve as standards for nutritional adequacy, to aid in diet planning, or to improve nutritional status, they are also useful as standards for evaluating the amounts and proportions of macronutrients, micronutrients, and various food components consumed by individuals and groups.

The primary impetus in the development of early dietary standards was the public's need for simple guidance on how to achieve nutritional adequacy from low-cost, readily available foods. During the millennia of human history prior to the mechanization of food production (which, historically speaking, is a relatively recent phenomenon), obtaining food was very labor intensive and subject to failure because of such conditions as drought and flooding, crop damage from pests, communicable diseases in humans, poverty, civil strife, and war. During this era hunger, nutrient deficiency, and starvation were common, and tragically, these conditions continue to plague sizable numbers of people, particularly in developing nations. However, more recently the most pressing problem has been the increasing prevalence of chronic disease due in large part to the disproportionate consumption of total fats, saturated and *trans* fats, refined sugars, refined grains, sodium, and heavily processed foods and the imbalance between energy intake and energy expenditure. Consequently, the focus of more recently developed dietary standards has shifted to what some refer to as our "food toxic environment," which contributes to the high prevalence of chronic disease such as obesity, heart disease, cancer, stroke, and type 2 diabetes.

Recognition of diet's role in health and disease has led to numerous efforts in the past several decades to formulate dietary guidelines and goals to promote health and prevent disease. A clear consensus has developed among most dietary guidelines and goals: dietary patterns are important factors in several of the leading causes of death, and dietary modifications can, in a number of instances, reduce one's risk of premature disease and death. Nutritional assessment is pivotal to improving dietary intake, thus reducing disease risk and improving health.

EARLY DIETARY STANDARDS AND RECOMMENDATIONS

The earliest formal dietary standard was established in the British Merchant Seaman's Act of 1835. The act made the provision of lemon juice (known as "lime juice") compulsory in the rations of British merchant sailors. This action followed the 1753 treatise by British naval surgeon James Lind (1716–1794) stating that citrus fruits cure scurvy and the introduction in 1796 of lemon juice for the British Navy.[1] Throughout the remainder of the 19th century, dietary standards for protein, carbohydrates, and fat were proposed by scientists in Europe, the United Kingdom, and North America. These dietary standards had two things in common. First, the catalyst for their development was the occurrence of starvation and the

diseases associated with it, resulting from economic dislocation and unemployment.[1,2] Second, they were, for the most part, **observational standards** because they were based on *observed* intakes rather than *measured* needs.[1]

Observational Standards

Carl Voit (1831–1908), a distinguished German physiologist of the late 1800s, made extensive observations of the amounts and kinds of foods eaten by German laborers and soldiers. Based on his observations, Voit concluded that the nutritional needs of a 70-**kilogram (kg)** male of his day doing moderate work would be met by a diet containing 118 g of protein, 500 g of carbohydrate, and 56 g of fat—a total of approximately 3000 **kilocalories (kcal).**[3] In 1895, Wilber Olin Atwater (1844–1907), a notable American physiologist and nutrition researcher who studied in Germany under Voit, observed the dietary habits of Americans. He recommended that men weighing 70 kg (154 lb) consume 3400 kcal and 125 g of protein each day.[2,3] For men engaged in more strenuous occupations, Voit and Atwater recommended 145 g and 150 g of protein per day, respectively. Rather than representing the actual physiological needs of the body, these recommendations were based on observations of what people eat when guided by their appetites and financial resources.[3]

One notable exception to the observational nature of dietary standards of the nineteenth century was the work of Edward Smith (1819–1874), a British physician, public health advocate, social reformer, and scientist who advocated better living conditions for Britain's lower classes, including prisoners. Smith conducted a dietary survey of unemployed British workers to determine what kind of diet would maintain health at the lowest cost.[2] His suggested allowances for protein, carbohydrate, and fat were based on actual laboratory measurements of caloric need and nitrogen excretion, as well as clinical observations that included absence of edema and anemia, "firmness of muscle, elasticity of spirits, capability for exertion."[1] Smith recommended approximately 3000 kcal of energy and 81 g of protein per day and believed that a diet adequate in calories and protein also would provide sufficient quantities of other necessary nutrients.[1,2]

Beginnings of Scientifically Based Dietary Standards

Advances in the early 20th century in the ability to more accurately estimate actual energy and nutrient needs led to recommendations based on physiologic requirements for protein, carbohydrate, and fat. At the same time, tremendous strides were made in understanding the role of vitamins and minerals in human nutrition. This led to a reassessment and scaling down of protein recommendations in standards established during the 1920s and 1930s by the United Kingdom, the United States, and the League of Nations. There was also an effort to include recommendations for vitamins and minerals and to make allowances for nutritional needs during pregnancy, lactation, and growth.[2]

Concern about limited resources worldwide and food shortages in European countries during World War I led the British Royal Society to appoint a committee to establish a standard for human energy needs. After reviewing the energy expenditure data of several scientists, the Royal Society Committee accepted the results of calorimetry research conducted by the nutrition scientist Graham Lusk (1866–1932) as applicable to the population of the United Kingdom. Lusk recommended 3000 kcal/day as an average energy requirement for adult males, with an appropriate adjustment for the needs of women and children. This standard also was used in estimating food requirements for the United Kingdom, France, and Italy as a basis for American food exports to these countries during World War I. In addition, the Royal Society Committee recommended that daily protein intake for adult males not fall below 70 g to 80 g, with no less than 25% of calories coming from fat. The committee made no specific recommendation for vitamins and minerals, but it recommended that "processed" foods should not be allowed to constitute a large proportion of the diet and that all diets should include a "certain proportion" of fresh fruits and green vegetables.[1]

The economic depression following the stock market crash in 1929 was the impetus for several dietary standards developed by the United Kingdom, the League of Nations, and the United States. Foremost among these was the standard proposed by Dr. Hazel Katherine Stiebeling (1896–1989) of the USDA in 1933 (see Figure 2.1). Hers was the first dietary standard to make deliberate recommendations for minerals and vitamins and maintenance of health rather than maintenance of work capacity.[2,4] In addition to energy and protein, the desirable amounts of calcium, phosphorus, iron, and vitamins A and C were stated. In 1939, these recommendations were expanded to include thiamin and riboflavin.[1,4]

Beginning in 1935, the League of Nations Technical Commission issued a series of dietary recommendations that were less concerned with defining requirements of food constituents than with outlining desirable allowances of the "protective" foods that had been lacking in so many diets.[1] Consumption of such foods as fruits, leafy vegetables, milk, eggs, fish, and meat was encouraged. These were among what outstanding American biochemist E.V. McCollum termed "protective foods," because of his early observations that they tend to protect against nutritional deficiencies. The recommendations also raised questions about the use of refined sugar, milled grain, and other foods low in vitamins and minerals.[2]

In 1938, the Canadian Council on Nutrition adopted the *Dietary Standard for Canada,* the first set of dietary standards intended specifically for use in Canada. Based

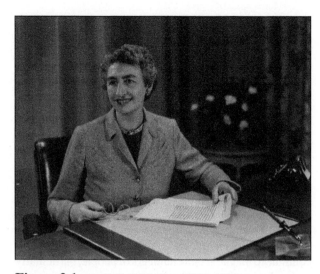

Figure 2.1 Hazel K. Stiebeling (1896–1989).
Stiebeling served in the U.S. Department of Agriculture from 1930 to 1963 as a research scientist and administrator. She was a pioneer in studying the food consumption patterns and dietary intakes of families in the United States and was instrumental in the development of the first edition of the Recommended Dietary Allowances.
Source: Special Collections, National Agricultural Library, USDA.

in part on the recommendations of the League of Nations and on information collected by the Canadian Council on Nutrition, it initially included recommendations for calories, protein, fat, calcium, iron, iodine, ascorbic acid, and vitamin D. The *Dietary Standard for Canada* was revised in 1950, 1963, and 1975. In 1983, Health Canada published the *Recommended Nutrient Intakes (RNIs) for Canadians.* As the links between diet and chronic disease risk became increasingly apparent, Canadian researchers realized the need for dietary recommendations that not only ensured adequate intake of all essential nutrients but also reduced the risk of chronic conditions such as atherosclerotic heart disease, cancer, obesity, hypertension, osteoporosis, and dental caries (tooth decay). In 1990, Health Canada published *Nutrition Recommendations: The Report of the Scientific Review Committee.* In addition to the RNIs, which were intended to ensure adequate nutrient intake to prevent deficiency, the report recommended an energy intake consistent with maintaining a healthy body weight, restricting total fat to no more than 30% of energy and saturated fat to no more than 10% of energy, reducing sodium in the diet, ensuring adequate intake of potassium, consuming alcoholic and caffeinated beverages in moderation, and fluoridating community water supplies to the level of 1 mg/liter.

RECOMMENDED DIETARY ALLOWANCES

In 1940, the U.S. federal government established the Committee of Food and Nutrition under the National Research Council of the National Academy of Sciences in Washington, DC. In 1941, this committee was established on a permanent basis and renamed the Food and Nutrition Board.[2] The role of the committee was to advise government agencies on problems relating to food and nutrition of the people and on nutrition problems in connection with national defense.[5] In 1941, the committee prepared the first Recommended Dietary Allowances (RDAs), "to serve as a guide for planning adequate nutrition for the civilian population of the United States."[7] The RDAs first appeared in print in 1941 in an article in the *Journal of the American Dietetic Association.*[7] However, it was not until 1943 that the first officially published edition of the RDAs appeared in book form.[2,4] To reflect advances in nutritional science, the RDAs were revised approximately every five years until 1989, when the 10th and last edition of *Recommended Dietary Allowances* was released.[8] The 10th edition of the RDAs provided recommendations for energy, protein, 3 electrolytes, 13 vitamins, and 12 minerals.

In essence, the RDAs have served as recommendations for nutrient intakes for 18 life stage and gender groups (life stage considers age and, when appropriate, pregnancy and lactation). The RDAs have accounted for individual differences in nutrient requirements and have included a fairly large margin of safety (i.e., they were set at a level considerably greater than the average requirement necessary to prevent deficiency disease).[9] They have been defined as "the levels of intake of essential nutrients that, on the basis of scientific knowledge, are judged by the Food and Nutrition Board to be adequate to meet the known nutrient needs of practically all healthy persons."[8] The first edition of *Recommended Dietary Allowances* was published with the objective of "providing standards to serve as a goal for good nutrition" and to serve as a guide for advising "on nutrition problems in connection with national defense."[8] However, since their inception, the RDAs have been used for a variety of other purposes for which they were not originally intended. These include use in labeling food, evaluating dietary survey data, planning and procuring food supplies for groups, planning food and nutrition information and education programs, and serving as a nutritional benchmark in the Food Stamp Program (renamed the Supplemental Nutrition Assistance Program, or SNAP, in October 2008), the Special Supplemental Food Program for Women, Infants, and Children (WIC), and the National School Lunch Program.

For more than five decades, the RDAs served as the premier nutrient standard, not only for the United States but also for many other countries throughout the developed and developing world. However, as knowledge of human nutrition increased and as nutritional concerns changed over time, limitations in the RDAs became apparent. For example, an underlying intent of the RDAs was to prevent deficiency disease. In recent decades, as chronic degenerative diseases have supplanted infectious

and nutrient-deficiency diseases as the leading causes of death, there has been growing interest in the role of diet and nutrition in decreasing chronic disease risk, conditions that the RDAs fail to adequately address. For example, the RDAs provided no recommendations for carbohydrate, dietary fibers, total fat, saturated fat, or cholesterol. There were no nutrient recommendations for older persons and no recommendations for food components that are not traditionally defined as nutrients (e.g., phytochemicals, aspartame, caffeine, and alcohol).[10] In addition, the recommended nutrient intake levels of the RDAs were generally limited to amounts obtainable through diet alone, and there was no guidance on the safe and effective use of vitamin, mineral, and other nutrient supplements, despite considerable public interest in use of such supplements.

Consequently, there arose a need for a more comprehensive set of nutritional and dietary standards that adequately addressed more contemporary nutritional concerns. In response, the Food and Nutrition Board, working in conjunction with scientists from the Canadian Institute of Nutrition and Health Canada, developed a new and expanded set of nutrient intakes known as the Dietary Reference Intakes.[10–15]

DIETARY REFERENCE INTAKES

The Dietary Reference Intakes (DRIs) are defined as "reference values that are quantitative estimates of nutrient intakes to be used for planning and assessing diets for apparently healthy people."[12] As shown in Box 2.1, they include four nutrient-based reference values—the Estimated Average Requirement, the Recommended Dietary Allowance, the Adequate Intake, and the Tolerable Upper Intake Level—and a recommendation for dietary energy intake known as the Estimated Energy Requirement. The DRIs attempt to address the weaknesses of the RDAs and to expand on the original Recommended Dietary Allowances by adding three new reference values and a recommendation for dietary energy intake.

The initiative to develop the DRIs formally began in June 1993, when the Food and Nutrition Board (FNB) organized a symposium and public hearing entitled "Should the Recommended Dietary Allowances Be Revised?"[9,10] This was followed by several symposia at nutrition-related professional meetings, at which the FNB discussed its tentative plans and invited input from interested nutrition professionals. From these activities arose a clear consensus that a more comprehensive set of nutritional and dietary standards was needed.

During this time period, Health Canada and Canadian scientists were reviewing the need to revise the Recommended Nutrient Intakes.[16] In April 1995, at a symposium cosponsored by the Canadian National

Box 2.1   The Dietary Reference Intakes

Estimated Average Requirement (EAR): The daily dietary intake level that is estimated to meet the nutrient requirement of 50% of healthy individuals in a particular life stage and gender group.

Recommended Dietary Allowance (RDA): The average daily dietary intake level that is sufficient to meet the nutrient requirement of nearly all (97% to 98%) healthy individuals in a particular life stage gender group.

Adequate Intake (AI): The recommended daily dietary intake level that is assumed to be adequate and that is based on experimentally determined approximations of nutrient intake by a group (or groups) of healthy people. The AI is an observational standard that is used when insufficient data is available to determine an RDA.

Tolerable Upper Intake Level (UL): The highest level of daily nutrient intake that is likely to pose no risk of adverse health affects to almost all apparently healthy individuals in the general population. As intake increases above the UL, the risk of adverse (toxic) effects increases.

Estimated Energy Requirement (EER): The average dietary energy intake that is predicted to maintain energy balance in a healthy adult of a defined age, gender, weight, height, and level of physical activity, consistent with good health. In children and in pregnant and lactating women, the EER includes the needs associated with the deposition of tissues or the secretion of milk consistent with good health.

Panel on Macronutrients, Panel on the Definition of Dietary Fiber, Subcommittee on Upper Reference Levels of Nutrients, Subcommittee on Interpretation and Uses of Dietary Reference Intakes, Standing Committee on the Scientific Evaluation of Dietary Reference Intakes. 2002. *Dietary Reference Intakes for Energy, Carbohydrate, Fiber, Fat, Fatty Acids, Cholesterol, Protein, and Amino Acids.* Washington, DC: National Academies Press, used with permission.

Institute of Nutrition and Health Canada, Canadian scientists reached a consensus that the Canadian government should investigate working with the FNB in developing a set of nutrient-based recommendations that will serve, where appropriate, the needs of both countries. In December 1995, the FNB began a close collaboration with the Canadian government and appointed a Standing Committee on the Scientific Evaluation of Dietary Reference Intakes (DRI Committee) composed of scientists from Canada and the United States to conduct and oversee the project. Consequently, the DRIs supersede not only the 10th edition of the *Recommended Dietary Allowances*[8] but also the Canadian Recommended Nutrient Intakes, which were last published in 1990.

The DRI Committee began its work by grouping the various nutrients and food components into eight categories and assigning each nutrient group to a panel of experts on those nutrients. The DRI Committee also formed two subcommittees: a Subcommittee on Upper Reference Levels of Nutrients to assist each panel in the development of the Tolerable Upper Intake Levels and a Subcommittee on Interpretation and Uses of Dietary Reference Intakes to determine appropriate examples for using the DRIs.[10–15] Box 2.2 shows the tasks of each panel.

The first DRI report was released in August 1997 and covered calcium, phosphorus, magnesium, vitamin D, and fluoride.[10] Subsequent reports have provided recommendations for the remaining vitamins and elements as well as for electrolytes, water, energy, physical activity, dietary fiber, and the macronutrients.[11–15] In 2011, the DRIs for calcium and vitamin D were updated in response to concerns that calcium intake might be inadequate in some groups and that calcium supplementation use was

increasing, particularly among older persons, and the uncertainty about what levels of calcium intake were optimal or excessive. In recent years there has been increasing interest in the potential role of vitamin D in a variety of health outcomes, such as increasing immunity and preventing cancer, diabetes, and preeclampsia during pregnancy.[16] In addition, the DRI Committee has released three reports that provide guidance on applying the DRIs in dietary assessment, dietary planning, and the nutrition labeling and fortification of foods.[17–19] Table 2.1 shows the Estimated Average Requirements (EARs) for the 22 different life stage and gender groups, which are shown in the column at the extreme left of the table. Tables 2.2 and 2.3 show the Recommended Dietary Allowances (RDAs) and the Adequate Intakes (AIs) for vitamins and elements, respectively. In these two tables, the values in bold type are RDAs, and those values in ordinary type and followed by an asterisk are AIs. Tables 2.4 and 2.5 show the Tolerable Upper Intake Levels (ULs) for vitamins and elements, respectively. The DRIs use different life stage and gender groups for the ULs than those used for the RDAs, AIs, and the EARs.

Estimated Average Requirement

The Estimated Average Requirement (EAR) is defined as "the daily intake value that is estimated to meet the requirement, as defined by the specified indicator of adequacy, in half of the apparently healthy individuals in a life stage or gender group."[12] The EAR serves as the basis for setting the Recommended Dietary Allowance (RDA). If an EAR cannot be established, then an RDA cannot be set. The currently established EARs are shown in Table 2.1.

Box 2.2   Tasks of the DRI Panels

- Review the scientific literature for each nutrient or food component under consideration for each of the sex, age, and condition groups.
- Consider the roles of each nutrient or food component in decreasing risk of chronic and other diseases and conditions.
- Interpret the current nutrient or food component intake data for each of the sex, age, and condition groups in North America.
- Develop criteria or indicators of adequacy for each nutrient or food component and provide substantive rationale for each criterion or indicator.
- Establish the Estimated Average Requirement (EAR) for each nutrient or food component (assuming that sufficient data are available) and the Recommended Dietary Allowance (RDA) for each life stage and gender group. If data are insufficient for establishing the EAR/RDA, set the Adequate Intake (AI).

- Establish an Estimated Energy Requirement (EER) at four levels of energy expenditure for each of the sex, age, and condition groups in North America, recommend physical activity levels (PAL) for children and adults to decrease chronic disease risk, and establish Acceptable Macronutrient Distribution Ranges (AMDRs) for carbohydrate, total fat, n-6 and n-3 polyunsaturated fatty acids, and protein for children and adults.
- Participate with the Subcommittee on Upper Reference Levels of Nutrients in estimating the level of nutrient or food component intake above which there is increased risk of toxicity or an adverse reaction—the Tolerable Upper Intake Level (UL).
- Participate with the Subcommittee on Interpretation and Uses of the DRIs in developing practical information and guidance on appropriately using the DRIs.

Standing Committee on the Scientific Evaluation of Dietary Reference Intakes, Food and Nutrition Board, Institute of Medicine. 1997. *Dietary Reference Intakes for Calcium, Phosphorus, Magnesium, Vitamin D, and Fluoride.* Washington, DC: National Academies Press, and from Panel on Macronutrients, Panel on the Definition of Dietary Fiber, Subcommittee on Upper Reference Levels of Nutrients, Subcommittee on Interpretation and Uses of Dietary Reference Intakes, Standing Committee on the Scientific Evaluation of Dietary Reference Intakes. 2002. *Dietary Reference Intakes for Energy, Carbohydrate, Fiber, Fat, Fatty Acids, Cholesterol, Protein, and Amino Acids.* Washington, DC: National Academies Press, used with permission.

Because of individual biological variation in nutrient absorption and metabolism, some individuals have a relatively low (lower than average) requirement for a nutrient, while others have a relatively high (higher than average) requirement. If the requirement of nutrient X in a given life stage and gender group (e.g., 19- to 30-year-old females who are neither pregnant nor lactating) were plotted as shown in Figure 2.2, a normal, or Gaussian, distribution might result, creating a bell-shaped curve. Although it is usually assumed that nutrient requirements are normally distributed, this is not always the case. In some instances, the nutrient requirements of a particular group may not be known because of insufficient data or, in the case of infants, because it would be unethical to perform the types of studies on infants that would be necessary to determine their nutrient requirements.[10–16] The EARs are sometimes, of necessity, based on scanty data or data drawn from studies with design limitations.[10–16] As seen in Figure 2.2, some individuals have a requirement for nutrient X that is much less than average, but the proportion of these people in a particular life stage and gender group is small, as indicated by the height of the curve above the horizontal axis. Likewise, the proportion having a requirement much greater than average is also small.

The DRI Committee defines requirement as "the lowest continuing intake level of a nutrient that, for a specified indicator of adequacy, will maintain a defined level of nutriture in an individual."[10–16] When setting the EAR, a specific criterion (or criteria) of adequacy must first be selected based on a thorough review of the scientific literature.[10–16] The DRI reports clearly identify the criterion or criteria used in establishing the EAR for each nutrient.[10–15] In some instances, the criterion differs for individuals at different life stages. Criteria used in establishing the EAR include the amount needed to prevent classic deficiency diseases, amounts of the nutrient or its metabolites measured in various tissues during depletion-repletion studies or during induced deficiency states in healthy adult volunteers, and the amount needed to adequately maintain a certain metabolic pathway that is dependent on the nutrient in question. When necessary because of insufficient data on the nutrient requirements of children, adolescents, and pregnant or lactating females, the DRI Committee may choose, when appropriate, to adjust the adult EAR on the basis of differences in reference weights of younger persons or to account for the increased nutrient requirements of the fetus and placenta and for milk production.[10–16] When selecting the criterion to be used, reduction of chronic degenerative disease risk is considered. But despite the intense interest in dietary modification of chronic disease risk, data related to the effects of nutrient intakes on morbidity and mortality from chronic disease in the United States and Canada are limited.

Recommended Dietary Allowance

The Recommended Dietary Allowance (RDA) is defined as "the average daily dietary intake level that is sufficient to meet the nutrient requirement of nearly all (97% to 98%) apparently healthy individuals in a particular life stage and gender group."[12] This is essentially the same

TABLE 2.1 | Dietary Reference Intakes (DRIs): Estimated Average Requirements
Food and Nutrition Board, Institute of Medicine, National Academies

Life Stage Group	Calcium (mg/d)	CHO (g/d)	Protein (g/kg/d)	Vit A (µg/d)[a]	Vit C (mg/d)	Vit D (µg/d)	Vit E (mg/d)[b]	Thiamin (mg/d)	Riboflavin (mg/d)	Niacin (mg/d)[c]	Vit B6 (mg/d)	Folate (µg/d)[d]	Vit B12 (µg/d)	Copper (µg/d)	Iodine (µg/d)	Iron (mg/d)	Magnesium (mg/d)	Molybdenum (µg/d)	Phosphorus (mg/d)	Selenium (µg/d)	Zinc (mg/d)
Infants																					
0 to 6 mo																					2.5
6 to 12 mo			1.0													6.9					2.5
Children																					
1–3 y	500	100	0.87	210	13	10	5	0.4	0.4	5	0.4	120	0.7	260	65	3.0	65	13	380	17	2.5
4–8 y	800	100	0.76	275	22	10	6	0.5	0.5	6	0.5	160	1.0	340	65	4.1	110	17	405	23	4.0
Males																					
9–13 y	1,100	100	0.76	445	39	10	9	0.7	0.8	9	0.8	250	1.5	540	73	5.9	200	26	1,055	35	7.0
14–18 y	1,100	100	0.73	630	63	10	12	1.0	1.1	12	1.1	330	2.0	685	95	7.7	340	33	1,055	45	8.5
19–30 y	800	100	0.66	625	75	10	12	1.0	1.1	12	1.1	320	2.0	700	95	6	330	34	580	45	9.4
31–50 y	800	100	0.66	625	75	10	12	1.0	1.1	12	1.1	320	2.0	700	95	6	350	34	580	45	9.4
51–70 y	800	100	0.66	625	75	10	12	1.0	1.1	12	1.4	320	2.0	700	95	6	350	34	580	45	9.4
>70 y	1,000	100	0.66	625	75	10	12	1.0	1.1	12	1.4	320	2.0	700	95	6	350	34	580	45	9.4
Females																					
9–13 y	1,100	100	0.76	420	39	10	9	0.7	0.8	9	0.8	250	1.5	540	73	5.7	200	26	1,055	35	7.0
14–18 y	1,100	100	0.71	485	56	10	12	0.9	0.9	11	1.0	330	2.0	685	95	7.9	300	33	1,055	45	7.3
19–30 y	800	100	0.66	500	60	10	12	0.9	0.9	11	1.1	320	2.0	700	95	8.1	255	34	580	45	6.8
31–50 y	800	100	0.66	500	60	10	12	0.9	0.9	11	1.1	320	2.0	700	95	8.1	265	34	580	45	6.8
51–70 y	1,000	100	0.66	500	60	10	12	0.9	0.9	11	1.3	320	2.0	700	95	5	265	34	580	45	6.8
>70 y	1,000	100	0.66	500	60	10	12	0.9	0.9	11	1.3	320	2.0	700	95	5	265	34	580	45	6.8
Pregnancy																					
14–18 y	1,000	135	0.88	530	66	10	12	1.2	1.2	14	1.6	520	2.2	785	160	23	335	40	1,055	49	10.5
19–30 y	800	135	0.88	550	70	10	12	1.2	1.2	14	1.6	520	2.2	800	160	22	290	40	580	49	9.5
31–50 y	800	135	0.88	550	70	10	12	1.2	1.2	14	1.6	520	2.2	800	160	22	300	40	580	49	9.5
Lactation																					
14–18 y	1,000	160	1.05	885	96	10	16	1.2	1.3	13	1.7	450	2.4	985	209	7	300	35	1,055	59	10.9
19–30 y	800	160	1.05	900	100	10	16	1.2	1.3	13	1.7	450	2.4	1,000	209	6.5	255	36	580	59	10.4
31–50 y	800	160	1.05	900	100	10	16	1.2	1.3	13	1.7	450	2.4	1,000	209	6.5	265	36	580	59	10.4

Reprinted with permission from the National Academies Press, Copyright 2011, National Academy of Sciences.

Sources: Dietary Reference Intakes for Calcium, Phosphorous, Magnesium, Vitamin D, and Fluoride (1997); *Dietary Reference Intakes for Thiamin, Riboflavin, Niacin, Vitamin B₆, Folate, Vitamin B₁₂, Pantothenic Acid, Biotin, and Choline* (1998); *Dietary Reference Intakes for Vitamin C, Vitamin E, Selenium, and Carotenoids* (2000); *Dietary Reference Intakes for Vitamin A, Vitamin K, Arsenic, Boron, Chromium, Copper, Iodine, Iron, Manganese, Molybdenum, Nickel, Silicon, Vanadium, and Zinc* (2001); *Dietary Reference Intakes for Energy, Carbohydrate, Fiber, Fat, Fatty Acids, Cholesterol, Protein, and Amino Acids* (2002/2005); and *Dietary Reference Intakes for Calcium and Vitamin D* (2011). These reports may be accessed via www.nap.edu.

Note: An Estimated Average Requirement (EAR) is the average daily nutrient intake level estimated to meet the requirements of half of the healthy individuals in a group. EARs have not been established for vitamin K, pantothenic acid, biotin, choline, chromium, fluoride, manganese, or other nutrients not yet evaluated via the DRI process.

[a] As retinol activity equivalents (RAEs). 1 RAE = 1 µg retinol, 12 µg β-carotene, 24 µg α-carotene, or 24 µg β-cryptoxanthin. The RAE for dietary provitamin A carotenoids is two-fold greater than retinol equivalents (RE), whereas the RAE for preformed vitamin A is the same as RE.

[b] As α-tocopherol. α-Tocopherol includes *RRR*-α-tocopherol, the only form of α-tocopherol that occurs naturally in foods, and the 2*R*-stereoisomeric forms of α-tocopherol (*RRR*-, *RSR*-, *RRS*-, and *RSS*-α-tocopherol) that occur in fortified foods and supplements. It does not include the 2*S*-stereoisomeric forms of α-tocopherol (*SRR*-, *SSR*-, *SRS*-, and *SSS*-α-tocopherol), also found in fortified foods and supplements.

Food and Nutrition Board, Institute of Medicine, National Academies

Life Stage Group	Vitamin A (µg/d)[a]	Vitamin C (mg/d)	Vitamin D (µg/d)[b,c]	Vitamin E (mg/d)[d]	Vitamin K (µg/d)	Thiamin (mg/d)	Riboflavin (mg/d)	Niacin (mg/d)[e]	Vitamin B6 (mg/d)	Folate (µg/d)[f]	Vitamin B12 (µg/d)	Pantothenic Acid (mg/d)	Biotin (µg/d)	Choline (mg/d)[g]
Infants														
0 to 6 mo	400*	40*	10*	4*	2.0*	0.2*	0.3*	2*	0.1*	65*	0.4*	1.7*	5*	125*
6 to 12 mo	500*	50*	10*	5*	2.5*	0.3*	0.4*	4*	0.3*	80*	0.5*	1.8*	6*	150*
Children														
1–3 y	300	15	15	6	30*	0.5	0.5	6	0.5	150	0.9	2*	8*	200*
4–8 y	400	25	15	7	55*	0.6	0.6	8	0.6	200	1.2	3*	12*	250*
Males														
9–13 y	600	45	15	11	60*	0.9	0.9	12	1.0	300	1.8	4*	20*	375*
14–18 y	900	75	15	15	75*	1.2	1.3	16	1.3	400	2.4	5*	25*	550*
19–30 y	900	90	15	15	120*	1.2	1.3	16	1.3	400	2.4	5*	30*	550*
31–50 y	900	90	15	15	120*	1.2	1.3	16	1.3	400	2.4	5*	30*	550*
51–70 y	900	90	15	15	120*	1.2	1.3	16	1.7	400	2.4[h]	5*	30*	550*
>70 y	900	90	20	15	120*	1.2	1.3	16	1.7	400	2.4[h]	5*	30*	550*
Females														
9–13 y	600	45	15	11	60*	0.9	0.9	12	1.0	300	1.8	4*	20*	375*
14–18 y	700	65	15	15	75*	1.0	1.0	14	1.2	400[i]	2.4	5*	25*	400*
19–30 y	700	75	15	15	90*	1.1	1.1	14	1.3	400[i]	2.4	5*	30*	425*
31–50 y	700	75	15	15	90*	1.1	1.1	14	1.3	400[i]	2.4	5*	30*	425*
51–70 y	700	75	15	15	90*	1.1	1.1	14	1.5	400	2.4[h]	5*	30*	425*
>70 y	700	75	20	15	90*	1.1	1.1	14	1.5	400	2.4[h]	5*	30*	425*
Pregnancy														
14–18 y	750	80	15	15	75*	1.4	1.4	18	1.9	600[j]	2.6	6*	30*	450*
19–30 y	770	85	15	15	90*	1.4	1.4	18	1.9	600[j]	2.6	6*	30*	450*
31–50 y	770	85	15	15	90*	1.4	1.4	18	1.9	600[j]	2.6	6*	30*	450*
Lactation														
14–18 y	1200	115	15	19	75*	1.4	1.6	17	2.0	500	2.8	7*	35*	550*
19–30 y	1300	120	15	19	90*	1.4	1.6	17	2.0	500	2.8	7*	35*	550*
31–50 y	1300	120	15	19	90*	1.4	1.6	17	2.0	500	2.8	7*	35*	550*

Reprinted with permission from the National Academies Press, Copyright 2011, National Academy of Sciences.

Sources: Dietary Reference Intakes for Calcium, Phosphorous, Magnesium, Vitamin D, and Fluoride (1997); Dietary Reference Intakes for Thiamin, Riboflavin, Niacin, Vitamin B6, Folate, Vitamin B12, Pantothenic Acid, Biotin, and Choline (1998); Dietary Reference Intakes for Vitamin C, Vitamin E, Selenium, and Carotenoids (2000); Dietary Reference Intakes for Vitamin A, Vitamin K, Arsenic, Boron, Chromium, Copper, Iodine, Iron, Manganese, Molybdenum, Nickel, Silicon, Vanadium, and Zinc (2001); Dietary Reference Intakes for Water, Potassium, Sodium, Chloride, and Sulfate (2005); and Dietary Reference Intakes for Calcium and Vitamin D (2011). These reports may be accessed via www.nap.edu.

Note: This table (taken from the DRI reports, see www.nap.edu) presents Recommended Dietary Allowances (RDAs) in **bold type** and Adequate Intakes (AIs) in ordinary type followed by an asterisk (*). An RDA is the average daily dietary intake level; sufficient to meet the nutrient requirements of nearly all (97–98 percent) healthy individuals in a group. It is calculated from an Estimated Average Requirement (EAR). If sufficient scientific evidence is not available to establish an EAR, and thus calculate an RDA, an AI is usually developed. For healthy breastfed infants, an AI is the mean intake. The AI for other life stage and gender groups is believed to cover the needs of all healthy individuals in the groups, but lack of data or uncertainty in the data prevent being able to specify with confidence the percentage of individuals covered by this intake.

[a] As retinol activity equivalents (RAEs). 1 RAE = 1 µg retinol, 12 µg β-carotene, 24 µg α-carotene, or 24 µg β-cryptoxanthin. The RAE for dietary provitamin A carotenoids is two-fold greater than retinol equivalents (RE), whereas the RAE for preformed vitamin A is the same as RE.

[b] As cholecalciferol. 1 µg cholecalciferol = 40 IU vitamin D.

[c] Under the assumption of minimal sunlight.

[d] As α-tocopherol. α-Tocopherol includes RRR-α-tocopherol, the only form of α-tocopherol that occurs naturally in foods, and the 2R-stereoisomeric forms of α-tocopherol (RRR-, RSR-, RRS-, and RSS-α-tocopherol) that occur in fortified foods and supplements. It does not include the 2S-stereoisomeric forms of α-tocopherol (SRR-, SSR-, SRS-, and SSS-α-tocopherol), also found in fortified foods and supplements.

[e] As niacin equivalents (NE). 1 mg of niacin = 60 mg of tryptophan; 0–6 months = preformed niacin (not NE).

[f] As dietary folate equivalents (DFE). 1 DFE = 1 µg food folate = 0.6 µg of folic acid from fortified food or as a supplement consumed with food = 0.5 µg of a supplement taken on an empty stomach.

[g] Although AIs have been set for choline, there are few data to assess whether a dietary supply of choline is needed at all stages of the life cycle, and it may be that the choline requirement can be met by endogenous synthesis at some of these stages.

[h] Because 10 to 30 percent of older people may malabsorb food-bound B12, it is advisable for those older than 50 years to meet their RDA mainly by consuming foods fortified with B12 or a supplement containing B12.

[i] In view of evidence linking folate intake with neural tube defects in the fetus, it is recommended that all women capable of becoming pregnant consume 400 µg from supplements or fortified foods in addition to intake of food folate from a varied diet.

[j] It is assumed that women will continue consuming 400 µg from supplements or fortified food until their pregnancy is confirmed and they enter prenatal care, which ordinarily occurs after the end of the periconceptional period—the critical time for formation of the neural tube.

TABLE 2.5 — Dietary Reference Intakes (DRIs): Tolerable Upper Intake Levels, Elements
Food and Nutrition Board, Institute of Medicine, National Academies

Life Stage Group	Arsenic[a]	Boron (mg/d)	Calcium (mg/d)	Chromium	Copper (μg/d)	Fluoride (mg/d)	Iodine (μg/d)	Iron (mg/d)	Magnesium (mg/d)[b]	Manganese (mg/d)	Molybdenum (μg/d)	Nickel (mg/d)	Phosphorus (g/d)	Selenium (μg/d)	Silicon[c]	Vanadium (mg/d)[d]	Zinc (mg/d)	Sodium (g/d)	Chloride (g/d)
Infants																			
0 to 6 mo	ND[e]	ND	1000	ND	ND	0.7	ND	40	ND	ND	ND	ND	ND	45	ND	ND	4	ND	ND
6 to 12 mo	ND	ND	1500	ND	ND	0.9	ND	40	ND	ND	ND	ND	ND	60	ND	ND	5	ND	ND
Children																			
1–3 y	ND	3	2500	ND	1000	1.3	200	40	65	2	300	0.2	3	90	ND	ND	7	1.5	2.3
4–8 y	ND	6	2500	ND	3000	2.2	300	40	110	3	600	0.3	3	150	ND	ND	12	1.9	2.9
Males																			
9–13 y	ND	11	3000	ND	5000	10	600	40	350	6	1100	0.6	4	280	ND	ND	23	2.2	3.4
14–18 y	ND	17	3000	ND	8000	10	900	45	350	9	1700	1.0	4	400	ND	ND	34	2.3	3.6
19–30 y	ND	20	2500	ND	10,000	10	1100	45	350	11	2000	1.0	4	400	ND	1.8	40	2.3	3.6
31–50 y	ND	20	2500	ND	10,000	10	1100	45	350	11	2000	1.0	4	400	ND	1.8	40	2.3	3.6
51–70 y	ND	20	2000	ND	10,000	10	1100	45	350	11	2000	1.0	4	400	ND	1.8	40	2.3	3.6
>70 y	ND	20	2000	ND	10,000	10	1100	45	350	11	2000	1.0	3	400	ND	1.8	40	2.3	3.6
Females																			
9–13 y	ND	11	3000	ND	5000	10	600	40	350	6	1100	0.6	4	280	ND	ND	23	2.2	3.4
14–18 y	ND	17	3000	ND	8000	10	900	45	350	9	1700	1.0	4	400	ND	ND	34	2.3	3.6
19–30 y	ND	20	2500	ND	10,000	10	1100	45	350	11	2000	1.0	4	400	ND	1.8	40	2.3	3.6
31–50 y	ND	20	2500	ND	10,000	10	1100	45	350	11	2000	1.0	4	400	ND	1.8	40	2.3	3.6
51–70 y	ND	20	2000	ND	10,000	10	1100	45	350	11	2000	1.0	4	400	ND	1.8	40	2.3	3.6
>70 y	ND	20	2000	ND	10,000	10	1100	45	350	11	2000	1.0	3	400	ND	1.8	40	2.3	3.6
Pregnancy																			
14–18 y	ND	17	3000	ND	8000	10	900	45	350	9	1700	1.0	3.5	400	ND	ND	34	2.3	3.6
19–30 y	ND	20	2500	ND	10,000	10	1100	45	350	11	2000	1.0	3.5	400	ND	ND	40	2.3	3.6
31–50 y	ND	20	2500	ND	10,000	10	1100	45	350	11	2000	1.0	3.5	400	ND	ND	40	2.3	3.6
Lactation																			
14–18 y	ND	17	3000	ND	8000	10	900	45	350	9	1700	1.0	4	400	ND	ND	34	2.3	3.6
19–30 y	ND	20	2500	ND	10,000	10	1100	45	350	11	2000	1.0	4	400	ND	ND	40	2.3	3.6
31–50 y	ND	20	2500	ND	10,000	10	1100	45	350	11	2000	1.0	4	400	ND	ND	40	2.3	3.6

Reprinted with permission from the National Academies Press, Copyright 2011, National Academy of Sciences.

Sources: Dietary Reference Intakes for Calcium, Phosphorous, Magnesium, Vitamin D, and Fluoride (1997); Dietary Reference Intakes for Thiamin, Riboflavin, Niacin, Vitamin B₆, Folate, Vitamin B₁₂, Pantothenic Acid, Biotin, and Choline (1998); Dietary Reference Intakes for Vitamin C, Vitamin E, Selenium, and Carotenoids (2000); Dietary Reference Intakes for Vitamin A, Vitamin K, Arsenic, Boron, Chromium, Copper, Iodine, Iron, Manganese, Molybdenum, Nickel, Silicon, Vanadium, and Zinc (2001); Dietary Reference Intakes for Water, Potassium, Sodium, Chloride, and Sulfate (2005); and Dietary Reference Intakes for Calcium and Vitamin D (2011). These reports may be accessed via www.nap.edu.

Note: A Tolerable Upper Intake Level (UL) is the highest level of daily nutrient intake that is likely to pose no risk of adverse health effects to almost all individuals in the general population. Unless otherwise specified, the UL represents total intake from food, water, and supplements. Due to a lack of suitable data, ULs could not be established for vitamin K, thiamin, riboflavin, vitamin B₁₂, pantothenic acid, biotin, and carotenoids. In the absence of a UL, extra caution may be warranted in consuming levels above recommended intakes. Members of the general population should be advised not to routinely exceed the UL. The UL is not meant to apply to individuals who are treated with the nutrient under medical supervision or to individuals with predisposing conditions that modify their sensitivity to the nutrient.

[a]Although the UL was not determined for arsenic, there is no justification for adding arsenic to food or supplements.

[b]The ULs for magnesium represent intake from a pharmacological agent only and do not include intake from food and water.

[c]Although silicon has not been shown to cause adverse effects in humans, there is no justification for adding silicon to supplements.

[d]Although vanadium in food has not been shown to cause adverse effects in humans, there is no justification for adding vanadium to food and vanadium supplements should be used with caution. The UL is based on adverse effects in

28

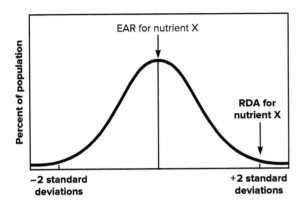

Figure 2.2 **The distribution of the requirement for nutrient X for a life stage and gender group.**
The Estimated Average Requirement (EAR) and the Recommended Dietary Allowance (RDA) are shown. The nutrient requirement level that is 2 standard deviations greater than the EAR is generally selected for the RDA.

Source: Otten JJ, Hellwig JP, Meyers LD. 2006. *Dietary Reference Intakes: The essential guide to nutrient requirements.* Washington, DC: National Academy Press.

definition as that used in the 10th edition of the *Recommended Dietary Allowances.*[8]

The RDA for a particular nutrient can be set only if the EAR for that nutrient is established. If the requirement for the nutrient among individuals in the life stage and gender group is normally distributed and if data about the variability in requirements are sufficient to calculate the **standard deviation (SD)** of the EAR (SD$_{EAR}$), the RDA is set at 2 standard deviations above the EAR, as illustrated in Figure 2.2. This is shown mathematically by the following equation:

$$RDA = EAR + 2\ SD_{EAR}$$

Obviously, if the RDA were set at the EAR, the RDA would meet the needs of only half the individuals in a life stage and gender group—those individuals having a requirement equal to or less than the EAR. The requirement for nutrient X for the other half of individuals in the group—those with a requirement greater than the EAR—would not be met. Thus, to meet the needs of nearly all apparently healthy individuals in a particular life stage and gender group, the RDA is set at 2 standard deviations above the EAR. The standard deviation indicates the degree of variation from the mean; in this case, it indicates how different the nutrient requirements of individual group members are from the group mean. At 2 standard deviations above the mean, the requirement for nutrient X would be met for nearly 98% of individuals in a life stage and gender group.

If data about variability in nutrient requirements are insufficient to calculate a standard deviation, a **coefficient of variation (CV)** for the EAR (CV$_{EAR}$) of 10% is generally assumed and used in place of the standard deviation.[10–16] The coefficient of variation is the standard

deviation divided by the mean, as shown in the following equations:

$$CV_{EAR} = SD_{EAR} \div EAR,$$
$$SD_{EAR} = CV_{EAR} \times EAR$$

In this situation, the RDA can be calculated as follows:

$$RDA = EAR + 2(CV_{EAR} \times EAR),\ or$$
$$RDA = EAR + 2(0.1 \times EAR),\ or$$
$$RDA = 1.2 \times EAR$$

If the nutrient requirement for a particular group is known to be skewed, other approaches can be used to find the intake level sufficient to meet the nutrient requirement of 97% to 98% of healthy persons in a particular life stage and gender group in order to set the RDA.[10–16]

A safety margin also is built into the RDA of a nutrient to compensate for its incomplete use by the body and to account for variations in the levels of the nutrient provided by various food sources. Adjustment also is made in some RDAs to account for the consumption of certain dietary components that are subsequently converted within the body to an essential nutrient. For example, the amino acid tryptophan can be converted to niacin within the body.[11] Examples of RDAs that have been included as part of the DRIs were shown in bold type in Tables 2.2 and 2.3.

Adequate Intake

If insufficient data are available to calculate an EAR, and thus an RDA cannot be set for a particular nutrient, a separate reference intake, known as Adequate Intake (AI), is used instead of the RDA. Adequate Intake is defined as "a value based on experimentally derived intake levels or approximations of observed mean nutrient intakes by a group (or groups) of healthy people."[10–16] For example, as was shown in Tables 2.2 and 2.3, most nutrient intake levels for infants (birth to 12 months of age) are expressed as AIs instead of RDAs because the types of studies necessary to determine the nutrient requirements of infants (e.g., depletion-repletion studies) cannot ethically be done. The AIs for infants from birth to 6 months of age were calculated based on the mean nutrient intakes of healthy, full-term infants 2 to 6 months of age who were exclusively breast-fed.[10–16] By weighing these infants before and after breast-feeding, researchers determined that the average volume of milk intake was 780 ml/day. Based on the nutritional composition of human milk, researchers could then determine the average nutritional intake of these infants. For infants 7 to 12 months of age, the AIs are based on the average nutrient intakes of 7- to 12-month-old infants fed a combination of human milk and typical complementary weaning foods used in North America.

As shown in Tables 2.2 and 2.3, the recommended intakes for vitamin D, vitamin K, pantothenic acid, biotin, choline, calcium, chromium, fluoride, manganese, potassium, sodium, and chloride are expressed as AIs for all life stages and gender groups. This is because there are insufficient data on the requirements of these nutrients, resulting in an inability to establish an EAR and an RDA. As future research provides additional data on the requirements for these nutrients, an EAR and RDA can be set.

It is important to note that the AI is an observational standard—it is based on observed or experimentally derived approximations of average nutrient intake that appear to maintain a defined nutritional state or criterion of adequacy in a group of people.[10–16] Defined nutritional states include normal growth, maintenance of normal circulating nutrient values, and other indicators of nutritional well-being and general health. Because it is set using presumably healthy groups of individuals, the AI is expected to meet or exceed the actual nutrient requirement in practically all healthy members of a specific life stage and gender group. Like the RDA, the AI is intended to serve as a goal for the nutrient intake of healthy individuals. When nutrient requirements are altered due to injury, disease, or some other special health need, the RDA and AI should serve as the basis for an individual's nutrient recommendations, which, depending on the situation, may then need to be adjusted by a registered dietitian or qualified health professional to accommodate the individual's increased or decreased nutrient needs.[10–16] Unlike the RDA, however, the AI is used when data on nutrient requirements are lacking, and consequently greater uncertainty surrounds the AI.[10–16] Its use indicates a need for additional research on the requirements for that particular nutrient or food component.

Tolerable Upper Intake Level

The Tolerable Upper Intake Level (UL) is defined as "the highest average daily nutrient intake level that is likely to pose no risk of adverse health effects in almost all individuals in the specified life stage group."[10–16] Examples of these were shown in Tables 2.4 and 2.5. The UL is not intended to be a recommended level of nutrient intake but, rather, an indication of the maximum amount of a nutrient that can, with a high degree of probability, be taken on a daily basis without endangering one's health—in other words, the maximum amount that likely can be *tolerated* by the body when consumed on a daily basis. The term *adverse effect* is defined as "any significant alteration in the structure or function of the human organism" or any "impairment of a physiologically important function that could lead to a health effect that is adverse."[10] To determine the UL, the DRI Committee uses a risk assessment model, which is discussed at length in the DRI reports.[10–16]

The UL was created in response to concerns about the potential for excessive nutrient intakes resulting from recent increases in consumption of nutrient-fortified foods and dietary supplements. Just as inadequate nutrient intake can adversely affect health (e.g., result in nutrient-deficiency disease), so can excessive nutrient intake. As illustrated in Figure 2.3, when a nutrient's level of intake is low, risk of inadequacy increases, as indicated by the curve on the left side of the figure. At a very low intake level, the curve is at its highest point, signifying that risk of inadequacy is 100% (indicated as 1.0 in Figure 2.3). When nutrient intake is very high, there is increased risk of excess nutrient intake (what the DRI Committee calls

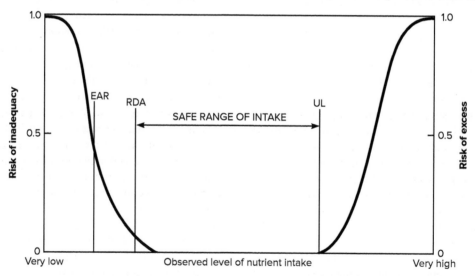

Figure 2.3 The risk of inadequate or excess intake varies according to the level of nutrient intake. When nutrient intake is very low, the risk of inadequacy is high. When nutrient intake is very high, the risk of excessive intake is high. Between the RDA and UL is a safe range of intake associated with a very low probability of either inadequate or excessive nutrient intake. EAR = Estimated Average Requirement; RDA = Recommended Dietary Allowance; UL = Tolerable Upper Intake Level.

Source: Otten JJ, Hellwig JP, Meyers LD. 2006. *Dietary Reference Intakes: The essential guide to nutrient requirements.* Washington, DC: National Academy Press.

"risk of adverse effects"), as indicated by the curve on the right side of the figure. An intake level at the UL is unlikely to pose a risk of excessive nutrient intake for most (but not necessarily all) individuals in a specific group. However, as nutrient intake increases above the UL, the risk of adverse health effects increases. When nutrient intake is at the EAR, risk of inadequacy is considered 50% (indicated as 0.5 in Figure 2.3). At the RDA, 97% to 98% of healthy individuals will have their requirement met. Between the RDA and UL is a safe range of intake associated with a very low probability of either inadequate or excessive nutrient intake. However, setting a UL does not suggest that a nutrient intake level greater than the RDA or AI is of any benefit to an individual.

Figure 2.3 does not show the AI because it is an observational standard and set without being able to estimate the requirement. However, the AI is intended to meet or exceed the actual nutrient requirement in practically all healthy members of a specific life stage and gender group and, thus, should be fairly close to the RDA for that nutrient and life stage and gender group, if the RDA is known. Once additional research provides data on the distribution of the requirement for a nutrient and the AI can be replaced with an EAR and RDA, it is likely that the RDA will be slightly less than, if not greater than, the RDA.[10–16]

Prior to the development of the DRIs, the Recommended Dietary Allowances failed to provide any guidance on the safe use of nutritional supplements and addressed the issue of supplement use only by recommending that the RDAs be met by consuming a diet ". . . composed of a *variety* of foods that are derived from diverse food groups rather than by supplementation or fortification. . . ."[8] It is important to note that this remains an excellent recommendation for a variety of reasons. For example, given the complexity of nutrients and other components in food (some of which we know little or nothing about) it is clear that we cannot solely rely on nutritional supplements as a source of these nutrients and other components and must depend primarily on food to obtain them.[12] However, there is need for information on the maximum amounts of supplemental nutrients that can be safely consumed, given the recent proliferation of nutrient-fortified foods in the marketplace, the increased interest in and use of nutritional and dietary supplements by North Americans, and a growing body of scientific evidence demonstrating that in some instances nutrient intakes in excess of the amounts typically obtained solely from diets can reduce chronic disease risk. The ULs help provide this information and fill an important niche. The ULs are not intended to apply to persons receiving nutrient or other dietary supplements under medical supervision.[12]

If adverse effects of excess nutrient consumption are associated with total nutrient intake, the ULs are based on total nutrient intake from food, water, and supplements. If adverse effects are associated only with intakes from supplements or fortified foods, the ULs are based on nutrient intakes from those sources.[12] For many nutrients, there are insufficient data available to set a UL. But the absence of a UL does not imply that a high intake of that nutrient is risk-free. On the contrary, it may suggest that greater caution is warranted when intakes exceed the RDA or AI.[12]

Estimated Energy Requirement

The Estimated Energy Requirement (EER) is the average dietary energy intake that is predicted to maintain energy balance in a healthy person of a defined age, gender, weight, height, and level of physical activity consistent with good health.[14] For infants, children, and adolescents the EER includes the energy needed for a desirable level of physical activity and for optimal growth, maturation, and development at an age- and gender-appropriate rate that is consistent with good health, including maintenance of a healthy body weight and appropriate body composition. For females who are pregnant or lactating, the EER includes the energy needed for physical activity, for maternal and fetal development, and for lactation at a rate that is consistent with good health.[14]

The EER is calculated using prediction equations developed by the DRI Committee for healthy-weight individuals age 0 to 100 years based on the 24-hour total energy expenditures of more than 1200 subjects measured using the doubly labeled water technique.[14] The doubly labeled water method (described in Chapter 7) is considered the most accurate approach for determining total energy expenditure (TEE) in free-living individuals (i.e., research subjects who are not restricted to a laboratory and who are able to go about their normal daily routines unencumbered by breathing equipment or any other laboratory apparatus). Using the measured 24-hour total energy expenditure data obtained from these healthy-weight subjects, the DRI Committee developed a series of regression equations that best predict the energy requirement of healthy-weight individuals using such variables as age, gender, life stage (pregnant or lactating), body weight, height, and physical activity level. A separate set of prediction equations were developed for adults (age 19 years and older) who are overweight or obese and for children and adolescents (age 3 to 18 years) who are at risk of overweight or who are overweight.[14] The equations for calculating EER are discussed at length in Chapter 7.

There is no Recommended Dietary Allowance or Tolerable Upper Intake Level for energy. By definition, the RDA is generally set at 2 standard deviations greater than the EAR for a given nutrient (e.g., vitamins, elements, and protein) and an energy intake 2 standard deviations greater than the average energy requirement would result in weight gain. Likewise, the UL is set at a nutrient intake level in excess of even the RDA, and an energy intake at such a high level would result in an undesirable and potentially unhealthy weight gain.[14]

Recommendations for Macronutrients

The DRI Committee has developed recommendations for the consumption of macronutrients and various food components. Table 2.6 shows the RDAs (values in bold type) and AIs (values in ordinary type followed by an asterisk) for **total water,** carbohydrate, **total fiber,** total fat, linoleic acid, α-linolenic acid, and protein for the 22 different life stage and gender groups.[14,15] Total water includes drinking water, water in other beverages, and water (moisture) in foods.[15] The values for carbohydrates

are based on the minimum amount of glucose needed by the brain and are typically exceeded in order for a person to meet the energy needs of the body while consuming an acceptable proportion of energy from fats and protein.[14]

The AI for total fiber in Table 2.6 is based on research findings showing that risk of coronary heart disease is reduced in adults consuming 14 g of total fiber/1000 kilocalories (kcal). Except for infants, the AI for total fiber was set by multiplying the recommendation for total fiber (i.e., 14 g of total fiber/1000 kcal) by the median energy intake

TABLE 2.6	Dietary Reference Intakes (DRIs): Recommended Dietary Allowances and Adequate Intakes, Total Water and Macronutrients
	Food and Nutrition Board, Institute of Medicine, National Academies

Life Stage Group	Total Water[a] (L/d)	Carbohydrate (g/d)	Total Fiber (g/d)	Fat (g/d)	Linoleic Acid (g/d)	α-Linolenic Acid (g/d)	Protein[b] (g/d)
Infants							
0 to 6 mo	0.7*	60*	ND	31*	4.4*	0.5*	9.1*
6 to 12 mo	0.8*	95*	ND	30*	4.6*	0.5*	**11.0**
Children							
1–3 y	1.3*	**130**	19*	ND[c]	7*	0.7*	**13**
4–8 y	1.7*	**130**	25*	ND	10*	0.9*	**19**
Males							
9–13 y	2.4*	**130**	31*	ND	12*	1.2*	**34**
14–18 y	3.3*	**130**	38*	ND	16*	1.6*	**52**
19–30 y	3.7*	**130**	38*	ND	17*	1.6*	**56**
31–50 y	3.7*	**130**	38*	ND	17*	1.6*	**56**
51–70 y	3.7*	**130**	30*	ND	14*	1.6*	**56**
> 70 y	3.7*	**130**	30*	ND	14*	1.6*	**56**
Females							
9–13 y	2.1*	**130**	26*	ND	10*	1.0*	**34**
14–18 y	2.3*	**130**	26*	ND	11*	1.1*	**46**
19–30 y	2.7*	**130**	25*	ND	12*	1.1*	**46**
31–50 y	2.7*	**130**	25*	ND	12*	1.1*	**46**
51–70 y	2.7*	**130**	21*	ND	11*	1.1*	**46**
> 70 y	2.7*	**130**	21*	ND	11*	1.1*	**46**
Pregnancy							
14–18 y	3.0*	**175**	28*	ND	13*	1.4*	**71**
19–30 y	3.0*	**175**	28*	ND	13*	1.4*	**71**
31–50 y	3.0*	**175**	28*	ND	13*	1.4*	**71**
Lactation							
14–18	3.8*	**210**	29*	ND	13*	1.3*	**71**
19–30 y	3.8*	**210**	29*	ND	13*	1.3*	**71**
31–50 y	3.8*	**210**	29*	ND	13*	1.3*	**71**

Reprinted with permission from the National Academies Press, Copyright 2011, National Academy of Sciences.

Source: Dietary Reference Intakes for Energy, Carbohydrate, Fiber, Fat, Fatty Acids, Cholesterol, Protein, and Amino Acids (2002/2005) and *Dietary Reference Intakes for Water, Potassium, Sodium, Chloride, and Sulfate* (2005). The report may be accessed via www.nap.edu.

Note: This table (taken from the DRI reports, see www.nap.edu) presents Recommended Dietary Allowances (RDA) in **bold type** and Adequate Intakes (AI) in ordinary type followed by an asterisk (*). An RDA is the average daily dietary intake level; sufficient to meet the nutrient requirements of nearly all (97–98 percent) healthy individuals in a group. It is calculated from an Estimated Average Requirement (EAR). If sufficient scientific evidence is not available to establish an EAR, and thus calculate an RDA, an AI is usually developed. For healthy breastfed infants, an AI is the mean intake. The AI for other life stage and gender groups is believed to cover the needs of all healthy individuals in the groups, but lack of data or uncertainty in the data prevent being able to specify with confidence the percentage of individuals covered by this intake.

[a]Total water includes all water contained in food, beverages, and drinking water.

[b]Based on g protein per kg of body weight for the reference body weight, e.g., for adults 0.8 g/kg body weight for the reference body weight.

[c]Not determined.

for each of the life stage and gender groups.[14] Human milk, which contains no **dietary fiber,** is considered the optimal source of nourishment for infants throughout at least the first year of life and is recommended as the only source of nourishment for the first four to six months of life. As solid foods are gradually introduced during the second six months of life, dietary fiber intake will increase. However, there are no data on dietary fiber intake for infants and no functional criteria for fiber status available upon which to establish an AI for total fiber for infants. Total fiber is defined as the sum of dietary fiber and **functional fiber.**[14] Dietary fibers are nondigestible carbohydrates and lignin that are naturally present in plant foods and that are consumed in their natural, intact state (i.e., in an unmodified form) as part of an unrefined food. Functional fibers are nondigestible carbohydrates that have beneficial physiological effects in humans but that have been isolated or extracted (i.e., removed) from foods and then added as an ingredient to food or taken as a dietary supplement. Although functional fibers are predominantly of plant origin, a few are of animal origin, such as the animal-derived connective tissues chitin and chitosan, which are found in the exoskeletons of arthropods such as crabs and lobsters. In essence, what distinguishes functional fiber from dietary fiber is the source of the fiber. Functional fibers have been removed from their original source and then added to another food or are consumed as a nutritional supplement. Dietary fibers are naturally present in plant foods that are eaten.[14] For example, the pectin consumed when an apple is eaten would be considered a dietary fiber. When the pectin is industrially extracted from fruits and then added as a gelling agent to jams, it is considered a functional fiber.[14]

Except for infants, no RDA or AI has been established for total fat because there are insufficient data available to determine a level of total fat intake associated with risk of inadequacy or prevention of chronic disease. There is no UL established for total fat because no level has been identified that is associated with an averse effect.[14] The AI for total fat for infants birth to 6 months is set at the mean

intake of fat by infants of this age who are exclusively breast-fed. The AI for total fat for infants 7 to 12 months of age is based on the mean fat intake of infants of this age who are fed human milk and age-appropriate complementary foods.[14] Linoleic acid (an *n*-6 fatty acid) and α-linolenic acid (an *n*-3 fatty acid) are necessary for optimal health, and an insufficient intake of either can result in adverse clinical symptoms such as a scaly skin rash, neurological abnormalities, and poor growth. Because neither linoleic acid nor α-linolenic acid is synthesized by the human body and because both are necessary for optimal health, they are considered essential fatty acids and an AI has been established for each.[14] For infants birth to 6 months of age, the AIs for linoleic acid and α-linolenic acid are set at the mean intakes of these fatty acids by infants of this age who are exclusively breast-fed. The AIs for linoleic acid and α-linolenic acid for infants 7 to 12 months of age are based on the mean intakes of these fatty acids by infants of this age who are fed human milk and age-appropriate complementary foods.[14] For the remaining life stage and gender groups, the AIs for linoleic acid and α-linolenic acid are set at the median intake of these fatty acids in the diets of Americans who have no apparent deficiency of these essential fatty acids.[14] The AI for protein for infants birth to 6 months of age is set at the mean protein intake of infants of this age who are exclusively breast-fed. The RDA for protein (grams of protein per day) for the remaining life stage and gender groups are shown in Table 2.6.[14] Although there were insufficient data available to establish a UL for protein, the DRI Committee has cautioned against the consumption of any single amino acids at levels greater than those normally found in foods.[14]

Acceptable Macronutrient Distribution Ranges (AMDRs) provide guidance to individuals on the consumption of total fat, *n*-6 polyunsaturated fatty acids (linoleic acid), *n*-3 polyunsaturated fatty acids (α-linolenic acid), carbohydrate, and protein to ensure adequate intake and to decrease risk of chronic disease. The AMDRs, shown in Table 2.7, are expressed in terms of percent of

TABLE 2.7	**Dietary Reference Intakes (DRIs): Acceptable Macronutrient Distribution Ranges** Food and Nutrition Board, Institute of Medicine, National Academies		
	Range (percent of energy)		
Macronutrient	**Children, 1–3 y**	**Children, 4–18 y**	**Adults**
Fat	30–40	25–35	20–35
n-6 polyunsaturated fatty acids[a] (linoleic acid)	5–10	5–10	5–10
n-3 polyunsaturated fatty acids[a] (α-linolenic acid)	0.6–1.2	0.6–1.2	0.6–1.2
Carbohydrate	45–65	45–65	45–65
Protein	5–20	10–30	10–35

Reprinted with permission from the National Academies Press, Copyright 2011, National Academy of Sciences.

Source: Dietary Reference Intakes for Energy, Carbohydrate, Fiber, Fat, Fatty Acids, Cholesterol, Protein, and Amino Acids (2002/2005). The report may be accessed via www.nap.edu.

[a]Approximately 10 percent of the total can come from longer-chain *n*-3 or *n*-6 fatty acids.

TABLE 2.8	Dietary Reference Intakes (DRIs): Acceptable Macronutrient Distribution Ranges
	Food and Nutrition Board, Institute of Medicine, National Academies

Macronutrient	Recommendation
Dietary cholesterol	As low as possible while consuming a nutritionally adequate diet
Trans fatty acids	As low as possible while consuming a nutritionally adequate diet
Saturated fatty acids	As low as possible while consuming a nutritionally adequate diet
Added sugars[a]	Limit to no more than 25% of total energy

Reprinted with permission from the National Academies Press, Copyright 2011, National Academy of Sciences.

Source: Dietary Reference Intakes for Energy, Carbohydrate, Fiber, Fat, Fatty Acids, Cholesterol, Protein, and Amino Acids (2002/2005). The report may be accessed via www.nap.edu.

[a]Not a recommended intake. A daily intake of added sugars that individuals should aim for to achieve a healthful diet was not set.

energy from each of these macronutrients for three different age ranges: 1 to 3 years of age, 4 to 18 years of age, and 19 years of age and older. No other distinctions are made with regard to life stage or gender.[14] Additional macronutrient recommendations for the prevention of chronic disease are shown in Table 2.8. These recommendations address concerns related to the health implications of diets containing excessive quantities of dietary cholesterol, *trans* fatty acids, saturated fatty acids, and added sugars. It is important to note that while it is suggested that consumption of added sugars be *limited to no more than 25% of total energy,* this is not a recommended level of intake. The 2015–2020 Dietary Guidelines for Americans recommend that individuals consume less than 10% of calories per day from added sugars. This will be reviewed later in this chapter.

Uses of the DRIs

The suggested uses of the DRIs fall into two broad categories: assessing nutrient intakes and planning for nutrient intakes. Each of the two categories is further divided into uses pertaining to individuals and uses pertaining to groups. The uses of the DRIs for assessing and planning the intakes of apparently healthy individuals and groups are outlined in Boxes 2.3 and 2.4, respectively.

The DRIs are not intended to serve as the only means of assessing the nutritional adequacy of an individual's diet. An individual's actual nutrient requirement can vary widely from the group average (the EAR), and without various biochemical and physiologic measures it is impossible to determine whether an individual's actual nutrient requirement is close to the group EAR, greater than the EAR, or less than the EAR. In addition, intake of most nutrients varies considerably from one day to the next,

requiring many days of measurement to estimate *usual* nutrient intake, as discussed in Chapter 3. Consequently, when assessing the adequacy of an individual's diet, use of multiple nutritional assessment methods—dietary, anthropometric, biochemical, and clinical—must be considered.

If an individual's usual intake of a nutrient is equal to or greater than the RDA or AI, it is unlikely that intake is inadequate. When usual intake is less than the EAR, there is a high likelihood that intake is inadequate. However, if usual intake falls between the EAR and RDA, the likelihood of inadequate intake will be difficult to determine, and in such instances use of other assessment techniques is important in determining nutrient adequacy.[17] If an individual's usual intake of a nutrient is less than the UL, there is little risk of excessive intake. Risk of adverse health effects from excessive intake increases when usual intake rises above the UL.[17] When planning a healthy individual's diet, the RDAs and AIs are intended to serve as a goal for average daily nutrient intake over time (over several days to several weeks, depending on the turnover rate of the nutrient in question).[18]

Assessing the adequacy of a group's nutrient intake involves comparing the distribution of usual intakes among group members with the distribution of the requirement for the nutrient.[17] A "cutpoint approach" is typically used to estimate the percentage of group members whose usual intakes are less than the EAR. The RDA is not intended to be used for estimating the prevalence of inadequate intakes in groups.[17] In the absence of an EAR, it may be necessary to use the AI to assess the adequacy of a group's intake, but greater care must be exercised than when using the EAR, given the fact that the AI is an observational standard.[17] The proportion of the population with usual intakes above the UL is likely to be at some risk of adverse effects due to overconsumption, while the proportion below the UL is likely to be at no risk.[17]

Data from the *What We Eat in America,* NHANES 2013–2014, indicate that about 38% of the population has a usual intake of vitamin C below the EAR. The 2015–2020 Dietary Guidelines for Americans (DGA) have identified vitamin C as a nutrient of concern. The EAR standard was used by DGA to also identify vitamin A, vitamin D, vitamin E, folate, calcium, and magnesium as nutrients of concern, as reviewed later in this chapter. Estimating the prevalence of inadequate nutrient intakes in a population requires accurate, quantitative information on usual nutrient intake by the group. Both the U.S. Department of Health and Human Services and the U.S. Department of Agriculture participate in the National Health and Nutrition Examination Survey, or NHANES, which provides data on the food and nutrient intake of Americans as well as data on various health determinants such as height, weight, blood pressure, blood cholesterol levels, and so on. NHANES and the other nutritional monitoring activities of these two agencies are discussed in Chapter 4.

The EAR is used in planning or making recommendations for the nutrient intake of groups. The group's mean

Box 2.3 **Uses of DRIs for Assessing Intakes of Individuals and Groups**

FOR AN INDIVIDUAL

EAR: Use to examine the probability that usual intake is inadequate.

RDA: Usual intake at or above this level has a low probability of inadequacy.

AI: Usual intake at or above this level has a low probability of inadequacy.

UL: Usual intake above this level may place an individual at risk of adverse effects from excessive nutrient intake.

EAR = Estimated Average Requirement

RDA = Recommended Dietary Allowance

AI = Adequate Intake

UL = Tolerable Upper Intake Level

FOR A GROUP

EAR: Use to estimate the prevalence of inadequate intakes within a group.

RDA: Do not use to assess intakes of groups.

AI: Mean usual intake at or above this level implies a low prevalence of inadequate intakes.[a]

UL: Use to estimate the percentage of the population at potential risk of adverse effects from excessive nutrient intake.

[a]When the AI for a nutrient is not based on mean intakes of healthy populations, this assessment is made with less confidence.

Reprinted with permission from the National Academies Press, Copyright 2000, National Academy of Sciences.

 Box 2.4 **Uses of DRIs for Planning Intakes of Apparently Healthy Individuals and Groups**

FOR AN INDIVIDUAL

EAR[a]: Do not use as an intake goal for the individual.

RDA: Plan for this intake; usual intake at or above this level has a low probability of inadequacy.

AI: Plan for this intake; usual intake at or above this level has a low probability of inadequacy.

UL: Plan for usual intake below this level to avoid potential risk of adverse effects from excessive nutrient intake.

[a]In the case of energy, an EER is provided. The EER is the dietary energy intake that is predicted (with variance) to maintain energy balance in a healthy adult of a defined age, gender, weight, height, and level of physical activity. In children and in pregnant and lactating women, the EER includes the needs associated with deposition of tissues or secretion of milk at rates consistent with good health. For individuals, the EER represents the midpoint of a range within which an individual's energy requirements are

FOR A GROUP

EAR[a]: Use to plan for an acceptably low prevalence of inadequate intakes within a group.

RDA: Do not use to plan intakes of groups.

AI[b]: Plan for mean intake at this level; mean usual intake at or above this level implies a low prevalence of inadequate intakes.

UL: Use in planning to minimize the proportion of the population at potential risk of excessive nutrient intake.

likely to vary. As such, it is below the needs of half the individuals with the specified characteristics, and it exceeds the needs of the other half. Body weight should be monitored and energy intake adjusted accordingly.

[b]The AI should be used with less confidence if it has not been established as a mean intake of a healthy group.

Reprinted with permission from the National Academies Press, Copyright 2003, National Academy of Sciences.

nutrient intake should be high enough so that only a small percentage of group members have an intake less than the EAR but not so high that too many group members have intakes above the UL. If the prevalence of nutrient inadequacy is too high, an appropriate intervention should be undertaken to increase intakes by those at greatest risk of inadequacy while maintaining an acceptably low prevalence of group members with intake above the UL.

NUTRIENT DENSITY

Nutrient density refers to a food's vitamin and mineral content relative to its energy content.[20–22] A nutrient-dense food is a good source of vitamins, minerals, and

other food components that may have positive health effects but is relatively low in energy. Nutrient-dense foods are lean or low in solids fats (fats that are solid at room temperature and that are major sources of saturated and *trans* fats) and are low in added sugars and refined starches, all of which add kilocalories but few essential nutrients or dietary fiber. Nutrient-dense foods also minimize or exclude added salt or other components that are high in sodium.[23]

Box 2.5 compares high-nutrient-dense foods with low-nutrient-dense foods. Although the low-nutrient-dense foods share similarities with the high-nutrient-dense foods, they differ in that they are higher in kilocalories because of fats and sugars, most of which are

Box 2.5

Foods having a high nutrient density (the left column) are good sources of essential nutrients but are relatively low in kilocalories compared to similar foods having a low nutrient density (the right column), which are relatively high in kilocalories because of the fats and sugars added during processing or preparation.

HIGH-NUTRIENT-DENSE FOODS	LOW-NUTRIENT-DENSE FOODS
Broccoli, steamed, served with lemon wedges	Broccoli, batter dipped, deep-fat fried
Potato, baked	Potato, french fried
Turkey breast, skinless, broiled	Hamburger patty, fried
Salad dressing, low-calorie	Salad dressing, regular
Milk, nonfat, plain	Milk, whole, plain
Orange juice, unsweetened, calcium-fortified	Soft-drink, orange-flavored, sugar-sweetened
Yogurt, nonfat, unsweetened	Yogurt, fruit-flavored, sweetened

added during processing, during preparation, or at the table. For example, broccoli that is served with a cheese sauce or is dipped in batter and deep-fat fried will have many of the same vitamins and minerals as the steamed broccoli, but the cheese sauce or deep-fat frying will add extra kilocalories that many people want to avoid to prevent unnecessary weight gain. Furthermore, a person can eat a liberal amount of the steamed broccoli served with lemon wedges without consuming excessive energy.

Figure 2.4 illustrates the difference in the number of calories in a food that is not nutrient-dense as opposed to a nutrient-dense form of the food. For example, a regular ground beef patty (75% lean) that weighs 3 ounces after

cooking contains 236 calories, whereas a cooked 3-ounce extra lean beef patty (90% lean) contains 184 calories. By choosing the extra lean beef instead of the regular ground beef, a person would consume less beef fat, amounting to 52 fewer calories. Breaded fried chicken strips weighing 3 ounces contain 246 calories, whereas a 3-ounce baked chicken breast contains only 138 calories. In this instance, a relatively simple change in the method of preparation and cooking the chicken has eliminated 108 calories that were added by the breading and frying fat. According to the 2010 Dietary Guidelines for Americans, nutrient-dense foods include all vegetables, fruits, whole grains, fat-free or low-fat milk and milk products, beans and

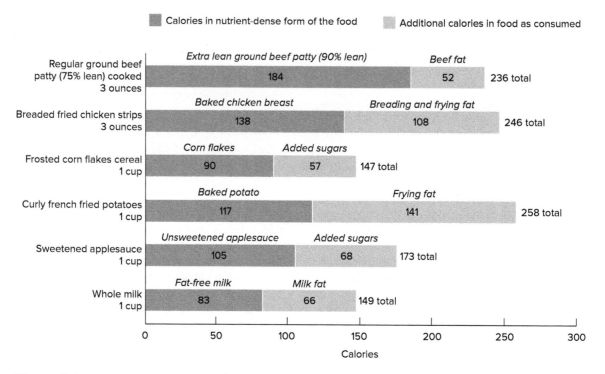

Figure 2.4 Examples of the calories in food choices that are not in nutrient-dense forms and the calories in nutrient-dense forms of these foods.

Source: U.S. Department of Health and Human Services and U.S. Department of Agriculture. 2010. *Dietary Guidelines for Americans, 2010.* Washington, DC: U.S. Government Printing Office. www.dietaryguidelines.gov.

peas, nuts and seeds, eggs, seafood, and lean poultry and meats that are prepared without added solid fats, sugars, refined grains, and salt and other sources of sodium.[23]

Nutrient density is not a new concept. Forty years ago it was initially defined as the ratio of the amount of a nutrient in a food to the energy provided by the same food, and was expressed as the amount of a nutrient per 1000 kcal.[24] A basic premise of nutrient density was that if the quantity of nutrients per 1000 kcal was great enough, the nutrient needs of a person would be met when his or her energy needs were met. In recent years there has been renewed interest in nutrient density as a useful approach to help people plan diets that maintain adequate nutrient intake while minimizing consumption of unnecessary kilocalories and reducing the intake of sodium, solid fats, dietary cholesterol, added sugars, and refined grains.[23] A key recommendation of the 2010 Dietary Guidelines for Americans is that individuals choose nutrient-dense foods, a recommendation that is widely supported by health professionals and nutrition organizations.[23,25] The diets of many North Americans are energy dense but nutrient poor.[22] Nutrient density addresses the issue that many people need to manage their body weight by controlling their energy intake while ensuring that they consume adequate nutrients and reduce their consumption of those food components that should be limited.[23] There is consistent scientific evidence that dietary patterns emphasizing nutrient-dense foods improve weight loss and weight management among adults and decrease the risk of developing type 2 diabetes among adults.[26] As emphasized later in this chapter, the 2015–2020 Dietary Guidelines for Americans shifted the focus from nutrient density to dietary patterns.

Nutrient Profiling

Using the concept of nutrient density to select nutritious foods and to plan healthy diets is hindered by the fact that there is no valid or scientific method for defining the nutrient density of foods and no specific standard or criteria for consistently identifying nutrient-dense foods.[25,27] Nutrient profiling can be used to address this problem. Nutrient profiling is the science of ranking or classifying foods based on their nutrient composition.[25,27,28] In recent years, numerous nutrient profiling models (sometimes referred to as nutrition quality indices) have been developed by a variety of groups, including food manufacturers, food retailers, government agencies, nonprofit organizations, and groups of experts not related to the food industry.[29,30] Nutrient profiling models use a mathematical formula or algorithm to calculate a score using a certain set of nutrient values to include as variables in the algorithm. Some models include those nutrients and food components that should be consumed more frequently, other models use only those nutrients and food components that should be consumed less frequently, while other models use a

combination of both.[25,30] The algorithms of some models are not available to the public or scientific community but are proprietary (i.e., copyrighted, patented, or kept a trade secret), whereas the algorithms of other models are freely available to the public and scientific community.[31] Unfortunately, few of the models have been studied to determine whether they actually improve the food choices of consumers to result in measurable improvements in health.[28] In recent years there has been considerable interest in using nutrient profiling models as one approach for rating the nutritional value of foods in front-of-package labeling systems.[29,31] Front-of-package labeling systems are discussed later in this chapter within the context of the nutrition labeling of food.

INDICES OF DIET QUALITY

Numerous indices of diet quality have been proposed and reported in the scientific literature.[32–34] How these indices define diet quality varies considerably, depending on the attributes selected by the creator of the particular index and by the era in which the index was developed. For example, earlier indices tend to define a high-quality diet as one supplying adequate protein and selected micronutrients for a given energy level. More recent indices define diet quality in terms of proportionality (eating more servings of certain food groups and fewer of others), moderation (limiting intake of foods and beverages contributing to excess intake of fat, dietary cholesterol, added sugars, sodium, and alcohol), and variety (thus increasing exposure to a wide range of nutritive and other food components).[32–34] Reflecting the nutritional era in which they were developed, earlier indices tend to focus on prevention of deficiency diseases, while more recent ones tend to address risk of chronic disease.

Diet quality indices are typically based on one of three approaches to assessing diet: comparing intake of certain nutrients and food components to a standard, comparing intake of foods or food groups to a standard, or evaluating both nutrient intake and foods or food groups.[32–34] The Diet Quality Index and the Healthy Eating Index evaluate intake of various nutrients and food components and assess consumption of foods and food groups.

Diet Quality Index

The Diet Quality Index (DQI) is an instrument used to assess the overall diet quality of groups and to evaluate risk for chronic disease related to dietary pattern.[32,35] It was originally published in 1994 and was based on eight dietary recommendations from the National Academy of Sciences publication *Diet and Health: Implications for Reducing Chronic Disease Risk.*[36] It was revised in 1999 to reflect the development of the Food Guide Pyramid in 1992, revisions in the *Dietary Guidelines for Americans,* and the creation of the Dietary Reference Intakes. Table 2.9

TABLE 2.9	Diet Quality Index Components and Scoring Guidelines*

Component	Scoring Criteria	
Total fat ≤ 30% of energy intake	≤ 30%	10 points
	31% to 40%	5 points
	> 40%	0 points
Saturated fat ≤ 10% of energy intake	≤ 10%	10 points
	11% to 13%	5 points
	> 13%	0 points
Dietary cholesterol < 300 mg per day	≤ 300 mg	10 points
	300 to 400 mg	5 points
	> 400 mg	0 points
2–4 servings of fruit per day	10–0 points, proportional to percent of recommended number of servings*	
3–5 servings of vegetables per day	10–0 points, proportional to percent of recommended number of servings	
6–11 servings of grains per day	10–0 points, proportional to percent of recommended number of servings	
Calcium intake as a percentage of Adequate Intake for life stage and gender group	10–0 points, proportional to percentage of Adequate Intake for life stage and gender group	
Iron intake as percent of Recommended Dietary Allowance for life stage and gender group	10–0 points, proportional to percentage of Recommended Dietary Allowance for life stage and gender group	
Dietary diversity score	10–0 points, proportional to consumption of foods across 23 food group categories	
Dietary moderation score	10–0 points, based on intake of added sugars, discretionary fat,† sodium, and alcohol in excess of recommended levels of intake	

Source: Haines PS, Siega-Riz AM, Popkin BM. 1999. The Diet Quality Index Revised: A measurement instrument for populations. *Journal of the American Dietetic Association* 99:697–704.

*Serving recommendations based on energy intake according to the Food Guide Pyramid.

†Discretionary fat is defined as all excess fat from the five major food groups beyond that which would be consumed if only the lowest fat forms of a given food were eaten. It includes fats added to food in preparation or at the table, including margarine, cheese, oil, meat drippings, and chocolate.

shows the revised Diet Quality Index (what its creators call the Diet Quality Index Revised). The Diet Quality Index scores diet on the basis of 10 indicators of diet quality. The first 3 indicators reflect macronutrient intake, the next 3 reflect the 1992 Food Guide Pyramid's recommendations for fruit, vegetable, and grain consumption, and the 2 recommendations for calcium and iron are based on the Dietary Reference Intakes. The last 2 indicators address the importance of consuming foods from a variety of food groups and having a moderate intake of sugar,

discretionary fat, sodium, and alcoholic beverages.[32] Each of the 10 components contributes a maximum of 10 points to the total DQI score, which has a maximum of 100 points. The higher the score, the higher the diet quality.

The DQI has been shown to be a useful instrument in evaluating dietary patterns. Healthier maternal dietary patterns during gestation as measured by the DQI were shown to be associated with offspring having a reduced risk of neural tube defects and orofacial clefts.[37] In an intervention designed to promote and evaluate dietary change among older cancer survivors enrolled in a home-based intervention trial, the DQI was shown to be an effective instrument in developing an intervention to improve the diet quality as well as in evaluating overall diet quality.[38]

Healthy Eating Index

The Healthy Eating Index (HEI) is an instrument developed by researchers at the U.S. Department of Agriculture for assessing how well the diets of Americans adhere to U.S. federal dietary guidance.[39] When originally developed in 1995, it was designed to determine adherence to the Food Guide Pyramid's serving recommendations. It was revised in 2005 and then again in 2010 following the release of the 2005 and 2010 editions of the *Dietary Guidelines for Americans* (discussed later in this chapter), which made several important changes in federal dietary guidance.[40,41] The 2015 version of the Healthy Eating Index will reflect the 2015–2020 Dietary Guidelines for Americans. Among these were encouraging adequate consumption of whole grains, whole fruit instead of fruit juice, and vegetables, particularly dark green and orange vegetables, and encouraging moderate consumption of sodium, saturated fat, and calories from alcoholic beverages and foods containing solid fats and added sugars. The current version, known as the Healthy Eating Index-2010 (HEI-2010), is used by the U.S. Department of Agriculture to assess diet quality as defined by the 2010 Dietary Guidelines for Americans.[41] The HEI-2010 is the only index issued by the U.S. federal government and computed on a regular basis for gauging the overall diet quality of Americans.

Table 2.10 summarizes the standards for HEI-2010. The various components are grouped into two categories: adequacy and moderation. The "adequacy components" were established to ensure adequacy of nutrient intake, while the "moderation components" are those whose intake should be limited.

The HEI-2010, which assesses diet quality as specified by the 2010 Dietary Guidelines for Americans, is made up of 12 components, as shown in Table 2.10. All of the components are assessed on a density basis (amounts per 1000 calories) to allow a common standard to be applied to individual diets or any other mix of foods. For each component, the HEI-2010 designates a certain amount as the standard (the best possible). A maximum

TABLE 2.10	Healthy Eating Index-2010 (HEI-2010) Components and Standards for Scoring.		
HEI-2010[1] Component	Maximum	Standard for Maximum Score	Standard for Minimum Score of Zero
Δ **Adequacy** *(Higher score indicates higher consumption)*			
Total fruit[2]	5	≥ 0.8 cup equiv. / 1000 kcal[10]	No fruit
Whole fruit[3]	5	≥ 0.4 cup equiv. / 1000 kcal	No whole fruit
Total vegetables[4]	5	≥ 1.1 cup equiv. / 1000 kcal	No vegetables
Green and beans[4]	5	≥ 0.2 cup equiv. / 1000 kcal	No dark-green vegetables, beans, or peas
Whole grains	10	≥ 1.5 once equiv. / 1000 kcal	No whole grains
Dairy[5]	10	≥ 1.3 cup equiv. / 1000 kcal	No dairy
Total protein foods[6]	5	≥ 2.5 once equiv. / 1000 kcal	No protein foods
Seafood and plant proteins[6,7]	5	≥ 0.8 once equiv. / 1000 kcal	No seafood or plant proteins
Fatty acids[8]	10	(PUFAs + MUFAs) / SFAs ≥ 2.5	(PUFAs + MUFAs) / SFAs ≤ 1.2
∇ **Moderation** *(higher score indicates lower consumption)*			
Refined grains	10	≤ 1.8 ounce equiv. / 1000 kcal	≥ 4.3 ounce equiv. / 1000 kcal
Sodium	10	≤ 1.1 gram / 1000 kcal	≥ 2.0 grams / 1000 kcal
Empty calories[9]	20	≤ 19% of energy	≥ 50% of energy

[1]Intakes between the minimum and maximum standards are scored proportionately.

[2]Includes 100% fruit juice.

[3]Includes all forms except juice.

[4]Includes any beans and peas not counted as Total Protein Foods.

[5]Includes all milk products, such as fluid milk, yogurt, and cheese, and fortified soy beverages.

[6]Beans and peas are included here (and not with vegetables) when the Total Protein Foods standard is otherwise not met.

[7]Includes seafood, nuts, seeds, soy products (other than beverages) as well as beans and peas counted as Total Protein Foods.

[8]Ratio of poly- and monounsaturated fatty acids (PUFAs and MUFAs) to saturated fatty acids (SFAs).

[9]Calories from solid fats, alcohol, and added sugars; threshold for counting alcohol is > 13 grams/1000 kcal.

[10]Equiv. = equivalent, kcal = kilocalories.

Further details on the HEI-2010 and scores for the U.S. population are available at http://www.cnpp.usda.gov/HealthyEatingIndex.htm and http://riskfactor. cancer.gov/tools/hei/.

Authors: Patricia M. Guenther, PhD, RD[1]; Kellie O. Casavale, PhD, RD[2]; Jill Reedy, PhD, RD[3]; Sharon l. Kirkpatrick, PhD, RD[3]; Hazel A.B. Hiza, PhD, RD[1]; Kevin J. Kuczynski, MS, RD[1]; Lisa L. Kahle, BA[4]; Susan M. Krebs-Smith, PhD, RD.[3]

[1]Center for Nutrition Policy and Promotion, U.S. Department of Agriculture; [2]Office of Disease Prevention and Health Promotion, U.S. Department of Health and Human Services; [3]National Cancer Institute, U.S. Department of Health and Human Services; [4]Information Management Services, Inc.

score—5, 10, or 20 points depending on the component— is given to amounts that meet the standard. Amounts that don't meet the standard get fewer points, with zero being the minimum score. The total HEI-2010 score is the sum of the component scores and has a maximum of 100 points.[41]

According to the Center for Nutrition Policy and Promotion (CNPP), the HEI can be used to monitor the quality of American diets, to examine relationships between diet and health-related outcomes and between diet cost and diet quality, to determine the effectiveness of nutrition intervention programs, and to assess the quality of food assistance packages, menus, and the U.S. food supply. The HEI-2010 is appropriate for all segments of the U.S. population to which the USDA Food Patterns apply, including women who are pregnant or lactating. It does not apply to children younger than 2 years of age or to older children who are consuming breast milk or infant formula.[41]

Table 2.11 summarizes the total and component scores for the U.S. total population, children ages 2–17 years, and adults ages 65 years and older. As a group, older adults have a higher total HEI score (68) than children (55). Areas of greatest concern regarding diet quality include low intake of whole grains, high intake of sodium, and quality

of fatty acid intake. The HEI-2015 will more than likely place more of a focus on added sugar intake.

The HEI-2010 scoring system reflects the vegetarian and vegan versions of the USDA Foods Pattern as well as the omnivore version. The National Cancer Institute maintains a website, http://epi.grants.cancer.gov/hei/, that provides an overview of the types of research that can be done using the HEI, gives step-by-step instructions on calculating scores and provides sample code for various types of analyses, and provides a list of papers and other resources on the HEI-2010 and how they have been used in research to assess diet quality at various levels, including food supply, community, and individual levels.

DIETARY GUIDELINES

Dietary guidelines or goals can be defined as statements from authoritative scientific bodies translating nutritional recommendations into practical advice to consumers about their eating habits. Rather than merely ensuring adequate nutrient intake, *they are primarily intended to address the more common and pressing nutrition-related health problems, such as heart disease, certain cancers,*

TABLE 2.11	HEI-2010 Total and Component Scores[1] for the U.S. Total Population, Children and Older Adults, NHANES 2011–2012

HEI-2010 Dietary Component (maximum score)	Total Population ≥ 2 Years (n = 7933)	Children 2–17 Years (n = 2857)	Older Adults ≥ 65 Years (n = 1032)
	Mean Score (standard error)		
Total fruit (5)	3.00 (0.11)	3.91 (0.18)	3.84 (0.22)
Whole fruit (5)	4.01 (0.17)	4.78 (0.22)	4.99 (0.05)
Total vegetables (5)	3.36 (0.08)	2.10 (0.09)	4.16 (0.19)
Greens and beans (5)	2.98 (0.15)	0.70 (0.09)	3.58 (0.47)
Whole grains (10)	2.86 (0.13)	2.50 (0.10)	4.23 (0.34)
Dairy (10)	6.44 (0.14)	9.03 (0.22)	5.99 (0.16)
Total protein foods (5)	5.00 (0.00)	4.44 (0.13)	5.00 (0.00)
Seafood and plant proteins (5)	3.74 (0.20)	3.05 (0.17)	4.91 (0.18)
Fatty acids (10)	4.66 (0.14)	3.29 (0.18)	5.60 (0.36)
Refined grains (10)	6.19 (0.15)	4.91 (0.16)	7.34 (0.31)
Sodium (10)	4.15 (0.06)	4.85 (0.25)	3.66 (0.26)
Empty calories (20)	12.60 (0.23)	11.50 (0.28)	14.99 (0.44)
Total HE1 score (100)	**59.00 (0.95)**	**55.07 (0.72)**	**68.29 (1.76)**

[1]Calculated using the population ratio method.

stroke, hypertension, and diabetes. They often are expressed as nonquantitative changes from the present average national diet or from people's typical eating habits. Examples of guidelines are "consume a variety of nutrient dense foods and beverages within and among the basic food groups while choosing foods that limit the intake of saturated and *trans* fats, cholesterol, added sugars, salt, and alcohol" and "choose fiber-rich fruits, vegetables, and whole grains often." Table 2.12 contrasts the DRIs with dietary guidelines.

Early Dietary Guidelines

Informal dietary guidelines have existed since time immemorial in the form of cultural practices, taboos, and religious teachings. The first formal set of dietary guidelines of modern times, however, was developed by nutrition professors from Sweden, Finland, Norway, and Denmark and published in 1968.[42] Several factors influenced the creation of this set of guidelines for the Nordic countries (Sweden, Finland, Norway, Denmark, and Iceland).[42] Dietary surveys showed that the proportion of calories from fat in the Swedish diet had increased from an average of about 29% at the end of the 19th century to 42% by the mid-1960s. There was concern over the high intakes of saturated fat, calories, and refined sugars and low intakes of fruits, vegetables, cereal products, lean meats, and nonfat dairy products. Swedish health authorities were concerned about the association between such dietary practices and obesity, coronary heart disease, hypertension, stroke, and tooth decay.

The Swedish guidelines called for a reduced energy intake (when appropriate) to prevent overweight; decreased consumption of total fat, saturated fat, sugar, and sugar-containing products; increased consumption of

TABLE 2.12	The Dietary Reference Intakes (DRIs) and Dietary Guidelines Contrasted

DRIs	Dietary Guidelines
Developed earlier	Developed more recently
Only one set per country	Multiple (sometimes incongruent) sets possible in a country
Expressed in quantitative terms as weight of nutrient per day	Often expressed as nonquantitative change from present average national diet
Primarily intended to ensure adequate nutrient intake	Primarily intended to help reduce risk of developing chronic degenerative disease
More firmly established scientifically	More provisional, based more on epidemiologic data
More concerned with micronutrients	Primarily deal with macronutrients but may also address micronutrient intake
Specific recommendations for each life stage and gender group	Generally the same advice for all in the defined target group
Expressed in technical language	Technical language avoided, better understood by the public

Source: Truswell AS. 1999. Dietary goals and guidelines: National and international perspectives. In Shils ME, Olson JA, Shike M, Ross AC, eds. *Modern nutrition in health and disease,* 9th ed. Baltimore: Williams & Wilkins.

vegetables, fruits, potatoes, nonfat milk, fish, lean meat, and cereal products; and regular physical activity, especially for those with sedentary occupations.[42]

These dietary trends were recognized in other Western nations, such as Australia, New Zealand, The Netherlands, the United Kingdom, Germany, and Canada, which, in the early 1970s, issued dietary guidelines of their own.[43]

During this time, a similar situation existed in the United States. Scientists were concerned about trends in the eating habits of Americans. Data from the USDA showed that the distribution of calories from carbohydrate and fat had changed significantly between 1909 and the 1970s. Based on the *disappearance* of food from the marketplace (see Chapter 4), the USDA concluded that the percent of calories provided by fats had increased from 32% to about 43%, while calories provided by carbohydrate had declined from 57% to 46%. The percent of calories from fats obtained from meat and dairy products had risen sharply, while carbohydrate from fruits, vegetables, and grains had fallen precipitously.[36] At the same time, there was increasingly convincing evidence linking dietary habits to the major causes of death in America: heart disease, cancer, and stroke. Although scientists recognized that heredity, age, and numerous environmental factors besides diet were involved in the causation of these diseases, diet was one factor over which people had a certain amount of control. This led private agencies, such as the American Medical Association, the American Heart Association, and the American Health Foundation, to publish dietary guidelines.

U.S. Dietary Goals

In February 1977, the report *Dietary Goals for the United States* was issued by the U.S. Senate Select Committee on Nutrition and Human Needs.[43] This was the first of several government reports setting prudent dietary guidelines for Americans.

In its introduction, the Senate Select Committee made this statement:

> The overconsumption of foods high in fat, generally, and saturated fat in particular, as well as cholesterol, refined and processed sugars, salt and/or alcohol has been associated with the development of one or more of six to ten leading causes of death: heart disease, some cancers, stroke and hypertension, diabetes, arteriosclerosis and cirrhosis of the liver.[43]

The committee then submitted seven goals, listed in Box 2.6. The Dietary Goals were to be accomplished through the changes in food selection and preparation listed in Box 2.7.

 Box 2.6   **Dietary Goals for the United States**

1. To avoid overweight, consume only as much energy (calories) as is expended; if overweight, decrease energy intake and increase energy expenditure.
2. Increase the consumption of complex carbohydrates and "naturally occurring" sugars from about 28% of energy intake to about 48% of energy intake.
3. Reduce the consumption of refined and processed sugars by about 45% to account for about 10% of total energy intake.
4. Reduce overall fat consumption from approximately 40% to about 30% of energy intake.
5. Reduce saturated fat consumption to account for about 10% of total energy intake and balance that with polyunsaturated and monounsaturated fats, which should account for about 10% of energy intake each.
6. Reduce cholesterol consumption to about 300 milligrams per day.
7. Limit the intake of sodium by reducing the intake of salt to about 5 grams a day.

Source: Select Committee on Nutrition and Human Needs. 1977. *Dietary goals for the United States.* Washington, DC: U.S. Senate.

 Box 2.7   **Recommendations from Dietary Goals for the United States**

1. Increase consumption of fruits, vegetables, and whole grains.
2. Decrease consumption of refined and other processed sugars and foods high in such sugars.
3. Decrease consumption of foods high in total fat and partially replace saturated fats, whether obtained from animal or vegetable sources, with polyunsaturated fats.
4. Decrease consumption of animal fat and choose meats, poultry, and fish, which will reduce saturated fat intake.
5. Except for young children, substitute low-fat and nonfat milk for whole milk and low-fat dairy products for high-fat dairy products.
6. Decrease consumption of butterfat, eggs, and other high-cholesterol sources. Some consideration should be given to easing the cholesterol goal for premenopausal women, young children, and the elderly to obtain the nutritional benefit of eggs in the diet.
7. Decrease consumption of salt and foods high in salt content.

Source: Select Committee on Nutrition and Human Needs. 1977. *Dietary goals for the United States.* Washington, DC: U.S. Senate.

The reaction to *Dietary Goals for the United States* from U.S. nutrition scientists and professionals was swift, strong, and polarized.[31] *Nutrition Today* published opinions about the goals from some leading nutrition scientists and professionals.[33,34] Some felt the goals were "hastily conceived and based on fragmentary evidence," "premature . . . because the diet has not yet been tested," "blatant sensationalism," "speculation," and "a nutritional debacle." One professional declared that the "Senate Select Committee has perpetrated a hoax." Other scientists believed the goals were "long overdue," "a giant step forward in improving the health of our citizens," "a valid criticism of our current diet," and "a significant achievement" and deserved "the broadest support from all who are concerned with the health and well-being of American citizens." Who was right? Time would tell.

It was immediately clear, however, that, to meet the goals, Americans would need to change the way they ate. Figure 2.5 compares the 1977 U.S. Dietary Goals with the diet of that time and highlights the necessary changes.

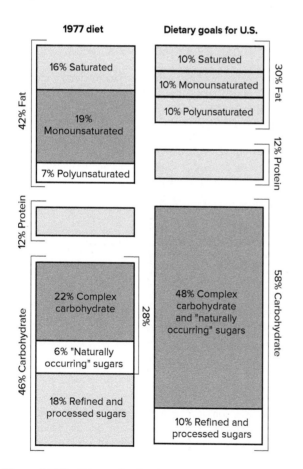

Figure 2.5 The *Dietary Goals for the United States*, established in 1977 (outlined in the column on the right), compared with the diet of the typical American adult of that time (outlined in the column on the left).

Source: U.S. Department of Health and Human Services and U.S. Department of Agriculture. 2010. *Dietary Guidelines for Americans, 2010.* Washington, DC: U.S. Government Printing Office. www.dietaryguidelines.gov.

The Dietary Guidelines for Americans

In 1980, the U.S. Department of Agriculture and U.S. Department of Health and Human Services jointly published the first edition of *Dietary Guidelines for Americans.*[46] Since then, the Dietary Guidelines for Americans (DGAs) have been revised every five years, with editions in 1985, 1990, 1995, 2000, 2005, 2010, and 2015. Since their inception, the DGAs have remained relatively consistent in terms of their recommendations for variety, proportionality, and moderation in healthful eating and in their focus on preventing chronic disease. Their ultimate goal has always been to "improve the health of our Nation's current and future generations by facilitating and promoting healthy eating and physical activity choices so that these behaviors become the norm among all individuals."[23] A basic premise of each edition has been that nutrient needs should be met primarily by consuming naturally occurring foods as opposed to relying on fortified foods or dietary supplements. Because of its remarkably complex nature, food provides a vast array of nutrients, food components, and phytochemicals that have beneficial effects on health. However, the DGAs recognize that in some instances, fortified foods and dietary supplements may be useful.[23,26]

Over the course of eight editions spanning over three decades, the Dietary Guidelines for Americans have evolved considerably. As shown in Table 2.13, the first edition, published in 1980, had 7 guidelines. This number was increased to 10 guidelines in the 2000 edition. The 2005 edition had a total of 41 recommendations grouped in 9 "focus areas." There were 23 key recommendations intended for the general population as well as 18 key recommendations for specific population groups such as women who are pregnant or breast-feeding, children and adolescents, and older persons. The 2010 edition had a total of 29 recommendations grouped under 5 "major themes." There were 23 key recommendations for the general public and 6 additional recommendations for specific population groups. In 2015, the Dietary Guidelines for Americans changed the focus to dietary patterns. Previous editions of the Dietary Guidelines focused mainly on individual components of the diet, such as food groups and nutrients. While important, researchers had focused more of their efforts on the relationship among overall eating patterns, health, and risk of chronic disease. This literature base was sufficiently well established to support recommendations on healthy eating patterns. The 2015–2020 Dietary Guidelines for Americans include three main chapters: Chapter 1: Key Elements of Healthy Eating Patterns; Chapter 2: Shifts Needed to Align with Healthy Eating Patterns; Chapter 3: Everyone Has a Role in Supporting Healthy Eating Patterns. The chapters are built around five guidelines and include 13 key recommendations with more details on what makes up healthy eating patterns. Box 2.8 summarizes the guidelines and recommendations in the 2015–2020 DGAs. An eating pattern is defined as the combination of foods and beverages that

TABLE 2.13 Dietary Guidelines for Americans, 1980 to 2015

1980 7 Guidelines	1985 7 Guidelines	1990 7 Guidelines	1995 7 Guidelines	2000 10 Guidelines	2005 9 Focus Areas	2010 5 Major Themes	2015-20 5 Guidelines
Eat a variety of foods.	Eat a variety of foods.	Eat a variety of foods.	Eat a variety of foods.	Let the Pyramid guide your food choices.	Adequate nutrients within caloric needs	Balancing calories to manage weight	Follow a healthy eating pattern across the lifespan
Maintain ideal weight.	Maintain desirable weight.	Maintain healthy weight.	Balance the food you eat with physical activity—maintain or improve your weight.	Aim for a healthy weight.	Weight management	Foods and food components to reduce	Focus on variety, nutrient density, and amount
				Be physically active each day.	Physical activity	Foods and nutrients to increase	
Avoid too much fat, saturated fat, and cholesterol.	Avoid too much fat, saturated fat, and cholesterol.	Choose a diet low in fat, saturated fat, and cholesterol.	Choose a diet low in fat, saturated fat, and cholesterol.	Choose a diet that is low in saturated fat and cholesterol and moderate in total fat.	Food groups to encourage	Building healthier eating patterns	Limit calories from added sugars and saturated fats and reduce sodium intake
					Fats	Helping Americans make healthy choices	
Eat foods with adequate starch and fiber.	Eat foods with adequate starch and fiber.	Choose a diet with plenty of vegetables, fruits, and grain products.	Choose a diet with plenty of grain products, vegetables, and fruits.	Choose a variety of grains daily, especially whole grains.	Carbohydrates		Shift to healthier food and beverage choices
				Choose a variety of fruits and vegetables daily.	Sodium and potassium		Support healthy eating patterns for all
Avoid too much sugar.	Avoid too much sugar.	Use sugars only in moderation.	Choose a diet moderate in sugars.	Choose beverages and foods to moderate your intake of sugars.	Alcoholic beverages		
Avoid too much sodium.	Avoid too much sodium.	Use salt and sodium only in moderation.	Choose a diet moderate in salt and sodium.	Choose and prepare foods with less salt.	Food safety		
If you drink alcohol, do so in moderation.	If you drink alcoholic beverages, do so in moderation.	If you drink alcoholic beverages, do so in moderation.	If you drink alcoholic beverages, do so in moderation.	If you drink alcoholic beverages, do so in moderation.			
				Keep food safe to eat.			
					41 Recommendations in total	29 Recommendations in total	13 Recommendations applied in their entirety to reflect an overall healthy eating pattern
					23 Key recommendations for the general public	23 Key recommendations for the general public	
					18 Recommendations for special populations	6 Recommendations for special populations	

Source: USDA.

Box 2.8   2015–2020 Dietary Guidelines for Americans

The primary focus of the 2015–2020 Dietary Guidelines for Americans is a HEALTHY EATING PATTERN, and this will require shifts in food and beverage choices by many individuals. About half of all American adults—117 million individuals—have one or more preventable chronic diseases, many of which are related to poor quality eating patterns and physical inactivity. These include cardiovascular disease, high blood pressure, type 2 diabetes, some cancers, and poor bone health. More than two-thirds of adults and nearly one-third of children and youth are overweight or obese. These high rates of overweight and obesity and chronic disease have persisted for more than two decades.

The 2015–2020 Dietary Guidelines provides **five general Guidelines** that encourage healthy eating patterns and the appropriate food and beverage choices. The full report can be downloaded at: https://health.gov/dietaryguidelines/2015/resources/2015-2020_Dietary_Guidelines.pdf

THE 5 GUIDELINES

1. **Follow a healthy eating pattern across the lifespan.** All food and beverage choices matter. Choose a healthy eating pattern at an appropriate calorie level to help achieve and maintain a healthy body weight, support nutrient adequacy, and reduce the risk of chronic disease.
2. **Focus on variety, nutrient density, and amount.** To meet nutrient needs within calorie limits, choose a variety of nutrient-dense foods across and within all food groups in recommended amounts.
3. **Limit calories from added sugars and saturated fats and reduce sodium intake.** Consume an eating pattern low in added sugars, saturated fats, and sodium. Cut back on foods and beverages higher in these components to amounts that fit within healthy eating patterns.
4. **Shift to healthier food and beverage choices.** Choose nutrient-dense foods and beverages across and within all food groups in place of less healthy choices. Consider cultural and personal preferences to make these shifts easier to accomplish and maintain.
5. **Support healthy eating patterns for all.** Everyone has a role in helping to create and support healthy eating patterns in multiple settings nationwide, from home to school to work to communities.

An underlying premise of the Dietary Guidelines is that nutritional needs should be met primarily from eating healthy foods not supplements. Here are the **key recommendations** to meet the five Guidelines and achieve a healthy eating pattern.

KEY RECOMMENDATIONS

1. **Consume a healthy eating pattern that accounts for all foods and beverages within an appropriate calorie level.**
   A primary goal of the Dietary Guidelines is that individuals throughout all stages of the lifespan have eating patterns that promote good health, a healthy

body weight, and disease prevention. An eating pattern represents what individuals habitually eat and drink, and is a better predictor of long-term health than individual foods or nutrients. Individuals should focus on eating patterns that emphasize nutrient-dense foods that are high in vitamins, minerals, polyphenols (i.e., food molecules that provide color), and fiber. Eating patterns can be tailored to one's socio-cultural and personal preferences.

The 2015–2020 Dietary Guidelines for Americans focus on three examples of healthy eating patterns:

1. The Healthy U.S.-Style Eating Pattern
2. The Healthy Mediterranean-Style Eating Pattern
3. The Healthy Vegetarian Eating Pattern

A. **A healthy eating pattern includes:**
   - A variety of vegetables from all of the subgroups—dark green, red and orange, legumes (beans and peas), starchy, and other
   - Fruits, especially whole fruits
   - Grains, at least half of which are whole grains
   - Fat-free or low-fat dairy, including milk, yogurt, cheese, and/or fortified soy beverages
   - A variety of protein foods, including seafood, lean meats and poultry, eggs, legumes (beans and peas), and nuts, seeds, and soy products
   - Oils

B. **A healthy eating pattern limits saturated fats and *trans* fats, added sugars, and sodium**
   - Consume less than 10 percent of calories per day from added sugars
   - Consume less than 10 percent of calories per day from saturated fats
   - Consume less than 2300 milligrams (mg) per day of sodium
   - If alcohol is consumed, it should be consumed in moderation—up to one drink per day for women and up to two drinks per day for men—and only by adults of legal drinking age.

C. **Meet the *Physical Activity Guidelines for Americans* (150–300 minutes per week).**
   - Adults need at least 150 minutes of moderate-intensity physical activity and should perform muscle-strengthening exercises on 2 or more days each week.
   - Youth ages 6 to 17 years need at least 60 minutes of physical activity per day, including aerobic, muscle-strengthening, and bone-strengthening activities.
   - Just as individuals can achieve a healthy eating pattern in a variety of ways that meet their personal and cultural preferences, they can engage in regular physical activity in a variety of ways throughout the day and by choosing activities they enjoy.

Source: U.S. Department of Health and Human Services and U.S. Department of Agriculture. December 2015. *2015–2020 Dietary Guidelines for Americans.* 8th ed.

makes up an individual's complete dietary intake over time.[47] An eating pattern is more than the sum of its parts because it represents the totality of what individuals habitually eat and drink. Over the long term, these dietary components act synergistically to support health. A healthy eating pattern is based on an individual's food budget and personal, cultural, and traditional preferences. The calorie level is adapted to the individual to achieve and maintain a healthy body weight, support nutrient adequacy, and reduce risk for chronic disease.

Originally, the Dietary Guidelines for Americans were targeted to the general public, but beginning with the 2005 edition they became more technical in nature and oriented toward policy makers, nutrition educators, nutritionists, and health-care providers for use in developing educational materials and in designing and implementing nutrition-related programs, including federal food, nutrition education, and information programs. The recommendations shown in Box 2.8 are based on sound scientific evidence collected through a thorough review of the best available scientific research and are considered authoritative statements to be used in developing federal nutrition policy. Because they are interrelated and mutually dependent, they should be used together when planning healthful diets.

The current DGAs are designed for professionals to help all individuals ages 2 years and older consume a healthy, nutritionally adequate diet. The information in the DGAs is used in developing federal food, nutrition, and health policies and programs and is the basis for nutrition education materials, programs, and policies at all levels of government, businesses, schools, community groups, media, and the food industry. In practice, aligning with the current DGAs at the population level requires broad coordination and collaboration to create a new model in which healthy lifestyle choices at home, school, and work and in the community are easy, accessible, affordable, and normative. In this model, everyone has a role in helping individuals shift their food, beverage, and physical activity choices to align with the DGAs.[47]

The Surgeon General's Report on Nutrition and Health

In 1988, *The Surgeon General's Report on Nutrition and Health* was issued.[48] This was a landmark publication summarizing the scientific evidence linking specific dietary factors to health maintenance and disease prevention and presenting recommendations for dietary change to improve the health of the American people.[49] The report recognized that what we eat can affect our risk for several of the leading causes of death and identified, as of primary importance, the need to reduce consumption of fat, especially saturated fat. It served as an authoritative source of information on which to base nutrition policy decisions and distinguished recommendations appropriate for the general public from those for special populations.[50]

Diet and Health

In 1989, the book *Diet and Health: Implications for Reducing Chronic Disease Risk* was published by the Committee on Diet and Health of the National Research Council.[36] It represented the view that dietary recommendations should go beyond the prevention of nutrient deficiencies to the prevention of chronic disease. From their extensive review of the scientific literature, the committee members concluded that, in addition to genetic and environmental factors, "dietary patterns are important factors in the **etiology** of several major chronic diseases and that dietary modifications can reduce such risks." The influence of diet is "very strong" for coronary heart disease and hypertension and "highly suggestive" for certain cancers (esophagus, stomach, large bowel, breast, lung, and prostate). The committee stated that dietary habits also play a role in dental caries, chronic liver disease, and obesity, which increases the risk of **type 2 diabetes mellitus.** Of particular concern was the need for Americans to reduce consumption of fats, saturated fats, and cholesterol and increase intake of fruits, vegetables, legumes, and whole-grain cereals.

Other Dietary Guidelines

Since the U.S. Dietary Goals were issued in 1977, numerous scientific organizations and professional groups have studied the impact of American dietary practices on health and disease and have issued their own dietary guidelines.

Although the various dietary recommendations span more than three decades, there is a remarkable degree of similarity in their major tenets. There is common agreement across all published guidelines that a healthy eating pattern is focused on (1) calorie control and regular physical activity to maintain a healthy weight, (2) intake of fat-free or low-fat dairy products, lean meats and seafood, and nutrient-dense and fiber-rich plant foods (a variety of fresh fruits and vegetables, whole grains, legumes, nuts, seeds), and (3) limited use of saturated and *trans* fats, added sugars, sodium, refined starches, and alcohol.

NUTRITION LABELING OF FOOD

Nutrition labeling of food in the United States began in 1973, when the U.S. Food and Drug Administration (FDA) established the U.S. Recommended Daily Allowances (U.S. RDAs) and instituted specific regulations for food labeling. In 1990, food labeling regulations in the United States were extensively revised by the Nutrition Labeling and Education Act of 1990. It should be noted that the U.S. Recommended Daily Allowances (U.S. RDAs) are not the same as the Recommended Dietary Allowances (RDAs).

U.S. Recommended Daily Allowances

In 1973, the FDA issued regulations requiring the nutrition labeling of any food containing one or more added nutrients or whose label or advertising included claims about the food's nutritional properties or its usefulness in the daily diet. Nutrition labeling was voluntary for almost all other foods. The *U.S. Recommended Daily Allowances (U.S. RDAs)* were nutrient standards developed by the FDA at that time for use in regulating the nutrition labeling of food. They replaced the Minimum Daily Requirement, which had been in use since 1940 for labeling vitamin and mineral supplements, breakfast cereals, and some special foods.

The Nutrition Labeling and Education Act

Between 1973 and 1993, there was growing awareness that the major nutritional problem facing North Americans was overconsumption of foods rich in total fat, saturated fat, and cholesterol and low in complex carbohydrates. There were also major breakthroughs in our knowledge of essential nutrient requirements (for example, the RDAs had been revised three times during this time). Despite these advances, the U.S. RDAs had not been updated, and food labeling regulations remained virtually unchanged. During the same period, the public and various professional and consumer interest groups called for food labels that were easily understood, that were truthful, and that reflected awareness of the relationship between diet and health. In 1990, the FDA's Nutrition Labeling and Education Act (NLEA) was passed, mandating nutrition labeling for almost all processed foods regulated by the FDA and authorizing appropriate health claims on the labels of such products. It brought about the most extensive food labeling reform in U.S. history. The NLEA also called for activities to educate consumers about nutrition information on the label and the importance of using that information in maintaining healthful dietary practices. The NLEA's final regulations were published in the January 6, 1993, *Federal Register;* August 8, 1994, was the final deadline for manufacturers to comply. The USDA's Food Safety and Inspection Service, responsible for the inspection of meat and poultry, issued parallel regulations that governed the labeling of meat and poultry.

The NLEA requires virtually all processed foods to carry nutrition information on the label. Foods exempted from the regulations include plain coffee and tea, some spices and flavorings, and other foods having insignificant nutritional value; ready-to-eat food prepared primarily on-site, such as deli and bakery items; foods in very small packages; restaurant food; bulk food that is not resold; and foods produced by businesses with food sales of less than $50,000 per year or total sales less than $500,000 per year unless the food item contains a nutrition claim. Nutrition labeling is voluntary for most raw foods.

On May 20, 2016, the FDA announced the new Nutrition Facts label for packaged foods. Major manufacturers will need to use the new label by July 26, 2018. The new label reflects scientific discoveries regarding diet and chronic diseases and makes it easier for consumers to make better-informed food choices. Figure 2.6 compares the standard Nutrition Facts label without or with voluntary components, and Figure 2.7 shows the labels for young children. Table 2.14 lists allowable nutrient content claims and Table 2.15 provides a comprehensive list of the Daily Values. Here is a summary of key updates to the Nutrition Facts label that are mandated by summer of 2018.

- Increase the type size for "Calories," "servings per container," and the "Serving size" declaration, and bold the number of calories and the "Serving size" declaration to highlight this information.
- Declare the actual amount, in addition to percent Daily Value of vitamin D, calcium, iron and potassium. The gram amounts for other vitamins (including vitamins A and C) and minerals can be voluntarily declared.
- List the footnote as follows: The % Daily Value tells you how much a nutrient in a serving of food contributes to a daily diet. 2000 calories a day is used for general nutrition advice.
- Include "added sugars," in grams and as percent Daily Value.
- Include "Total Fat," "Saturated Fat," and "*Trans Fat*" on the label. "Calories from Fat" is no longer required because research shows the type of fat is more important than the amount.
- Use updated Daily Values (Table 2.15) for nutrients like sodium (reduced to 2300 mg), dietary fiber (increased to 28 g), calcium (increased to 1300 mg), potassium (increased to 4700 mg), and vitamin D (increased to 20 mcg). These changes are based on current scientific evidence.
- Serving sizes must be based on amounts of foods and beverages that people are actually eating, not what they should be eating. For packages that are between one and two servings, such as a 20-ounce soda or a 15-ounce can of soup, the calories and other nutrients must be labeled as one serving because people typically consume it in one sitting. For certain products that are larger than a single serving but that could be consumed in one sitting or multiple sittings, provide "dual column" labels to indicate the amount of calories and nutrients on both a "per serving" and "per package"/"per unit" basis.

A list of all ingredients must appear on all processed and packaged foods. When appropriate, ingredient lists must include any FDA-certified color additives, the sources of any protein hydrolysates, a declaration that caseinate is a milk derivative when caseinate is found in foods claiming to be nondairy, and a declaration of the total percentage of juice in any beverage claiming to contain juice.

An important feature of the NLEA is that it regulates nutrient content claims and health claims on food labels or other labeling of food, such as advertisements. Nutrient content claims are those describing the amount of nutrients in foods, such as "cholesterol free," "low fat," "light," or "lean." Examples of these are shown in Table 2.14. In

Standard vertical

Nutrition Facts

8 Servings per container

Serving size	**2/3 cup (55g)**

Amount per serving

Calories	**230**

	% Daily Value*
Total Fat 8g	**10%**
Saturated Fat 1g	**5%**
Trans Fat 0g	
Cholesterol 0mg	**0%**
Sodium 160mg	**7%**
Total Carbohydrate 37g	**13%**
Dietary Fiber 4g	**14%**
Total Sugars 12g	
Includes 10g Added Sugars	**20%**
Protein 3g	
Vitamin D 2mcg	10%
Calcium 260mg	20%
Iron 8mg	45%
Potassium 235mg	6%

*The % Daily Value (DV) tells you how much a nutrient in a serving of food contributes to a daily diet. 2,000 calories a day is used for general nutrition advice.

Standard vertical (w/voluntary)

Nutrition Facts

17 Servings per container

Serving size	**3/4 cup (28g)**

Amount per serving

Calories	**140**

	% Daily Value*
Total Fat 1.5g	**2%**
Saturated Fat 0g	**0%**
Trans Fat 0g	
Polyunsaturated Fat 0.5g	
Monounsaturated Fat 0.5g	
Cholesterol 0mg	**0%**
Sodium 160mg	**7%**
Total Carbohydrate 22g	**8%**
Dietary Fiber 2g	
Soluble Fiber <1g	
Insoluble Fiber 1g	
Total Sugars 9g	
Includes 8g Added Sugars	**16%**
Protein 9g	**18%**
Vitamin D 2mcg (80 IU)	10%
Calcium 130mg	10%
Iron 4.5mg	25%
Potassium 115mg	2%
Vitamin A 90mcg	10%
Vitamin C 9mg	10%
Thiamin 0.3mg	25%
Riboflavin 0.3mg	25%
Niacin 4mg	25%
Vitamin B_6 0.4mg	25%
Folate 200mcg DFE (120mcg folic acid)	50%
Vitamin B_{12} 0.6mcg	25%
Phosphorus 100mg	8%
Magnesium 25mg	6%
Zinc 3mg	25%

*The % Daily Value (DV) tells you how much a nutrient in a serving of food contributes to a daily diet. 2000 calories a day is used for general nutrition advice.

Calories per gram:

Fat 9   •   Carbohydrates 4   •   Protein 4

Figure 2.6 Key concepts of the 2016 Nutrition Facts label without and with voluntary components.

Infants through 12 months of age

Nutrition Facts

4 Servings per container

Serving size	1 pack (70g)

Amount Per Serving
Calories **25**

	% Daily Value
Total Fat 0g	0%
Saturated Fat 0g	
Trans Fat 0g	
Cholesterol 0mg	
Sodium 74mg	
Total Carbohydrate 5g	5%
Dietary Fiber 1g	
Total Sugars 3g	
Includes 0g Added Sugars	
Protein 0g	0%
Vitamin D 0mcg	0%
Calcium 5mg	2%
Iron 1mg	10%
Potassium 230mg	35%

(A)

Children 1–3 years

Nutrition Facts

1 Serving per container

Serving size	1 container (85g)

Amount Per Serving
Calories **70**

	% Daily Value*
Total Fat 1.5g	4%
Saturated Fat 0.5g	5%
Trans Fat 0g	
Cholesterol 10mg	3%
Sodium 240mg	16%
Total Carbohydrate 11g	7%
Dietary Fiber 1g	7%
Total Sugars 1g	
Includes 1g Added Sugars	4%
Protein 3g	23%
Vitamin D 0mcg	0%
Calcium 35mg	6%
Iron 0.6mg	8%
Potassium 30mg	0%

*The % Daily Value (DV) tells you how much a nutrient in a serving of food contributes to a daily diet. 1000 calories a day is used for general nutrition advice.

(B)

Figure 2.7 Nutrition Facts labels for foods designed for children less than 12 months of age (A) and for foods intended for children 1 to 3 years of age (B).

addition to the nutrient claims shown in Table 2.14 are those using the word *reduced* or *less*. A food making the claim "reduced or less sodium" has to contain at least 25% less sodium per serving than an appropriate food used for comparison purposes. For example, potato chips labeled "low sodium" must contain at least 25% less sodium than comparable potato chips (the "reference food").

The FDA defines a health claim as any claim on the package label or other labeling of a food that characterizes the relationship of any nutrient or other substance in the food to a disease or health-related condition. According to FDA regulations, health claims are allowed only under certain circumstances and must be scientifically based and standardized. Allowable health claims are shown in Box 2.9. The NLEA stipulates that foods bearing health claims must not contain any nutrient or substance in an amount that increases the risk of a disease or a health condition. Foods bearing health claims must contain 20% or less of the Daily Value of fat, saturated fat,

cholesterol, and sodium per serving. For example, whole milk (which is high in calcium) may not bear a calcium-osteoporosis claim because its fat content exceeds 20% of the Daily Value for fat. Skim and 1% fat milk easily qualify for the calcium-osteoporosis claim. According to FDA regulation, claims that a substance will prevent a disease are drug claims. Health claims on food labels are limited to saying that a food "may" or "might" reduce the risk of a disease or health condition.

Front-of-Package Labeling

A relatively new approach to nutrition labeling is to use front-of-package (FOP) labeling systems displaying symbols or icons, typically printed on the front of the label, to summarize key nutritional aspects or characteristics of foods.[29] Some FOP systems are based on a nutrition profiling model (discussed earlier in this chapter). Some show the percent Daily Value for select nutrients or food components, whereas others highlight that the food is a good

TABLE 2.14	Examples and Meanings of Some Allowable Nutrient Content Claims

Example of Nutrient Content Claim	Meaning of Nutrient Content Claim
Sugar free	Less than 0.5 g sugars per serving
Calorie free	Less than 5 kcal per serving
Low calorie	40 kcal or less per serving
Fat free	Less than 0.5 g fat per serving
Saturated fat free	Less than 0.5 g saturated fat and less than 0.5 g *trans* fat per serving
Low fat	3 g or less per serving
Low saturated fat	1 g or less of saturated fat and less than 0.5 g *trans* fat per serving
Trans fat free	Less than 0.5 g *trans* fat and less than 0.5 g saturated fat per serving
Cholesterol free	Less than 2 mg of cholesterol and 2 g or less of both saturated fat and *trans* fat
Low cholesterol	20 mg or less of cholesterol and 2 g or less of both saturated fat and *trans* fat
Sodium free	Less than 5 mg sodium per serving
Low sodium	140 mg or less per serving
Very low sodium	35 mg or less per serving
Lean meat or poultry	Less than 10 g total fat, less than 4.5 g of saturated and *trans* fat combined, and less than 95 mg cholesterol per serving and per 100 g for individual foods
Extra lean meat or poultry	Less than 5 g total fat, less than 2 g saturated and *trans* fat combined, and less than 95 mg cholesterol per serving and per 100 g for individual foods
High, rich in	20% or more of Daily Value to describe protein, vitamins, minerals, dietary fiber, or potassium per serving
Good source of More, added	10% to 19% or more of Daily Value per serving
	Contains a nutrient that is at least 10% percent of Daily Value more than the reference food, regardless of whether the food is altered (fortified or enriched)
Light, lite	One-third fewer calories or half the fat of the reference food; if the food derives 50% or more of its calories from fat, the reduction must be 50% of the fat; can also mean that sodium content has been reduced by at least 50%

Source: U.S. Food and Drug Administration, Center for Food Safety and Applied Nutrition.

TABLE 2.15	Daily Values (including Daily Reference Values and Reference Daily Intakes) based on a caloric intake of 2000 calories, for adults and children four or more years of age. Updated in 2016.

Food Component	Daily Value	Food Component	Daily Value
Total Fat	78 grams (g)	Niacin, NE	16 mg
Saturated Fat	20 g	Vitamin B6	1.7 mg
Cholesterol	300 milligrams (mg)	Folate, DFE	400 µg
Total Carbohydrate	275 g	Vitamin B12	2.4 µg
Added sugars	50 g	Biotin	30 µg
Sodium	2300 mg	Pantothenic acid	5 mg
Potassium	4700 mg	Phosphorus	1250 mg
Dietary Fiber	28 g	Iodine	150 µg
Protein	50 g	Magnesium	420 mg
Vitamin A, RAE	900 micrograms (µg)	Zinc	11 mg
Vitamin C	90 mg	Selenium	55 µg
Calcium	1300 mg	Copper	0.9 mg
Iron	18 mg	Manganese	2.3 mg
Vitamin D	20 µg	Chromium	35 µg
Vitamin E	15 mg	Molybdenum	45 µg
Vitamin K	120 µg	Chloride	2300 mg
Thiamin	1.2 mg	Choline	550 mg
Riboflavin	1.3 mg		

Source: Food and Drug Administration. https://www.regulations.gov/document?D=FDA-2012-N-1210-0875.

Box 2.9   **Nutrient–Disease Relationship Claims Allowed on the Nutrition Facts Label**

- Calcium and risk of osteoporosis
- Sodium and risk of hypertension
- Dietary saturated fat and cholesterol and risk of coronary heart disease
- Dietary fat and risk of cancer
- Fiber-containing grain products, fruits, and vegetables and risk of cancer
- Fruits, vegetables, and grain products that contain fiber, particularly soluble fiber and risk of coronary heart disease

- Fruits and vegetables and risk of cancer
- Folic acid and risk of neural tube defects
- Sugar alcohols and risk of dental caries
- Soluble fiber and risk of coronary heart disease
- Soy protein and risk of coronary heart disease
- Plant sterol and stanol esters and risk of coronary heart disease

Source: U.S. Food and Drug Administration, Center for Food Safety and Applied Nutrition.

source of a particular food group, such as whole grains or vegetables. A recent review of 20 different FOP systems representative of those in the marketplace found wide variation in the criteria used for ranking foods and some cases where various systems conflicted with each other.[29] Some FOP systems cannot be evaluated because the evaluation criteria they use are not publicly available. The large number of widely different FOP systems and the lack of transparency in how the nutritional value of foods are rated contribute to confusion among consumers.[54,55] Although such systems ostensibly are intended to help consumers easily identify nutritious foods, concerns have been raised about the use of FOP systems in marketing foods that are of questionable nutritional value.[54,55] For example, some FOP systems selectively focus on a product's vitamin and mineral fortification while ignoring its high content of salt and added sugars. Concerns have been raised that some FOP systems and health claims made by manufacturers have violated Food and Drug Administration regulations prohibiting food labeling from bearing statements that are "false and misleading in any particular."[54] One FOP system developed by a group of several food manufacturers was voluntarily withdrawn after the Connecticut attorney general began an investigation into whether the system violated that state's consumer protection law.[56]

The need for a scientifically based FOP system that not only informs consumers but encourages healthier food choices and purchasing behaviors prompted the U.S. Congress to direct the Centers for Disease Control and Prevention and the Food and Drug Administration (FDA) to work with the Institute of Medicine (IOM) to examine some of the existing FOP systems and develop recommendations for an FOP nutrition rating system and symbols.[29,31] This led to a recommendation for the development of a "single, standardized system that is easily understood by most age groups"—focusing on those nutrients or food components "most strongly associated with diet-related health risks affecting the greatest number of Americans"—and that is regulated by the FDA.[31] The IOM recommended that one, standard symbol be

used to display calories per serving and to assign zero to three nutritional "points" for the content of saturated fat, *trans* fat, and added sugars.[31] The symbol should appear on all grocery products, appearing in a consistent location across all products. The criteria for scoring foods should be freely available to the public (nonproprietary) and consistent with and linked to the Nutrition Facts panel.[31]

Daily Values

The **Daily Values** are dietary reference values intended to help consumers use food label information to plan healthy diets. They serve as the basis for quantifying the amounts of various nutrients and food components on food labels. They are to be used for regulatory purposes only and are not intended to serve as recommended intakes. The basis for calculating the Daily Values are two separate sets of nutrient reference values: the **Daily Reference Values (DRVs)** and the **Reference Daily Intakes (RDIs).** These values assist consumers in interpreting information about the amount of a nutrient that is present in a food and in comparing nutritional values of food products. DRVs are established for adults and children 4 or more years of age, as are RDIs, with the exception of protein. DRVs are provided for total fat, saturated fat, cholesterol, total carbohydrate, sodium, dietary fiber, protein, and added sugars. RDIs are provided for vitamins and minerals. In order to limit consumer confusion, however, the label includes a single term (i.e., Daily Value [DV]), to designate both the DRVs and RDIs. Specifically, the label includes the % DV, except that the % DV for protein is not required unless a protein claim is made for the product or if the product is to be used by infants or children under 4 years of age. Table 2.16 provides the most current standards for Daily Values used in the Nutrition Facts food label.

FOOD GUIDES

A food guide is a nutrition education tool translating scientific knowledge and dietary standards and recommendations into an understandable and practical form for use by those who have little or no training in nutrition.[40,57]

TABLE 2.16 | **Major USDA Food Guides (1916–1995), Showing Food Groups and Numbers of Servings***

Food Guide	Number of Food Groups	Protein-Rich Foods — Milk	Meat	Breads	Vegetables	Fruits	Other — Fats	Sugars
Caroline Hunt buying guides (1916)	5	Meats and other protein-rich foods 10% of energy from milk 10% of energy from other foods 1 c milk + 2–3 svgs of other foods based on 3-oz svg		Cereals and other starchy foods 20% of energy 9 svgs based on 1 oz or ¾ c dry cereal	Vegetables and fruits 30% of energy 5 svgs based on average 8-oz svg		Fatty foods 20% of energy 9 svgs based on 1-Tbsp svg	Sugars 10% of energy 10 svgs based on 1-Tbsp svg
H. K. Stiebeling buying guide (1930s)	12	Milk 2 c	Lean meat, poultry, fish 9–10 svgs/wk; Dry, mature beans, peas, nuts 1 svg/wk; Eggs 1	Flours, cereals as desired	Leafy green, yellow 11–12 svgs per wk; Potato, sweet potato 1 svg; Other vegetables and fruit 3 svgs	Tomato and citrus 1 svg	Butter; Other fats	Sugars
Basic Seven foundation diet (1940s)	7	Milk and milk products 2 or more svgs svg = 1 c	Meat, poultry, fish, eggs, dried beans, peas, nuts 1–2 svgs	Breads, flour, and cereals every day	Leafy green, yellow 1 or more svgs; Potato and other fruits and vegetables 2 or more svgs	Citrus, tomato, cabbage, salad greens 1 or more svgs	Butter, fortified margarine some daily	
Basic Four foundation diet (1956–1970s)	4	Milk group 2 or more svgs	Meat group 2 or more svgs 2–3 oz svgs	Bread, cereal 4 or more svgs 1 oz dry, 1 slice ½–¾ c cooked	Vegetable-fruit group 4 svgs include dark green/yellow vegetables frequently ½ c or typical portion			
Hassle-Free foundation diet (1979)	5	Milk-cheese group 2 svgs 1 c, 1½ oz cheese	Meat, poultry, fish, and bean group 2 svgs 2- to 3-oz svg	Bread-cereal group 4 or more svgs 1 oz dry, 1 slice ½–¾ c cooked	Vegetable-fruit group 4 svgs include vitamin C source daily and dark-green/yellow vegetables frequently ½ c or typical portion		Fats, sweets, alcohol group use dependent on calorie needs	
Food Guide Pyramid total diet (1984)	6	Milk, yogurt, cheese 2–3 svgs 1 c, 1½ oz cheese	Meat, poultry, fish eggs, dry beans, nuts 2–3 svgs 5–7 oz total/day	Breads, cereals rice pasta 6–11 svgs whole-grain and enriched 1 slice, ½ c cooked	Vegetable 3–5 svgs dark green deep yellow starchy/legumes other ½ c raw ½ c cooked	Fruit 2–4 svgs citrus other ½ c or average	Fats, oils, sweets total fat not to exceed 30% of energy sweets vary according to energy need	

Source: USDA.

*Number of servings are daily unless noted otherwise; svg = serving.

Food guides are problem oriented and address specific nutritional problems identified within the targeted population. Typically, foods are classified into basic groups according to similarity of nutrient content or some other criteria. If a certain number of servings from each group is consumed, a balanced and adequate diet is thought likely to result.

The USDA has been at the forefront of food guide development in the United States. The major food guides developed by the USDA from 1916 through development of the Food Guide Pyramid are outlined in Table 2.16. The USDA's first food guides are credited to Caroline Hunt (1865–1927), a nutrition specialist in USDA's Bureau of Home Economics.[57] In 1916, she developed *Food for Young Children,* followed in 1917 by *How to Select Foods.* In these, foods were categorized into five groups—milk and meat; cereals; vegetables and fruits; fats and fat foods; and sugars and sugary foods. These "buying guides" were designed to ensure adequate energy intake from fat, carbohydrate, and protein while encouraging sufficient variety for minerals and some of the newly discovered body-regulating substances we now know as vitamins. The financial constraints imposed by the economic depression of the early 1930s led to the development of food guides providing advice to families for purchasing foods at various cost levels. Hazel Stiebeling (1896–1989), a food economist in USDA's Bureau of Home Economics, led in the development of these buying guides. She emphasized a balance between high-energy foods (e.g., fats and sweets) and "protective" or nutrient-dense foods supplying essential nutrients. Among the protective foods are milk, which supplies calcium, and fruits and vegetables, which supply vitamins A and C.[57]

Hunt's and Stiebeling's buying guides gave way to food guides promoting "foundation diets." These food guides recommended a minimum number of servings from different food groups, which provided a foundation diet supplying a major portion of the RDAs. It was assumed that, to meet their energy needs, most people would consume more food than the guide specified. This extra food would provide not only necessary energy but additional nutrients as well. It was further assumed that such a diet would meet requirements for all essential nutrients, not just those included in the RDAs.[45,46] During the mid-1940s, the USDA developed the "Basic Seven," which was widely used for many years. Its complexity and lack of specific serving sizes led to the development of the "Basic Four" in 1956.[57,58] The assumption underlying development of the Four Food Groups was that eating the specified numbers of servings from the different food groups would supply approximately 1200 kcal, approximately 100% of the RDAs for vitamins A and C and calcium, and at least 80% of the RDAs for the remaining five nutrients of the 1953 revision of the RDAs.[58] Vitamins A and C and calcium were given priority status because they were shown to be **shortfall nutrients** (nutrients whose intakes were below recommended levels among a significant part of the population).[58]

In 1979, the USDA issued the Hassle-Free Guide to a Better Diet. This was a revision of the Four Food Groups that gave more attention to micronutrients in food groups and included a fifth food group: fats, sweets, and alcohol. The purpose of including this fifth group was to help consumers recognize fats, sweets, and alcohol as empty calories and to draw attention to the need for considering them in meal planning, since no servings from this group were recommended. The Hassle-Free Guide highlighted the need to use fat, sugars, and alcohol moderately and gave special attention to calories and dietary fiber.[57]

Publication of the *Dietary Goals for the United States* in 1977 (review Figure 2.4 and Box 2.6) was a turning point for dietary guidance and food guides. Following this landmark event, the USDA and USDHHS published the *Dietary Guidelines for Americans* in 1980, with revisions following every five years. In 1980, the USDA began working on a new food guide to replace the Basic Four. This led to development of the food guide shown in Table 2.17. Three key messages of this guide were variety (eating a selection of foods of various types that together meet nutritional needs); proportionality (eating appropriate amounts of various types of foods to meet nutritional needs); and moderation (avoiding too much of food components in the total diet that have been linked to diseases).[57] Despite dissemination of the food guide in several publications developed by the USDA and other groups (including the 1990 edition of *Dietary Guidelines for Americans*), the perception remained among the public and professionals that the USDA was still using the Basic Four developed in the 1950s.[57,58] This led the USDA to develop a separate publication explaining the food guide and containing an appealing illustration conveying the key messages of the guide.

TABLE 2.17	**Daily Food Guide Developed by the USDA to Replace the Basic Four**

Food Group	Suggested Servings*
Vegetables	3–5
Fruits	2–4
Breads, cereals, rice, and pasta	6–11
Milk, yogurt, and cheese	2–3
Meats, poultry, fish, dry beans and peas, eggs, and nuts	2–3

Source: From USDA/USDHHS. 1990. *Nutrition and Your Health: Dietary Guidelines for Americans,* 3rd ed. Washington, DC: U.S. Government Printing Office.

*Eat a variety of foods daily, choosing different foods from each group. Most people should have at least the lower number of servings suggested from each food group. Some people may need more because of their body size and activity levels. Young children should have a variety of foods but may need small servings.

FOOD GUIDE PYRAMID

The Food Guide Pyramid was released in 1992 and designed to serve as a graphic outline of what constituted a healthy diet and to convey the concepts of variety, proportionality, and moderation. As shown in Figure 2.8, five food groups (cereals and grains, vegetables, fruits, dairy products, and protein-rich foods) were arranged horizontally, with cereals and grains at the base of the pyramid to indicate that foods from this group should compose the largest portion of the diet. At the apex of the pyramid were fats, oils, and sweets, to indicate that these were to be consumed sparingly. The recommended number of servings from each of the five groups was expressed as a range: persons consuming the number of servings at the low end of the range would consume approximately 1600 kcal per day, while those consuming the number of servings at the high end of the range would consume approximately 2800 kcal per day.

The Food Guide Pyramid has been criticized by some as representing "a mix of well-supported findings, educated guesses, and political compromises with powerful economic interests such as the dairy and meat industries."[59] Some felt that the recommended number of servings of meat (two to three per day) may be unhealthy

and that the Food Guide Pyramid ignored important differences in types of fat, such as saturated and *trans* fatty acids, as opposed to monounsaturated fatty acids.[59] Others objected to the USDA's approach to grouping foods—for example, grouping nonfat dairy products (skim milk or nonfat yogurt, for example) with higher-fat dairy products, such as ice cream and many cheeses, or grouping legumes with meat, many of which are high in fat. The USDA's failure to emphasize sources of calcium other than dairy products was regarded by some as insensitive to individuals of African, Asian, or Hispanic descent, who are more likely to experience lactose malabsorption than are those of Northern European descent. In response to these and other concerns, alternative pyramids were developed. Among these were the Mediterranean Pyramid, the Vegetarian Pyramid, and a variety of Asian Pyramids.[59]

MyPyramid

In 2005, the USDA released an updated and revised food guide graphic called "MyPyramid" that replaced the Food Guide Pyramid released in 1992. The USDA's stated motives for developing the MyPyramid graphic was to increase consumer use of its food guidance system,

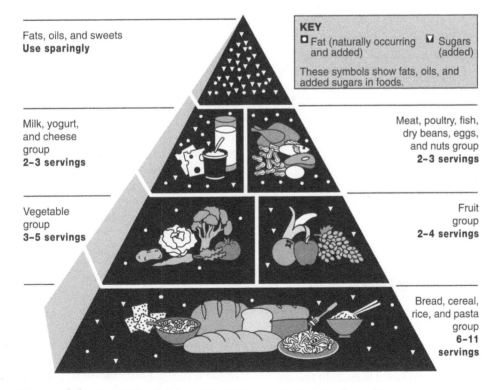

Figure 2.8 The U.S. Department of Agriculture's Food Guide Pyramid.
Source: The U.S. Department of Agriculture's Food Guide Pyramid.

better motivate consumers to make healthier food choices, more effectively address the increasing prevalence of overweight and obesity in America, and ensure that its food guidance system reflected recent advances in nutritional science. The new graphic was accompanied by an online system of interactive, consumer-friendly tools that provided advice on diet and physical activity that was specific and tailored to the needs of the individual user. With access to a computer and the Internet, an individual could develop a detailed set of dietary recommendations suitable for one's age, sex, and physical activity level.

In general, MyPyramid was part of an overall food guidance system from the federal government that emphasized the need for a more individualized approach to improving diet and lifestyle. MyPyramid supported accumulating scientific evidence that individuals could dramatically improve their overall health by making modest dietary improvements and by incorporating regular physical activity into their daily lives.

MYPLATE

In June 2011, the USDA released the MyPlate graphic as part of the federal government's efforts to develop a comprehensive approach to effectively communicate the 2010 Dietary Guidelines for Americans (DGAs). Shown in Figure 2.9, MyPlate uses a familiar mealtime symbol as a simple visual cue and reminder to eat healthfully at mealtimes by incorporating healthier choices among the food groups, with particular emphasis on increasing intake of vegetables and fruits.[60] The graphic was deliberately

designed to be simple in order to grab consumers' attention and be recognized by a wide variety of audiences. It is intended not to provide a specific message but to serve as a beginning point for the efforts of educators to help people of all age groups, cultures, and learning levels better understand how to make healthier choices at mealtimes. It is also intended to serve as a reminder of healthful eating, reinforcing what has been conveyed through educational efforts.[61]

The graphic and accompanying educational materials are the result of a multiyear research and development program by the USDA in response to what many in the nutrition community felt was a need for a new image to refocus attention on healthy eating that would replace the Pyramids. From this research program, two apparently opposing needs emerged: a need to simplify nutrition messaging and the need for more information. It also became apparent that no single message or graphic would be sufficient to meet the needs of all consumers and that a comprehensive and layered approach would be necessary to effectively communicate the 2010 DGAs. After studying the responses of consumers to several different potential images, researchers decided that a plate graphic best conveyed a positive yet simple visual message emphasizing the need to increase consumption of vegetables and fruits and to eat healthfully. To meet consumers' desire for more information, a variety of new educational resources are available to the public and to educators to be used in conjunction with the MyPlate graphic.[60,61]

To help consumers understand their energy, food, and nutrient requirements, the USDA has developed an innovative online feature called SuperTracker, which is discussed in Chapter 5 and can be accessed at www.choosemyplate.gov/tools-supertracker. One feature of SuperTracker provides meal plans and sample menus based on an individual's recommended energy level, which is based on the individual's age, sex, height, weight, physical activity level, and so forth. Box 2.10 outlines the MyPlate Daily Checklist at the 2000-calorie-per-day level. Checklists are available at www.choosemyplate.gov/MyPlate-Daily-Checklist and include specific plans for 1000 to 3200 calories per day. The food plans can be personalized based on age, sex, height, weight, and physical activity level using SuperTracker (see www.supertracker.usda.gov).

The New American Plate

The concept of using a graphic image of vegetables, fruits, and other plant products covering half or more of a dinner plate is not unique to MyPlate. The New American Plate (see www.aicr.org/new-american-plate/) is a food guide based on the recommendations of the research report *Food, Nutrition, and the Prevention of Cancer: A Global Perspective,* which was published by the American Institute for Cancer Research (AICR) and

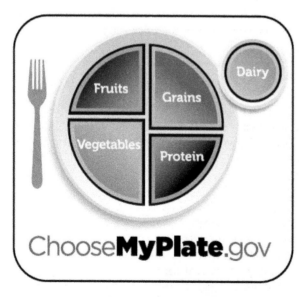

Figure 2.9 In 2011, the U.S. Department of Agriculture released the MyPlate graphic, which provides a visual representation of the advice contained in the 2010 Dietary Guidelines for Americans.

Source: USDA Center for Nutrition Policy and Promotion.

Box 2.10   USDA Meal Planning Guide for 12 Different Levels of Energy Expenditure

United States Department of Agriculture

MyPlate Daily Checklist
Find your Healthy Eating Style

Everything you eat and drink matters. Find your healthy eating style that reflects your preferences, culture, traditions, and budget—and maintain it for a lifetime! The right mix can help you be healthier now and into the future. The key is choosing a variety of foods and beverages from each food group—*and making sure that each choice is limited in saturated fat, sodium, and added sugars.* Start with small changes—"MyWins"—to make healthier choices you can enjoy.

Food Group Amounts for 2,000 Calories a Day

Fruits	Vegetables	Grains	Protein	Dairy
2 cups	**2 1/2 cups**	**6 ounces**	**5 1/2 ounces**	**3 cups**
Focus on whole fruits	Vary your veggies	Make half your grains whole grains	Vary your protein routine	Move to low-fat or fat-free milk or yogurt
Focus on whole fruits that are fresh, frozen, canned, or dried.	Choose a variety of colorful fresh, frozen, and canned vegetables—make sure to include dark green, red, and orange choices.	Find whole-grain foods by reading the Nutrition Facts label and ingredients list.	Mix up your protein foods to include seafood, beans and peas, unsalted nuts and seeds, soy products, eggs, and lean meats and poultry.	Choose fat-free milk, yogurt, and soy beverages (soy milk) to cut back on your saturated fat.

 Limit Drink and eat less sodium, saturated fat, and added sugars. Limit:
- Sodium to **2300 milligrams** a day.
- Saturated fat to **22 grams** a day.
- Added sugars to **50 grams** a day.

Be active your way: Children 6 to 17 years old should move **60 minutes** every day. Adults should be physically active at least **2 1/2 hours** per week.
Use SuperTracker to create a personal plan based on your age, sex, height, weight, and physical activity level.
SuperTracker.usda.gov

Source: USDA.

its affiliate, the World Cancer Research Fund located in the United Kingdom. The report (available at http://www.aicr.org), first published in 1997 and updated in 2007, is an exhaustive review of the scientific literature relating to the influence of diet and nutrition on the risk of cancer. The report's key finding is that 30% to 40% of all cancers could be prevented by eating healthfully and being physically active. The New American Plate encourages healthful eating by illustrating that plant foods such as vegetables, fruits, whole grains, and beans should cover two-thirds (or more) of one's plate. Animal foods such as fish, poultry, lean meats, or low-fat dairy products should cover one-third (or less) of the plate. The report encourages variety, moderation, and proportionality and emphasizes eating more plant foods and moderate amounts of lean meats and low-fat dairy products. There is overwhelming scientific evidence that

diets emphasizing nutrient-dense plant foods increase a person's daily consumption of vitamins, minerals, dietary fiber, and phytochemicals and tend to be lower in calories. Such diets are associated with a substantially lower risk of cancer and obesity. Furthermore, eating smaller portions of low-fat dairy products and lean meats, especially fish and chicken, is also linked to lower risk of cancer and obesity. A key recommendation from the AICR is to eat at least five servings of vegetables and fruits each day. This one dietary change alone has the potential to prevent at least 20% of all cancers. A standard serving of vegetables is 1/2 cup of cooked vegetables or 1 cup of raw vegetables such as salad. An example of a serving of fruit is a medium-size apple, orange, pear, or banana or 1/2 cup of chopped fruit. It is important to eat a variety of vegetables, including dark green, leafy vegetables and those that are deep orange in color.

TABLE 2.18	Average Macronutrient and Kilocalorie Content in One Serving from Each of the Food Lists			
Food List	Carbohydrate (grams)	Protein (grams)	Fat (grams)	Kilocalories
Carbohydrates				
Starch: breads, cereals and grains, starchy vegetables, crackers, snacks, and beans, peas, and lentils	15	3	1	80
Fruits	15	0	0	60
Milk				
Fat-free, low-fat, 1%	12	8	0–3	100
Reduce-fat, 2%	12	8	5	120
Whole	12	8	8	160
Sweets, desserts, and other carbohydrates	15	varies	varies	varies
Nonstarchy vegetables	5	2	0	25
Proteins				
Lean	0	7	2	45
Medium-fat	0	7	5	75
High-fat	0	7	8+	100
Plant-based	varies	7	varies	varies
Fats	0	0	5	45
Alcohol	varies	0	0	100

© Academy of Nutrition and Dietetics, reprinted with permission

A variety of whole fruits (as opposed to juice) should be eaten as well, including citrus fruits and those that are good sources of vitamin C. In addition, the AICR recommends eating at least seven servings per day of other plant-based foods such as brown rice, whole-wheat pasta, whole-wheat bread, crushed buckwheat (kasha), millet, lentils, black-eyed peas, and various beans such as black, pinto, kidney, navy, and garbanzo.

FOOD LISTS AND CHOICES

The "Choose Your Foods" **system** is a method of planning meals that simplifies controlling energy consumption (particularly from carbohydrate), helps ensure adequate nutrient intake, and allows considerable variety in food selection. Also, once a person becomes familiar with the system, he or she can use it to quickly approximate kilocalorie and macronutrient levels in individual foods or an entire meal.

The food exchange system originally was developed in 1950 by the Academy of Nutrition and Dietetics (formerly known as the American Dietetic Association) and the American Diabetes Association in cooperation with the U.S. Public Health Service for use in planning the diets of persons who have diabetes.[62] Before then, no standardized method for planning diabetic diets existed, and many health professionals and people with diabetes complained that meal planning often was laborious and difficult to adapt to individual food preferences.

The system categorizes foods and beverages according to their carbohydrate, protein, fat, alcohol, and energy content and lists them in four categories—carbohydrates, meat and meat substitutes, fat, and alcoholic beverages—as shown in Table 2.18. The carbohydrate group includes foods that supply most of their energy in the form of carbohydrate: starchy foods, fruits, milk and other dairy products, other carbohydrates, and nonstarchy vegetables. The milk and dairy products are further divided into three categories on the basis of their fat and energy content. The proteins include foods that serve as good protein sources and supply variable amounts of fat and no carbohydrate except for the plant-based meat substitutes. The meat and meat substitutes are further divided into four categories, primarily on the basis of their fat and energy content. According to this system, an alcoholic beverage is one providing 100 kilocalories, variable amounts of carbohydrate, and no protein or fat.

A detailed listing of foods within each of the groups and the serving size for each food are given in materials published jointly by the American Dietetic Association and the American Diabetes Association.[63] In 2014,

TABLE 2.19	**Food Lists and Basic Choices for Meal Planning**

Starch List

One starch choice contains 15 g carbohydrate, 3 g protein, 1 g fat, and 80 calories. Foods that are considered starches include cereals, grains, pasta, breads, crackers, starchy vegetables, and cooked dried beans, peas, and lentils (cooked dried beans, peas, and lentils are also found on the proteins list). For health benefits, at least half of the servings of grains each day should be whole grains. In general, one starch exchange is
- 1/2 cup of cooked cereal, grain, or starchy vegetable
- 1/3 cup of cooked rice or pasta
- 1 ounce of bread, such as one slice of bread 3/4 to 1 oz of most snack foods (some snack foods may also have extra fat)

Fruit List

One fruit choice contains 15 g carbohydrate, 0 g protein, 0 g fat, and 60 calories. Fresh, frozen, canned, and dried fruits and fruit juices are on this list. Fresh, frozen, and dried fruits are good sources of fiber. Fruit juices contain very little fiber. Citrus fruits, berries, and melons are good sources of vitamin C. In general, one fruit choice is
- 1 small fresh fruit (3/4 to 1 cup)
- 1/2 cup of canned or frozen fruit
- 2 tablespoons of dried fruit 1/2 cup of unsweetened fruit juice

Milk and Milk Substitutes

One exchange of milk contains 12 g carbohydrate and 8 g protein with the number of grams of fat and the number of calories varying, as shown in Table 2.18. In general one milk choice is
- 1 cup or 8 fluid oz, or 2/3 cup yogurt, or 1/2 cup evaporated milk

Nonstarchy Vegetables

One choice of a nonstarchy vegetable (those containing small amounts of carbohydrate) provides 5 g carbohydrate, 2 g protein, 0 g fat, and 25 calories. Aim for a variety of vegetables and eat at least 2 to 3 nonstarchy vegetable choices daily. One choice of a nonstarchy vegetable is
- 1/2 cup cooked vegetables or vegetable juice
- 1 cup raw vegetables

Proteins

One choice of meat contains 0 g carbohydrate, 7 g protein, with the number of grams of fat and the number of calories varying, as shown in Table 2.18. One choice of a meat substitute provides 7 g protein with variable amounts of carbohydrate, fat, and energy, as shown in Table 2.18. One choice of a protein substitute is
- 1 oz cooked or canned meat, poultry, or fish
- 1 oz cheese
- 2 egg whites
- 1 whole egg 1/2 cup beans or tofu

Fats

One choice of fat contains 0 g carbohydrate, 0 g protein, 5 g fat, and 45 calories. Limit fried foods, and choose unsaturated fats instead of saturated and *trans* fats whenever possible. Nuts and seeds are good sources of unsaturated fats. One fat choice is
- 1 teaspoon of oil
- 1 teaspoon stick butter, margarine, shortening, or lard
- 1 tablespoon cream cheese, regular
- 8 large black olives
- 1 tablespoon seeds
- 6 mixed nuts

© Academy of Nutrition and Dietetics, Choose Your Foods: Exchange Lists for Diabetes. Copyright ©2014, reprinted with permission.

"exchange" was dropped in favor of "choice," which is now used to describe a certain quantity of food within a group of similar foods. Table 2.19 provides a basic summary of common amounts of food that are included in each type of food list. When planning a meal, food choices within a group can be substituted, for any other food within that group without varying the approximate amount of carbohydrate, protein, fat, and energy supplied by the meal, as long as the serving size of the food adheres to that specified in the food choice list. At breakfast, for example, a person could substitute one slice of bread for 3/4 cup of unsweetened, ready-to-eat cereal because each of these foods is considered one choice from the starch group, and as such, each has the same amount of macronutrients and the same number of kilocalories. The American Dietetic Association and the American Diabetes Association have also developed lists for foods commonly eaten by various ethnic and regional groups.

Ideally, when diabetes is diagnosed in a patient, a dietitian works with the patient to design a meal plan

TABLE 2.20	Sample Meal Patterns Using the Food Choice Lists for Meal Planning

1500-Kilocalorie Diet with Two Snacks

	Breakfast	Lunch	Snack	Dinner	Snack
Starch	2	2	½	2	½
Meat, medium-fat	1	2	1	2	
Vegetable		1		1	
Fruit	1	1		1	
Milk, skim	½	½			½
Fat	1	1		1	

	Kcal	Carbohydrate	Protein	Fat
Total	1510	178 g	79 g	45 g
Percent of energy		50%	22%	28%

2000-Kilocalorie Diet with Two Snacks

	Breakfast	Lunch	Snack	Dinner	Snack
Starch	2	2	½	3	½
Meat, medium-fat	1	2	1	2	1
Vegetable		1		2	
Fruit	2	2		2	
Milk, skim	1	1		1	
Fat	1	1		1	

	Kcal	Carbohydrate	Protein	Fat
Total	2005	261 g	103 g	50 g
Percent of energy		55%	22%	23%

2500-Kilocalorie Diet with Two Snacks

	Breakfast	Lunch	Snack	Dinner	Snack
Starch	3	3	1	4	1
Meat, medium-fat	1	3	1	3	1
Vegetable		2		2	
Fruit	2	2		2	
Milk, skim	1	1		1	
Fat	1	1		1	

	Kcal	Carbohydrate	Protein	Fat
Total	2500	326 g	131 g	60 g
Percent of energy		55%	22%	23%

Source: USDA

individualized to the patient's dietary preferences, daily schedule, medications, body weight, serum lipid levels, and exercise habits. This meal plan is sometimes expressed in terms of the number of foods from the lists. Many weight management programs and meal plans for people with diabetes are based on the food choice system because it simplifies the task of counting calories. An outstanding feature of the food choice system is that, rather than specifying a particular food, it gives a person an almost unlimited variety of foods from which to choose in planning meals. A person following one of the meal patterns in Table 2.20 can select a number of different foods from the starch list to get his or her choices from that list. The same is true for the protein, fruit, milk, and fat selections. The important thing is to select the specified *number* of food choices and the correct *serving size* from each list.[63]

SUMMARY

1. A number of tools and methods are available for nutrition professionals to use in evaluating dietary intakes of individuals and groups. Included among these are standards of recommended nutrient intake, measurements of nutrient density, dietary guidelines or goals, and food guides.

2. With a few exceptions, dietary standards up until the 20th century were observational and lacked a firm scientific base. Advances in metabolic, vitamin, and mineral research during the early 20th century led to the establishment of scientifically based estimates of human nutrient requirements by the League of Nations and several European countries, Canada, and the United States.

3. One of the earliest and most familiar of the dietary standards is the Recommended Dietary Allowance (RDA), developed by the Food and Nutrition Board of the National Research Council. The RDAs provided specific nutrient recommendations for healthy persons in each life stage and gender group. They were originally developed in 1941 and revised about every five years. Their primary focus was prevention of micronutrient deficiency. The last edition of the RDAs was published in 1989.

4. Limitations in the RDAs became apparent as nutritional science advanced and as the primary nutrition concern of North America changed from nutrient deficiency to food and nutrient overconsumption, with an attendant increase in chronic disease risk. In addition, the RDAs had no recommendations for carbohydrate, fiber, fat, cholesterol, and food components not traditionally regarded as nutrients (e.g., phytochemicals). They failed to address the role of nutrition in reducing chronic disease risk and gave no guidance on use of nutritional supplements.

5. In response to the RDAs' limitations, scientists from the Food and Nutrition Board, the Canadian Institute of Nutrition, and Health Canada developed a new set of nutrient reference values, known as the Dietary Reference Intakes (DRIs). The DRIs include four reference values: Estimated Average Requirement (EAR), Adequate Intake (AI), Tolerable Upper Intake Level (UL), and Recommended Dietary Allowance (RDA). In addition, the DRIs include an Estimated Energy Requirement and Acceptable Macronutrient Distribution Ranges that suggest the percent of kilocalories to be obtained from total fat, essential fatty acids, carbohydrate, and protein.

6. EAR is the daily dietary intake level estimated to meet the nutrient requirement of 50% of healthy individuals in a particular life stage and gender group. The EAR is the basis for establishing the RDA, which, as traditionally defined, is an intake level sufficient to meet the nutrient requirement of nearly all healthy individuals in a particular life stage and gender group.

7. If there are insufficient data to establish an EAR, then the AI is used instead of the RDA. The AI is actually an observational standard and is defined as a recommended intake level that is assumed to be adequate and that is based on experimentally determined approximations of nutrient intake by a group (or groups) of healthy people. The UL is the highest level of daily nutrient intake that is likely to pose no risk of adverse health effects to almost all apparently healthy individuals in the general population.

8. The suggested uses of the DRIs are clearly delineated and fall into two broad categories: assessing nutrient intakes of individuals and groups and planning for nutrient intakes of individuals and groups. The DRIs address health promotion and the prevention of both chronic and deficiency disease. They also provide guidance on using nutritional supplements. They are intended to be used in conjunction with other nutritional assessment approaches, rather than as the only means of assessing nutrient adequacy.

9. A nutrient-dense food is a good source of vitamins, minerals, and other food components that may have positive health effects but is relatively low in energy. Nutrient-dense foods are lean or low in solids fats and are low in added sugars and refined starches, all of which add kilocalories but few essential nutrients or little dietary fiber. Nutrient-dense foods also minimize or exclude added salt or other components that are high in sodium.

10. Dietary guidelines, or goals, are dietary standards primarily intended to address the more common and pressing nutrition-related health problems of chronic disease. They often are expressed as nonquantitative change from the present average national diet or from people's typical eating habits.

11. Since the late 1960s, numerous dietary guidelines have been issued by governments and various health organizations. Overall, they have consistently called for maintenance of healthy body weight, decreased

consumption of saturated fat, *trans* fat, and added sugars, increased consumption of complex carbohydrates, and use of alcoholic beverages in moderation, if at all.

12. Nutrition labeling in the United States began in 1973, when the Food and Drug Administration established the U.S. Recommended Daily Allowances (U.S. RDAs). In 1990, Congress passed the Nutrition Labeling and Education Act, which made sweeping changes in nutrition labeling regulations, replaced the U.S. RDAs with the Reference Daily Intakes (RDIs), and established the Daily Reference Values (DRVs). The RDIs and DRVs are collectively referred to as the Daily Values.

13. Food guides are nutrition education tools that translate dietary standards and recommendations into understandable and practical forms for use by those who have little or no training in nutrition. Generally, foods are classified into groups according to their similarity in nutrient content. If a certain amount of food from each group is consumed, a balanced and adequate diet is thought likely to result. A familiar example of a food guide is MyPlate.

14. The food choice system simplifies meal planning for persons limiting energy consumption and helps ensure adequate nutrient intake. Originally developed to facilitate meal planning for persons with diabetes, it is easily adapted to personal food preferences and is useful for quickly approximating kilocalorie and macronutrient levels in foods. The specified serving sizes of foods within each food choice list are approximately equal in their contribution of energy and macronutrients.

REFERENCES

1. Leitch I. 1942. The evolution of dietary standards. *Nutrition Abstracts and Reviews* 11:509–521.

2. Harper AE. 1985. Origin of Recommended Dietary Allowances: An historic overview. *American Journal of Clinical Nutrition* 41:140–148.

3. McCollum EV. 1957. *A history of nutrition.* Boston: Houghton Mifflin.

4. Harper AE. 2003. Contributions of women scientists in the U.S. to the development of Recommended Dietary Allowances. *Journal of Nutrition* 133:3698–3702.

5. Roberts LJ. 1958. Beginnings of the Recommended Dietary Allowances. *Journal of the American Dietetic Association* 34:903–908.

6. Otten JJ, Hellwig JP, Meyers LD, editors. 2006. *Dietary Reference Intakes: The essential guide to nutrient requirements.* Washington, DC: National Academies Press.

7. Committee on Food and Nutrition, National Research Council. 1941. Recommended allowances for the various dietary essentials. *Journal of the American Dietetic Association* 17:565–567.

8. Food and Nutrition Board, National Research Council. 1989. *Recommended Dietary Allowances,* 10th ed. Washington, DC: National Academies Press.

9. Food and Nutrition Board, Institute of Medicine. 1994. *How should the Recommended Dietary Allowances be revised?* Washington, DC: National Academies Press.

10. Standing Committee on the Scientific Evaluation of Dietary Reference Intakes, Food and Nutrition Board, Institute of Medicine. 1997. *Dietary Reference Intakes for calcium, phosphorus, magnesium, vitamin D, and fluoride.* Washington, DC: National Academies Press.

11. Standing Committee on the Scientific Evaluation of Dietary Reference Intakes, Food and Nutrition Board, Institute of Medicine. 1998. *Dietary Reference Intakes for thiamin, riboflavin, niacin, vitamin B6, folate, vitamin B12, pantothenic acid, biotin, and choline.* Washington, DC: National Academies Press.

12. Standing Committee on the Scientific Evaluation of Dietary Reference Intakes, Food and Nutrition Board, Institute of Medicine. 2000. *Dietary Reference Intakes for vitamin C, vitamin E, selenium, and carotenoids.* Washington, DC: National Academies Press.

13. Panel on Micronutrients, Subcommittee on Upper Reference Levels of Nutrients and of Interpretation and Uses of Dietary Reference Intakes, Standing Committee on the Scientific Evaluation of Dietary Reference Intakes. 2001. *Dietary Reference Intakes for vitamin A, vitamin K, arsenic, boron, chromium, copper, iodine, iron, manganese, molybdenum, nickel, silicon, vanadium, and zinc.* Washington, DC: National Academies Press.

14. Panel on Macronutrients, Panel on the Definition of Dietary Fiber, Subcommittee on Upper Reference Levels of Nutrients, Subcommittee on Interpretation and Uses of Dietary Reference Intakes, Standing Committee on the Scientific Evaluation of Dietary

Reference Intakes. 2002. *Dietary Reference Intakes for energy, carbohydrate, fiber, fat, fatty acids, cholesterol, protein, and amino acids.* Washington, DC: National Academies Press.

15. Panel on Dietary Reference Intakes for Electrolytes and Water, Standing Committee on the Scientific Evaluation of Dietary Reference Intakes, Food and Nutrition Board. 2004. *Dietary Reference Intakes for water, potassium, sodium, chloride, and sulfate.* Washington, DC: National Academies Press.

16. Committee to Review Dietary Reference Intakes for Vitamin D and Calcium, Food and Nutrition Board. Ross AC, Taylor CL, Yaktine AL, Del Valle HB, editors. 2011. *Dietary Reference Intakes for calcium and vitamin D.* Washington, DC: National Academies Press.

17. Subcommittee on Interpretation and Uses of Dietary Reference Intakes, Standing Committee on the Scientific Evaluation of Dietary References Intakes, Food and Nutrition Board. 2000. *Dietary Reference Intakes: Applications in dietary assessment.* Washington, DC: National Academies Press.

18. Subcommittee on Interpretation and Uses of Dietary Reference Intakes, Standing Committee on the Scientific Evaluation of Dietary References Intakes. 2003. *Dietary Reference Intakes: Applications in dietary planning.* Washington, DC: National Academies Press.

19. Committee on Use of Dietary Reference Intakes in Nutrition Labeling, Food and Nutrition Board. 2003. *Dietary Reference Intakes: Guiding principles for nutrition labeling and fortification.* Washington, DC: National Academies Press.

20. Backstrand JR. 2003. Quantitative approaches to nutrient density for public health nutrition. *Public Health Nutrition* 6:829–837.

21. Drewnowski A. 2009. Defining nutrient density: Development and validation of the Nutrient Rich Foods index. *Journal of the American College of Nutrition* 28:421S–426S.

22. Kennedy E, Racsa P, Dallal G, Lichtenstein AH, Goldberg J, Jacques P, Hyatt R. 2008. Alternative approaches to the calculation of nutrient density. *Nutrition Reviews* 66:703–709.

23. U.S. Department of Health and Human Services and U.S. Department of Agriculture. 2010. *Dietary Guidelines for Americans, 2010.* Washington, DC: U.S. Government Printing Office.

24. Hansen RG, Wyse BW. 1980. Expression of nutrient allowances per 1,000 kilocalories. *Journal of the American Dietetic Association* 76:223–227.

25. Nicklas TA. 2009. Nutrient profiling: The new environment. *Journal of the American College of Nutrition* 28:416S–420S.

26. Dietary Guidelines Advisory Committee. 2010. *Report of the Dietary Guidelines Advisory Committee on the Dietary Guidelines for Americans, 2010.* Washington, DC: U.S. Department of Agriculture, Agricultural Research Service.

27. Drenowski A, Fulgoni V. 2008. Nutrient profiling of foods: Creating a nutrient-rich food index. *Nutrition Today* 66:23–39.

28. Chiuve SE, Sampson L, Willett WC. 2011. The association between a nutritional quality index and risk of chronic disease. *American Journal of Preventive Medicine* 40:505–513.

29. Institute of Medicine. 2010. *Examination of front-of-package nutrition rating systems and symbols: Phase I report.* Washington, DC: National Academies Press.

30. Fulgoni VL, Keast DR, Drewnowski A. 2009. Development and validation of the Nutrient-Rich Foods index: A tool to measure nutritional quality of foods. *Journal of Nutrition* 139:1549–1554.

31. Institute of Medicine. 2012. *Front-of-package nutrition rating systems and symbols: Promoting healthier choices.* Washington, DC: National Academies Press.

32. Haines PS, Siega-Riz AM, Popkin BM. 1999. The Diet Quality Index Revised: A measurement instrument for populations. *Journal of the American Dietetic Association* 99:697–704.

33. Waijers PMCM, Feskens EJM, Ocke MC. 2007. A critical review of predefined diet quality scores. *British Journal of Nutrition* 97:219–231.

34. Fransen HP, Ocke MC. 2008. Indices of diet quality. *Current Opinion in Clinical Nutrition and Metabolic Care* 11:559–565.

35. Patterson RE, Haines PS, Popkin BM. 1994. Diet Quality Index: Capturing a multidimensional behavior. *Journal of the American Dietetic Association* 94:57–64.

36. Food and Nutrition Board, National Research Council. 1989. *Diet and health: Implications for reducing chronic disease risk.* Washington, DC: National Academies Press.

37. Carmichael SL, Yang W, Feldkamp ML, Munger RG, Siega-Riz AM, Botto LS, Shaw G. 2012. Reduced risks of neural tube defects and orofacial clefts with higher diet quality. *Archives of Pediatric and Adolescent Medicine* 166:121–126.

38. Snyder DC, Sloane R, Haines PS, Miller P, Clipp EC, Morey MC, Pieper C, Cohen H, Demark-Wahnefried W. 2007. The Diet Quality Index-Revised: A tool to promote and evaluate dietary change among older cancer survivors enrolled in a home-based intervention trial. *Journal of the American Dietetic Association* 107:1519–1529.

39. Kennedy ET, Ohls J, Carlson S, Fleming K. 1995. The Healthy Eating Index: Design and applications. *Journal of the American Dietetic Association* 95:1103–1108.

40. Guenther PM, Reedy J, Krebs-Smith SM, Reeve BB, Basiotis PP. 2007. *Development and evaluation of the Healthy Eating Index–2005, Technical Report.* Washington, DC: Center for Nutrition Policy and Promotion, U.S. Department of Agriculture.

41. Guenther PM, Kirkpatrick SI, Reedy J, Krebs-Smith SM, Buckman DW, Dodd KW, Casavale

KO, Carroll RJ. 2014. The Healthy Eating Index–2010 is a valid and reliable measure of diet quality according to the 2010 Dietary Guidelines for Americans. *Journal of Nutrition* 144:399–407.

42. Truswell AS. 1987. Evolution of dietary recommendations, goals, and guidelines. *American Journal of Clinical Nutrition* 45:1060–1072.

43. Select Committee on Nutrition and Human Needs, U.S. Senate. 1977. *Dietary goals for the United States.* Washington, DC: U.S. Government Printing Office.

44. Twenty commentaries. 1977. *Nutrition Today* 12(6):10–27.

45. Additional commentaries. 1978. *Nutrition Today* 13(1):30–32.

46. U.S. Department of Agriculture/ U.S. Department of Health and Human Services. 1980. *Nutrition and your health: Dietary Guidelines for Americans.* Washington, DC: U.S. Government Printing Office.

47. U.S. Department of Health and Human Services and U.S. Department of Agriculture. December 2015. *2015–2020 Dietary Guidelines for Americans,* 8th ed. Available at http:// health.gov/dietaryguidelines/ 2015/guidelines/.

48. U.S. Department of Health and Human Services. 1988. *The surgeon general's report on nutrition and health.* Washington, DC: U.S. Government Printing Office.

49. Nestle M. 1988. The surgeon general's report on nutrition and health: New federal dietary guidance policy. *Journal of Nutrition Education* 20:252–254.

50. McGinnis JM, Nestle M. 1989. The surgeon general's report on nutrition and health: Policy implications and implementation strategies. *American Journal of Clinical Nutrition* 49:23–28.

51. Kushi LH, Doyle C, McCullough M, Rock CL, Demark-Wahnefried W, Bandera EV, Gapstur S, Patel AV, Andrews K, Gansler T. 2012. American Cancer Society guidelines on nutrition and physical activity for cancer prevention. *CA: A Cancer Journal* 62:30–67.

52. Eckel RH, Jakicic JM, Ard JD, de Jesus JM, Houston Miller N, Hubbard VS, Lee IM, Lichtenstein AH, Loria CM, Millen BE, Nonas CA, Sacks FM, Smith SC Jr, Svetkey LP, Wadden TA, Yanovski SZ, American College of Cardiology/American Heart Association Task Force on Practice Guidelines. 2014. 2013 AHA/ACC guideline on lifestyle management to reduce cardiovascular risk: A report of the American College of Cardiology/American Heart Association Task Force on Practice Guidelines. *Journal of the American College of Cardiology* 63(25 Pt B):2960–2984.

53. Evert AB, Boucher JL, Cypress M, Dunbar SA, Franz MJ, Mayer-Davis EJ, Neumiller JJ, Nwankwo R, Verdi CL, Urbanski P, Yancy WS Jr, American Diabetes Association. 2013. Nutrition therapy recommendations for the management of adults with diabetes. *Diabetes Care* 36:3821–3842.

54. Nestle M, Ludwig DS. 2010. Front-of-package food labels: Public health or propaganda? *Journal of the American Medical Association* 303:771–772.

55. Brownell KD, Koplan JP. 2011. Front-of-package nutrition labeling: An abuse of trust by the food industry? *New England Journal of Medicine* 364:2373–2375.

56. Neuman W. 2009. Food label program to suspend operations. *New York Times,* October 24, B1.

57. Welsh S, Davis C, Shaw A. 1992. A brief history of food guides in the United States. *Nutrition Today* 27(6):6–11.

58. Welsh SO, Davis C, Shaw A. 1993. *USDA's Food Guide: Background and development.* Hyattsville, MD: U.S. Department of Agriculture, Human Nutrition Information Service.

59. Willett WC. 1994. Diet and health: What should we eat? *Science* 264:532–537.

60. Post R, Haven J, Maniscalco S. 2012. Putting MyPlate to work for nutrition educators. *Journal of Nutrition Education and Behavior* 44:98–99.

61. U.S. Department of Agriculture. 2011. *Development of 2010 Dietary Guidelines for Americans consumer messages and new food icon: Executive summary of formative research.* Alexandria, VA: USDA Center for Nutrition Policy and Promotion.

62. Caso EK. 1950. Calculation of diabetic diets. *Journal of the American Dietetic Association* 26:575–583.

63. American Dietetic Association. 2014. *Choose your foods: Food lists for diabetes.* Chicago: American Dietetic Association.

ASSESSMENT ACTIVITY 2.1

Using Standards to Evaluate Nutrient Intake

Nutrient standards are indispensable in establishing a benchmark from which to assess adequacy of nutrient intake. This assessment activity will help you become familiar with the Daily Values established by the U.S. Food and Drug Administration (FDA) for food labeling purposes: the Daily Reference Values (DRVs) and the Reference Daily Intakes (RDIs). The activity asks you to

		Dietary Reference Intakes (Tables 2.1, 2.2, 2.3)		Daily Value (Table 2.16)	
Nutrient	**Mean Intake***	**Standard**	**Percent of Standard**	**Standard**	**Percent of Standard**
Vitamin B6	1.91 mg	_____	_____	_____	_____
Vitamin C	72 mg	_____	_____	_____	_____
Vitamin D	4.0 µg	_____	_____	_____	_____
Calcium	872 mg	_____	_____	_____	_____
Magnesium	248 mg	_____	_____	_____	_____
Choline	275 mg	_____	_____	_____	_____
Zinc	9.4 mg	_____	_____	_____	_____
Sodium	3210 mg	_____	_____	_____	_____

TABLE 2.21 — **Mean Intakes of Selected Nutrients and Energy of U.S. Females 20–29 Years Old and How They Compare with the Daily Values and Reference Daily Intakes**

*From What We Eat in America, NHANES 2013–2014 (https://www.ars.usda.gov/) (click on "Nutrient Data Tools").

use the Daily Value standard to assess the intake levels of eight nutrients and to compare results from these standards.

Table 2.21 shows mean intakes for eight nutrients by U.S. females age 20 to 29 years from the What We Eat in America, National Health and Nutrition Examination Survey (NHANES). What We Eat in America, NHANES (discussed in detail in Chapter 4) is a national food survey conducted as a partnership between the U.S. Department of Health and Human Services and the U.S. Department of Agriculture. The data were averaged from 24-hour dietary recalls.

1. Locate the recommended intakes of the eight nutrients for females from the appropriate DRI table found in this chapter and the Daily Value from Table 2.16. Record these in Table 2.21 in the appropriate "Standard" columns.

2. Calculate how intakes compare with each standard by using the following formula. Enter the percent of standard value in the appropriate "Percent of Standard" columns in Table 2.21.

$$\text{Percent of standard} = \left(\frac{\text{Intake}}{\text{Standard}} \right) \times 100$$

3. Which of the average nutrient intakes are greater than recommended? Which are lower than recommended?

ASSESSMENT ACTIVITY 2.2

Go to SuperTracker (www.supertracker.usda.gov), and log in. If you have not done so already, create an account and profile. You will perform additional assessment activities from this website later in this course.

Next click on "my plan" to see your daily food group targets (what and how much to eat within your calorie allowance).

Fill in the following information from your personalized plan.

Your Name _____

Your total calorie per day allowance: _____

FOOD GROUP	Food Group Amount (list exact amount recommended)	What Counts As... (list 3 examples with portion amounts)	2 Recommended Tips (list 2 recommended tips from list)
Grains >Whole grains	_____ _____	**1 ounce of grains** 1. _____ 2. _____ 3. _____	1. _____ _____ 2. _____ _____
Vegetables >Dark green >Red and orange >Beans and peas >Starchy >Other	_____ _____ _____ _____ _____	**1 cup of vegetables** 1. _____ 2. _____ 3. _____	1. _____ _____ 2. _____ _____
Fruits	_____	**1 cup of fruit** 1. _____ 2. _____ 3. _____	1. _____ _____ 2. _____ _____
Dairy	_____	**1 cup of dairy** 1. _____ 2. _____ 3. _____	1. _____ _____ 2. _____ _____
Protein Foods >Seafood	_____ _____	**1 ounce protein food** 1. _____ 2. _____ 3. _____	1. _____ _____ 2. _____ _____

MEASURING DIET

STUDENT LEARNING OUTCOMES

After studying this chapter, the student will be able to:

1. Discuss why measuring diet is important in assessing nutritional status and in nutritional epidemiology.

2. Explain how research design considerations, characteristics of study participants, and available resources influence the selection of the dietary measurement method.

3. Describe the strengths and limitations of the methods for measuring dietary intake.

4. Discuss the strengths and limitations of using telephone interviews to obtain 24-hour recalls.

5. Discuss how technology is changing how dietary intake data are collected.

6. Describe the use of biologic markers in measuring food and nutrient intake.

7. Explain how estimation or measurement of energy requirements and energy expenditure can be used in validating dietary measurement methods.

INTRODUCTION

Measurement of nutrient intake is probably the most widely used indirect indicator of nutritional status. It is used routinely in national nutrition monitoring surveys, epidemiologic studies, nutrition studies of free-living participants (those living outside a controlled setting), and various federal and state health and nutrition program evaluations. To the uninitiated, measurement of nutrient intake may appear to be straightforward and fairly easy. However, estimating an individual's usual dietary and nutrient intake is difficult. The task is complicated by weaknesses of data-gathering techniques, human behavior, the natural tendency of an individual's nutrient intake to vary considerably from day to day, and the limitations of nutrient composition tables and databases. Despite these weaknesses, nutrient intake data are valuable in assessing nutritional status when used in conjunction with anthropometric, biochemical, and clinical data. The USDA National Agricultural Library (NAL), Food and Nutrition Information Center (FNIC), maintains a website on nutritional assessment that provides good support information: https://fnic.nal.usda.gov/dietary-guidance/individual-dietary-assessment.

This chapter discusses the reasons for measuring diet and different ways of approaching the topic. Techniques for measuring diet are described along with their strengths and weaknesses. The issues of accuracy and validity are examined, and the number of days of individual dietary intake required to characterize the usual nutrient intake of groups and individuals is discussed.

In some instances, data on the kinds and amounts of food eaten by groups or individuals are important because they allow the estimation of nutrient intake. However, conversion of dietary intake data to nutrient intake data requires information on the nutrient content of foods. This is provided by food composition tables and nutrient databases, which are subject to certain limitations and potential sources of error.

Reasons for Measuring Diet

Assessing dietary status includes considering the types and amounts of foods consumed and the intake of the nutrients and other components contained in foods. When food consumption data are combined with information on the nutrient composition of food, the intake of particular nutrients and other food components can be estimated.[1]

Why measure diet? The ultimate reason is to improve human health.[2,3] Nutritional problems are at the root of the leading causes of death, particularly in developed nations. Food and nutrient intake data are critical for investigating the relationships between diet and these diseases, identifying groups at risk for nutrient deficiency or excess, and formulating food and nutrition policies for disease reduction and health promotion. In general, however, there are four major uses of dietary intake data: assessing and monitoring food and nutrient intake, formulating and evaluating government health and agricultural policy, conducting epidemiologic research, and using the data for commercial purposes.[4] These are outlined in Box 3.1.

Planning national and international food and nutrition programs depends on estimates of per capita (per person) food, energy, and nutrient consumption. Although per capita consumption cannot easily be measured directly, estimates of food disappearance (or availability) (discussed in detail in Chapter 4) are frequently used indirect indicators of consumption. Food consumption data are used in formulating public and private agricultural policies for the production, distribution, and consumption of food.

Repeated surveys estimating food disappearance, such as those conducted by the U.S. Department of Agriculture (USDA), suggest important trends in overall patterns of food consumption over time. Among these are changes in the American diet since the early 1900s in sources of energy, composition of foods, consumption of specific food groups, and eating patterns (such as snacking and eating away from home), all of which can have profound health, social, and economic implications. Dietary assessment is used in determining the extent of malnutrition in a population, developing nutrition intervention and consumer education programs, constructing food guides, devising low-cost food plans, and providing a basis for food and nutrition legislation. Comparisons of dietary practices and nutritional intake with the distribution of disease have demonstrated important links between diet and disease and have shown how dietary changes can modulate disease risk and enhance health.

Approaches to Measuring Diet

Various methods for collecting food consumption data are available. It is important to note, however, that no single best method exists, and diet measurement will always be accompanied by some degree of error.[5] Each method has its own advantages and disadvantages. Despite these disadvantages and the inevitability of error, properly collected and analyzed, dietary intake data have considerable value, as summarized in Box 3.1. Being informed about the strengths and weaknesses of the methods available will better enable researchers and others to scrutinize nutrition research and to draw their own conclusions about a study's results. It will also allow researchers to choose the approach best suited for the task and enable them to use the methods in ways that improve data quality. Selecting the appropriate measurement method, correctly applying it, and using proper data analysis techniques can make the difference between data showing a diet-disease relationship and data showing no relationship where one may actually exist. Choosing the appropriate method for measuring diet depends on such considerations as the research design, characteristics of the study participants, and available resources.

Research Design Considerations

Let's consider five types of research designs: ecological, cross-sectional, case-control, prospective cohort, and experimental. **Ecological** or **correlational studies** compare the level of some factor (e.g., saturated fat intake) with the level of another factor (e.g., coronary heart disease mortality) in the same population. They are useful only for generating hypotheses regarding associations between suspected risk factors and disease outcome and are incapable of testing hypotheses to determine whether a cause-and-effect relationship

| Box 3.1 | Reasons for Measuring Diet |

ASSESSING AND MONITORING FOOD AND NUTRIENT INTAKE

Ensuring adequacy of the food supply

Data from national surveys and food disappearance indicate the adequacy of food, energy, and nutrient supply.

Estimating the adequacy of dietary intakes of individuals and groups

What We Eat in America (WWEIA) is the dietary intake interview component of the National Health and Nutrition Examination Survey (NHANES). WWEIA is conducted as a partnership between the U.S. Department of Agriculture (USDA) and the U.S. Department of Health and Human Services (DHHS). DHHS is responsible for the sample design and data collection, and USDA is responsible for the survey's dietary data collection methodology, maintenance of the databases used to code and process the data, and data review and processing. USDA also funds the collection and processing of Day 2 dietary intake data, which are used to develop variance estimates and calculate usual nutrient intakes.

Monitoring trends in food and nutrient consumption

Trends in percent of energy from fat, carbohydrate, and protein per person can be derived from dietary surveys and food disappearance data.

Estimating exposure to food additives and contaminants

The FDA's Total Diet Study is an ongoing FDA program that monitors levels of about 800 contaminants and nutrients in the average U.S. diet.

FORMULATING AND EVALUATING GOVERNMENT HEALTH AND AGRICULTURAL POLICY

Planning food production and distribution

Data indicating a marginal or an inadequate supply of energy and/or nutrients can provide direction for planning food production, regulating food imports and exports, and setting priorities for food aid.

Food consumption data allow certain groups or income levels to be targeted for food assistance programs, such as WIC, SNAP, and the school lunch program.

Establishing food and nutrition regulations

National and individual consumption data allow identification of potential problems to be addressed by food regulations (e.g., labeling) and programs for food enrichment or fortification.

Establishing programs for nutrition education and disease risk reduction

NHLBI-sponsored Expert Panels/Work Groups work with the American Heart Association (AHA), the American College of Cardiology (ACC), The Obesity Society (TOS), and other professional societies to develop new cardiovascular disease prevention clinical practice guidelines for lifestyle, risk assessment, cholesterol, and obesity.

Evaluating the success and cost-effectiveness of nutrition education and disease risk reduction programs

The decline in the average serum total cholesterol of Americans suggests that cholesterol-lowering campaigns have been successful.

CONDUCTING EPIDEMIOLOGIC RESEARCH

Studying the relationships between diet and health

The purpose of many studies is to investigate the relationship between dietary and nutritional intake and health and disease— for example, the relationships between diet and coronary heart disease, cancer, hypertension, and anemia.

Identifying groups at risk of developing diseases because of their diet and/or nutrient intake

Nutrient consumption data show that women of childbearing age often have low folate intake, which increases the risk of their children being born with neural tube defects.

COMMERCIAL PURPOSES

Data from national nutrition surveys are used by food manufacturers to develop advertising campaigns or new food products.

Source: Sabry JH. 1988. Purposes of food consumption surveys. In *Manual on methodology for food consumption studies,* Cameron ME, Van Staveren WA, eds. New York: Oxford University Press.

exists between two variables. It is important to keep in mind that correlation is not necessarily causation. The data used in ecological studies often are only a rough estimate of dietary intake derived from food disappearance studies (discussed in Chapter 4) and are not based on actual dietary intake measurements obtained by the methods discussed in this chapter. Much of these data are readily available from national and international agencies. Using such data, early researchers into the causes of coronary heart disease (CHD) showed that saturated fat consumption was positively correlated with risk of CHD. This association led to more definitive studies that demonstrated a cause-and-effect relationship between high saturated fat intake and increased risk of CHD. An example of an ecological study is shown in Figure 3.1, which illustrates the relationship between per capita (per person) meat consumption in various countries and the annual incidence of cases of colon cancer in women. Such research does not establish that a cause-and-effect relationship exists between meat consumption and risk of colon cancer in women, but it does suggest that this is a question worth investigating further using a research method better capable of testing hypotheses.

Cross-sectional studies provide a "snapshot" of the health of a population at a specific point in time. Figure 3.2 illustrates data collected by NHANES between 2011 and 2014 that show how the prevalence of hypertension (here defined as a systolic blood pressure ≤140 mm Hg or a diastolic blood pressure ≤90 mm Hg) increases as

Americans age. Various health and dietary measurements are performed on a relatively small group of people that is representative of the larger general population. The much smaller "sample" is selected from the "population" using statistical sampling techniques to ensure that it is representative of the larger population. Analysis of the data collected from the sample allows conclusions to be drawn about the health and dietary habits of the population from which the sample has been taken. Examples of surveys include the National Health and Nutrition Examination Survey, the National Health Interview Survey (NHANES), the Behavioral Risk Factor Surveillance System, and the Diet and Health Knowledge Survey, all of which are discussed in Chapter 4. The goal is to collect information on the current diet or dietary habits in the immediate past. The 24-hour recall is the most common method used in surveys, although food records (or food diaries) and food frequency questionnaires are sometimes used.

Case-control studies compare levels of *past exposure* to some factor of interest (e.g., some nutrient or dietary component) in two groups of study participants (cases and controls) to determine how the past exposure relates to a currently existing disease. *Cases* are those study participants who are diagnosed with a disease being studied (e.g., coronary heart disease, cancer, or osteoporosis). *Controls* are people very similar to the cases except that they do not have the disease of interest. The investigators then look *retrospectively* (backward in time) to measure each group's level of exposure to the factor of interest to determine whether differences in the

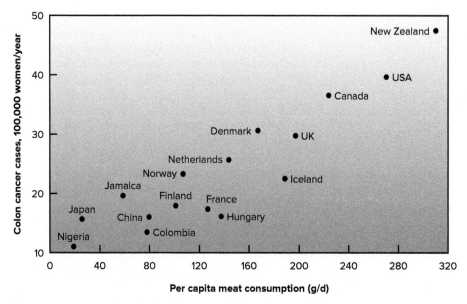

Figure 3.1 In this ecological study, an association was shown between per capita meat consumption and annual incidence of colon cancer per 100,000 women in various countries. Although useful at generating hypotheses, ecological studies are not capable of testing hypotheses.

Source: Armstrong B, Doll R. 1975. Environmental factors and cancer incidence and mortality in different countries, with special reference to dietary practices. *International Journal of Cancer* 15:617–631.

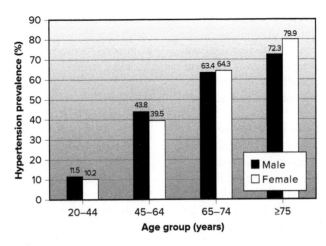

Figure 3.2 Cross-sectional data collected by the National Health and Nutrition Examination Survey between 2011 and 2014 show how the prevalence of hypertension increases as Americans age.

Source: National Center for Health Statistics. 2016. *Health, United States, 2015: With Special Feature on Racial and Ethnic Health Disparities.* Hyattsville, MD: NCHS.

level of exposure are related to the reasons cases have the disease and controls do not. Thus, case-control studies require methods that measure dietary intake in the recent past (e.g., the year before diagnosis) or in the distant past (e.g., 10 years ago or in childhood). Methods that focus on current behavior, such as the 24-hour recall and food records, are not suitable. The only good choices for case-control studies are food frequency questionnaires, which assess diet in the past.

Time and budgetary constraints are major factors influencing the choice of dietary measurement methods, particularly with cohort studies having tens of thousands of subjects who may be followed for decades. In some cohort studies, subjects are asked to submit information about their diets every three to four years, in which case relying on food records that are labor intensive and costly to analyze would be impractical and cost-prohibitive. Traditionally, 24-hour recalls have been labor intensive to collect and analyze, but technology has changed that. The National Cancer Institute developed an Internet-based automated self-administered 24-hour dietary recall (ASA24) application to collect and code dietary intake data (https://asa24.nci.nih.gov/).[6–8] Based on the USDA's Automated Multiple-Pass Method of collecting a 24-hour recall (discussed later in this chapter), the ASA24 allows subjects to report foods consumed by either typing the name of the food into a text box or browsing through a list of foods and clicking on the desired option. Subjects are then asked to provide information on portion size for each food reported.[7] The self-administered food frequency questionnaire has generally been the dietary assessment method of choice for studies involving large numbers of subjects. Traditionally, these have been paper-and-pencil questionnaires, designed to be optically scanned, that are mailed to subjects, completed at home, and then mailed back to the researchers for data entry and processing. More recently, researchers have been moving to entirely Web-based data collection systems in which food frequency questionnaires are administered online and other relevant data are collected via the Internet.[6]

Experimental or **intervention studies** can range from tightly controlled clinical studies involving relatively small numbers of subjects, who may be housed in a metabolic ward of a hospital, to studies involving large numbers of subjects receiving some intervention. Experimental studies are similar to prospective cohort studies in that they generally begin with disease-free subjects who undergo some exposure of interest and are then followed forward in time and observed to determine whether the exposure of interest (or lack of exposure) affects risk of disease. Unlike cohort studies, in experimental studies subjects are randomly assigned to at least two different groups, one or more experimental groups and a control group. The experimental group receives the exposure of interest (the intervention), which could be a special diet, a pharmaceutical agent, or a nutritional supplement. The control group receives a placebo (an ineffectual treatment), which allows it to serve as a comparison group because it is treated in the same way as the experimental group(s) with the exception that the control group does not receive the exposure of interest.

In experimental studies, researchers may assess diet for initial screening purposes to determine whether subjects meet the design protocol, or they may periodically measure the diets of subjects to determine whether the intervention has an impact on diet and nutritional status. The choice of the assessment methodology depends on the design protocol and the number of subjects in the study. Any of the available methods would be suitable for studies having a small number of subjects. Large population studies necessitate more efficient data collection methods, such as the food frequency questionnaire or the 24-hour recall, especially a Web-based food frequency questionnaire or an automated self-administered 24-hour recall.[6,9]

Prospective cohort studies or simply **cohort studies** compare *future exposure* to various factors in a large group or *cohort* of study participants in an attempt to determine how exposure to the factors relates to diseases that may develop. Consequently, cohort studies require methods that measure current diet or dietary habits in the immediate past, such as 24-hour recalls, food records, and food frequency questionnaires.[6]

The Framingham Heart Study is an example of a longitudinal study. Initiated in 1949, the original cohort consisted of more than 5000 30- to 62-year-old residents of Framingham, Massachusetts. Since joining the study, the participants have undergone regular examinations and dietary assessments in an attempt to identify factors contributing to the subsequent development of coronary heart disease and high blood pressure. This and other prospective studies have shown that reducing fat intake, controlling body weight and blood pressure, avoiding smoking, and exercising regularly can reduce risk for coronary heart disease and stroke.

Sometimes the goal of dietary assessment is to quickly screen a group of people for probable dietary risk. In these instances, a brief targeted food frequency questionnaire identifying people with a high intake of fat, cholesterol, or sodium or a low intake of dietary fiber, fruits, or vegetables can be administered. Two such instruments—the "fat screener," developed by researchers at the National Cancer Institute, and the MEDFICTS questionnaire—are discussed in the section on food frequency questionnaires. The food frequency questionnaire and the 24-hour recall are also suitable for this purpose.[6]

A case-control study investigated whether the quality of the diets of mothers in the year prior to pregnancy was associated with the risk of neural tube defects (e.g., spina bifida or anencephaly) and orofacial clefts (e.g., cleft lip or cleft palate) in their offspring.[5] Using a food frequency questionnaire, researchers evaluated the diets of 936 mothers who had given birth to an infant with a neural tube defect and 2475 mothers who had given birth to an infant with an orofacial cleft. These were the cases. The same food frequency questionnaire was used to evaluate the diets of 6147 mothers who shared many characteristics with the cases but who did not give birth to an infant with one of the malformations being studied. These were the controls. Using data from the food frequency questionnaires, the quality of the mothers' diets was scored using the Diet Quality Index (discussed in Chapter 2). The data analysis showed that mothers having the highest scores on

the Diet Quality Index (those in the top quartile) were much less likely to have an offspring with a malformation compared to mothers having the lowest scores (in the bottom quartile).[5]

Characteristics of Study Participants

Factors influencing the selection of a dietary measurement technique include literacy, memory, commitment, age, ability to communicate, and culture of the participants. If some study participants are likely to be unable to read and/or write, the best methods would be a 24-hour recall or a food frequency questionnaire administered by a member of the research team. The food record, the automated self-administered 24-hour recall, or the self-administered food frequency questionnaire would not be recommended. The 24-hour recall and food frequency questionnaire require the ability to remember past eating habits. Food records, the automated self-administered 24-hour recall, and the self-administered food frequency questionnaire require the training and active participation of the study participants. In the case of the food record, the level of effort required can also lead participants to change their dietary patterns during the recording period. Consequently, there is concern about response rates, the comparability of recording skills among participants, and the quality of dietary intake results.[1,6]

The ability to communicate may be limited in study participants who are very young, elderly, developmentally disabled, victims of stroke or Alzheimer's disease, or deceased. In these instances, dietary intake data may have to be collected from another person familiar with the study participant, such as a parent, spouse, child, or sibling. This other person is known as a **surrogate source.** Surrogate sources are discussed later in this chapter in the section "Surrogate Sources." A food inventory method can be useful for older persons living at home. Direct observation of eating habits of persons in institutional care facilities can also be done.[1] The eating habits of children have been assessed using the 24-hour recall, food records, and food frequency questionnaires. Assessing the diets of younger children may require information from surrogates or use of the "consensus recall method," in which the child and both parents give combined responses on a 24-hour recall. This approach has been shown to give more accurate information than a recall from either parent alone.[1]

Assessing the diets of ethnic populations requires modification of existing methods. If participants are interviewed, it is preferable that these be done by persons of the same ethnic or cultural background, so that dietary information can be gathered more effectively. Nutrient analyses of ethnic foods and dishes will likely require changes in food composition databases. Food frequency questionnaires will have to be modified to include food common to the ethnic group being studied.[1,6]

Available Resources

Some methods for measuring diet are more expensive and labor intensive to administer than others. Before a study begins, the budget must be carefully considered, so that the costs entailed will match the available resources. Except in the case of the automated self-administered 24-hour recall, the 24-hour recall must be administered by a trained interviewer. If the food record is used, study participants should be trained to properly record their diets. Considerable labor is required to enter data from conventional 24-hour recalls and food records into a computer for analysis. Food frequency questionnaires can be self-administered, and responses can be marked on a form, which is then optically scanned. Data can then be downloaded into a computer for analysis, thus saving considerable time, effort, and expense. Food records and 24-hour recalls tend to be more feasible methods to use in research with smaller numbers of participants. Food frequency questionnaires, on the other hand, are often preferred by researchers studying large numbers of people.

TECHNIQUES IN MEASURING DIET

Measurement of dietary intake usually is conducted for one of three purposes: to compare average nutrient intakes of different groups, to rank individuals within a group, and to estimate an individual's usual intake. Dietary measurement techniques can be categorized as daily food consumption methods (food record and 24-hour recall) and recalled "usual" or average food consumption methods (diet history and food frequency questionnaire).[1,6] These techniques have also been categorized as meal-based (food record and 24-hour recall) and list-based (food frequency questionnaire).[5]

24-Hour Recall

In the traditional dietary recall method, a trained interviewer asks the respondent to recall in detail all the food and drink consumed during a period of time in the recent past. The interviewer then records this information for later coding and analysis. (In coding, a number is assigned to each kind of food, allowing it to be identified easily for computer analysis.) In most instances, the time period is the previous 24 hours. Thus, the method is most commonly known as the **24-hour recall**.[1,6] Occasionally, however, the time period is the previous 48 hours, the past 7 days, or, in rare instances, even the preceding month. However, memories of intake may fade rather quickly beyond the most recent day or two, so that loss in accuracy may exceed gain in representativeness.[1,6]

In addition to recording responses, the interviewer helps the respondent remember all that was consumed during the period in question and assists the respondent in estimating portion sizes of foods consumed. A common technique of the 24-hour recall is to begin by asking what the respondent first ate or drank on last awakening. The recall proceeds from the morning of the present day to the current moment. The interviewer then begins at the point exactly 24 hours in the past and works forward to the time of awakening. Some researchers ask respondents to recall their diet from midnight to midnight of the previous day. Asking the respondent about his or her activities during the day and inquiring how they might have been associated with eating or drinking can help in recalling food intake. An inquiry about the previous evening's activities, for example, will stimulate the respondent's memory and may help him or her recall the snack eaten while watching a favorite television program.

After the interview, the recall is checked for omissions and/or mistakes. A respondent may have to be contacted later by telephone or mail to clarify an entry or to obtain information such as brand names, preparation methods, and serving sizes. The recall can then be analyzed using a computerized diet analysis program.

The 24-hour recall has several strengths. It is inexpensive, it is quick to administer (20 minutes or less), and it can provide detailed information on specific foods, especially if brand names can be recalled.[1,6] It requires only short-term memory. It is well accepted by respondents because they are not asked to keep records, and their expenditure of time and effort is relatively low. Thus, probability sampling within populations and individuals is possible. The method is considered by some to be more objective than the dietary history and food frequency questionnaire, and its administration does not alter the usual diet.[1,6–8]

Recalls have several limitations. Respondents may withhold or alter information about what they ate because of poor memory or embarrassment or to please or impress the interviewer and researchers. Respondents tend to underreport binge eating, consumption of alcoholic beverages, and consumption of foods perceived as unhealthful. Respondents also tend to overreport consumption of name-brand foods, expensive cuts of meat, and foods considered healthful.[1,6] Foods eaten but not reported are known as **missing foods,** while foods not eaten but reported are known as **phantom foods.** Several researchers report that, when respondents' actual food consumption is low, they have a tendency to overestimate the amount recalled, and, when their actual consumption is high, they underestimate the amount recalled. Some researchers call this phenomenon the "flat-slope syndrome."[10,11] Energy intake often is underestimated if drinks, sauces, and dressings are not reported.

Underreporting can be limited by using a *multiple-pass 24-hour recall method,* in which the interviewer and respondent review the previous day's eating episodes several times to obtain detailed and accurate information about food intake.[1,6] In one version of the method, a *quick list* of foods eaten in the previous 24 hours is initially compiled. In the second pass, a *detailed description* of foods on the quick list is obtained. The respondent is asked to clarify the description and preparation methods of foods on the quick list. For example, if a respondent reports eating breakfast cereal, the interviewer will ask whether milk was used on the cereal and, if so, what kind of milk and how much was used. In the third pass, called the *review,* the interviewer reviews the data collected, probes for additional eating occasions, and clarifies food portion sizes using household dishes and measures (e.g., cups, bowls, glasses, spoons), geometric shapes (e.g., circles, triangles, rectangles), and food labels.

A computer-assisted, five-step, multiple-pass 24-hour recall system is the primary instrument for measuring dietary intake in the National Health and Nutrition Examination Survey (NHANES), which is discussed in Chapter 4.[6] This computer-assisted interview system was developed by the USDA and is known as the USDA Automated Multiple-Pass Method (AMPM). The AMPM is being used in large national surveys in the United States and Canada including What We Eat in America, NHANES (yearly since 2002, with two 24-hour recalls each for 5000 individuals), and the Canadian Community Health Survey. In the first pass, a quick list of foods and beverages consumed the previous day is collected. In the second pass, potential foods forgotten during the quick list step are probed. In the third pass, the time and eating occasion for each food are collected. In the fourth pass, a detailed description, amount, and additions are collected for each food during a review of the 24-hour day. In the fifth and final step, a final probe for anything else consumed is conducted.[6] A 24-hour recall using this method typically takes 30 to 45 minutes to complete.[6] Use of the AMPM, thorough training and retention of interviewers, and use of other quality-control measures should assure collection of accurate data from this national survey.[6]

Another technological advancement in dietary assessment methodology has been the creation of an Internet-based automated self-administered 24-hour dietary recall application known as the ASA24. Developed by the National Cancer Institute, the ASA24 uses technology drawn from the USDA's Automated Multiple-Pass Method to provide a Web-based tool to researchers, educators, and the public for collecting multiple automated self-administered 24-hour recalls.[6-8] During the first pass of the interview, respondents are asked to report each eating occasion and time of consumption, with queries about where the meals or snacks were eaten, whether the food was eaten while alone or in the presence of others, and whether there was television and/or computer use while eating. The ASA24 allows subjects to report foods consumed by either typing the name of the food into a text box or browsing through a list of food and drink terms derived from the National Health and Nutrition Examination Survey (discussed in Chapter 4). Respondents are asked detailed questions about food preparation, portion size, and additions to foods and beverages so that food codes from USDA's Food and Nutrient Database for Dietary Studies

(discussed in Chapter 5) can be assigned. Respondents are able to modify food and drink choices at multiple points during the interview and are asked to provide information about the use of dietary supplements. The system uses a variety of images of foods on plates, in bowls, and in beverage containers to help respondents estimate portion sizes. The ASA24 has visual cues with an optional animated guide and optional audio cues to instruct respondents, enabling the system to be used by low-literacy individuals and those with speech and hearing impairments, and is available in a variety of languages. A "child friendly" version for use by school-age children was released in 2012, with updates provided every two years.[6-8] The ASA24 can be accessed at the website of the National Cancer Institute at http://epi.grants.cancer.gov/asa24/.

The primary limitation of the 24-hour recall is that data on a *single day's diet,* no matter how accurate, are a very poor descriptor of an individual's *usual* nutrient intake because of day-to-day or **intraindividual variability.**[1,6] Even if several 24-hour recalls are collected from one person, it may be impossible to measure intake of infrequently eaten foods, such as liver. However, a sufficiently large number of 24-hour recalls may provide a reasonable estimate of the mean nutrient intake of a group.[1,6] Depending on the purpose for which data are used, multiple 24-hour recalls performed on an individual and spaced over various seasons may provide a reasonable estimate of that person's usual nutrient intake.[6] Two separate multiple-pass 24-hour recalls are obtained from most NHANES participants using the USDA's AMPM. The first recall is obtained by a trained staff member in a face-to-face interview with the respondent. The second recall is obtained 3 to 10 days later by telephone, which research shows is a feasible and valid method for obtaining 24-hour recalls.[6]

The necessary number of days of data collection depends on several factors: whether estimates of usual intake are for individuals or groups, the nutrients of interest, sample size, and degree of intraindividual and interindividual variability. Twenty-four-hour recalls can provide reasonably accurate data about the preceding day's dietary intake, but reports of diet for the preceding week or month do not accurately characterize dietary intake during those periods.[1,6] Box 3.2 summarizes the strengths and limitations of the 24-hour recall method.

Food Record, or Diary

In this method, the respondent records, at the time of consumption, the identity and amounts of all foods and beverages consumed for a period of time, usually ranging from one to seven days. An example of a food record form is given in Appendix A. Food and beverage consumption can be quantified by estimating portion sizes, using household measures, or weighing the food or beverage on scales. In many instances, household measures such as cups, tablespoons, and teaspoons or measurements made with a ruler are used to quantify portion size. Certain items, such as eggs, apples, or 12-oz cans of soft drinks, may be thought of as units and simply counted. This method is sometimes referred to as the **estimated food record** because portion sizes are estimated (that is, in terms of coffee cups, dippers, bowls, glasses, and so on), or household measures are used. When food is weighed, the record may be referred to as a **weighed food record.** Box 3.3 compares these two methods. The use of food scales is preferred by European nutrition researchers, who consider it more accurate than using household measures, as is typically done by North American researchers. The degree of accuracy from household measures appears acceptable for most research purposes, especially considering the fact that some respondents may find it burdensome to accurately record their diet if they have to weigh everything they eat and drink.

The food record does not depend on memory because the respondent ideally records food and beverage consumption (including snacks) at the time of eating. In addition, it can provide detailed food intake data and important information about eating habits (for example, when, where, and with whom meals are eaten and the respondent's mood when choosing certain foods). Data from a

---

 Box 3.2   **Strengths and Limitations of the 24-Hour Recall**

STRENGTHS

Requires less than 20 minutes to administer

Inexpensive

Easy to administer

Can provide detailed information on types of food consumed

Low respondent burden

Probability sampling possible

Can be used to estimate nutrient intake of groups

Multiple recalls can be used to estimate nutrient intake of individuals

More objective than dietary history

Does not alter usual diet

Useful in clinical settings

LIMITATIONS

One recall is seldom representative of a person's usual intake

Underreporting/overreporting occurs

Relies on memory

Omissions of dressings, sauces, and beverages can lead to low estimates of energy intake

May be a tendency to overreport intake at low levels and underreport intake at high levels of consumption

Data entry can be very labor intensive

Source: Bingham SA, Nelson M, Paul AA, et al. 1988. Methods for data collection at an individual level. In Cameron ME, Van Staveren WA (eds.), *Manual on methodology for food consumption studies.* New York: Oxford University Press.

 Box 3.3   **Comparison of the Estimated Food Record and the Weighed Food Record**

ESTIMATED FOOD RECORD

Amounts of food and leftovers are measured in household measures (cups, tablespoons, teaspoons) or estimated using such measures as coffee cups, bowls, glasses, and dippers

The researchers then quantify these measures by volume and weight

Considered less accurate than the weighed food record

Considered an acceptable method for collecting group intake data

Puts less burden on the respondent than the weighed food record and thus cooperation rates are likely to be higher, especially over long recording periods

As effective in ranking subjects into thirds and fifths as weighed records

WEIGHED FOOD RECORD

Food and leftovers are weighed using scales or computerized techniques supplied by researchers

Considered more accurate than the estimated food record

Preferred by some researchers for gathering data on individuals

Requires a greater degree of subject cooperation than the estimated food record and thus is likely to have a greater impact on eating habits than the estimated food record

Cost of scales may be prohibitive in some instances

Source: Bingham SA, Nelson M, Paul AA, et al. 1988. Methods for data collection at an individual level. In Cameron ME, Van Staveren WA (eds.), *Manual on methodology for food consumption studies.* New York: Oxford University Press.

Box 3.4   **Strengths and Limitations of the Food Record**

STRENGTHS

Does not depend on memory

Can provide detailed intake data

Can provide data about eating habits

Multiple-day data more representative of usual intake

Reasonably valid up to five days

LIMITATIONS

Requires high degree of cooperation

Response burden can result in low response rates when used in large national surveys

Subject must be literate

Takes more time to obtain data

Act of recording may alter diet

Analysis is labor intensive and expensive

---

multiple-day food record also is more representative of usual intake than are single-day data from either a 24-hour recall or a 1-day food record. However, multiple food records from nonconsecutive, random days (including weekends) covering different seasons are necessary to arrive at useful estimates of usual intake.[1,6]

Food records have several limitations. They require a literate and cooperative respondent who is able and willing to expend the time and effort necessary to record dietary intake. However, such a respondent may not be representative of the general population. The act of recording food intake after several days can lead even motivated respondents to reduce the number of foods and snacks eaten and to decrease the complexity of their diets to simplify the recording process.[1,6] When asked directly about recording their food intake, 30% to 50% of respondents have reported changing their eating habits while keeping a food record.[6] Thus, the food record may significantly underreport energy and nutrient intakes.[1,6] Box 3.4 summarizes the strengths and limitations of the food record.

Food Frequency Questionnaires

Food frequency questionnaires assess energy and/or nutrient intake by determining how frequently a person consumes a limited number of foods that are major sources of nutrients or of a particular dietary component in question. The questionnaires consist of a list of approximately 150 or fewer individual foods or food groups that are important contributors to the population's intake of energy and nutrients. Respondents indicate how many times a day, week, month, or year that they usually consume the foods.[1,6] In some food frequency questionnaires, a choice of portion size is not given. These generally use "standard" portion sizes (the amounts customarily eaten per serving for various age/sex groups) drawn from large-population data. An example of this format is given in Figure 3.3A. It simply asks how many times a year, month, week, or day a person eats dark bread or ice cream. This is sometimes referred to as a **simple,** or **nonquantitative, food**

frequency questionnaire format. The **semiquantitative food frequency questionnaire,** shown in Figure 3.3B, gives respondents an idea of portion size. It asks how many times a year, month, week, or day a person eats a slice of dark bread or a 1/2 cup serving of ice cream. In addition to asking the frequency of consumption, the **quantitative food frequency questionnaire,** shown in Figure 3.3C, asks the respondent to describe the size of his or her usual serving as small, medium, or large relative to a standard serving. Respondents mark their answers on an answer sheet, which can then be optically scanned, so that their responses can be directly downloaded into a computer for analysis, thus saving the researchers considerable time and money. This feature makes food frequency questionnaires a cost-effective approach for measuring diet in large epidemiologic studies that can have tens of thousands of subjects.

Targeted food frequency questionnaires known as "screeners" have been developed to assess intake of calcium, dietary fiber, fruits and vegetables, and percent energy from fat. Screeners are particularly useful in situations that do not require assessment of the total diet or quantitative accuracy in dietary estimates and in situations in which financial resources are limited. They are commonly used in epidemiologic research investigating the relationship between diet and such conditions as cancer and cardiovascular disease but are not considered substitutes for more definitive approaches to measuring diet, such as multiple 24-hour recalls.[1,6,12,13] Figure 3.4 shows a self-administered, machine-readable screener developed by the U.S. National Cancer Institute's Risk Factor Assessment Branch (http://epi.grants.cancer.gov/rfab/) to estimate an individual's usual intake of percent energy from fat. The foods asked about on the instrument were selected because they were the most important predictors of variability in percent energy from fat among adults in USDA's 1989–1991 Continuing Survey of Food Intakes of Individuals (discussed in Chapter 4). Procedures for scoring the screener are available at the Risk Factor Assessment Branch website (http://epi.grants.cancer.gov/diet/screeners/fat/).

A	Average Use During Past Year					
Food Item	<1 month	1–3 month	1–4 week	5–7 week	2–4 day	5+ day
coffee						
dark bread						
ice cream						

B	Average Use During Past Year								
Food Item	<1 month	1–3 month	1 week	2–4 week	5–6 week	1 day	2–3 day	4–5 day	6+ day
coffee (1 cup)									
dark bread (1 slice)									
ice cream (1/2 cup)									

C		Your Serving Size			How Often?				
Food Item	Medium Serving	S	M	L	Day	Week	Month	Year	Never
coffee	(1 cup)								
dark bread	(1 slice)								
ice cream	(1/2 cup)								

Figure 3.3 **Examples of three food frequency questionnaire formats: (A) the simple, or nonquantitative, format; (B) the semiquantitative format; (C) the quantitative format.**

Source: National Cancer Institute, Risk Factor Assessment.

The U.S. National Cancer Institute has also developed a variety of screeners for assessing intake of fruits and vegetables, fiber and whole grains, added sugars, dairy products, red meats and processed meats, and calcium, and percentage of energy from total fats. An example of a fruit and vegetable screener developed by the National Cancer Institute is shown in Appendix B. This self-administered, machine-readable instrument was designed to assess consumption of fruits and vegetables in the past month and can be completed in about 14 minutes. When compared to estimates of fruit and vegetable intake based on four telephone-administered 24-hour recalls, this screener and a similar one were shown to have potential for estimating median intake of fruits and vegetables but were less useful for accurately ranking the intakes of individuals.[13] Additional information on this screener and scoring procedures are available at the Risk Factor Assessment Branch website (http://epi.grants.cancer.gov/diet/screeners/).

A questionnaire developed to quickly estimate how frequently foods high in total fat, saturated fatty acids, and cholesterol are eaten is shown in Appendix C. It is called the MEDFICTS Dietary Assessment Questionnaire (**M**eats, **E**ggs, **D**airy, **F**ried foods, **I**n baked goods, **C**onvenience foods, **T**able fats, **S**nacks) and is recommended by the National Cholesterol Education Program as a simple approach to assess a person's intake of total fat, saturated fat, and dietary cholesterol.[14]

MEDFICTS focuses on foods that are major contributors of total fat, saturated fat, and cholesterol commonly eaten by North Americans. Within each of the questionnaire's eight categories, foods are placed into either a high-fat, high-cholesterol group (Group 1) or a low-fat, low-cholesterol group (Group 2). Group 1 foods are major contributors of dietary fat and cholesterol, and to the right of these groups is a series of boxes with numbers representing points under each box. Group 2 foods are minor contributors of fat and cholesterol. No points are given for Group 2 foods except if a respondent indicates a large portion size for Group 2 meats, in which case six points are given. In completing the questionnaire, the respondent simply checks the boxes representing his or her frequency of weekly consumption and typical serving size for each food group. The points for weekly consumption (shown below each box) are multiplied by the points for serving size and totaled in the score column. The points from each side of the questionnaire are totaled and compared with the key. A total score of 70 or more indicates a need for dietary change to reduce intake of total fat, saturated fat, and dietary cholesterol. A score between 40 and 69 suggests that the respondent is following a "heart-healthy diet" as defined by the National Cholesterol Education Program.[14] A score less than 40 suggests adherence to the National Cholesterol Education Program's therapeutic lifestyle changes diet, which is

National Cancer Institute Quick Food Scan

1. Think about your eating habits over the past 12 months. About how often did you eat or drink each of the following foods? Remember breakfast, lunch, dinner, snacks, and eating out. Blacken in only one bubble for each food.

Type of Food	Never	Less than Once Per Month	1–3 Times Per Month	1–2 Times Per Week	3–4 Times Per Week	5–6 Times Per Week	1 Time Per Day	2 or More Times Per Day
Cold cereal	○	○	○	○	○	○	○	○
Skim milk, on cereal or to drink	○	○	○	○	○	○	○	○
Eggs, fried or scrambled in margarine, butter, or oil	○	○	○	○	○	○	○	○
Sausage or bacon, regular-fat	○	○	○	○	○	○	○	○
Margarine or butter on bread, rolls, pancakes	○	○	○	○	○	○	○	○
Orange juice or grapefruit juice	○	○	○	○	○	○	○	○
Fruit (not juices)	○	○	○	○	○	○	○	○
Beef or pork hot dogs, regular-fat	○	○	○	○	○	○	○	○
Cheese or cheese spread, regular-fat	○	○	○	○	○	○	○	○
French fries, home fries, or hash brown potatoes	○	○	○	○	○	○	○	○
Margarine or butter on vegetables, including potatoes	○	○	○	○	○	○	○	○
Mayonnaise, regular-fat	○	○	○	○	○	○	○	○
Salad dressings, regular-fat	○	○	○	○	○	○	○	○
Rice	○	○	○	○	○	○	○	○
Margarine, butter, or oil on rice or pasta	○	○	○	○	○	○	○	○

2. Over the past 12 months, when you prepared foods with margarine or ate margarine, how often did you use a reduced-fat margarine?

○ Didn't use Margarine   ○ Almost never   ○ About 1/4 of the time   ○ About 1/2 of the time   ○ About 3/4 of the time   ○ Almost always or always

3. Overall, when you think about the foods you ate over the past 12 months, would you say your diet was high, medium, or low in fat?

○ High   ○ Medium   ○ Low

Figure 3.4 **A short food frequency questionnaire known as a "screener" developed by the National Cancer Institute to estimate an individual's usual intake of percent of energy from fat.**

Source: National Cancer Institute, Risk Factor Assessment Branch.

discussed in Chapter 8 and outlined in the *Third Report of the Expert Panel on Detection, Evaluation, and Treatment of High Blood Cholesterol in Adults.*[1] Studies suggest that the MEDFICTS does a good job of estimating intake of total fat, saturated fat, and cholesterol, compared with intake estimates based on multiple food records.[15,16]

Numerous food frequency questionnaires have been developed and tested. Three of the more common ones used in nutritional epidemiology research are those developed by Walter Willett and coworkers at Harvard University School of Public Health, Gladys Block and Amy Subar, Frances Thompson, and coworkers at the National Cancer Institute.

Willett Questionnaire

Beginning in 1979, a team of Harvard University nutritionists and epidemiologists headed by Walter C. Willett developed a series of self-administered semiquantitative food frequency questionnaires to conduct epidemiologic research on the relationships between nutrient and food intake and risk of chronic disease. Over the years, their original 61-item questionnaire was modified several times.[17–19] A 131-item questionnaire was designed to classify individuals according to levels of average daily intake of nutrients and certain foods and food components during the past year.[20] Its format is similar to that shown in Figure 3.3B. It is self-administered and machine readable, thus making it convenient for use in large epidemiologic studies. Foods included in the questionnaire are those that are major sources of the nutrients, foods, and food components of interest to the researchers. Open-ended questions are also included to identify specific brands of margarine, ready-to-eat cereals, cooking oils, vitamin/mineral supplements, and other foods eaten at least once per week.[20] For each item on the questionnaire, respondents are given nine choices ranging from less than once per month to six or more times per day. Nutrient values are calculated by multiplying nutrient content of each item by frequency of use.

The Willett questionnaire has been designed to be self-administered by nurses and other health professionals in such epidemiologic studies as the Nurses' Health Study and the Health Professionals Follow-up Study with populations of more than 120,000 female nurses and nearly 50,000 male health professionals, respectively.[45,46] A similar food frequency questionnaire is being used successfully in the Iowa Women's Health Study, a prospective cohort study involving a socioeconomically diverse group of older women living in Iowa.[21]

Researchers at Harvard University Medical School and Brigham and Women's Hospital in Boston have adapted the Willett food frequency questionnaire for assessing the diets of children and adolescents ages 9 to 18. Known as the Youth/Adolescent Questionnaire (YAQ), it is self-administered and includes a list of 151 foods. According to reproducibility studies, it has a reasonable ability to assess the eating habits of children and adolescents.

Block Questionnaires

Over the past three decades, Dr. Gladys Block has developed a series of self-administered, scannable quantitative food frequency questionnaires and screeners that are based on an earlier food frequency questionnaire known as the Block Health Habits and History Questionnaire (HHHQ), which was developed by Block and coworkers at the National Cancer Institute in 1992.[6] The HHHQ was designed to collect data on diet and well-established risk factors for cancer and total mortality, and it has proven useful in assessing total dietary intake.[6] In 1993, Block founded the firm NutritionQuest (NutritionQuest.com), which develops and markets a number of products and services to health professionals and researchers. Included among these are a series of food frequency questionnaires for children, adolescents, and adults, food screeners for adults, and physical activity surveys and screeners for adolescents and adults. All of NutritionQuest's questionnaires and screeners are available in "paper-and-pencil" format and electronic format. With the paper-and-pencil format, the respondent completes a printed questionnaire, which is then mailed to NutritionQuest for processing, and the results are then returned to the researchers. With the electronic format, respondents complete the questionnaire or screener online or the questionnaire can be downloaded onto a computer and completed "off-line" and then submitted electronically for analysis. The food frequency questionnaires from NutritionQuest are variable in length, ranging from 70 to 110 food items and are available in English and Spanish. There are screeners for fat, sugar, fruits, vegetables, soy products, dietary fiber, vitamin D, and folic acid, which range in length from 7 to 50 questions. Block questionnaires have been used in a number of research projects, including studies conducted by the National Aeronautic and Space Administration (NASA) and the National Institutes of Health.

Diet History Questionnaire

The Diet History Questionnaire (DHQ) is a freely available, self-administered food frequency questionnaire developed by staff at the U.S. National Cancer Institute's Risk Factor Assessment Branch. It can be used by researchers, clinicians, or teachers without permission. The original DHQ I had 124 food items and included information about portion sizes and dietary supplement use. It took about one hour to complete and was designed, based on cognitive research findings, to be easy to use.[22,23] The DHQ II has an updated list of 134 food items based on more recent dietary data from national surveys and has eight questions about dietary supplement uses. The DHQ II is available in four versions: assessment of the past year's dietary intake with questions about portion sizes (the standard version), past-year assessment without portion sizes, past-month assessment with portion sizes, and past-month assessment without portion sizes.[24] The DHQ II is available in a paper-based form and in an identical Web-based form referred to as DHQ*Web. The paper-based DHQ II and its analysis software are available for downloading at no charge from the website of the National Cancer Institute. The DHQ*Web is an automated, electronic food frequency questionnaire allowing respondents to log in at any time and to complete the questionnaire in one sitting or to save their responses, log out, and then to return to the questionnaire later to begin where they left off. The software prompts respondents to correct or modify any missing or inconsistent entries and to completely answer all questions before proceeding to the next question. The DHQ II is shown in Appendix D. The questionnaire can be downloaded from the National Cancer Institute's website at http://epi.grants.cancer.gov/dhq2/. The DHQ II software provides quantitative data on the intake of many nutrients, dietary constituents, and food groups, as shown in Table 3.1. Data on food groups are also available. The primary databases used to compute nutrient and food group estimates are the U.S. Department of Agriculture's (USDA) Food and Nutrient Database for Dietary Studies (FNDDS) and USDA's MyPyramid Equivalents. Additional nutrients have been added from the Nutrition Data System for Research (NDS-R). New foods and nutrients can be added to the database, and other modifications can be made in the DHQ software with relative ease.[24]

TABLE 3.1	Nutrients and Food Components Analyzed by the Diet History Questionnaire II

Primary Energy

Energy (kilocalories)	% calories from fat
Energy (kilojoules)	% calories from carbohydrate
Total fat	% calories from protein
Total carbohydrate	% calories from alcohol
Available carbohydrate	
Total protein	
Animal protein	
Vegetable protein	
Alcohol	

Fat and Cholesterol

Cholesterol	% calories from SFA
Solid fats	% calories from MUFA
Total saturated fatty acids (SFA)	% calories from PUFA
Total monounsaturated fatty acids (MUFA)	Polyunsaturated to saturated fat ratio
Total molyunsaturated fatty acids (PUFA)	Cholesterol to saturated fatty acid index
Trans-fatty acids (TRANS)	
Conjugated linoleic acid (18:2)	
Omega-3 fatty acids	

Carbohydrates

Total sugars	Added sugars (by total sugars)
Fructose	Added sugars (by available carbohydrate)
Galactose	
Glucose	
Lactose	
Maltose	
Sucrose	
Starch	

Fiber

Total dietary fiber
Soluble dietary fiber
Insoluble dietary fiber
Pectins

Vitamins

Total vitamin A activity (retinol equivalents)	Beta-tocopherol
Total vitamin A activity (International Units)	Gamma-tocopherol
Total vitamin A activity (retinol activity equivalents)	Delta-tocopherol
Beta-carotene equivalents (derived from provitamin A carotenoids)	Vitamin K (phylloquinone)
Retinol	Vitamin C (ascorbic acid)
Vitamin D (calciferol)	Thiamin (vitamin B1)
Vitamin D2 (ergocalciferol)	Riboflavin (vitamin B2)
Vitamin D3 (cholecalciferol)	Niacin (vitamin B3)
Vitamin E (International Units)	Niacin equivalents
Vitamin E (total alpha-tocopherol)	Pantothenic acid
Natural alpha-tocopherol (RRR-alpha-tocopherol or d-alpha-tocopherol)	Vitamin B6 (pyridoxine, pyridoxyl, and pyridoxamine)
Synthetic alpha-tocopherol (all rac-alpha-tocopherol or dl-alpha-tocopherol)	Total folate
	Dietary folate equivalents
	Natural folate (food folate)
	Synthetic folate (folic acid)
Total alpha-tocopherol equivalents	Vitamin B12 (cobalamin)

Carotenoids

Beta-carotene (provitamin A carotenoid)
Alpha-carotene (provitamin A carotenoid)
Beta-cryptoxanthin (provitamin A carotenoid)
Lutein + zeaxanthin
Lycopene

Minerals

Calcium	Manganese
Phosphorus	Selenium
Magnesium	Sodium
Iron	Potassium
Zinc	
Copper	

Fatty Acids

SFA 4:0 (butyric acid)	PUFA 18:3 n-3 (alpha-linolenic acid [ALA])
SFA 6:0 (caproic acid)	PUFA 18:4 (parinaric acid)
SFA 8:0 (caprylic acid)	PUFA 20:4 (arachidonic acid)
SFA 10:0 (capric acid)	PUFA 20:5 (eicosapentaenoic acid [EPA])
SFA 12:0 (lauric acid)	
SFA 14:0 (myristic acid)	
SFA 16:0 (palmitic acid)	PUFA 22:5 (docosapentaenoic acid [DPA])
SFA 17:0 (margaric acid)	
SFA 18:0 (stearic acid)	PUFA 22:6 (docosahexaenoic acid [DHA])
SFA 20:0 (arachidic acid)	
SFA 22:0 (behenic acid)	TRANS 16:1 (trans-hexadecenoic acid)
MUFA 14:1 (myristoleic acid)	
MUFA 16:1 (palmitoleic acid)	TRANS 18:1 (trans-octadecenoic acid)
MUFA 18:1 (oleic acid)	
MUFA 20:1 (gadoleic acid)	TRANS 18:2 (trans-octadecadienoic acid)
MUFA 22:1 (erucic acid)	
PUFA 18:2 (linoleic acid)	CLA cis-9, trans-11
PUFA 18:3 (linolenic acid)	CLA trans-10, cis-12

Amino Acids

Tryptophan	Arginine
Threonine	Histidine
Isoleucine	Alanine
Leucine	Aspartic acid
Lysine	Glutamic acid
Methionine	Glycine
Cystine	Proline
Phenylalanine	Serine
Tyrosine	
Valine	

Isoflavones and Similar

Daidzein	Coumestrol
Genistein	Biochanin A
Glycitein	Formononetin

Sugar Alcohols (Polyols)

Erythritol	Mannitol
Inositol	Pinitol
Isomalt	Sorbitol
Lactitol	Xylitol
Maltitol	

Other Food Components

Acesulfame potassium
Aspartame
Saccharin
Sucralose
Tagatose
Caffeine
Phytic acid
Oxalic acid
3-Methylhistidine
Sucrose polyester
Choline
Betaine
Glycemic index (glucose reference)
Glycemic index (bread reference)
Glycemic load (glucose reference)
Glycemic load (bread reference)
Nitrogen
Ash
Water

Source: National Cancer Institute, Risk Factor Assessment.

NHANES Food Frequency Questionnaire

The NHANES Food Frequency Questionnaire (NHANES FFQ) is a food frequency questionnaire that is based on the Diet History Questionnaire and Cancer Institute have developed a statistical method for estimating usual dietary intake by combining data from two 24-hour recalls with data collected by the NHANES FFQ and other data about a subject's gender, age, and race.[26,27]

The 24-hour recall, the primary dietary data collection instrument used in NHANES, is capable of collecting a considerable amount of detail about when, with what, and how much a person eats and drinks for each day that the recall is obtained. But because the diet of an individual varies greatly from one day to the next (known as intraindividual variability, as discussed earlier in this chapter), the 24-hour recall is incapable of adequately measuring the usual intake of foods that are not consumed nearly every day. Measuring the intake of these infrequently consumed foods requires multiple 24-hour recalls, which is impractical, given the respondent burden and the expense involved in obtaining a large number of recalls. A strength of the FFQ is that it provides good data on the probability of an individual's intake of foods, including those that are infrequently consumed, because it asks how often a person consumes those foods and beverages over a relatively long period of time, usually over the course of a year. A shortcoming of the FFQ is that it does not provide good data about how much of the food and beverage a person consumes. By knowing how frequently a food or beverage is consumed over the course of a year and by knowing how much of the food or beverage is consumed (or is likely to be consumed) each day or every time it is consumed, researchers can estimate usual food and nutrient intake with reasonable accuracy.[25–27] The NHANES FFQ is designed to collect information about frequency of food intake during the past year but does not ask about portion size, which reduces the respondent burden compared to that of a quantitative food frequency questionnaire. Studies suggest that the National Cancer Institute's statistical approach of combining data from two 24-hour recalls with data from the NHANES FFQ and other data on a subject's gender, age, and race can be effective in estimating the usual dietary intake of infrequently consumed foods.[26,27] The entire questionnaire can be downloaded from the National Cancer Institute's website at http://epi.grants.cancer.gov/diet/usualintakes/. The NHANES FFQ is shown in Appendix E.

Strengths and Limitations

Food frequency questionnaires have several strengths. They place a modest demand on the time and energy of respondents and generate estimates of food and nutrient intake that may be more representative of usual intake than a few days of diet records. They are relatively quick to administer. Approximately 30 minutes are required to complete the diet section of the Block Dietary Questionnaire and about 60 minutes are needed to complete the DHQ. They can be self-administered, machine read, or administered online and thus are relatively economical to use in large-scale studies.[6,19,23,28,29] However, data quality may be better when the questionnaire is administered by a trained interviewer. Estimates of nutrient and food intake from repeat administrations of food frequency questionnaires generally compare favorably, showing reasonable reproducibility (see the section "Reproducibility" later in this chapter).[6,17–20]

There are questions about how well food frequency questionnaires estimate the actual average nutrient intakes of individuals and groups—what is called validity. Studies comparing nutrient or food intake estimates obtained from food frequency questionnaires with estimates obtained from "criterion methods," such as multiple food records or 24-hour recalls, suggest that food frequency questionnaires are appropriate for estimating mean intakes of energy and some nutrients for groups and for ranking persons as having a low, average, or high consumption of energy and certain nutrients.[1,6,17–23] Some investigators, however, challenge these conclusions.[30,31] Pooled data using doubly labeled water as the standard for energy assessment showed that FFQ underreported energy intake by 24% to 33%.[32] In comparison, 24-hour recalls underreported energy intake by 6% to 16% for young and middle-aged adults.[32]

Food frequency questionnaires have definite limitations. Because the food list is limited to approximately 100 to 150 foods and food groups, these must be representative of the most common foods consumed by respondents in the sample. Short questionnaires are faster and easier to administer but lack comprehensiveness. Long questionnaires may do a better job of assessing nutrient intake but also require respondents to make an almost overwhelming number of decisions. Longer food frequency questionnaires have the disadvantage of being tedious to complete. Individual foods listed on the questionnaire are more likely to be remembered than foods grouped under such headings as "any other fruit" or "any other vegetable" unless a trained interviewer carefully probes the respondent. Grouping foods under broad categories precludes the ability to collect information about specific food items.[30] Portion sizes allow limited choices as well, and they must be the most typical of what is usually eaten. Questionnaires lacking portion size selections or having poorly chosen ones may identify only individuals at the extremes of the nutrient-intake distribution. However, the usefulness of such portion size information is questioned by research suggesting that defined portion sizes may not be meaningful to some respondents.[33] However, frequency is a more important determinant of nutrient intake than portion size.[34] Another limitation is reliance on the ability of the respondent to describe his or her diet.[1,6]

Box 3.5   **Strengths and Limitations of Food Frequency Questionnaires**

STRENGTHS

Can be self-administered

Machine readable

Modest demand on respondents

Relatively inexpensive for large sample sizes

May be more representative of usual intake than a few days of diet records

Design can be based on large population data

Considered by some as the method of choice for research on diet-disease relationships

LIMITATIONS

May not represent usual foods or portion sizes chosen by respondents

Intake data can be compromised when multiple foods are grouped within single listings

Depend on ability of subject to describe diet

It is important that food frequency questionnaires be culturally sensitive. Failure to include foods commonly eaten by groups with unique dietary habits may result in underestimates of nutrient intake, particularly if the foods are major sources of certain nutrients or food components. The Block and Willett questionnaires address this shortcoming by providing space for respondents to write in foods that they at least occasionally eat but that are not included in the food list. Food lists also must be periodically updated to keep pace with the thousands of new food products entering the marketplace each year.

Despite these limitations, the food frequency questionnaire is used in NHANES and in other large population surveys to collect data on how frequently food is consumed, especially those foods consumed infrequently, for use in statistical models to estimate usual food intake. The food frequency questionnaire is considered by some as the method of choice for research on relationships between diet and disease, on both the macronutrient and the micronutrient levels, especially in large prospective cohort studies involving tens of thousands of subjects. Box 3.5 summarizes the strengths and limitations of food frequency questionnaires.

Diet History

Diet history is used to assess an individual's usual dietary intake over an extended period of time, such as the past month or year.[1,6] Traditionally, the diet history approach has been associated with the method of assessing a respondent's usual diet developed by B. S. Burke during the 1940s.[35]

Burke's original method involved four steps: (1) collect general information about the respondent's health habits, (2) question the respondent about his or her usual eating pattern, (3) perform a cross-check on the data given in step 2, and (4) have the respondent complete a three-day food record.[35]

A trained nutritionist begins the interview by asking questions about the number of meals eaten per day; appetite; food dislikes; presence or absence of nausea and vomiting; use of nutritional supplements; cigarette smoking; habits related to sleep, rest, work, and exercise; and so on. This allows the interviewer to become acquainted with the respondent in ways that may be helpful in obtaining further information. This is followed by a 24-hour recall, in which the interviewer also inquires about the respondent's usual pattern of eating during and between meals, beginning with the first food or drink of the day. The interviewer records the respondent's description of his or her usual food intake, including types of food eaten, serving sizes, frequency and timing, and significant seasonal variations.

With the respondent's stated usual dietary practices recorded, the interviewer then cross-checks the data by asking specific questions about the respondent's dietary preferences and habits. For example, the respondent may have said that he or she drinks an 8-oz glass of milk every morning. The interviewer then should inquire about the participant's milk-drinking habits to clarify and verify the information given about the respondent's milk intake. Finally, the participant is asked to complete a three-day food record, which serves as an additional means of checking the usual intake. Burke admits that this is the least helpful part of the method, and it generally is omitted by the few researchers who currently use this method.

The strengths of the diet history approach are that it assesses the respondent's usual nutrient intake, including seasonal changes, and data on all nutrients can be obtained.[1,6] The method is one of the preferred methods for obtaining estimates of usual nutrient intake.[1,6] Estimates of protein intake by the method correlate well with measures of nitrogen excretion. If what is needed for research purposes is a list of items that is typical of an individual's diet rather than a specific list of items eaten during a certain period of time, the diet history appears adequate to determine the typical diet. Most people are able to report what they typically eat, even if they cannot report exactly what they ate during a specific period of time.[33]

Among the method's limitations are that one to two hours are required to conduct the interview, highly trained interviewers are needed, coding is difficult and expensive, and nutrient intake tends to be overestimated.[1,6,35] The method also requires a cooperative respondent with the ability to recall his or her usual diet.

Box 3.6 summarizes the strengths and limitations of the diet history method.

Duplicate Food Collections

Collection of food consumption data generally is not an end in itself but, rather, a means of eventually arriving at an estimate of nutrient intake. The limitations of using food consumption data to arrive at nutrient intake are the incompleteness of food composition tables, mistakes in coding and entering data, and nutrient losses during food storage and preparation that may not be accounted for in food composition tables.[1,3] A more direct method of calculating nutrient intake that avoids these particular problems is **duplicate food collections.**

When performing duplicate food collections, participants place in collection containers identical portions of all foods and beverages consumed during a specified period.[36] This then is chemically analyzed at a laboratory for nutrient content. To prevent bacterial decomposition of the duplicate samples, they should be kept refrigerated and delivered to the laboratory daily.

This method has the strength of potentially providing a more accurate determination of actual nutrient intake, compared with calculations based on food composition data. Values in composition tables may not be representative of nutrient levels in the particular foods that respondents consume because of seasonal or regional differences, agricultural practices, and losses during marketing and preparation. A participant may have eaten a food that was introduced recently into the marketplace that is not listed in a food composition table or database. Among the method's limitations are the necessity of preparing the additional amount of food to be collected and the work involved in measuring or weighing exactly duplicate portions of food and beverage. In a one-year dietary intake study conducted by researchers at the USDA Human Nutrition Research Center in Beltsville, Maryland, respondents kept daily food records throughout the one-year period and provided duplicate food collections for one week during each of the four seasons of the year.[36,37] The participants' mean calculated nutrient intake was 12.9% less during the four weeks when duplicate food collections were done. Reductions were greatest for foods rich in fat and protein—often the most expensive foods. The respondents may have felt guilty about "wasting" food that went into the collection jar or were concerned about the food's expense, despite receiving payment for their participation in the study. Thus, intakes during food collection periods may not be representative of habitual nutrient intake.

Box 3.7 summarizes the strengths and limitations of the duplicate food collection method.

 Box 3.6   **Strengths and Limitations of the Diet History Method**

STRENGTHS	LIMITATIONS
Assesses usual nutrient intake	Lengthy interview process
Can detect seasonal changes	Requires highly trained interviewers
Data on all nutrients can be obtained	Difficult and expensive to code
Can correlate well with biochemical measures	May tend to overestimate nutrient intake
	Requires cooperative respondent with ability to recall usual diet

---

 Box 3.7   **Strengths and Limitations of the Duplicate Food Collection Method**

STRENGTHS	LIMITATIONS
Can provide more accurate measurements of actual nutrient intake than calculations based on food composition tables	Expense and effort of preparing more food
	Effort and time to collect duplicate samples
	May underestimate usual intake

Food Accounts

Food accounts are used to measure dietary intake within households and institutions where congregate feeding is practiced, such as penal institutions, nursing homes, military bases, and boarding schools.[38] The method accounts for all food on hand in the home or institution at the beginning of the survey period, all that is purchased or grown throughout the period, and all that remains by the end of the survey. Inventories establish amounts of food on hand at the beginning and ending of the survey period, and invoices or other accounting methods provide records of food purchased or obtained from a farm or garden. Trained personnel make site visits at the beginning and ending of the survey period and as necessary throughout the period to assist in recordkeeping. The daily mean consumption per person is calculated for each food item from the total amount of food consumed during the survey period and the number of people in the household or institution.[38]

When used to measure household food consumption, the usual survey period is two to four weeks. To capture seasonal variations, some researchers may record consumption over different seasons for shorter periods. In addition to the amounts of different foods consumed by family members, it is necessary to account for the number of people present at each meal, the number of meals eaten away from home, and the number served to visitors.[38]

The strengths of the method are that the survey can include a large sample size, food consumption can be monitored for a relatively long period of time, and data on the annual mean consumption and general food patterns and habits of the population can be obtained. The likelihood that the method will alter the diet is less than with the food record method. The method is also relatively economical because personnel need only make periodic visits for supervising and controlling the recording.[38]

Included among the limitations of the method are its inability to account for food that is given to animals, thrown away due to spoilage, or discarded as plate waste or for other reasons. Because respondent literacy and cooperation are necessary, families or institutions willing to keep food accounts may not be representative of the population of interest. Accuracy may suffer due to forgetfulness or lack of faithfulness in maintaining food accounts. The method provides information only on the mean daily consumption of the whole family; it does not indicate how food is distributed among the various family members. Thus, it is only appropriate for measuring food consumption of groups.[38]

Box 3.8 summarizes the strengths and limitations of the food account method.

Food Balance Sheets

The **food balance sheet** is a method of indirectly estimating the amounts of food consumed by a country's population at a certain time. It provides data on food *disappearance* (sometimes referred to as *food availability*) rather than actual food consumption. It is calculated using beginning and ending inventories, figures on food production, imports and exports, and adjustments for nonhuman food consumption (for example, cattle feed, pet food, seed, and industrial use). Food disappearance can be thought of as the amount of food that "disappears" from the food distribution system. Much of this is purchased by consumers at supermarkets; however, a considerable amount is lost due to spoilage.

Mean per capita annual amounts are calculated by dividing total disappearance of food by the country's population.[38] This method has been valuable for detecting trends in the amount of food that disappears from the food distribution system within a country over time and thus has been used to roughly indicate likely trends in consumption as well. It is useful for promoting agricultural production in various parts of the world and for encouraging a more even distribution of food among different countries.[38] Because these data are collected in a roughly similar manner in countries around the world, they are useful in epidemiologic research across countries. Food disappearance data will be discussed in greater detail in Chapter 4 in connection with national surveys.

The strengths of the method are that it can give a total view of the food supplies of a country, can be used in drawing conclusions about general food habits and

---

 Box 3.8   **Strengths and Limitations of the Food Account Method**

STRENGTHS

Suitable for use with large sample sizes

Can be used over relatively long periods

Gives data on dietary patterns and habits of families and other groups

Less likely to lead to alterations in diet than some other methods

Relatively economical

LIMITATIONS

Does not account for food losses

Respondent literacy and cooperation necessary

Not appropriate for measuring individual food consumption

dietary trends within a country, and is valuable in planning international nutrition policy and formulating food programs.[38] In some instances, information on food disappearance may be the only accessible data representing a country's food consumption practices.

The method has a number of limitations. The accuracy of data depends on available statistics, the quality of which can vary greatly, depending on a country's level of development. The data represent only the total amount of food that reportedly leaves the food distribution system, apparently for consumption. Note that it is not an estimate of what was actually consumed. It also does not show how food was distributed among individuals or groups within a particular country. The method also does not account for food that is wasted or fed to animals (for example, pets).[38]

Box 3.9 summarizes the strengths and limitations of the food balance sheet.

Telephone Interviews

Telephone interviewing is an accepted and widely used method for collecting dietary intake data. Investigators have used the technique to administer 24-hour recalls and food frequency questionnaires, particularly to follow up on face-to-face interviews. In NHANES, two computer-assisted, multiple-pass 24-hour recalls are obtained from each participant; the first is collected during an in-person interview, and the second is obtained by telephone 3 to 10 days later.[4] Telephone interviews are a principal method of collecting dietary intake data for the USDA.[39,40] Preadolescent children were shown to be able to provide 24-hour recall data during telephone interviews that compared favorably with written records of their intake unobtrusively collected by parents.[41] Recalls obtained by telephone interview showed good agreement with the observed intake of both college students and elderly participants.[42] Telephone reporting has been shown to be an acceptable method of collecting food record data, whether the data are reported directly to an individual or left on a recording device, such as a telephone answering machine.

Telephone interviews have several strengths. Cost of the method has been reported to be approximately one-fourth to one-half that of comparable personal interviews. They also have the potential of easing the time, logistical, and personnel constraints associated with nutrition surveys.[39,42,43] Telephone surveys have higher response rates than mail surveys.[43] The respondent burden may be somewhat lower with this method, compared with personal interviews. In an era of pervasive suspicion of strangers resulting from rising crime rates, some respondents may find this method more conducive to personal safety than interviews within their homes.

The use of telephone interviewing has been complicated in recent years by the growth of call-screening technologies and heightened privacy concerns resulting from an increased number of telemarketing calls and by changes in personal communication technologies, most notably the dramatic increase in the percentage of cellular-telephone-only households. About one-half of American homes in 2015 had only wireless telephones (also known as cellular, cell, or mobile phones). Compared to those who still have landlines, persons living in cellular-telephone-only households are more likely to be renters, live with unrelated adult roommates, be young adults under age 30 years, live in poverty, and be Latino.[43] This can result in lower response rates and undercoverage bias. A further complication is the fact that approximately 3% of U.S. households have no telephone service of any type. To improve the quality and validity of data collected by surveys that have traditionally relied on data collected by telephone interviews, surveys are increasingly turning to multiple modes of collecting data, including contacting more subjects via cellular phone and using mail to follow up with nonrespondents.[43]

Twenty-four-hour recall or food frequency data collected over the telephone are subject to the same limitations as that collected in personal interviews. The problem of estimating portion sizes can be addressed by providing respondents with measuring cups, spoons, rulers, two-dimensional and three-dimensional measuring guides, and photographic atlases of food portion sizes.[6–8,18,44] NHANES participants are given a set of measuring guides after the first 24-hour recall is obtained during the in-person interview and are instructed on how to use them when the second 24-hour recall is obtained during a

---

 Box 3.9   **Strengths and Limitations of the Food Balance Sheet**

STRENGTHS

Can give a total view of a country's food supplies

Indicates food habits and dietary trends

Used to plan international nutrition policies and food programs

May be the only data available on a country's food consumption practices

LIMITATIONS

Accuracy of data may be questionable

Only represents food available for consumption

Does not represent food actually consumed

Does not indicate how food was distributed

Does not account for wasted food

Box 3.10   **Strengths and Limitations of Telephone Interviews**

STRENGTHS

One-quarter to one-half the cost of a comparable personal interview

Fewer time, logistical, and personnel constraints

Lower respondent burden

Give respondent more personal security

LIMITATIONS

Subject to many of the same disadvantages of collecting 24-hour recall and food record data

Estimating portion sizes in recalls may be difficult unless steps are taken to address the problem

subsequent telephone interview.[6–8] The tendency of 24-hour recalls to underestimate energy and nutrient intake can be ameliorated by using the multiple-pass 24-hour recall method.[6–8,45] For the Automated Multiple-Pass Method (AMPM) 24-hour recall method used in NHANES, data show that mean energy intake is under-reported by only 10% in males, 12% in females, and 3% in normal-weight individuals.[45]

Box 3.10 summarizes the strengths and limitations of telephone interviews.

Technological Innovations in Assessment

An area of active research and development in dietary assessment methodology is the use of technology to improve dietary measurement by reducing respondent burden, increasing the validity of dietary intake data, and reducing costs.[9,46,47] Examples of technological innovations previously mentioned in this chapter include the Automated Multiple-Pass Method (AMPM) 24-hour recall, the Internet-based automated self-administered 24-hour dietary recall (ASA24), and the Web-based version of the food frequency questionnaire known as DHQ*Web. In the early 1990s, researchers at the USDA's Western Human Nutrition Research Center developed a dietary measurement system utilizing an electronic scale interfaced with a handheld computer.[48–50] Called the Nutrition Evaluation Scale System, the respondent entered into the computer the identity of foods to be eaten, and the computer then guided the respondent through the steps of weighing the foods and any leftovers after the meal. The software used icons, sounds, and on-screen prompts to guide respondents through the process of entering data. The identity and weights of foods consumed were saved in the computer's memory. These data then could be transferred to another computer for review by a dietitian and eventual analysis using a food composition database.

More recently, there has been considerable interest in using digital images to simplify the process of recording, identifying, and quantifying meals and snacks.[51–55] This could be thought of as a digital image food record, an example of which is shown in Figure 3.5. One common approach being investigated is to have a respondent use a digital camera to capture images of foods and beverages

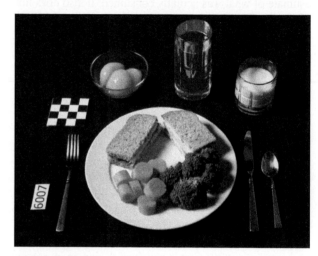

Figure 3.5

Digital images of a meal such as this one can be taken by respondents and electronically sent to researchers who can analyze the images to identify and quantify the foods and beverages in the meal. The fiducial marker on the left side of the image assists researchers in accurately estimating portion sizes of food items.

©McGraw-Hill Education/Jesselyn Zbytowski, photographer

before and after eating. These images are then electronically sent to researchers, who analyze them to identify and quantify the foods in the images. Some researchers are using mobile phones equipped with high-resolution digital cameras to capture images that can be automatically sent to researchers for analysis.[51–53] Others are investigating the use of proprietary devices specifically designed to capture images.[54,55] One system uses a miniature camera attached to a lanyard that can be worn around the neck to capture images of food that can then be provided to researchers.[54] Another uses a handheld personal digital assistant with an integrated camera and mobile telephone card that respondents can use to capture images of foods and beverages, which are then sent to researchers for analysis.[55]

Advantages of these systems include a relatively low respondent burden and the potential for image analysis software to automatically record, identify, and quantify the volume of foods and beverages in the image. However, if there is uncertainty about the identity and volume of the food, the technology allows the respondent to fairly easily provide detailed information that might be requested by researchers. A lower respondent burden may lead to fewer alterations in diet that inevitably result from maintaining several days of food records. Research suggests that this technology may be particularly valuable for use by adolescents, who are generally adept at using technology but have poor compliance when asked to report their food intake using more traditional diet measurement techniques.[52] Studies support that the magnitude of underreporting is reduced with wearable camera-assisted 24-hour recall compared to multiple-pass 24-hour dietary recalls using traditional methods.[56,57] These systems are limited by their higher cost relative to the more traditional methods and image quality, which can be degraded by room lighting and poor camera resolution and focus. There is also the need for an object of known dimensions and markings (referred to as a *fiducial marker*) to be in the image as a size reference in order to accurately estimate portion size. Fiducial markers can include a checkered tablecloth provided by the researchers, a dinner plate of known diameter, or some other object of known dimension. Distinguishing between visually similar foods (such as skim milk versus whole milk, or premium ice cream versus ice milk) can be problematic. Some form of written or verbal records will continue to be necessary to document preparation methods and identify visually similar foods. Estimates of food consumption based on the analysis of photographs and digital images of the meals of respondents have been compared with weighed food records made on the same meals. When performed by trained observers, these estimates compared favorably to the weighed food records, supporting the validity of digital images as methods for measuring food intake and estimating food portion size.[55–57]

Box 3.11 summarizes the strengths and limitations of the digital imaging methods.

Surrogate Sources

There are times when a respondent may not be able to provide the dietary intake data that investigators desire. In some instances, a respondent may have a problem with hearing, speech, or memory due to disease, trauma, or advanced age. This is especially a problem with elderly respondents participating in case-control studies. In such instances, obtaining information from **surrogate sources** may improve information quality and provide data otherwise unavailable from deceased or incompetent participants. Potential surrogate respondents include the respondent's spouse or partner, children, other close relatives, and friends.[1,6,58]

Several investigators have studied the use of surrogate sources of dietary intake. A review of these studies demonstrates that "surrogate respondents can provide dietary information, but that incomplete responses must be anticipated."[58] In some cases, surrogate respondents provide more valid data than the respondents themselves. Surrogate sources often can provide good information on specific foods or nutrients. The availability of data from surrogate respondents varies with the surrogate's relationship to the participant, the surrogate's sex (e.g., females provide more accurate data about the eating habits of males than males do about the eating habits of females), and the number of shared meals. There may be considerable difference in the quality of surrogate data between spouses or partners of deceased participants and spouses or partners of living participants.[6]

Surrogate sources are good in studies in which there is rapid mortality of study participants, in which there is concern about biased recall from participants, or in which participants have problems with memory impairment or difficulty communicating because of such causes as stroke or Alzheimer's disease. In some instances, data from surrogates are good enough for ranking persons in quintiles (one of five levels) in terms of their nutrient intake (i.e., as having an intake that is very low, low, average, high, or very high). In any event, surrogate sources must be carefully selected and data closely scrutinized because misclassification of dietary intake can occur easily when relying on surrogate sources alone.[1,6,58]

 Box 3.11   **Strengths and Limitations of Digital Imaging Methods**

STRENGTHS

Digital imaging method has good validity

Recording food intake takes less time than 24-hour recalls or food records

Respondent burden is less

Methods appear to be acceptable to subjects

Eating habits may be less affected by recording

LIMITATIONS

Large initial expense is involved, but this may be offset by lower long-term costs

Periodic revalidations are recommended

Unable to distinguish visually similar foods or document preparation methods

Subject to technical problems caused by sophisticated equipment

CONSIDERATIONS FOR CERTAIN GROUPS

Adaptations in dietary measurement can be made for certain groups, such as young persons, the reading-impaired, individuals having problems recalling their diet, persons who are visually or hearing-impaired, and the obese. These considerations, summarized in Box 3.12, facilitate collection of intake data from persons who otherwise might have difficulty participating in surveys.

ISSUES IN DIETARY MEASUREMENT

Validity

Validity is the ability of an instrument to actually measure what it is intended to measure.[1,6] In most instances, investigators are interested in knowing what a respondent's *usual intake* is or has been. Thus, validating an instrument involves comparing estimates of intake obtained by that instrument with a respondent's usual intake. Because it is difficult if not impossible to know a person's true usual intake, investigators must turn to *relative,* or *criterion, validity.* Relative, or criterion, validity is defined as the comparison of a new instrument with another instrument (a so-called gold standard), which has a greater degree of *demonstrated,* or *face, validity.*[1,6] However, if the two instruments fail to compare favorably, the question must be asked, "Which instrument (if any) gives the best estimate of usual intake?" The failure of one instrument to compare favorably with another may not lie in the instrument's being validated; it actually may have given the best estimate of usual intake. The fault may lie in the criterion instrument.

The validity of food frequency questionnaires has been examined by comparing estimates of food and nutrient intake obtained from food frequency questionnaires with estimates obtained from multiple food records or 24-hour recalls, which are thought to give a more detailed and quantitative estimate of dietary intake over an extended period.[1,6] Researchers at Harvard University, for example, collected four one-week weighed-diet records over the course of a year from 173 participants.[17] These served as an estimate of usual intake during the one-year period and the criterion against which intake data from the food frequency questionnaire were compared. Results of the study showed that a simple self-administered food frequency questionnaire can provide useful information about individual nutrient intakes over a one-year period. To study the questionnaire's ability to assess diet in the recent past, the researchers administered it to the same group of participants three to four years after the weighed food records were collected, and they concluded that the questionnaire was useful in estimating nutrient intake four years in the past.[18] A number of other validation studies have been done as well.[1,6,20,21] Nutrient estimates derived from food frequency questionnaires compared favorably with those derived from criterion methods, suggesting that food frequency questionnaires can be appropriate to use in epidemiologic research. Overall, these studies support the use of food frequency questionnaires for estimating a group's average intake for energy and some nutrients. They also suggest that the method is appropriate for ranking individuals in terms of nutrient intake (e.g., categorizing individuals as having a low, average, or high intake of some nutrient).[1,6,17] Other investigators, however, question the use of food frequency questionnaires in epidemiologic research with data suggesting that energy intake is underreported by 24% to 33% for both men and women relative to doubly labeled water.[30-32]

The validity of a food frequency questionnaire depends in large part on items included in the food list and assumptions about portion size and nutrient content of the various groups.[1,6] Another important consideration in validation studies is the appropriateness of the criterion instrument. Given the weaknesses of food records and 24-hour recalls in characterizing usual intake, how appropriate are they to use as a truth measure against which to judge another instrument, such as the food frequency questionnaire? If, in a validation study, data from food frequency questionnaires compare unfavorably to data from a criterion method, is it necessarily the fault of the food frequency questionnaire? A proposal for circumventing this dilemma is to include a biological marker as a *third* criterion method in the validation process.[6,34] Biological markers are discussed in the section "Use of Biological Markers."

Some investigators have compared estimates of dietary intake using various methods with respondents' *actual* intake, which the investigators observed surreptitiously.[10,11] Usually, the respondents ate all or at least most of their meals in a cafeteria or residential metabolic research facility where their food intake could be observed. Different assessment methods then could be used to measure respondents' intake during the period when their diet was observed. Among these were the 24-hour recall, food records, and food frequency questionnaires. However, such comparisons over relatively short periods of time in monitored or controlled situations fail to adequately validate a method intended to assess the usual, self-selected diets of free-living persons.[1,6,11]

Use of Biological Markers

Another approach to validating dietary measurement methods is to compare intake data with certain biological markers associated with dietary intake.[1,6,19,34,62,63] Biological markers offer the advantages of being easily accessible (urine, feces, blood, tissue samples) and providing a validity check of dietary intake independent of respondents' accuracy and truthfulness. A major problem, however, is that many factors other than dietary intake can affect nutrient concentrations in tissues, even

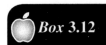

| **Box 3.12** | **Considerations When Measuring Diet in Certain Groups** |

GROUP	CONSIDERATIONS
Young persons	Dietary intake data on children under 8 years of age are best obtained from the person responsible for meals. For information on food eaten away from home, interview the child in the presence of the parent or guardian. Data on meals eaten at school, kindergarten, or day care center can be obtained from those responsible for their meals. Reliable data on intake in the previous 24 hours can be obtained from children 8 years of age and older.
Persons with recall problems	There appears to be no firm evidence that memory of past diet is impaired during aging despite popular belief to the contrary. The ability to recall past diet may be more a function of how much attention is paid to what is eaten.[1,6] Diet recall can be helped through the use of checklists and visual aids, such as food models and photographs.[1,6] Information obtained from surrogates (spouse, sibling, or caregiver) can improve the quality of data.[6,58] Reproducibility of recall of diet many years in the past by older persons has been shown to be good but is reduced by older age, cognitive impairment, and male sex.[1,6]
Persons with impaired vision or hearing	Intake measurement instructions can be communicated to the visually impaired through large-print materials, tape recordings, radio, telephone, personal interview, and Braille. Some visually impaired persons have video equipment that will enlarge print to a readable size. Data can be collected through personal interview, by telephone or tape recorder, or over specially equipped computer systems. Communication of instructions to and collection of data from hearing-impaired persons is easily done with self-explanatory and well-prepared printed materials. Use of an interpreter of sign language and visual aids, such as food models or photographs, can be helpful. Verbal responses to an interviewer can facilitate collection of data.
Persons who cannot read well	Personal and telephone interviews, digital imaging methods, and computerized or Web-based systems with visual and audio prompts can all be used in collecting dietary intake data from the reading-impaired. Persons with limited reading ability may be able to use printed materials having an appropriate vocabulary. Food models, photographs, and digital images are especially helpful.
The obese	Several studies have questioned the validity of reported energy intake in obese persons, indicating a tendency to underreport energy intake using the dietary history and food records.[59–61]

Source: Cameron ME, Van Staveren WA. 1988. *Manual on methodology for food consumption studies.* New York: Oxford University Press, and other indicated sources.

in well-fed persons.[1,6,19] Although many biological markers have potential for use, only a limited number have been investigated. Among these are urinary nitrogen, sodium, and potassium; plasma levels of carotenoids, vitamin E, and vitamin C; fatty acids in adipose tissue; changes in serum triglyceride; and assessment of energy expenditure and body weight.[6,19,34,62,63]

Analysis of nitrogen in multiple 24-hour urine samples, a well-known biological marker, has been used to verify protein intake in dietary surveys.[6,19,34,64,65] If acceptable agreement exists between urinary nitrogen excretion and estimated protein intake, it can be assumed that intake of other nutrients is fairly well represented. Use of this method depends on several assumptions: that respondents are in nitrogen balance (there is no accumulation of protein for growth or repair or unusual losses due to starvation or injury); that estimates of extrarenal nitrogen excretion sufficiently cover losses through the feces, hair, skin, and other routes; and that all urine has been collected over the course of the collection period.[66]

Urinary sodium is a useful measure of dietary sodium intake, especially because amounts used at the table and in cooking are difficult to assess. Fecal sodium losses are minimal, and in temperate climates it is assumed that amounts in sweat are negligible. Differences in urinary sodium and estimated dietary intakes have been shown to be as low as 5%. Although fecal losses of potassium are greater and more variable than with sodium, urinary potassium has been used for validating dietary potassium intake.[19,65,66]

A potential problem with measurements of nitrogen, sodium, and potassium in 24-hour urine samples is the necessity of obtaining a *complete* 24-hour urine sample—a requirement some participants have difficulty adhering to. One approach to checking on the completeness of 24-hour urine samples is use of the para-amino-benzoic acid (PABA) marker. Participants take one PABA tablet three times a day with their meals. The PABA is excreted in the urine. A 24-hour urine collection containing less than 85% of the PABA marker is considered unsatisfactory, either because the participant did not take all the PABA tablets or one or more urine specimens were omitted from the collection.[65,66]

Plasma levels of total carotenoids, α-carotene, β-carotene, lycopene, vitamin C, and vitamin E have been shown to compare favorably with intakes of these substances based on administration of a food frequency questionnaire.[64,67] Changes in plasma triglyceride levels have been shown useful in estimating total fat intake.[62,63] This measurement is based on the observation that as intake of total fat (except for *trans* fatty acids) increases, plasma triglyceride decreases and, to a lesser extent, plasma high-density lipoprotein cholesterol increases.

Linoleic acid in adipose tissue can be used as an index of dietary intake of linoleic acid over the past two to three years, whereas the linoleic acid content of erythrocytes (red blood cells) can be an index of dietary linoleic acid during the past six to eight weeks.[62] A small piece of adipose tissue can be easily removed from beneath the skin and measured for linoleic acid. This can be an independent way of estimating intake of specific fatty acids that are not endogenously synthesized. Such measurements have been shown to compare favorably with estimates of usual intake based on two weeks of weighed food records and a food frequency questionnaire.[19,62]

Energy Expenditure and Weight Maintenance

Another approach to validating dietary measurement methods is to compare reported energy intake with body weight and energy expenditure calculated from an equation or measured using the doubly labeled water method. Self-reported energy intake has been compared with energy expenditure determined through use of the doubly labeled water method (discussed in greater detail in Chapter 8). Briefly, participants drink a known amount of water labeled with deuterium (^{2}H) and oxygen-18 (^{2}H$_2$^{18}O).[61,68,69] They provide periodic samples of urine or saliva over the next two weeks or so, which allows monitoring of the body's elimination of deuterium and oxygen-18. Knowledge of the rates at which these isotopes are eliminated allows researchers to calculate energy expenditure in free-living participants with considerable accuracy and precision, despite certain limitations discussed in Chapter 8.

During a 10-day field exercise in the Canadian Arctic, the self-reported energy intake of 20 infantry soldiers was 39% less than their actual energy expenditure measured by doubly labeled water.[70] Researchers from the Ontario Cancer Institute and the University of British Columbia studied the accuracy of reported energy intakes from 7 consecutive days of food records obtained from a subset of 29 women participating in the Canadian Diet and Breast Cancer Prevention Trial. The mean body mass index (BMI, weight in kilograms divided by height in meters squared, or kg/m^2) of the subjects was 23.1 ± 2.5 (mean ± standard deviation) and thus essentially within what is considered a healthy range for BMI. Reported energy intakes averaged 20% less than mean total energy expenditure determined by doubly labeled water.[71] Researchers from Maastricht University compared total energy expenditure measured by doubly labeled water with reported energy estimates from 7-day food records completed by 30 adult males. The subjects had a mean BMI (kg/m^2) of 34 ± 4 (mean ± standard deviation) and thus were considered obese. Reported energy intakes averaged 37% less than mean total energy expenditure. The researchers estimated that, during the week that subjects kept food records, their energy consumption averaged 26% less than the previous week, when subjects were not recording their intake. These results suggest that, not only do subjects underreport energy intake but they also are likely to eat less food during the recording period.[61,72]

Researchers from the University of Vermont compared total energy expenditure measured by doubly labeled water with estimates of energy intake based on four multiple-pass 24-hour recalls obtained over a two-week period in a group of 35 low-income adult females. Underreporting of energy intake averaged 17%. However, underreporting was greater in subjects who were obese and in those who had lower literacy (difficulty reading and spelling), compared with nonobese subjects and those who had a higher degree of literacy.[73] In another study, energy intake was measured in 118 fourth- and fifth-graders who kept eight-day food records with the help of parents and nutritionists. Average daily energy intake was found to range from 17% to 33% less than total energy expenditure measured by doubly labeled water.[74]

Researchers at the USDA Beltsville Human Nutrition Research Center compared self-reported energy intakes with the amount of energy the participants actually required to maintain their body weight to within ± 0.9 kg. The data, collected from 266 research participants over a 14-year period, showed that only 11% of self-reported energy intakes were accurate to within ± 100 kcal and that 81% of participants underreported their energy intake by 700 kcal ± 379 kcal (mean ± standard deviation).[75] Data combined from five large studies showed that energy intake from 24-hour recalls was only modestly underreported by 6% to 13% in young and middle-aged adults compared to doubly labeled water.[32,76] In the same pooling study, however, energy intake was underreported by 24% to 33%.

Another approach to check for underreporting is to compare reported usual energy intake with **resting energy expenditure** (REE), calculated using various equations, such as those shown in Table 3.2 and the Estimated Energy Requirement (EER) equations discussed in Chapter 7. A wide variety of ratios of reported intake to estimated REE have been used to categorize individuals into plausible or implausible reporters, and these can be adjusted for physical activity, sample size, the number of days of self-report, and variance in the data.[32] If a subject's reported usual energy intake is < 0.9 times his or her calculated REE, underreporting of energy, and therefore nutrient, intake is highly likely.[32] Using data from the third National Health and Nutrition Examination Survey, researchers at the National Center for Health Statistics compared reported energy intakes of nearly 8000 adult survey participants with their calculated resting energy expenditure.[77] About 18% of males and 28% of females were classified as underreporters using a range of cutoff values (0.9 to 1.54) based on sample size and the number of days of food recording. Underreporting was highest in females and in persons who were older,

overweight, or trying to lose weight. Researchers at the USDA Western Human Nutrition Research Center compared reported energy intakes from seven-day food records with energy intake necessary to maintain a stable body weight in 22 adult females of widely varying body weight.[78] The subjects completed a variety of behavioral questionnaires that measured hunger, restrained eating, emotional eating (excessive eating in response to anger, fear, or anxiety), anxiety, and depression. Cognitive performance tests were also administered to the subjects. These assessed mental acuity, the ability to sustain or focus attention, short-term memory, and manual dexterity. Underreporting of energy by nonobese females (mean BMI 21.3 kg/m^2) was estimated at 10%, while that of obese subjects (mean BMI 34.2 kg/m^2) was nearly 20%. In the obese group, the presence of emotional factors related to depression were linked to greater likelihood of underreporting.

The observation that underreporting of food intake is common led researchers at the Beltsville Human Nutrition Research Center to propose the hypothesis of the "uncertainty principle of food-intake measurements: the degree of deviation of reported from real intake is proportional to the degree of attention focused on the intake."[75] Although the task of maintaining food records resulted in an 18% underestimate of energy intake, collection of duplicate food portions resulted in a decline of an additional 13%.[75] Thus, although the collection of dietary data is critical to our

TABLE 3.2	**Equations for Calculating Resting Energy Expenditure***

World Health Organization		
Females	3–9 years old	22.5 W + 499
	10–17 years old	12.2 W + 746
	18–29 years old	14.7 W + 496
	30–60 years old	8.7 W + 829
	> 60 years old	10.5 W + 596
Males	3–9 years old	22.7 W + 495
	10–17 years old	17.5 W + 651
	18–29 years old	15.3 W + 679
	30–60 years old	11.6 W + 879
	> 60 years old	13.5 W + 487

Harris-Benedict (Values Rounded for Simplicity)	
Females	REE = 655 + 9.6W + 1.9S − 4.7A
Males	REE = 66 + 13.8W + 5S − 6.8A

*REE = resting energy expenditure; W = body weight in kg; S = stature in cm; A = age in years.

Source: National Cancer Institute, Risk Factor Assessment.

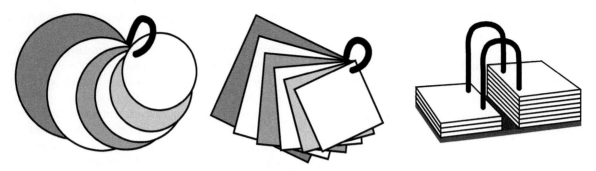

Figure 3.6 Simple geometric shapes representing foods are sometimes used to help survey participants estimate food portion size. Each piece has a known dimension (surface area or thickness) and is made from poster board or other materials.

understanding of nutrition, *dietary intake data must be interpreted with considerable caution,* whether self-reported or obtained by observers of whose presence respondents are aware.[75,79]

Despite the difficulty of accurately measuring usual dietary intake, our ability to quantify the degree of misreporting and to identify some of the characteristics of subjects related to misreporting represents progress toward the goal of accurately measuring diet. The potential exists for "targeting specific areas of dietary assessment techniques to prevent or at least to minimize the effect of each factor on collection of valid data."[80] The best example of this is the ASA24, a freely available Web-based tool that was developed to address these challenges by eliminating the need for an interviewer, utilizing the multiple-pass approach of the AMPM, and implementing automated coding.[8]

Reproducibility

Reproducibility, or **reliability,** can be defined as the ability of a method to produce the same estimate on two or more occasions, assuming that nothing has changed in the interim. Reproducibility is concerned only with whether a method is capable of providing the *same or similar answer* two or more times and does not necessarily indicate whether the answer is *correct.* Reproducibility studies can partially answer the validity question; a method cannot give a correct answer every time unless it gives approximately the same answer each time. Problems in instrument design, respondent instructions, or quality control also can be uncovered by reproducibility studies.

ESTIMATING PORTION SIZE

Accurate estimation of portion size is an important element in self-reports of dietary intake. Research shows that without training, individuals have difficulty

accurately estimating the portion sizes of foods eaten and that this is particularly the case with children.[6,7] A variety of approaches have been developed to help respondents estimate portion sizes. Among the simplest and least costly are "food models" composed of two-dimensional geometric shapes of various sizes cut out of poster board, as shown in Figure 3.6. Circles of various diameters can be used to help estimate the diameter of round foods, such as apples, oranges, tomato slices, hamburger patties, hamburger buns, and cookies. Square and rectangular pieces are useful in estimating the length and width of bread, cake, some cuts of meat, and cheese. Pie-shaped pieces of various radii can be used in estimating portion sizes of pie, round cake, watermelon, and pizza. Pieces of polyurethane foam 3 to 4 inches square and of varying thicknesses can be used to help respondents estimate the thickness of foods, providing a third dimension. Individual pieces can be used, or several can be stacked to achieve the desired thickness. An alternate approach is to have a number of pieces of cardboard cut 3 to 4 inches square, which can then be stacked to aid in estimating the thickness of food. Polystyrene balls of various diameters are useful in estimating sizes of round food objects. Bowls, plates, measuring cups and spoons, and drinking cups of various sizes also can be used to help respondents estimate serving sizes of soup, breakfast cereal, salad, beverages, sugar, and margarine. An increasingly common approach is using photographs or digital images to facilitate portion size estimation.[7,44,80–82] Photographs of actual foods illustrating three different serving sizes on a plate can be used, as shown in Figure 3.7. The plates used in Figure 3.7 are all the same size and are used to provide a sense of scale. Researchers at the USDA have developed a *Food Model Booklet* that contains a collection of life-size, two-dimensional images representing different shapes and sizes of foods, including life-size images of plates, bowls, cups, and glasses.[44] Figure 3.8 is an image from the *Food Model Booklet* showing a life-size dinner plate with four different-size

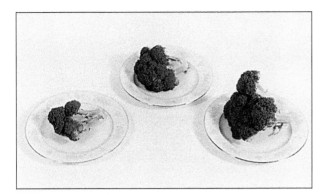

Figure 3.7
Some investigators use photographs to help respondents more accurately estimate food portion size.
Source: USDA.

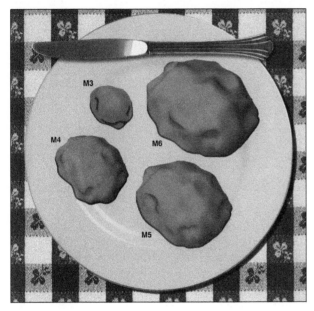

Figure 3.8
This two-dimensional image from the USDA's *Food Model Booklet* shows a life-size dinner plate with four different-size amorphous mounds representing different portion sizes of foods that mound on a plate. The knife lying across the top of the plate provides a size reference.
Source: USDA.

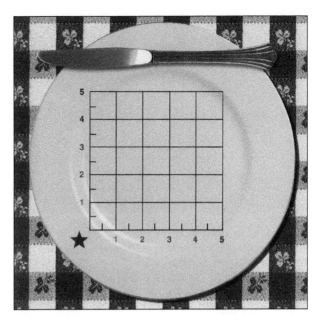

Figure 3.9
This two-dimensional image from the USDA's *Food Model Booklet* shows a grid superimposed on the dinner plate to assist survey respondents in estimating the length and width of square or rectangular foods.
Source: USDA.

amorphous mounds representing different portion sizes of foods that mound on a plate, such as casseroles, mashed potatoes, or rice. The knife lying across the top of the plate provides a size reference. The grid superimposed on the dinner plate in Figure 3.9 can be used to estimate the length and width of square or rectangular foods, such as lasagna, meat loaf, or sheet cake. As in Figure 3.8, the knife lying across the top of the plate and the checkered tablecloth serve as size references to improve portion size estimates.[44,45] Two-dimensional

food models and photographs or digital images have been shown to be as effective as three-dimensional models for estimating portion size in nutritional research.[6,7,81,82]

When, during an interview, identification of particular brand names of foods consumed is important, a notebook containing photographs of various foods, pictures cut from magazine advertisements, or actual food labels can be used. A photograph of a supermarket dairy case, for example, can help respondents identify the brand of margarine or similar spreads used at home. During the course of a 24-hour recall, for example, a child is likely to remember the brand of potato or corn chips he or she ate but perhaps not the particular bag size. Including in the notebook an assortment of snack food wrappers (for candy, chips, and chewing gum of various brands and sizes) can be helpful in collecting accurate intake data. Lifelike food models, such as those shown in Figure 3.10, also can be used to help respondents estimate food portion sizes. In addition, glasses, bowls, and cups of various sizes; household spoons; measuring spoons; and measuring cups can be used as aids in helping respondents estimate portion size, as shown in Figure 3.11.

The 24-hour recall is the principle dietary assessment method used in the National Health and Nutrition Examination Survey (discussed in Chapter 4) and most participants provide two 24-hour recalls, both using the

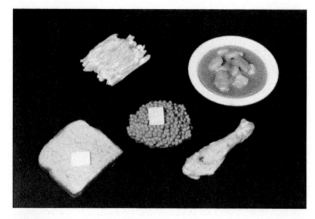

Figure 3.10
Lifelike food models can be used to improve accuracy in
estimating food portion sizes.
Source: USDA.

Automated Multiple-Pass Method (AMPM). The first
recall is administered in person and a variety of plates,
bowls, cups, glasses, and three-dimensional forms are
used to assist participants in estimating the portion sizes
of foods, as shown in Figure 3.11. During this initial
face-to-face interview, the participant is given a copy of
the *Food Model Booklet* and instructed in its use. The
second 24-hour recall is administered over the telephone
at a later, randomly selected time, also using the AMPM.
During the second 24-hour recall, the participant can use
the *Food Model Booklet* to help in accurately estimating
the portion sizes of foods. The ASA24 uses a dynamic
set of images to assist with the estimation of portion size,
greatly facilitating the assessment of actual food
consumed.

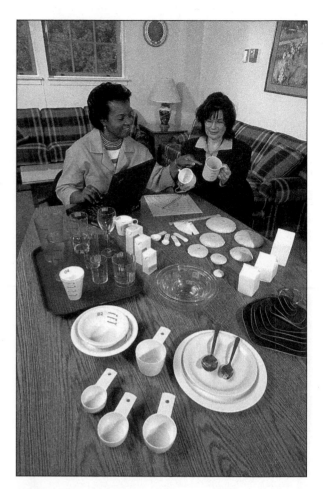

Figure 3.11
Using serving size aids during an in-home interview, USDA
nutritionist Grace Omolewa-Tomobi, left, helps a study
participant with her 24-hour recall of food portions.
Source: USDA/Photo by Stephen Ausmus.

SUMMARY

1. The ultimate reason for measuring diet is to improve
   human health. Other reasons include assessing and
   monitoring food and nutrient intake, formulating
   and evaluating government health and agricultural
   policy, conducting epidemiologic research, and
   using the data for commercial purposes.

2. No single best method exists for measuring dietary
   intake. Each method possesses certain advantages
   and disadvantages. The method used depends on
   research design considerations, characteristics of the
   study participants, available resources, and whether
   the intent is to estimate average group intake, rank

   individuals within a group, or estimate an
   individual's usual intake.

3. In the 24-hour recall method, a trained interviewer
   may ask the respondent to remember all foods and
   beverages consumed during the past 24 hours. The
   Automated Multiple-Pass Method (AMPM) and the
   Internet-based automated self-administered 24-hour
   recall (ASA24) have simplified and improved the
   collecting of dietary data using the 24-hour recall.
   The 24-hour recall is quickly administered, has a
   low respondent burden, but does not give data
   representative of an individual's usual intake.

4. When keeping a food record, or diary, the respondent records, at the time of consumption, the identity and amounts of all foods and beverages consumed during a one- to seven-day period. Foods can be either quantified using household measures or weighed, in which case the method is called weighed food recording. This method does not rely on memory, can provide detailed intake data, requires a high degree of respondent cooperation, and may result in alterations of diet.

5. A food frequency questionnaire assesses nutrient intake by determining the frequency of consumption of a limited number of foods known to be major sources of the dietary components of interest. Respondents indicate how many times a day, week, month, or year the foods usually are consumed. Relatively high-quality data can be gathered on large groups of respondents; data may be more representative of usual intake than a few days of diet records; respondents must be able to describe their diets; and foods and portion sizes included in questionnaires must be carefully chosen. An Internet-based food frequency questionnaire, the DHQ*Web, can be completed online, simplifying the collection and submission of questionnaire data.

6. Collection of duplicate food portions is a more direct method of assessing nutrient intake that avoids some of the problems associated with coding and entering data and the limitations of food composition tables, such as nutrient losses during food storage and preparation. Respondents collect identical portions of all foods and beverages consumed during a specified period, which are then analyzed for nutrient content. Respondent concern about the expense of duplicate portions can alter eating habits, resulting in underestimates of nutrient intake.

7. Food accounts estimate dietary intake within households and institutions where congregate feeding is practiced. The food inventory at the end of the survey period is subtracted from the sum of the beginning inventory and food obtained during the study period. Daily mean consumption per person is calculated by dividing total food consumed by number of meals served. This is a relatively economical method of assessing dietary intake of large groups. It does not account for food losses or meals eaten outside the group and cannot provide estimates of individual food intake.

8. The food balance sheet provides data on food disappearance (or availability) rather than actual food consumption. Mean per capita annual amounts are calculated by dividing total food disappearance by the country's population. It detects trends in food availability within a country over time and generates data that are useful in epidemiologic research across countries. The data represent only food that disappeared from the food distribution system and may be of questionable accuracy.

9. The high cost of research has led to innovations in the collection of dietary intake data. Included among these are telephone interviewing, analyzing images of meals submitted by respondents, and Internet-based administration of 24-hour recalls and food frequency questionnaires. Some of these methods have the potential for reducing respondent burden and increasing the validity of dietary intake data and the cost-effectiveness of collecting such data.

10. Surrogate sources are necessary when intake data are needed from persons unwilling or unable to provide them. Potential surrogate respondents include the spouse, partner, children, other close relatives, and friends of the respondent.

11. Validity is the ability of an instrument to measure what it is intended to measure. Validating a method involves comparing measurements of intake obtained by that method with estimates obtained using another method that is thought to have a greater degree of demonstrated, or face, validity. Some biological markers can provide a validity check of dietary intake independent of respondents' accuracy and truthfulness.

12. Reproducibility, or reliability, is the ability of a method to produce the same estimate on two or more occasions, assuming that nothing has changed in the interim. Reproducibility studies are important in partially answering the validity question; a method cannot give a correct answer every time unless it gives approximately the same answer each time.

13. Estimates of portion sizes can be sources of error in measuring dietary intake. A number of tools have been developed to assist respondents in accurately reporting amounts of foods consumed. These include photographs of food, geometric shapes of various sizes, measuring devices, and lifelike plastic food models.

REFERENCES

1. Van Saveren WA, Ocké MC. 2006. Estimation of dietary intake. In Bowman BA, Russell RM (eds.), *Present knowledge in nutrition,* 9th ed. Washington, DC: ILSI Press, 795–806.

2. Stamler J. 1994. Assessing diets to improve world health: Nutritional research on disease causation in populations. *American Journal of Clinical Nutrition* 59(suppl): 146S–156S.

3. Sabry JH. 1988. Purposes of food consumption surveys. In Cameron ME, Van Staveren WA (eds.), *Manual on methodology for food consumption studies.* New York: Oxford University Press.

4. Carroll RJ, Freedman LS, Hartman AM. 1996. Use of semiquantitative food frequency questionnaires to estimate the distribution of usual intake. *American Journal of Epidemiology* 143:392–404.

5. Carmichael SL, Yang W, Feldkamp ML, Munger RG, Siega-Riz AM, Botto LD, Shaw G. 2012. Reduced risks of neural tube defects and orofacial clefts with higher diet quality. *Archives of Pediatric and Adolescent Medicine* 166:121–126.

6. Thompson FE, Subar AF. 2008. Dietary assessment methodology. In Coulston AM, Boushey CJ (eds.), *Nutrition in the prevention and treatment of disease,* 2nd ed. San Diego: Academic Press, 3–39.

7. Subar AF, Crafts J, Zimmerman TP, Wilson M, Mittl B, Islam NG, McNutt S, Potischman N, Buday R, Hull SG, Baranowski T, Guenther PM, Willis G, Tapia R, Thompson FE. 2010. Assessment of the accuracy of portion size reports using computer-based food photographs aids in the development of an automated self-administered 24-hour recall. *Journal of the American Dietetic Association* 110:55–64.

8. Thompson FE, Dixit-Joshi S, Potischman N, Dodd KW, Kirkpatrick SI, Kushi LH, Alexander GL, Coleman LA, Zimmerman TP, Sundaram ME, Clancy HA, Groesbeck M, Douglass D, George SM, Schap TE, Subar AF. 2015. Comparison of interviewer-administered and automated self-administered 24-hour dietary recalls in 3 diverse integrated health systems. *American Journal of Epidemiology* 181:970–978.

9. Ngo J, Engelen A, Molag M, Roesle J, Garcia-Segovia P. 2009. A review of the use of information and communication technologies for dietary assessment. *British Journal of Nutrition* 101:S102–S112.

10. Johnson RK, Driscoll P, Goran MI. 1996. Comparison of multiple-pass 24-hour recall estimates of energy intake with total energy expenditure determined by the doubly labeled water method in young children. *Journal of the American Dietetic Association* 96:1140–1144.

11. McNutt S, Hall J, Cranston B, Soto P, Hults S. 2000. The 24-hour dietary recall data collection and coding methodology implemented for the 1999–2000 National Health and Nutrition Examination Survey. *FASEB Journal* 14:A759.

12. England CY, Andrews RC, Jago R, Thompson JL. 2015. A systematic review of brief dietary questionnaires suitable for clinical use in the prevention and management of obesity, cardiovascular disease and type 2 diabetes. *European Journal of Clinical Nutrition* 69:977–1003.

13. Thompson FE, Subar AF, Smith AF, Midthune D, Radimer KL, Kahle LL, Kipnis V. 2002. Fruit and vegetable assessment: Performance of 2 new short instruments and a food frequency questionnaire. *Journal of the American Dietetic Association* 102:1764–1772.

14. National Institutes of Health. 2001. *Third report of the Expert Panel on Detection, Evaluation, and Treatment of High Blood Cholesterol in Adults.* Washington, DC: National Institutes of Health, National Heart, Lung, and Blood Institute.

15. Kris-Etherton P, Eissenstat B, Jaax S, Srinath U, Scott L, Rader J, Pearson T. 2001. Validation for MEDFICTS: A dietary assessment instrument for evaluating adherence to total and saturated fat recommendations of the National Cholesterol Education Program step 1 and step 2 diets. *Journal of the American Dietetic Association* 101:81–86.

16. Srinath U, Shacklock F, Scott LW, Jaax S, Kris-Etherton PM. 1993. Development of MEDFICTS: A dietary assessment instrument for evaluating fat, saturated fat, and cholesterol intake. *Journal of the American Dietetic Association* 93:A105.

17. Willett WC, Sampson L, Stampfer MJ, Rosner B, Bain C, Witschi J, Hennekens CH, Speizer FE. 1985. Reproducibility and validity of a semiquantitative food frequency questionnaire. *American Journal of Epidemiology* 122:51–65.

18. Feskanich D, Rimm EB, Giovannucci EL, Colditz GA, Stampfer MJ, Litin LB, Willett WC. 1993. Reproducibility and validity of food intake measurements from a semiquantitative food frequency questionnaire. *Journal of the American Dietetic Association* 93:790–796.

19. Willett WC. 1998. *Nutritional epidemiology,* 2nd ed. New York: Oxford University Press.

20. Rimm EB, Giovannucci EL, Stampfer MJ, Colditz GA, Litin LB, Willett WC. 1992. Reproducibility and validity of an expanded self-administered semiquantitative food frequency questionnaire among male health professionals. *American Journal of Epidemiology* 135:1114–1126.

21. Munger RG, Folsom AR, Kushi LH, Kaye SA, Sellers TA. 1992. Dietary assessment of older Iowa women with a food frequency questionnaire: Nutrient intake, reproducibility, and

comparison with 24-hour dietary recall interviews. *American Journal of Epidemiology* 136:192–200.

22. Thompson FE, Subar AF, Brown CC, Smith AF, Sharbaugh CO, Jobe JB, Mittl B, Gibson JT, Ziegler RG. 2002. Cognitive research enhances accuracy of food frequency questionnaire reports: Results of an experimental validation study. *Journal of the American Dietetic Association* 102:212–218, 223–225.

23. Subar AF, Thompson FE, Kipnis V, Midthune D, Hurwitz P, McNutt S, McIntosh A, Rosenfeld S. 2001. Comparative validation of the Block, Willett, and National Cancer Institute food frequency questionnaires: The Eating at America's Table Study. *American Journal of Epidemiology* 154:1089–1099.

24. National Cancer Institute, Risk Factor Monitoring and Methods. http://riskfactor.cancer.gov/dhq2/.

25. Subar AF, Dodd KW, Guenther PM, Kipnis V, Midthune D, McDowell M, Tooze JA, Freedman LS, Krebs-Smith SM. 2006. The food propensity questionnaire: Concept, development, and validation for use as a covariate in a model to estimate usual food intake. *Journal of the American Dietetic Association* 106:1556–1563.

26. Tooze JA, Midthune D, Dodd KW, Freedman LS, Krebs-Smith SM, Subar AF, Guenther PM, Carroll RJ, Kipnis V. 2006. A new statistical method for estimating the usual intake of episodically consumed foods with application to their distribution. *Journal of the American Dietetic Association* 106:1575–1587.

27. Tooze JA, Kipnis V, Buckman DW, Carroll RJ, Freedman LS, Guenther PM, Krebs-Smith SM, Subar AF, Dodd KW. 2010. A mixed-effects model approach for estimating the distribution of usual intake of nutrients: The NCI method. *Statistics in Medicine* 29:2857–2868.

28. Byers T. 2001. Food frequency dietary assessment: How bad is good enough? *American Journal of Epidemiology* 154:1087–1088.

29. Willett W. 2001. Invited commentary: A further look at dietary questionnaire validation. *American Journal of Epidemiology* 154:1100–1102.

30. Archer E, Pavela G, Lavie CJ. 2015. The inadmissibility of What We Eat in America and NHANES dietary data in nutrition and obesity research and the scientific formulation of national dietary guidelines. *Mayo Clinics Proceedings* 90:911–926.

31. Schaefer EJ, Augustin JL, Schaefer MM, Rasmussen H, Ordovas JM, Dallal GE, Dwyer JT. 2000. Lack of efficacy of a food-frequency questionnaire in assessing dietary macronutrient intakes in subjects consuming diets of known composition. *American Journal of Clinical Nutrition* 71:746–751.

32. Subar AF, Freedman LS, Tooze JA, Kirkpatrick SI, Boushey C, Neuhouser MI, Thompson FE, Potischman N, Guenther PM, Tarasuk V, Reedy J, Krebs-Smith SM. 2015. Addressing current criticism regarding the value of self-report dietary data. *Journal of Nutrition* 145:2639–2645.

33. Smith AF. 1991. Cognitive processes in long-term dietary recall. *Vital and Health Statistics* 6(4). Hyattsville, MD: National Center for Health Statistics.

34. Willett WC. 1994. Future directions in the development of food-frequency questionnaires. *American Journal of Clinical Nutrition* 59(suppl):171S–174S.

35. Burke BS. 1947. The dietary history as a tool in research. *Journal of the American Dietetic Association* 23:1041–1046.

36. Kim WW, Mertz W, Judd JT, Marshall MW, Kelsay JL, Prather ES. 1984. Effect of making duplicate food collections on nutrient intakes calculated from diet records. *American Journal of Clinical Nutrition* 40:1333–1337.

37. Mertz W. 1992. Food intake measurements: Is there a "gold standard?" *Journal of the American Dietetic Association* 82:1463–1465.

38. Pekkarinen M. 1970. Methodology in the collection of food consumption data. *World Review of Nutrition and Dietetics* 12:145–171.

39. Casey PH, Goolsby SLP, Lensig SY, Perloff BP, Bogle ML. 1999. The use of telephone interview methodology to obtain 24-hour dietary recalls. *Journal of the American Dietetic Association* 99:1406–1411.

40. Tran KM, Johnson RK, Soultanakis RP, Matthews DE. 2000. In-person vs. telephone administered multiple-pass 24-hour recalls in women: Validation with doubly labeled water. *Journal of the American Dietetic Association* 100:777–780, 783.

41. Van Horn LV, Gernhofer N, Moag-Stahlberg A, Ferris R, Hartmuller G, Lasser VI, Stumbo P, Craddick S, Ballew C. 1990. Dietary assessment in children using electronic methods: Telephones and tape recorders. *Journal of the American Dietetic Association* 90:412–416.

42. Dubois S, Boivin JF. 1990. Accuracy of telephone dietary recalls in elderly subjects. *Journal of the American Dietetic Association* 90:1680–1687.

43. Blumberg SJ, Luke JV. December 2015. Wireless substitution: Early release of estimates from the National Health Interview Survey, January–June 2015. National Center for Health Statistics. Available from: http://www.cdc.gov/nchs/nhis.htm.

44. McBride J. 2001. Was it a slab, a slice, or a sliver? *Agricultural Research* 49(3):4–7.

45. Ahluwalia N, Dwyer J, Terry A, Moshfegh A, Johnson C. 2016. Update on NHANES dietary data: Focus on collection, release, analytical considerations, and uses to inform public policy. *Advances in Nutrition* 7(1):121–134.

46. Long JD, Littlefield LA, Estep G, Martin H, Rogers TJ, Boswell C, Shriver BJ, Roman-Shriver CR. 2010. Evidence review of technology and dietary assessment. *Worldviews on Evidence-Based Nursing* 7:191–204.

47. Thompson FE, Subar AF, Loria CM, Reedy JL, Baranowski T. 2010. Need for technological innovation in dietary assessment. *Journal of the American Dietetic Association* 110:48–51.

48. Fong AKH, Kretsch MJ. 1990. Nutrition evaluation scale system reduces time and labor in recording quantitative

dietary intake. *Journal of the American Dietetic Association* 90:664–670.

49. Kretsch MJ, Fong AKH. 1990. Validation of a new computerized technique for quantitating individual dietary intake: The Nutrition Evaluation Scale System (NESSy) vs. the weighed food record. *American Journal of Clinical Nutrition* 51:477–484.

50. Weiss R, Fong AKH, Kretsch MJ. 2003. Adapting ProNutra to interactively track food weights from an electronic scale using ProNESSy. *Journal of Food Composition and Analysis* 16:305–311.

51. Weiss R, Stumbo PJ, Divakaran A. 2010. Automatic food documentation and volume computation using digital imaging and electronic transmission. *Journal of the American Dietetic Association* 101:42–44.

52. Boushey CJ, Kerr DA, Wright J, Lutes KD, Ebert DS, Delp EJ. 2009. Use of technology in children's dietary assessment. *European Journal of Clinical Nutrition* 63:S50–S57.

53. Six BL, Schap TE, Zhu FM, Mariappan A, Bosch M, Delp EJ, Ebert DS, Kerr DA, Boushey CJ. 2010. Evidence-based development of a mobile telephone food record. *Journal of the American Dietetic Association* 110:74–79.

54. Sun M, Fernstrom JD, Jia W, Hackworth SA, Yao N, Li Y, Li C, Fernstrom MH, Sclabassi RJ. 2010. A wearable electronic system for objective dietary assessment. *Journal of the American Dietetic Association* 110:45–47.

55. Wang D, Kogashiwa M, Kira S. 2007. Development of a new instrument for evaluating individual's dietary intakes. *Journal of the American Dietetic Association* 106:1588–1593.

56. Gemming L, Rush E, Maddison R, Doherty A, Gant N, Utter J, Ni Mhurchu C. 2015. Wearable cameras can reduce dietary under-reporting: Doubly labelled water validation of a camera-assisted 24 h recall. *British Journal of Nutrition* 113:284–291.

57. Gemming L, Utter J, Ni Mhurchu C. 2015. Image-assisted dietary assessment: A systematic review of the evidence. *Journal of the Academy of Nutrition and Dietetics* 115:64–77.

58. Samet JM. 1989. Surrogate measures of dietary intake. *American Journal of Clinical Nutrition* 50:1139–1144.

59. Sudo N, Perry C, Reicks M. 2010. Adequacy of dietary intake information obtained from mailed food records differed by weight status and not education level of midlife women. *Journal of the American Dietetic Association* 101:95–100.

60. Scagliusi FB, Ferriolli E, Laureano C, Cunha CSF, Gualano B, Lourenco BH, Lancha AH. 2009. Characteristics of women who frequently under report their energy intake: A doubly labeled water study. *European Journal of Clinical Nutrition* 63:1192–1199.

61. Trabulsi J, Schoeller DA. 2001. Evaluation of dietary assessment instruments against doubly labeled water, a biomarker of habitual energy intake. *American Journal of Physiology—Endocrinology and Metabolism* 281:E891–E899.

62. Hodson L, Skeaff CM, Fielding BA. 2008. Fatty acid composition of adipose tissue and blood in humans and its use as a biomarker of dietary intake. *Progress in Lipid Research* 27:348–380.

63. Overby NC, Serra-Majem L, Andersen LF. 2009. Dietary assessment methods on n-3 fatty acid intakes: A systematic review. *British Journal of Nutrition* 102:S56–S63.

64. Satia-Abouta J, Patterson RE, King IB, Stratton KL, Shattuck AL, Kristal AR, Potter JD, Thornquist MD, White E. 2003. Reliability and validity of self-report of vitamin and mineral supplement use in the Vitamins and Lifestyle Study. *American Journal of Epidemiology* 157:944–954.

65. Day NE, McKeown, Yong MY, Welch A, Bingham S. 2001. Epidemiological assessment of diet: A comparison of a 7-day diary with a food frequency questionnaire using urinary markers of nitrogen, potassium, and sodium. *International Journal of Epidemiology* 30:309–317.

66. Bingham SA. 1994. The use of 24-h urine samples and energy expenditure to validate dietary assessments. *American Journal of Clinical Nutrition* 59(suppl):227S–231S.

67. McNaughton SA, Marks GC, Gaffney P, Williams G, Green A. 2005. Validation of a foodfrequency questionnaire of carotenoid and vitamin E intake using weighed food records and plasma biomarkers: The method of triads model. *European Journal of Clinical Nutrition* 59:211–218.

68. Speakman JR. 1998. The history and theory of doubly labeled water technique. *American Journal of Clinical Nutrition* 68(suppl):932S–938S.

69. Burrows TL, Martin RJ, Collins CE. 2010. A systematic review of the validity of dietary assessment methods in children when compared with the method of doubly labeled water. *Journal of the American Dietetic Association* 101:1501–1510.

70. Jones PJH, Jacobs I, Morris A, Duchmarme MB. 1993. Adequacy of food rations in soldiers during an Arctic exercise measured by doubly labeled water. *Journal of Applied Physiology* 75:1790–1797.

71. Martin LJ, Su W, Jones PJ, Lockwood GA, Tritchler DL, Boyd NF. 1996. Comparison of energy intakes determined by food records and doubly labeled water in women participating in a dietary-intervention trial. *American Journal of Clinical Nutrition* 63:483–490.

72. Goris AHC, Westerterp-Plantenga MS, Westerterp KR. 2000. Undereating and underrecording of habitual food intake in obese men: Selective underreporting of fat intake. *American Journal of Clinical Nutrition* 71:130–134.

73. Johnson RK, Soultanakis RP, Matthews DE. 1998. Literacy and body fatness are associated with underreporting of energy intake in US low-income women using the multiple-pass 24-hour recall: A doubly labeled water study. *Journal of the American Dietetic Association* 98:1136–1140.

74. Champagne CM, Baker NB, DeLany JP, Harsha DW, Bray GA. 1998. Assessment of energy intake underreporting by doubly labeled water and observations on reported energy intake in children. *Journal of the American Dietetic Association* 98:426–430, 433.

75. Mertz W, Tsui JC, Judd JT, Reiser S, Hallfirsch J, Morris ER, Steele PD, Lashley E. 1991. What are people really eating? The relation between energy intake derived from estimated diet records and intake determined to maintain body weight. *American Journal of Clinical Nutrition* 54:291–295.

76. Freedman LS, Commins JM, Moler JE, Arab L, Baer DJ, Kipnis V, Midthune D, Moshfegh AJ, Neuhouser ML, Prentice RL, Schatzkin A, Spiegelman D, Subar AF, Tinker LF, Willett W. 2014. Pooled results from 5 validation studies of dietary self-report instruments using recovery biomarkers for energy and protein intake. *American Journal of Epidemiology* 180:172–188.

77. Briefel RR, Sempos CT, McDowell MA, Chien S, Alaimo K. 1997. Dietary methods research in the third National Health and Nutrition Examination Survey: Underreporting of energy intake. *American Journal of Clinical Nutrition* 65(suppl):1203S–1209S.

78. Kretsch MJ, Fong AKH, Green MW. 1999. Behavioral and body size correlates of energy intake underreporting by obese and normal-weight women. *Journal of the American Dietetic Association* 99:300–306.

79. Schoeller DA. 1999. Recent advances from application of doubly labeled water to measurement of human energy expenditure. *Journal of Nutrition* 129:1765–1768.

80. Kubena KS. 2000. Accuracy in dietary assessment: On the road to good science. *Journal of the American Dietetic Association* 100:775–776.

81. Posner BM, Smigelski C, Duggal A, Morgan JL, Cobb J, Cupples A. 1992. Validation of two dimensional models for estimating portion size in nutrition research. *Journal of the American Dietetic Association* 92:738–741.

82. Toobert DJ, Strycker LA, Hampson SE, Westling E, Christiansen SM, Hurley TG, Herbert JR. 2011. Computerized portion-size estimation compared to multiple 24-hour dietary recalls for measurement of fat, fruit, and vegetable intake in overweight adults. *Journal of the American Dietetic Association* 111:1578–1583.

ASSESSMENT ACTIVITY 3.1

Collecting a 24-Hour Recall

The 24-hour recall is probably the most commonly used technique for measuring diet. Consequently, it is important that health professionals involved in nutritional assessment understand, practice, and master this technique. In this assessment activity, you will collect a 24-hour recall from a classmate and calculate that person's intake of kilocalories, protein, carbohydrate, total fat, calcium, and iron from a food composition table. Be sure to have a classmate collect a 24-hour recall from you, too. This will provide you with additional experience with recalls. You also will need your own 24-hour recall for an assessment activity in Chapter 5.

This assessment activity also will help you become more familiar with using food composition tables. Experience in using food composition tables is valuable. Sometimes it is faster and easier to refer to a food composition table for a nutrient value than to use a computer. Familiarity with food composition tables will also make that task easier.

1. For this assessment activity, we suggest you use a photocopy of the form provided with this activity. It not only provides space for recording the names and quantities of foods and beverages consumed, but it also allows you to easily record values for energy and nutrients for reported foods.

2. Familiarize yourself with the form *before* beginning your interview. Enter the name of the person being interviewed and the day and date.

3. After completing the recall form, manually calculate the intakes of kilocalories, protein, carbohydrate, total fat, calcium, and iron, using the food composition table in Home and Garden Bulletin 72. This can be downloaded free at: https://www.ars.usda.gov/ARSUserFiles/80400525/Data/hg72/hg72_2002.pdf. If you cannot find a particular food or beverage in the food composition table, use a similar food or beverage or refer to another food composition table.

4. As you do this assignment, think about the following questions:
   How representative of your respondent's usual dietary intake is this one day of intake data?
   Did you have any difficulty finding any foods in the food composition table?
   If you had to substitute one food for another, how do you think that substitution affected the total nutrient values?

24-Hour Recording Form for Assessment Activity 3.1

Name of person interviewed _____ **Date** _____ **Day of week** _____

Food/Drink	Type/How Prepared	Quantity	Kilocalories	Protein	Carbohydrate	Total Fat	Calcium	Iron
Total								

ASSESSMENT ACTIVITY 3.2

Completing a Three-Day Food Record

Obtaining dietary intake data that are representative of the usual intake of *individuals* requires data from multiple days.

In this assignment, you will complete a three-day food record on yourself using the food diary recording form in Appendix A or one provided by your professor.

1. Familiarize yourself with the form in Appendix A and accompanying instructions *before* beginning your diary.

2. Record your food and beverage intake for two weekdays (Monday through Friday) and one weekend day (Saturday or Sunday). Because most people eat differently on weekend days than on weekdays, this will make your record more representative of your usual intake throughout the entire week.

3. Do not alter your normal diet during the recording period. Provide responses that are as accurate as possible. Record your food and beverage intake as soon after eating as possible.

4. You may save your completed food record for later analysis using diet analysis software.

ASSESSMENT ACTIVITY 3.3

Diet History Questionnaire

Compared with other techniques for measuring diet, food frequency questionnaires are a recent development. There is considerable interest in food frequency questionnaires as a relatively simple and inexpensive approach to characterizing the usual food and nutrient intake of individuals. A food frequency questionnaire developed by researchers at the U.S. National Cancer Institute (NCI) and used in several epidemiologic studies sponsored by the NCI is the Diet History Questionnaire (DHQ). The DHQ is explained in greater detail in this chapter. The DHQ is shown in Appendix D, and the entire questionnaire can be downloaded from the website of the NCI (http://epi.grants.cancer.gov/dhq2/forms/). In addition, a Web-based version of the DHQ named the DHQ*Web is available for use by the public at no cost and can be accessed through the website of the NCI.

Instructors may wish to administer the DHQ to students and use the software to process the questionnaires to develop nutrient intake data for discussion purposes. Instructors can also have their students complete the DHQ online using the DHQ*Web version of the questionnaire. A request for a study must be made by the instructor two weeks before planned use of DHQ (dhq@imsweb.com). Data from either the paper-and-pencil or Web-based versions can then be compared with national averages. Output from multiple groups of students from different disciplines could be compared to see if significant differences in food and nutrient intake exist along different groups of students.

ASSESSMENT ACTIVITY 3.4

The Automated Self-Administered 24-Hour Recall (ASA24)

The Automated Self-Administered 24-hour Recall (ASA24) is an Internet-based automated self-administered 24-hour dietary recall application developed by the National Cancer Institute (http://epi.grants.cancer.gov/asa24/). The ASA24 uses technology drawn from the USDA's Automated Multiple-Pass Method to provide a Web-based tool to researchers, educators, and the public for collecting multiple automated self-administered

24-hour recalls. Anyone interested in seeing how the ASA24 works can enter a 24-hour recall at a demonstration website for respondents. The demonstration version will not save any recall data or provide any dietary analyses. The full version of ASA24 is available only to registered users at a researcher website, which allows researchers, clinicians, and teachers to register a study and obtain dietary analyses. For example, a teacher could register students in a nutritional assessment course who would be given the assignment of entering two or more 24-hour recalls over a specified period of time. This activity would provide real-life experience in the administration of 24-hour recalls and an exposure to how technology is changing the collection of dietary intake data. The ASA24 website can be found at https://asa24.nci.nih.gov/demo/.

ASSESSMENT ACTIVITY 3.5

Dietary Screeners

Brief dietary assessment tools, dietary screeners, or short, targeted food frequency questionnaires are quick and easy to use, are simple to score, and provide focused information that can be used in the management of obesity and chronic disease.

Go to the following website and fill in the "Fat Intake Screener" and "Fruit, Vegetable, and Fiber Screener."

https://fnic.nal.usda.gov/dietary-guidance/individual-dietary-assessment

Print out the two reports, bring them to class, and discuss them with your classmates and instructor.

NATIONAL DIETARY AND NUTRITION SURVEYS

STUDENT LEARNING OUTCOMES

After studying this chapter, the student will be able to:

1. Discuss the goals and objectives of the National Nutrition Monitoring and Related Research Program.

2. Compare and contrast the roles of the two U.S. federal agencies primarily involved in nutritional monitoring activities in the United States.

3. Distinguish between nutritional monitoring activities conducted by the HHS and those conducted by the USDA, when presented with a list of surveys.

4. Discuss the USDA's role in collecting data on food availability, individual food and nutrient consumption, and attitudes and knowledge about diet and health.

5. Discuss the HHS's role in collecting data on individual food and nutrient consumption, health status, and exposure to pesticide residues, industrial chemicals, and radionuclides.

6. Describe the concept of the Mobile Examination Center and how it is used in conducting NHANES.

7. Name the methods used to collect dietary intake data in NHANES.

8. Compare and contrast estimates of food consumption based on annual per capita food availability data and data collected by direct survey methods.

9. Discuss the role and significance of the survey What We Eat in America, NHANES.

10. Demonstrate the ability to access online sources of diet and health survey data.

INTRODUCTION

Nutritional monitoring is an important activity for any government serious about promoting its citizens' health. The principle goal of nutritional monitoring is to accurately measure the dietary and nutritional status of a population and the quality, quantity, and safety of the food it consumes.[1] Data on the nutritional and health status of a population that are generated by nutritional monitoring are used for many purposes. They can identify nutritional problems of the country as a whole (e.g., excessive fat and cholesterol consumption) and groups at nutritional risk (e.g., low calcium intake by adolescent females). These data are used to justify changes in government policy and the spending of billions of dollars for planning and implementing programs related to food, nutrition, and health promotion, such as the Special Supplemental Nutrition Program for Women, Infants, and Children (WIC) and the Supplemental Nutrition Assistance Program (SNAP). They are important in evaluating the cost-effectiveness of such programs, particularly when voters and legislators express concern about escalating budget deficits, controlling the high cost of government, cutting taxes, or limiting government involvement in issues related to diet and health. These data are also critical to research into the relationships between nutrition and health. This chapter discusses nutritional monitoring in the United States and the most important surveys comprising the federal government's nutrition and health surveillance activities. It also discusses the major findings of these surveys.

IMPORTANCE OF NATIONAL DIETARY AND NUTRITION SURVEYS

National dietary and nutrition surveys have a number of important functions. They can show how food supplies are distributed according to such demographic factors as region, income, sex, race, and ethnicity. Survey data are important in monitoring nutritional status of a country's population. By observing trends in the health and dietary practices of a population, relationships between diet and health can be elucidated. They identify groups that are at nutritional risk and that may benefit from food assistance programs. They are important for developing the Thrifty Food Plan, which forms the basis for determining benefit levels for participants of SNAP, formerly the Food Stamp program. They are also used for evaluating the effectiveness of various USDA food assistance programs. For example, a before-and-after comparison of food consumption practices by SNAP participants revealed that the program allowed families to purchase more nutritious foods and increased the market for surplus agricultural products. After analyzing nutritional and health survey data, the U.S. Government Accountability Office, or GAO, reported that women participating in the WIC

program had a 25% reduction in low birth weight births (under 2500 g, or 5.5 lb) and a 44% reduction in very low birth weight births (under 1500 g, or 3.3 lb) compared with similar women not participating in the WIC program.[2] The Government Accountability Office estimated that, for each tax dollar spent on WIC benefits, nearly $3.00 were saved within the first year by federal, state, and local governments and private insurance companies in reduced health-care costs and special education. These and other uses of data from nutrition and health surveys are summarized in Box 4.1.

Data from dietary surveys can be used to track food consumption trends over time, examine current dietary practices of specific groups of people, and monitor average intakes of pesticides, toxic substances, radioactive substances, and industrial chemicals. Studies of nutritional status allow monitoring of the general health of a population through health and medical histories, dietary interviews, physical examinations, and laboratory measurements.[3]

Dietary and nutrition surveys are important to government agencies that supervise their country's agriculture and food industries. Data from surveys provide a sound basis for developing policies and programs related to agricultural production, marketing agricultural products, projecting supply and demand, and determining the adequacy of the available food supply.[4] These data provide early warning of impending food shortages and can indicate how such crises may be prevented or alleviated.[5] They have been used to develop the Dietary Guidelines for Americans and the nutrition and related health objectives included in *Healthy People 2020*.

Using food balance sheets (see Chapter 3), a government can estimate the "disappearance" of food from its food distribution system and thus arrive at an indirect and rough estimate of food consumption by its citizens. Data on food disappearance or "availability" do not measure actual food consumption, only what enters and leaves the food distribution system. However, these data allow comparisons among different countries and the creation of a world food picture. These comparisons, in turn, can serve as the basis for the formulation of international policies designed to improve the world food and nutrition situation and prevent imbalances in dietary standards among countries.[6]

NUTRITIONAL MONITORING IN THE UNITED STATES

Nutritional monitoring can be defined as "the assessment of dietary or nutritional status at intermittent times with the aim of detecting changes in the dietary or nutritional status of a population."[7] It involves data collection and data analysis in five general areas:

- Nutritional and health status measurements
- Food consumption measurements

Box 4.1   **Uses of Data from Nutrition and Health Surveys**

PUBLIC POLICY

Monitoring Surveillance

- Identify high-risk groups and geographic areas with nutrition-related problems to facilitate implementation of public health intervention programs and food assistance programs
- Evaluate changes in agricultural policy that may affect the nutritional quality and healthfulness of the U.S. food supply
- Assess progress toward achieving the nutrition objectives in *Healthy People 2020*
- Evaluate the effectiveness of nutritional initiatives of military feeding systems
- Report health and nutrition data from state-based programs to comply with federal administrative program requirements
- Monitor food production and marketing

Nutrition-Related Programs

- Nutrition education and dietary guidance (Dietary Guidelines for Americans)
- Food assistance programs

- Nutrition intervention programs
- Public health programs

Regulatory

- Food labeling
- Food fortification
- Food safety
- Inform policy development (e.g., nutrients of public health concern such as sodium, added sugars, caffeine, *trans* fatty acids, saturated fat

SCIENTIFIC RESEARCH

- Nutrient requirements (Dietary Reference Intakes)
- Diet-health relationships
- Knowledge and attitudes and their relationship to dietary and health behavior
- Nutritional monitoring research—national and international
- Food composition analysis
- Economic aspects of food consumption
- Nutrition education research

Source: Ahluwalia N, Dwyer J, Terry A, Moshfegh A, Johnson C. 2016. Update on NHANES dietary data: Focus on collection, release, analytical considerations, and uses to inform public policy. *Advances in Nutrition* 7:121–134.

- Food composition measurement and nutrient data banks
- Dietary knowledge, behavior, and attitude assessments
- Food supply and demand determinations[1]

Since about the middle of the 20th century, the U.S. government has sought to obtain objective data on which to base decisions regarding nutrition-related public policies. Initially, this was done by the U.S. Department of Agriculture (USDA), which collected food disappearance data and began conducting national household food consumption surveys. In the latter part of the 20th century, the USDA abandoned household food consumption surveys and began conducting a cross-sectional survey of food intakes of individuals that eventually became known as the Continuing Survey of Food Intakes by Individuals. In the 1960s, the U.S. Department of Health and Human Services (DHHS) began conducting their own cross-sectional surveys of the health and nutritional status of the U.S. population, which evolved into the National Health and Nutrition Examination Surveys.[8] Some nutritional monitoring activities are conducted at the state level, providing state-specific data on nutritional and health status that may not be available from national surveys. Many of these state activities are supported and coordinated by federal agencies, such as the USDA, CDC, and HHS.

NATIONAL NUTRITIONAL MONITORING AND RELATED RESEARCH PROGRAM

As early as 1971, Congress, the nutrition community, various private groups, and expert panels expressed concern about problems with the federal government's nutritional monitoring program and the lack of coordination between the USDA and HHS. Issues were raised about the frequency and costs of data collected by the two agencies, delays in reporting data, the low response rates seen in some surveys, and, in certain instances, the poor quality of data.[1,8–10] Problems in the two agencies' nutritional monitoring activities were addressed by a number of reports by the National Research Council, the Federation of American Societies for Experimental Biology, and the Government Accountability Office (a research arm of Congress that audits government programs and highlights areas of waste and fraud). These reports called for the agencies to develop better methods for collecting dietary intake data, to use standardized data collection techniques that allow data to be compared across the different surveys, and to improve coverage of groups at nutritional risk, such as pregnant and lactating women, infants, preschool children, adolescents, and older persons.[1]

Recognition of the need to improve nutrition monitoring led to passage of the National Nutrition Monitoring and Related Research Act of 1990 (PL 101–445). This legislation required the secretaries of the USDA and HHS to prepare and implement a comprehensive 10-year plan for integrating the nutritional monitoring activities of the two agencies. This 10-year coordinated effort was called the National Nutrition Monitoring and Related Research Program (NNMRRP).[1,11] The legislation also calls for the creation of an Interagency Board for Nutrition Monitoring and Related Research and a National Nutrition Monitoring Advisory Council.

The NNMRRP coordinates the nutrition monitoring activities of numerous federal agencies under the joint direction of the USDA and HHS. The program encompasses a group of more than 50 surveys and surveillance activities assessing the health and nutritional status of the U.S. population.[12] The program's goal is to "establish a comprehensive nutrition monitoring and related research program for the federal government by collecting quality data that are continuous, coordinated, timely, and reliable; using comparable methods for data collection and reporting of results; and efficiently and effectively disseminating and exchanging information with data users."[11] Critical to the success of reaching this goal are three overall national objectives and three objectives addressing state and local nutrition monitoring efforts. The three national objectives are (1) to achieve continuous and coordinated data collection, (2) to improve the comparability and quality of data collected by the USDA and HHS, and (3) to improve the research base for nutrition monitoring. The three state and local objectives are (1) to develop and strengthen state and local capacities for continuous and coordinated data collection; (2) to improve methodologies to enhance comparability of NNMRRP data across federal, state, and local levels; and (3) to improve the quality of state and local nutrition monitoring data.[1,11] The NNMRRP also addresses the need for better nutrition monitoring information about selected population subgroups, more efficient and effective data dissemination to users, and better ways to meet the needs of data users.

To facilitate data dissemination, the National Nutrition Monitoring and Related Research Act of 1990 requires periodic publication of reports on the dietary, nutritional, and health-related status of the U.S. population. For example, every year the National Center for Health Statistics publishes *Health: United States.* This outstanding publication highlights and updates nutrition monitoring data, information, and research in a user-friendly format, using colorful graphics, extensive data tables, and brief narratives. To improve communication among data users, *The Directory of Federal and State Nutrition Monitoring and Related Research Activities* is periodically published by the Interagency Board for Nutrition Monitoring and Related Research. The directory contains information about federal and state nutrition monitoring activities, the sponsoring agency, contact persons, and the survey's purpose, date, target population, and design.[13]

Data collected through surveys are made available in a variety of forms, such as journal articles, government publications, and electronic files available for download from various government websites (see www.cdc.gov/nchs).

ROLE OF THE U.S. DEPARTMENT OF AGRICULTURE

The earliest efforts at nutritional monitoring in the United States were carried out by the USDA.[1,4,14] In the late 1800s and early 1900s, USDA researchers used the food inventory method to collect data on the amounts and costs of food consumed by a relatively small, nonrepresentative group of households. Between 1935 and 1948, the USDA conducted three nationwide, nonrepresentative surveys of food consumption at the household level. Beginning in 1955, the USDA began a series of four nationally representative surveys of food consumption at the household level. The first of these was the 1955 Household Food Consumption Survey (HFCS). This was followed by the 1965–66 HFCS, the 1977–78 Nationwide Food Consumption Survey (NFCS), and the 1987–88 NFCS; these three surveys also measured food intake by individual household members. Following the 1987–88 NFCS, the USDA discontinued the NFCS and its efforts to measure household food consumption and focused entirely on assessing individual food intake through the Continuing Survey of Food Intakes by Individuals (CSFII) and evaluating the dietary knowledge and attitudes of CSFII respondents through the Diet and Health Knowledge Survey. In 1998, the USDA initiated the Supplemental Children's Survey to the CSFII to provide a sample of sufficient size in order to adequately estimate exposure to pesticide residues in the diets of children. In 2002, the CSFII and the National Health and Nutrition Examination Survey (NHANES) were integrated, as discussed later in this chapter. The USDA also collects data on the amounts of food passing through the wholesale and retail food distribution system (called food availability data) and evaluates food security in America.

Food Availability

Since about the middle of the 20th century, the USDA has been developing annual estimates of the amount of food that is *available for consumption* from the U.S. food distribution system. Known as food availability data or per capita food availability, these data are based on the measurement of the amount of food moving through the domestic food production and distribution system from farms to all outlets: supermarkets, restaurants, and fast-food outlets.[15,16]

Per capita (per person) food availability is calculated by dividing the total amount of food available for consumption by the total number of people in the U.S. population.[16] These estimates have also been referred to as food disappearance data because they estimate the amount of food that disappears into the food marketing system.[15,16] It is important to note that food availability is not a direct measure of actual food consumption but, rather, an estimate of the amount of food that has left the wholesale and retail food distribution system, which includes foods eaten at home and away from home. Food availability data serve as a proxy, or substitute, for actual consumption and can only estimate the amount of food leaving the food distribution system. It is reasonable to assume that most, but not all, of the food leaving the food distribution system is consumed by people. Unless adjusted for losses due to food being discarded due to spoilage, or wasted or fed to animals, food availability data typically overstate the amount of foods and nutrients that people actually consume.[16,17]

Factors that led the USDA to begin compiling food availability data included a need to track food surpluses during World War I, legislation in the early 1930s to ensure an adequate food supply for domestic consumption during the Great Depression, and concerns about potential food shortages during the droughts of 1934 and 1936. Food availability data are valuable for monitoring the ability of the food supply to meet the nutritional needs of the U.S. population, for examining historical trends in food and nutrient consumption, and for evaluating changes in the American diet, especially in response to technological changes in agriculture and food processing. These data are helpful for determining whether federal enrichment and fortification standards are being met, monitoring how the food and agriculture industries are responding to the public's health concerns, and providing data for the development of dietary recommendations.[16] The USDA issued its first estimates of per capita food availability in 1941 to assess food requirements and supplies as America's entry into World War II was imminent. In 1949 the USDA was able to compile and publish data on per capita food availability for as far back as 1909, the first year for which reliable data were available.[4] Since then, estimates of per capita availability of major foods have been published annually with only a few exceptions. Historical series on per capita food availability were developed to analyze long-term trends, shifts in demand, and nutrients provided by foods.

Food availability data are derived using the **balance sheet approach** (discussed in Chapter 3) to track more than 250 agricultural commodities that are the major sources of food energy and nutrients for Americans. As shown in Figure 4.1, annual data on food exports, food not meant for human consumption (for example, livestock feed, seed, and food used for industrial purposes), military procurement, and year-end inventories are subtracted from data on beginning year inventories, total food production, and imports to arrive at an estimate of food available for domestic consumption.[3,4] This estimate then is divided by the U.S. population count to derive per capita availability of food. Per capita availability of energy and a number of nutrients is then calculated using food composition tables.[3,4] Food availability data reflect changes in overall patterns of food availability over time and have been the only source of information on food and nutrient trends since the beginning of the 20th century.[3,7,14,15] When used in conjunction with similar data developed in other countries, epidemiologists have been able to study the relationships between diet and disease. For example, scientists have investigated how different levels of dietary fat and cholesterol intake across countries relate to coronary heart disease death rates in those countries.[3] Food availability data also serve as a rough check on the reasonableness of results from household food consumption surveys.[4] Because data on per capita food availability are obtained directly from food producers and distributors instead of from individual consumers, they are not subject to the error in reporting that often is seen in consumer survey data. There are drawbacks to this approach, and per capita food availability data must be interpreted with care.[4,15,16] The estimates are largely based on data collected for purposes other than estimating food and nutrient intake and can vary considerably in adequacy, accuracy, and accessibility. They do not provide information relating to food consumption on a regional, household, or individual basis. Additionally, unless adjusted for losses, the estimates fail to account for food losses at the primary level (from farm to retail), losses at the retail level (for example, food at the supermarket that spoils or reaches its expiration date and is discarded), or losses at the consumer level, including at restaurants, at fast-food outlets, and in households (for example, disposal of inedible parts, spoiled food, plate waste, and food fed to pets and other animals).[16,17]

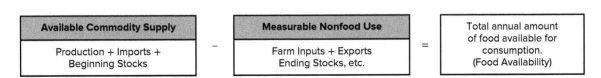

Figure 4.1 **How the food balance sheet approach is used to arrive at data on unadjusted food availability.**

Source: Gerrior S, Bente L, Hiza H. 2004. Nutrient content of the U.S. food supply, 1909–2000. *Home Economics Research Report No. 56.* Washington, DC: U.S. Department of Agriculture, Center for Nutrition Policy and Promotion.

ERS Food Availability (per Capita) Data System

The USDA's Economic Research Service (ERS) (www.ers. usda.gov) collects food availability data and makes them available to users through the ERS Food Availability (per Capita) Data System, which contains three related but separate series or sets of food availability data: Food Availability data, Loss-Adjusted Food Availability data, and Nutrient Availability data.[17] The Food Availability data series, which is the core set of data, is the only data set on the amount of food available for consumption in the United States, providing data extending as far back in time as 1909. In compiling these data, the ERS calculates the amounts of several hundred foods available for human consumption in the United States and provides estimates of per capita availability. For example, users can obtain data on pounds of red meat and poultry or gallons of fluid milk and cream available for domestic consumption per capita per year. Units of measurement depend on whether the commodity is a solid or a liquid. As shown in Figure 4.1, this series is compiled using data on production, imports, exports, beginning and ending stocks, and nonfood uses. Per capita estimates are arrived at by dividing the total amount of food available by the U.S. population for that year.[17]

In the mid-1990s, the ERS began an effort to make food availability data more useful by adjusting them for losses at the primary, retail, and consumer levels and converting the adjusted data into daily individual intake amounts and numbers of servings, which better represent what consumers actually eat.[17] Referred to as the Loss-Adjusted Food Availability data series, they are available in Excel spreadsheets from the ERS website beginning with data from 1970, the first year in the loss-adjusted data series. The spreadsheets provide estimated loss-adjusted data for per capita availability in pounds per year, calories available per day, and servings expressed as MyPyramid equivalents available per day. These estimates can then be compared with various dietary and nutrient intake standards to determine, for example, whether Americans are meeting the Dietary Guidelines for Americans for different food groups.[17] It is important to keep in mind that the loss-adjusted data do not directly measure actual consumption, but are useful for approximating what Americans eat on a daily basis.[17]

The process of adjusting the data for losses is based on several assumptions and limited research and documentation, which may result in the losses being understated or overstated. Food loss is difficult to measure, especially at the consumer level, given the fact that participants in household surveys on food waste often change their behavior during the survey period, failing to acknowledge or report the amount of food they typically discard or waste.[16,17]

The USDA Center for Nutrition Policy and Promotion (www.cnpp.usda.gov) is responsible for calculating nutrient availability data using the unadjusted food availability data from the ERS and data on the nutrient composition of foods from the USDA Nutrient Database for Standard Reference (discussed in Chapter 5). Nutrient availability data are provided in Excel spreadsheets from the ERS website for calories per capita per day of food energy and 27 nutrients and dietary components (for example, protein, carbohydrates, fats, vitamins, and minerals) in the U.S. food supply. Because these data are based on unadjusted food availability data, they likely overstate actual nutrient intake.[17] Per capita food and nutrient availability data are summarized in the "Dietary Trends" section of this chapter.

Continuing Survey of Food Intakes by Individuals

In 1985, the USDA began a national survey of individual dietary intake known as the *Continuing Survey of Food Intakes by Individuals (CSFII),* which was conducted during three time intervals, 1985–86, 1989–91, and 1994–96.[7,14] The CSFII replaced the NFCS as the USDA's primary survey for estimating individual food and nutrient intake.[1,14] The CSFII provided timely information on U.S. diets; allowed further study of the dietary habits of certain population groups thought to be at nutritional risk (e.g., low-income people); provided data on "usual" diets by measuring several days of data collected over the course of a year; and demonstrated how diets vary over time for individuals and groups of people.

In the 1985–86 CSFII, dietary intake data were collected using six 24-hour recalls that were obtained at approximately two-month intervals. This not only provided data somewhat more representative of usual dietary intake but also diminished seasonal influence on dietary intake because data were collected throughout the year. In the 1989–91 CSFII, data were collected using one 24-hour recall and a two-day food diary.

In the 1994–96 CSFII, popularly known as the *What We Eat in America* survey, data were collected using two multiple-pass 24-hour recalls administered in the home by trained interviewers. The recalls were conducted on 2 nonconsecutive days, 3 to 10 days apart.[7,14] A nationally representative sample of approximately 16,000 individuals of all ages from all 50 states participated in the survey. It sampled a disproportionately larger number of low-income people, young children, and older persons to better ascertain their dietary practices. This is known as "oversampling."

In 2002 the CSFII and the National Health and Nutrition Examination Survey (NHANES) were integrated, as discussed later in this chapter. Under the integrated framework, the USDA is responsible for the survey's dietary data collection methodology, maintenance of the database used to code and process the data, and data review and processing.[18]

Diet and Health Knowledge Survey

The Diet and Health Knowledge Survey (DHKS) measured the attitudes and knowledge of Americans about diet and health. It was initiated during the 1989–91 CSFII and conducted again during the 1994–96 CSFII but has not been conducted since then. The DHKS provided information about Americans' perceptions about the adequacy of their own food and nutrient intakes, the personal importance they placed on dietary guidance messages, their self-appraised weight status, the importance they placed on factors related to buying food, and the beliefs they held that influenced dietary behavior.[14] For example, 56% of respondents in the 1994–96 CSFII/DHKS reported that they thought their diet was "about right" in calcium. However, nearly two-thirds of these persons had a mean calcium intake less than the 1989 RDA for calcium. Among those adults reporting that their weight was "about right," 45% of adult males and 17% of adult females had a body mass index that placed them in the "overweight" or "obese" category, based on self-reported height and weight.

The DHKS was conducted after the CSFII was completed. For example, approximately two weeks after the second 24-hour recall was collected in the 1994–96 CSFII, a group of nearly 6000 persons ages 20 years and older were randomly selected by a computerized process from among all adults who had provided two days of dietary intake data. These persons were then contacted by telephone and asked to answer a series of questions on knowledge and attitudes about dietary guidance and health. Administering the DHKS shortly after the completion of the CSFII allowed individuals' attitudes and knowledge about healthy eating to be linked with their food choices and nutrient intakes.

The future of the DHKS has been uncertain after the integration of the CSFII and NHANES in 2002. Although some questions about health and diet behavior are included in the integrated survey, the DHKS has not been totally included in the current survey.

Supplemental Children's Survey

The purpose of the Supplemental Children's Survey was to collect dietary intake data from a representative group of children of sufficient size in order to estimate exposure to pesticide residues in the diets of American children. Between December 1997 and November 1998, two 24-hour recalls were collected from roughly 5000 children up to age 9 years. The recalls were obtained through in-person interviews on two nonconsecutive days. For infants and children under 6 years of age, a parent or knowledgeable caregiver was asked to provide the data. For children 6 to 9 years of age, the child was interviewed with adult assistance. In addition to the in-home 24-hour recall, interviewers contacted schools, baby-sitters, and day care providers for information about food eaten away from home.

The Supplemental Children's Survey was a response to concerns about pesticide residues in the diets of infants and children and the lack of good data to accurately assess youngsters' exposure to pesticide residues in the foods they were eating. Concerns about children's exposure to pesticides were heightened by a 1993 report of the National Academy of Sciences entitled "Pesticides in the Diets of Infants and Children." This report was instrumental in passage of the Food Quality Protection Act of 1996, which required the USDA to provide the Environmental Protection Agency with statistically valid information on the food consumption patterns of American infants and children, so that children's exposure to pesticide residues could be estimated with reasonable accuracy.

Food Insecurity and Hunger

Although hunger in North America does not compare in severity to that experienced by many in developing countries, it is a problem nevertheless. Hunger in North America has been a long-term concern of public health nutritionists on the continent and among some of the more enlightened and compassionate legislators and policy makers. However, it was only in the 1990s that the U.S. government actually developed a comprehensive national measure of the severity of food insecurity and hunger in the United States.[17] One of the mandates of the National Nutrition Monitoring and Related Research Program (NNMRRP) was that the USDA's Food and Nutrition Service and the DHHS's National Center for Health Statistics jointly develop "a standardized mechanism and instrument(s) for defining and obtaining data on the prevalence of 'food insecurity' or 'food insufficiency' in the U.S. and methodologies that can be used across the NNMRRP and at state and local levels." In response to this mandate, the USDA led a several-year collaborative effort to draft, pilot-test, and refine an instrument to measure the prevalence and severity of food insecurity and hunger in America, building on the prior work of several nongovernmental organizations.[5]

The USDA determines food security or food insecurity using responses to 18 questions (shown in Box 4.2) about conditions and behaviors known to characterize households having difficulty meeting basic food needs. Each question asks whether the condition or behavior occurred during the previous 12 months and whether the reason for the condition or behavior was a lack of money or other resources to obtain food.[19] For example, an interviewer would read the following statement: "We worried whether our food would run out before we got money to buy more." The interviewer would then ask whether, in the last 12 months, this was often, sometimes, or never true in the household. Or the interviewer would ask the following question: "In the last 12 months were you ever hungry, but didn't eat, because there wasn't enough money for food?"

Box 4.2

Questions Used by U.S. Department of Agriculture to Assess the Food Security of U.S. Households

1. "We worried whether our food would run out before we got money to buy more." Was that often, sometimes, or never true for you in the last 12 months?
2. "The food that we bought just didn't last and we didn't have money to get more." Was that often, sometimes, or never true for you in the last 12 months?
3. "We couldn't afford to eat balanced meals." Was that often, sometimes, or never true for you in the last 12 months?
4. In the last 12 months, did you or other adults in the household ever cut the size of your meals or skip meals because there wasn't enough money for food? (Yes/No)
5. (If yes to Question 4) How often did this happen—almost every month, some months but not every month, or in only 1 or 2 months?
6. In the last 12 months, did you ever eat less than you felt you should because there wasn't enough money for food? (Yes/No)
7. In the last 12 months, were you ever hungry, but didn't eat, because there wasn't enough money for food? (Yes/No)
8. In the last 12 months, did you lose weight because there wasn't enough money for food? (Yes/No)
9. In the last 12 months did you or other adults in your household ever not eat for a whole day because there wasn't enough money for food? (Yes/No)
10. (If yes to Question 9) How often did this happen—almost every month, some months but not every month, or in only 1 or 2 months?

(Questions 11–18 were asked only if the household included children age 0–17.)

11. "We relied on only a few kinds of low-cost food to feed our children because we were running out of money to buy food." Was that often, sometimes, or never true for you in the last 12 months?
12. "We couldn't feed our children a balanced meal, because we couldn't afford that." Was that often, sometimes, or never true for you in the last 12 months?
13. "The children were not eating enough because we just couldn't afford enough food." Was that often, sometimes, or never true for you in the last 12 months?
14. In the last 12 months, did you ever cut the size of any of the children's meals because there wasn't enough money for food? (Yes/No)
15. In the last 12 months, were the children ever hungry but you just couldn't afford more food? (Yes/No)
16. In the last 12 months, did any of the children ever skip a meal because there wasn't enough money for food? (Yes/No)
17. (If yes to Question 16) How often did this happen—almost every month, some months but not every month, or in only 1 or 2 months?
18. In the last 12 months, did any of the children ever not eat for a whole day because there wasn't enough money for food? (Yes/No)

Source: Coleman-Jensen A, Rabbitt MP, Gregory CA, and Singh A. September 2016. *Household food security in the United States in 2015, ERR-215,* U.S. Department of Agriculture, Economic Research Service.

Since 1995, the U.S. Bureau of the Census has administered this instrument as part of its annual Current Population Survey (CPS), thus providing statistically valid, nationally representative data on the prevalence and severity of food insecurity in America.[5,19] In 2006, the USDA introduced new terms to categorize the ranges of severity of food security and insecurity to ensure that the terms were objective, measurable, and scientifically sound and that they conveyed useful and relevant information to policy officials and to the public.[19] The change in terminology (outlined in Table 4.1) was made upon the recommendation of an independent panel of experts convened by the National Academy of Sciences at the USDA's request.[19,20] It is important to note that while the terms were changed, there was no change in the methods used to assess household food security and insecurity. As shown in Table 4.1, two general categories have consistently been used to describe the food security condition of U.S. households: "food security" and "food insecurity," and these categories did not change in 2006. Prior to 2006, households reporting food insecurity were further

categorized as having "food insecurity without hunger" or as having "food insecurity with hunger." Beginning in 2006, these two categories were changed to "low food security" and "very low food security," respectively. Box 4.3 defines these key terms.

While data on the prevalence of hunger is of considerable interest and value for policy and program design, the expert panel noted that the USDA's methodology did not measure "resource-constrained hunger" (i.e., physiological hunger resulting from food insecurity). The expert panel suggested that the term "hunger" should refer to a "potential consequence of food insecurity that, because of prolonged, involuntary lack of food, results in discomfort, illness, weakness, or pain that goes beyond the usual uneasy sensation."[19,20] To measure hunger in this sense would require collection of more detailed and extensive information on physiological experiences of individual household members than could be accomplished effectively in the context of the CPS. The panel recommended, therefore, that new methods be developed to measure hunger and that a national assessment of hunger be

TABLE 4.1	Terms to Categorize the Ranges of Food Security and Insecurity Used by the USDA before 2006 and since 2006		
	Detailed Categories		
General Categories (these did not change in 2006)	Name of Category Before 2006	Name of Category Since 2006	Description of Conditions in the Household
Food security	Food security	**High food security**	No reported indications of food access problems or limitations.
		Marginal food security	One or two reported indications—typically of anxiety over food sufficiency or shortage of food in the house. Little or no indication of changes in diets or food intake.
Food insecurity	Food insecurity without hunger	**Low food security**	Reports of reduced quality, variety, or desirability of diet. Little or no indication of reduced food intake.
	Food insecurity with hunger	**Very low food security**	Reports of multiple indications of disrupted eating patterns and reduced food intake.

Source: Economic Research Service, U.S. Department of Agriculture.

 Box 4.3 | **Definitions of Food Security, Food Insecurity, Low Food Security, Very Low Food Security, and Hunger**

FOOD SECURITY

Access by all people at all times to enough food for an active, healthy life. Food security includes at a minimum: (1) the ready availability of nutritionally adequate and safe foods, and (2) an assured ability to acquire acceptable foods in socially acceptable ways (e.g., without resorting to emergency food supplies, scavenging, stealing, or other coping strategies).

FOOD INSECURITY

Limited or uncertain availability of nutritionally adequate and safe food or limited or uncertain ability to acquire acceptable foods in socially acceptable ways.

LOW FOOD SECURITY

Households classified as having low food security report multiple indications of food access problems, but typically report few, if any, indications of reduced food intake.

These households reduced the quality, variety, and desirability of their diets, but the quantity of food intake and normal eating patterns were not substantially disrupted.

VERY LOW FOOD SECURITY

Households classified as having very low food security report that the food intake of one or more members was reduced and eating patterns were disrupted because of insufficient money or other resources for food. In most but not all of these households, one or more household members were hungry at some time during the year and did not eat because there was not enough money for food.

HUNGER

A potential consequence of food insecurity that, because of prolonged, involuntary lack of food, results in discomfort, illness, weakness, or pain that goes beyond the usual uneasy sensation.

Sources: Coleman-Jensen A, Rabbitt MP, Gregory CA, and Singh A. September 2016. *Household food security in the United States in 2015, ERR-215,* U.S. Department of Agriculture, Economic Research Service.

conducted using an appropriate survey of individuals rather than a survey of households.[20]

The USDA estimates that in 2015, 87.3% of all American households were food-secure and that 12.7% of all American households were food-insecure, as shown in Figure 4.2 and Table 4.2. Of the food-insecure households, 7.7% reported low food security and 5.0% reported very low food security. Figure 4.3 shows the prevalence of food security and insecurity in U.S. households with children in 2015. Of these households, 83.4% were classified

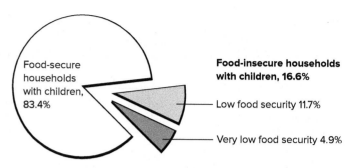

Figure 4.3 Food security of U.S. households with children in them in 2015.

Of U.S. households that had children in them, 83.4% were classified as food-secure in 2015 and 16.6% were classified as food-insecure.

Source: Coleman-Jensen A, Rabbitt MP, Gregory CA, and Singh A. September 2016. *Household food security in the United States in 2015, ERR-215,* U.S. Department of Agriculture, Economic Research Service.

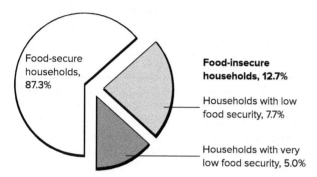

Figure 4.2 Food security of U.S. households in 2015.

An estimated 87.3% of American households were food-secure throughout the entire year in 2015, meaning that they had access at all times to enough food for an active, healthy life for all household members. The remaining households (12.7%) were food-insecure at least some time during the year, including 5.0% with very low food security, meaning that the food intake of one or more household members was reduced and their eating patterns were disrupted at times during the year because the household lacked money and other resources for food.

Source: Coleman-Jensen A, Rabbitt MP, Gregory CA, and Singh A. September 2016. *Household food security in the United States in 2015, ERR-215,* U.S. Department of Agriculture, Economic Research Service.

as food-secure and 16.6% were classified as food-insecure. As shown in Table 4.2, the prevalence of food insecurity in households with a female head and no spouse is nearly three times greater than in households headed by a married couple. Food insecurity among black non-Hispanic and Hispanic households is more than twice as great compared to white non-Hispanic households.[19]

ROLE OF THE U.S. DEPARTMENT OF HEALTH AND HUMAN SERVICES

The U.S. Department of Health and Human Services (HHS) has been involved in nutritional and health-related monitoring since the late 1950s, at which time it was

TABLE 4.2	Prevalence of Food Security, Food Insecurity, Low Food Security, and Very Low Food Security Among U.S. Households by Selected Characteristics, by Percent, 2015			
		Food-Insecure		
Category	**Food-Secure**	**Low Food Security**	**Very Low Food Security**	**All**
Income below poverty level	61.7	21.4	16.9	38.3
Female head, no spouse	69.7	20.9	9.4	30.3
Male head, no spouse	77.6	14.2	8.2	22.4
Black non-Hispanic	78.5	13.6	7.9	21.5
Hispanic	80.9	12.7	6.4	19.1
With children < 18y	83.4	11.7	4.9	16.6
All households	87.3	7.7	5	12.7
Married-couple families	89.8	7.7	2.5	10.2
White non-Hispanic	90	5.7	4.3	10

Source: Coleman-Jensen A, Rabbitt MP, Gregory CA, and Singh A. September 2016. *Household food security in the United States in 2015, ERR-215,* U.S. Department of Agriculture, Economic Research Service.

known as the Department of Health, Education, and Welfare. Its current name was adopted in 1979. The HHS's involvement in nutritional monitoring began in response to the National Health Survey Act of 1956, which mandated a continuing survey of the U.S. population for statistical data on amount, distribution, and effects of illness and disability in the United States. To comply with the 1956 act, HHS conducted a series of three National Health Examination Surveys. These were followed by the landmark Ten-State Nutrition Survey and then the National Health and Nutrition Examination Surveys, including the Hispanic Health and Nutrition Examination Survey. In addition to these, the HHS is responsible for a number of other surveys related to diet and nutrition, health, knowledge and attitudes, and food labeling. Included among these are the National Health Interview Survey, the Total Diet Study, the Health and Diet Study, the Behavioral Risk Factor Surveillance System, and the Food Label and Package Survey.

National Health Examination Surveys

The National Health Examination Surveys (NHES) were a series of three health surveys conducted by the National Center for Health Statistics of the HHS. NHES I was conducted from 1960 to 1962 and examined the prevalence of selected chronic diseases and health conditions in nearly 7000 Americans 18 to 79 years of age.[21] Using a variety of physical and physiologic measurements, such as blood pressure, serum cholesterol, skinfold measurements, height and weight, and electrocardiography, NHES I was able to focus on such conditions as coronary heart disease, arthritis, rheumatism, and diabetes.[21]

NHES II was conducted from 1963 to 1965 and sampled more than 7000 children 6 to 11 years old. From 1966 to 1970, NHES III studied nearly 7000 persons 12 to 17 years old. A primary task of NHES II and NHES III was to measure growth and development in American children and adolescents. This provided much of the data used by the National Center for Health Statistics in formulating its original growth charts, which have been updated using data from NHANES III (described in Chapter 6 and shown in Appendix H).

Ten-State Nutrition Survey

The Ten-State Nutrition Survey was the nation's first comprehensive survey to assess the nutritional status of a large segment of the U.S. population.[8] During the 1960s, concerns about hunger and malnutrition in America escalated, leading legislators, health professionals, and private citizens to investigate the problem. Their reports revealed "chronic hunger and malnutrition in every part of the United States"[22] and described the situation as "shocking" and having reached "emergency proportions."[8] Congress responded by mandating the Department of Health,

Education, and Welfare to conduct a "comprehensive survey of the incidence and location of serious hunger and malnutrition and health problems incident thereto in the United States."[8]

The Ten-State Nutrition Survey targeted geographic areas having high proportions of low-income persons, inner-city residents, and migrant workers. Between 1968 and 1970, data were collected in the following 10 states: California, Kentucky, Louisiana, Massachusetts, Michigan, New York (including New York City), South Carolina, Texas, Washington, and West Virginia.[8]

Although the survey helped reveal the extent and severity of hunger and malnutrition in America, groups surveyed were not representative of the general U.S. population, and consequently its findings could not be extrapolated to the overall population. The survey also demonstrated the difficulty and complexity of assessing nutritional status and recognized the need for additional data on the nutritional status of the U.S. population and the need for a continuing program of national nutritional surveillance. This led to the addition of a nutritional assessment component to the National Health Examination Survey and the beginning of the National Health and Nutrition Examination Survey.[8]

National Health and Nutrition Examination Survey

The **National Health and Nutrition Examination Surveys (NHANES)** were originally conducted by the National Center for Health Statistics (NCHS), an agency of the HHS. Since January 2002 the CSFII has been integrated into NHANES, and the operation of NHANES has been a joint effort of HHS and USDA. Its purpose is to monitor the overall nutritional status of the U.S. population through detailed interviews and comprehensive examinations. Interviews include dietary, demographic, socioeconomic, and health-related questions. Examinations consist of a medical and dental examination, physiologic measurements, and laboratory tests.[12,23,24]

First National Health and Nutrition Examination Survey (NHANES I)

NHANES I, conducted from 1971 to 1975, was designed to assess general health status, with particular emphasis on nutritional status and health of the teeth, skin, and eyes. Its target population was a representative sample of approximately 29,000 noninstitutionalized civilian Americans ages 1 to 74 years. The nutrition component of NHANES I consisted of four major parts: dietary intake based on a 24-hour recall and food frequency questionnaire; biochemical levels of various nutrients based on assays of whole blood, serum, and urine samples; clinical signs of nutrient-deficiency disease; and anthropometric measurements. Although NHANES I originally was designed to provide data on the population's health and nutritional status at the time of the survey (in other words, a **cross-sectional survey**), the NHANES I Epidemiologic Follow-up Study, conducted in 1982–84, allowed subjects to be reexamined to assess the influence of nutritional status on development of disease and death.

Second National Health and Nutrition Examination Survey (NHANES II)

NHANES II was conducted from 1976 to 1980. It targeted nearly 28,000 noninstitutionalized civilian Americans 6 months to 74 years of age, of which more than 25,000 (91%) were interviewed and more than 20,000 (73%) were examined. Examination components included dietary interviews, anthropometric measurements, a variety of biochemical assays on whole blood, serum, and urine, glucose tolerance tests, blood pressure measurement, electrocardiography, and radiography of the chest and cervical and lumbar spine.[7]

Hispanic Health and Nutrition Examination Survey (HHANES)

HHANES was the largest and most comprehensive Hispanic health survey ever conducted in the United States. Planning for the survey began in 1979, and the actual data were collected from 1982 to 1984 under the direction of the NCHS.[25] The survey collected health and nutritional data on the three largest subgroups of Hispanics living in the 48 contiguous states: nearly 9500 Mexican Americans residing in five southwestern states (Arizona, California, Colorado, New Mexico, and Texas); more than 2000 Cuban Americans living in Dade County, Florida; and more than 3500 Puerto Ricans residing in the New York City metropolitan area (selected counties in New York, New Jersey, and Connecticut).[25,26] Response rates ranged from 79% to 89% for interviews and from 61% to 75% for physical examinations. Because HHANES was not designed as a national Hispanic survey, its results do not necessarily apply to all Hispanics living in the United States. However, the sampled population included about 76% of the Hispanic-origin population of the United States as of 1980.[25]

Rather than providing a comprehensive picture of the health status or total health care needs of Hispanics, HHANES was designed to obtain basic data on certain chronic conditions and baseline health and nutritional information. As in NHANES, HHANES used five data-collecting techniques: interviews, physical examinations, diagnostic testing, anthropometrics, and laboratory tests.[25,27,28] Interviews were conducted at the homes of survey participants, followed by examinations at a mobile examination center, which consisted of three connected semitrailers, which were specially designed and equipped for testing.[27] The nutritional component included an evaluation of iron status and anemia, serum vitamin A levels, and food consumption as related to diabetes, digestive diseases, overweight, dental health, and alcohol consumption.[25]

Third National Health and Nutrition Examination Survey (NHANES III)

Data collection for NHANES III began October 1988 and ended October 1994.[12,24,29] The survey was conducted in two phases of equal length and sample size. A total of approximately 40,000 noninstitutionalized Americans ages 2 months and older were asked to complete an extensive examination and interview. The response rates for the interview and examination were 86% and 78%, respectively.[12] Four population groups were specially targeted for examination: children ages 2 months to 5 years, persons 60 years of age and older, black Americans, and Mexican Americans.[24] A disproportionately large number of persons in these four groups were examined to appropriately assess their nutritional and health status.

In planning for the survey in 1985, the NCHS intended it to provide several types of data: prevalence estimates of compromised nutritional status and trends in nutrition-related risk factors; data on the relationships among diet, nutritional status, and health; prevalence estimates of overweight and obesity in the U.S. population; and anthropometric data on children and adolescents, allowing revision of the original NCHS growth charts (see Chapter 6 and Appendix H), which were based on data collected before 1976.[30] Four areas received special emphasis: child health, health of older Americans, occupational health, and environmental health.

NHANES: A Continuous and Integrated Survey

In response to the recommendations of the National Nutrition Monitoring and Related Research Act of 1990, major changes have taken place in the operation of NHANES. In 1999 NHANES became a continuous, annual survey rather than one conducted periodically. Each year about 6000 persons from 15 counties across the United States are interviewed, and of these, approximately 5000 are examined in the NHANES mobile examination centers, which are discussed later in this section. All NHANES data collection methods are automated, and interview and examination data are recorded online, which results in rapid entry and transmittal of data.[18] Automated edit checks, quality control measures, and questionnaire sequencing have reduced data entry errors and improved interviewer performance. Every year, data are collected from a representative sample of the U.S. population, from newborns to older persons, and released in 2-year cycles, whereas previously it took as long as 6 years before a representative population sample was assessed. Results are now reported in a more timely manner; before this change, researchers sometimes had to wait as long as 10 years before gaining access to data that were representative of the entire U.S. population.

Another major change was the integration of the USDA Continuing Survey of Food Intakes by Individuals (CSFII) and NHANES in January 2002. Under the integrated framework, USDA is responsible for establishing

Box 4.4   NHANES Goals

The basic survey goal of NHANES is to monitor the health status of the U.S. population. Other current goals of the NHANES survey are to

- Estimate the number and percent of persons in the U.S. population, and designated subgroups, with selected diseases and risk factors
- Monitor trends in the prevalence, awareness, treatment, and control of selected diseases
- Monitor trends in risk behaviors and environmental exposures

- Analyze risk factors for selected diseases
- Study the relationship between diet, nutrition, and health
- Explore emerging public health issues and new technologies
- Establish a national probability sample of genetic material for future genetic research
- Establish and maintain a national probability sample of baseline information on health and nutritional status

Source: http://www.cdc.gov/nchs/nhanes/.

the dietary data collection methodology, maintaining the database on food composition, and coding and processing all dietary intake data, and HHS is responsible for the sample design and collecting all data.[18] Data from the integrated survey, sometimes referred to as *What We Eat in America, NHANES,* are available from the website of the National Center for Health Statistics, www.cdc.gov/nchs. By working cooperatively and combining the expertise of their respective staff, the two agencies provide more comprehensive and more accurate information on the health and nutrition characteristics of the U.S. population in a cost-effective and timely manner.

The Food and Drug Administration (FDA) uses data from NHANES to evaluate the need to change fortification regulations for the nation's food supply and to develop and evaluate the effectiveness of new regulations to improve food safety.[31] NHANES data are used in

developing and evaluating public education efforts. Many of the health objectives for the year 2020, including several in the nutrition priority area, rely on data from NHANES. The goals of NHANES are listed in Box 4.4.

Initial health interviews are conducted in the respondents' homes by specially trained staff members. Anthropometric measurements, physical examinations, testing, blood and urine collections, additional interviews, and the initial 24-hour recalls are performed in specially designed and equipped mobile examination centers (MECs), which travel to survey locations throughout the country. Each MEC consists of four trailers, each approximately 48 ft long by 8 ft wide, providing about 1570 sq ft of space. Several days before a survey is to begin at a particular location, the trailers are transported to the survey site, aligned, and leveled (as shown in Figure 4.4), and all connections of the passageways, electricity, water, and

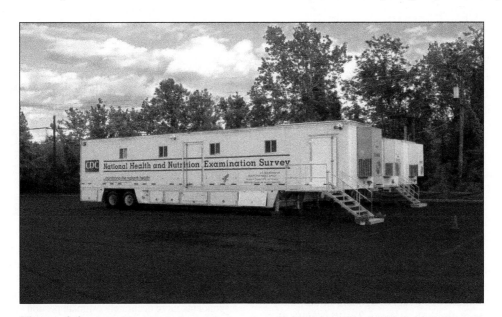

Figure 4.4 One of the Mobile Examination Centers (MEC) used in the National Health and Nutrition Examination Survey (NHANES).
Source: National Center for Health Statistics, U.S. Centers for Disease Control and Prevention.

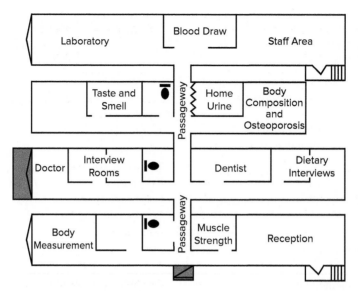

Figure 4.5 Floor plan of the Mobile Examination Centers used in the National Health and Nutrition Examination Survey (NHANES).
Source: National Center for Health Statistics.

sewer are made. Each MEC contains a laboratory; examination rooms for physical, dental, vision, hearing, bone density, and X-ray examinations and anthropometric measurements; a computer room; and other rooms for conducting interviews and collecting specimens.[24] The floor plan of the MEC is shown in Figure 4.5. There are three MECs and two separate examination teams. At any given time, two MECs are set up and fully operational, and one MEC is in the process of being moved from one survey site to another, parked, set up, and made ready by the time an examination team arrives. A link to the National Center for Health Statistics' narrated slide show tour of the MEC can be found at http://www.cdc.gov/nchs/nhanes/.

The 24-hour recall method is most often used for determining dietary intake in the NHANES (see Figure 4.6).[23] Since 2002, NHANES has been collecting food and nutrient intake data via two 24-hour recalls obtained with the AMPM method, updated nutrient databases, and sophisticated statistical modeling. These carefully developed procedures have significantly reduced underreporting. Targeted food frequency questionnaires focus on specific nutrition-health issues over varying NHANES cycles (e.g., fish/seafood and mercury, dairy and calcium, alcohol). Since 2007, detailed information on dietary supplement use has also been collected during the household interview for the past 30 days as well as during the two 24-hour recalls.[23] Dietary recall data for WWEIA-NHANES are collected on both weekdays and weekend days. Dietary interviews are announced to NHANES participants, and as a result, the possibility of self-reporting bias exists. For children 11 years of age and under, interviews are obtained through a proxy familiar with the child's intake. Since 2001, the USDA's Food and Nutrient Database for Dietary Studies (FNDDS) has been used to

assign codes to all foods and beverages and amounts reported by participants during their 24-hour dietary interviews.[23] The FNDDS is updated on an ongoing basis by the USDA to reflect changes in consumption and the marketplace for each survey period.

During the household screening interview, eligible household members participate in a detailed in-person interview (23). This includes questions on demographic, socioeconomic, dietary (including supplement use), and health-related areas. Depending on the NHANES

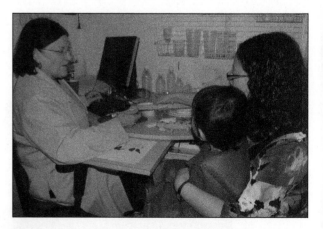

Figure 4.6
The first of the two automated multiple-pass 24-hour recalls collected from NHANES respondents is completed by a trained interviewer in the Mobile Examination Center (MEC). Two-dimensional and three-dimensional aids are used to help respondents more accurately estimate portion sizes. A variety of spoons, measuring spoons, bowls, plates, cups, and tumblers are used in the interview.
Source: Centers for Disease Control and Prevention.

TABLE 4.3	Components in NHANES Data 1999–Current (Household Interview and MEC Visit)

Sociodemographic status

Medical history

Medication use

Nutrition knowledge and behaviors

Infant feeding practices

Eating away from home

Weight history

Clinical exam, selected conditions

Anthropometric measurements

Body composition

Biological specimen collection, lab testing

Physical activity

24-hour recall

Dietary supplements use

Food frequency questionnaire

Source: Ahluwalia N, Dwyer J, Terry A, Moshfegh A, Johnson C. 2016. Update on NHANES dietary data: Focus on collection, release, analytical considerations, and uses to inform public policy. *Advances in Nutrition* 7:121–134.

TABLE 4.4	Examination Components During Various Phases of the Continuous NHANES Survey, 1999 to Current

	Age Group
Arthritis body measures	20–69 years
Audiometry	1/2 sample 20–69 years
Balance	1/2 sample 40–69 years
Bioelectrical impedance analysis	8–49 years
Blood pressure	8 years and over
Body measurements	Birth and over
Cardiovascular (CV) fitness	12–49 years
Dermatology	20–59 years
Dietary	Birth and over
Dietary supplement	Birth and over
Dual energy X-ray absorptiometry	8 years and over
Grip strength test	6 years and over
Lower extremity disease	40 years and over
Mental health	8–39 years
Ophthalmology	40 years and over
Oral health	2 years and over
Physical activity monitor	6 years and over
Physical functioning	50 years and over
Physician exam	Birth and over
Respiratory health	6–79 years
Taste and smell	40 years and over
Tuberculin skin test	1 year and over
Vision	12 years and over

Source: National Health and Nutrition Examination Survey 1999–2016 Survey Content Brochure.

cycle, information is collected on food security and nutrition knowledge, attitudes, and behaviors. The Flexible Consumer Behavior Survey, conducted in partnership with the Economic Research Service (ERS) of the USDA, includes topics such as participation in food and nutrition assistance programs, as well as family food expenditures at home and away from home. Data on nutritional knowledge, use of food labels and nutritional information, and importance of factors such as price, convenience, and taste while shopping for groceries or dining out have also been collected. Information on infant-feeding practices, eating away from home, and consumption of certain food groups (e.g., milk and dark green, leafy vegetables) is collected as part of the dietary behavior questionnaire.[23] Participants aged 16 years and older also report on weight history, perceived weight status, and methods used for weight control. In addition, data are collected on consumption of various types of dietary supplements, including vitamins, minerals, and non–vitamin-mineral supplements (e.g., botanical supplements and amino acids). Table 4.3 summarizes major components that have been measured in various cycles of the continuous NHANES, including diet and nutrition information.

Each of the two examination teams consists of a group of 16 persons who work and travel together: two dietary interviewers, a physician, a dentist, an ultrasonographer, four X-ray technicians, a phlebotomist, three medical technologists, a health interviewer, a home examiner, and a coordinator. Two locally hired staff supplement the team at each site. Most of the staff, especially the interviewers, are fluent in both Spanish and English. Although the interviewing staff are not required to have academic

credentials, most are experienced interviewers who represent a cross section of society. A large staff of interviewers conduct the household interviews. In each location, local health and government officials are notified of the upcoming survey. Households in the survey receive an advance letter and booklet to introduce the survey.

Participants are provided with transportation to and from the MEC. Participants receive reimbursement for completing the four-hour examination and an additional sum if they arrive at the MEC on time and, if requested, are fasting. Those unable to go to the MEC are given a less extensive examination in their homes. All participants receive a thorough physical examination, various anthropometric measurements, a dietary interview, and a private health interview and have their blood drawn for multiple analyses. Depending on the participant's age, additional examination components are performed. In general, the older the participant, the more extensive the examination. Table 4.4 shows the components of the NHANES examination by age range. A large number of analyses are performed on blood and urine samples

TABLE 4.5	Laboratory Components During Various Phases of the Continuous NHANES Survey, 1999 to Current

Acrylamide

Albumin

Aldehydes

Aromatic amines

Arsenic

Bone alkaline phosphatase

BV/trichomonas

Cadmium

Caffeine exposure

CD4/CD8

Celiac disease (tTG-EMA)

Chemistry panel

Chlamydia

Cholesterol (total), HDL, LDL, triglycerides, Lp(a), Apo B

Complete blood count

Cotinine

C-reactive protein (CRP)

Creatine phosphokinase

Creatinine

Cryptosporidium

Cytomegalovirus

Diisocyanates

Dust allergens

Environmental phenols

Erythrocyte protoporphyrin

Estradiol

Ferritin

Fibrinogen

Fluoride (plasma, water)

Folate (RBC, serum)

Follicle stimulating hormone/luteinizing hormone

Fungicides

Glucose

Glycohemoglobin

Gonorrhea

Halogenated phenolic compounds, pesticides

Helicobacter pylori

Hepatitis A, B, C, D, E

Herbicides—substituted ureas and others

Herpes 1 and antibody

Heterocylic aromatic amines (Tobacco Markers)

HLA-B7 (inflammatory arthritis)

Homocysteine

Human immunodeficiency virus (HIV) antibody

Human papillomavirus (HPV)

Hydroxylated polychlorinated biphenyls

Immunoglobulin E-allergens

Insulin/C-peptide

Latex

Minerals: chromium, cobalt, iodine, iron, manganese, selenium, copper, zinc

Measles/varicella/rubella

Metals, lead, mercury

Methicillin resistant staphlococcus aureus (MRSA)

Methylmalonic acid

Nicotine analogs

Nondioxin-like polychlorinated biphenyls

N-teleopeptide (NTX)

Oral glucose tolerance (OGTT)

Organophosphate insecticides

Osmolality

Parathyroid hormone

Perchlorate/thiocynate/nitrates

Pesticides

Phthalates

Phytoestrogens

Polyaromatic hydrocarbons (PAH)

Polychlorinated, polybrominated, polyfluorinated compounds

Polyunsaturated fatty acids

Prostate specific antigen (PSA)

Sex hormone binding globulin

Syphillis

Testosterone

Thyroid function testing

Tobacco-specific nitrosamines

Total iron binding capacity (TIBC)/transferrin saturation

Toxaphenes

Toxoplasma

Trans fatty acids

Transferrin receptor

Trichomonas

Tuberculosis

Urine flow rate calculation

Vitamin A, E, B6, B1, C, D, carotenoids

Volatile nitrosamines, organic compounds

White blood cells/deoxyribonucleic acid (WBC/DNA)

Source: National Health and Nutrition Examination Survey 1999–2016 Survey Content Brochure.

obtained from respondents, as shown in Table 4.5. These lab tests include a comprehensive diagnostic chemistry panel, lipid panel, complete blood count, and tests for sexually transmitted diseases, vitamin and minerals, iron status, hormones, environmental chemicals, metals, immune measures, and tobacco use.

NHANES uses a variety of measures to assess health and nutritional status, as illustrated in Figure 4.7.

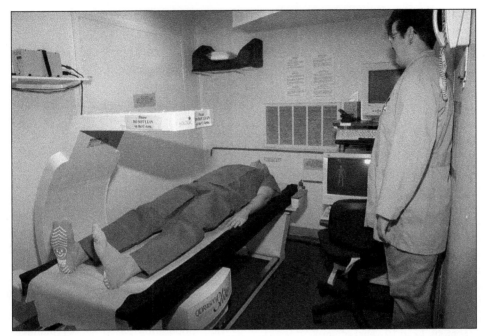

Figure 4.7
The use of dual-energy X-ray absorptiometry (DXA) for measuring bone mineral density to assess body composition is one example of the many different examination components used in the National Health and Nutrition Examination Survey (NHANES).

Source: National Center for Health Statistics, U.S. Centers for Disease Control and Prevention.

TABLE 4.6	**Anthropometric Measures by Age Category Performed in the Continuous NHANES 1999 to Current**		
Birth+	**2 months+**	**2 years+**	**8 years+**
Recumbent length	Recumbent length	Recumbent length (through 47 months)	
Head circumference	Head circumference (through 6 months)		
Weight	Weight	Standing height	Standing height
	Upper arm length	Weight	Weight
	Arm circumference	Upper arm length	Upper leg length
		Arm circumference	Upper arm length
		Waist circumference	Arm circumference
			Waist circumference
			Sagittal abdominal diameter

Source: National Health and Nutrition Examination Survey (NHANES). January 2016. Anthropometry Procedures Manual.

In addition to the numerous assays performed on respondents' blood and urine samples, several anthropometric measures are performed on participants, as shown in Table 4.6. Anthropometric measurements are a mainstay of the NHANES initiative, with some variations across NHANES testing cycles.[23] Anthropometric data are used to examine the relationships between body measures and body composition and activity, dietary patterns, and risk factors for cardiovascular disease, diabetes, and hypertension. They also allow growth and development in children to be monitored and provide nationally representative data on selected body measures and estimates of the prevalence of overweight and obesity. The recent increase in the prevalence of overweight and obesity among all sex, age, and racial and ethnic groups has been called an epidemic. NHANES is unique in collecting nationally representative measured data on body measures and composition. Body measures data from NHANES are used to provide representative reference data, set health objectives, and monitor trends. Anthropometry data have been collected with comparable methods since the first National Health Examination Survey, conducted between 1960 and 1962. NHANES is incorporating novel, validated assessment techniques as they become available, including measurement of the sagittal abdominal diameter as an indicator of abdominal obesity.[23]

In addition to the first 24-hour recall, two different interviews are administered to NHANES respondents while they are in the MEC. A computer-assisted personal interview (CAPI) asks about current health status, physical activity, urinary incontinence (persons 20 to 59 years of age), reproductive health (females age 12 years and older), and tobacco and alcohol use (persons 20 years of age and older). A more private audio computer-assisted personal self-interview (ACASI) seeks information about alcohol and tobacco use (persons 12 to 19 years of age), use of illegal drugs (persons 12 to 59 years of age), sexual behavior (persons 14 to 59 years of age), and instances of misconduct such as shoplifting, vandalism, cruelty to animals, and lying (persons 12 to 19 years of age).

The post-MEC data collection procedures vary across NHANES cycles and have included physical activity monitoring (with accelerometers), telephone-based 24-hour dietary recall, consumer behavior questionnaires, and home-collected urine samples.[23]

Other HHS Surveys

Other surveys that provide important data on health and on food and nutrient intake include the Total Diet Study, the Navajo Health and Nutrition Survey, the Pregnancy Nutrition Surveillance System, the Pediatric Nutrition Surveillance System, the Health and Diet Survey, the Behavioral Risk Factor Surveillance System, and the National Health Interview Survey.

Total Diet Study

The Total Diet Study (TDS) is an ongoing FDA program that monitors levels of about 800 contaminants and nutrients in the average U.S. diet.[32] Since it began in 1961, as a program to monitor for radioactive contamination of foods, the TDS has expanded to include pesticide residues, industrial and other toxic chemicals, and nutrient elements. An important aspect of the study is that the FDA buys foods from the same places that consumers do, and prepares the foods as consumers typically would, to provide realistic estimates. The ongoing nature of the study enables the FDA to track trends in the average American diet and inform the development of interventions to reduce or minimize risks, when needed.

To conduct the study, the FDA buys, prepares, and analyzes about 280 kinds of foods and beverages from representative areas of the country, four times a year. The TDS uses various methods to analyze foods and beverages for analytes in the following categories (Table 4.7):

- Toxic and nutrient chemical elements
- Pesticides
- Industrial chemicals
- Radionuclides

Using these data, the FDA estimates how much of the contaminants and nutrients the entire U.S. population, some subpopulations, and each person consumes annually, on average. Because eating patterns may change over time, the FDA updates the list of foods to be analyzed about every 10 years. This includes revising the list of foods to be tested, accounting for trends in what consumers eat, and using current data on how much of those foods consumers eat. The FDA uses the TDS results in various ways and, for example, suggests potential areas of focus for U.S. food-safety and nutrition programs.

Navajo Health and Nutrition Survey, 1991–1992

The Navajo Health and Nutrition Survey was a reservation-wide, population-based survey planned by the Indian Health Service to establish prevalence data on nutrition-related chronic diseases and to generate a valid description of the health and nutritional status and dietary behaviors of the Navajo people in general and for selected subgroups within that population.[11,33,34] A total of 985 people 12 years of age and older from 459 households participated in the survey. Data collection took place over a five-month period during 1991 to 1992. Information was collected on dietary intake, food

TABLE 4.7	**Total Diet Study Measurements**

The Food and Drug Administration's Total Diet Study (TDS) monitors the U.S. population's average annual dietary intake of more than 800 chemical contaminants and of certain nutrients. The chemical contaminants include radionuclides, pesticide residues, industrial chemicals, and toxic elements, either naturally occurring or resulting from human activity. The number of different kinds of foods analyzed in this long-term study has increased from 82, when it began in 1961, to about 280 currently. Categories of contaminants and nutrients include the following.

Toxic and Nutrient Elements

- Arsenic, cadmium, chromium, lead, mercury, iodine, and other elements in food

Pesticides and Industrial Chemicals

- Analysis of 400 pesticides, herbicides, and industrial chemicals

Radionuclides

- Strontium-90, gamma-ray emitting radionuclides

Source: U.S. Food and Drug Administration, Center for Food Safety and Applied Nutrition.

frequency, anthropometric measurements, lipid profiles, blood pressure, and full blood chemistries, including oral glucose tolerance tests.[11] The survey showed that obesity is a major problem among the Navajo, that 40% of Navajos age 45 years and older have diabetes (a third of these individuals are unaware of their condition), and that another 18% have impaired glucose tolerance and are, therefore, at risk of developing type 2 diabetes.[34] Among the Navajo, risk factors for cardiovascular disease are common, vegetable and fruit consumption is low, consumption of fats is high, and there is a lack of clinical services, particularly for managing diabetes and hypertension. Although reproductive health issues related to traditionally high parity (e.g., iron deficiency anemia) are problems among Navajo women, they do not appear to be as important as the high prevalence of obesity, diabetes, and coronary heart disease risk factors seen in Navajo women. The survey illustrates some of the critical health and nutrition concerns facing Native North American people and the need to better address those concerns.[34]

Pregnancy Nutrition Surveillance System (Ending 2012)

The Pregnancy Nutrition Surveillance System (PNSS), conducted by the U.S. Centers for Disease Control and Prevention (CDC), was designed to monitor the prevalence of nutrition-related problems and behavioral risk factors that are related to infant mortality and low birth weight among high-risk prenatal populations. These factors include overweight, underweight, smoking, alcohol consumption, anemia, lack of prenatal care, and adolescent pregnancy. The program was begun in 1979 when five states (Arizona, California, Kentucky, Louisiana, and Oregon) began working with the CDC in monitoring the prevalence of nutrition problems among infants born to high-risk pregnant women. In 2009, 31 states, the District of Columbia, 1 U.S. territory, and 5 Native American Tribal Organizations contributed data representing approximately 1,300,000 women. The system also studied the relationship of nutritional status to weight gain during pregnancy and birth outcome. Data were collected from the Special Supplemental Nutrition Program for Women, Infants, and Children (WIC) and the Title V Maternal and Child Health Program (MCH).[11,35]

Pediatric Nutrition Surveillance System (Ending 2012)

The Pediatric Nutrition Surveillance System (PedNSS), conducted by the CDC, was an ongoing child-based public health surveillance system whose goal was to collect, analyze, and disseminate data to guide public health policy and action.[11,36] Data from PedNSS were used for priority setting and for planning, implementing,

monitoring, and evaluating specific public health programs to improve the health and nutritional status of U.S. children. Data from the Ten-State Nutrition Survey (1968–1970) showed that the nutritional status of children from low-income families was unsatisfactory. Of particular concern were findings from the survey showing inadequate intakes of calories, calcium, iron, and vitamins A and C by low-income black and Hispanic children. In response, the CDC began working with five states (Arizona, Kentucky, Louisiana, Tennessee, and Washington) in 1973 to develop a system to continuously monitor the nutritional status of selected high-risk population groups, which was the beginning of PedNSS. In 2009, 47 states, 2 U.S. territories, 6 Native American Tribal Organizations, and the District of Columbia contributed data representing approximately 8,940,000 children < 5 years of age.[36] The data were routinely collected by health, nutrition, and food assistance programs, such as Special Supplemental Nutrition Program for Women, Infants, and Children (WIC), the Early and Periodic Screening, Diagnosis, and Treatment (EPSDT) Program, the Title V Maternal and Child Health Program, and Head Start. Examples of data collected by the PedNSS are shown in Figure 4.8 and Figure 4.9. Figure 4.8 shows trends in the prevalence of low birth weight (LBW) (a birth weight < 2500 grams or < 5.5 pounds) by race and ethnicity 2001–2010. American Indians, Alaska Natives, and Hispanics experience the lowest prevalence of LBW, whereas non-Hispanic blacks have the highest prevalence at approximately 13%. The average for all groups is approximately 9%, which is considerably higher than the year 2020 goal of reducing the prevalence of LBW to 7.8% or less.[36] Figure 4.9 shows the prevalence of obesity and overweight among children 2 to 5 years of age by race and ethnicity.

Non-Hispanic blacks and Asian/Pacific Islanders have the lowest prevalence of obesity and overweight, and American Indians/Alaska Natives and Hispanics experience the highest prevalence. In persons 2 to 20 years of age, obesity is defined as a BMI-for-age ≥ 95th percentile, and overweight is defined as a BMI-for-age ≥ 85th but to < 95th percentile using the 2000 CDC Growth Charts (as discussed in Chapter 6).[36]

Health and Diet Survey

The Health and Diet Survey is a random-digit dialed telephone survey of a nationally representative sample of American households conducted periodically by the U.S. Food and Drug Administration's Center for Food Safety and Applied Nutrition. Each survey contains a core set of questions relating to health and nutrition and additional questions that provide timely information on current health and diet issues or special topics. Participants are asked about topics that include knowledge and

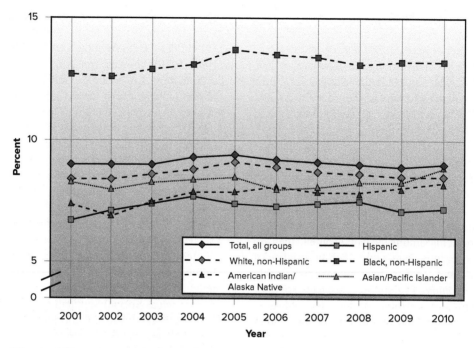

Figure 4.8 **Trends in the prevalence of low birth weight, by race and ethnicity, 2001–2010.**
Low birth weight is defined as a birth weight < 2500 g or < 5.5 lb.
Source: Pediatric Nutrition Surveillance System, U.S. Centers for Disease Control and Prevention.

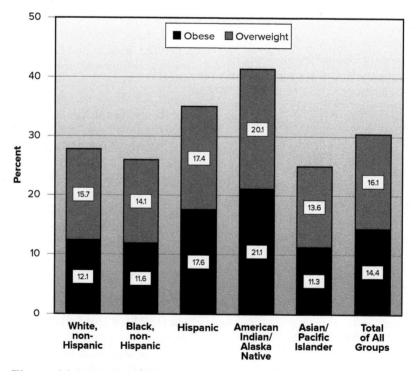

Figure 4.9 **Prevalence of obesity and overweight among U.S. children age 2 to 5 years, by race and ethnicity, 2010.**
Obesity is defined as a BMI-for-age ≥ 95th percentile and overweight is defined as a BMI-for-age ≥ 85th to < 95th percentile using the 2000 CDC Growth Charts, as discussed in Chapter 6.
Source: Pediatric Nutrition Surveillance System, U.S. Centers for Disease Control and Prevention.

perceptions about sodium, cholesterol, fats, and food labels; self-reported health-related behaviors, such as dieting, sodium avoidance, and efforts to lower blood pressure and blood cholesterol levels; and beliefs about the relationships between diet and cancer, high blood pressure, and heart disease. Survey data are used to evaluate the effectiveness of public education initiatives of various federal. For example, in the 2014 survey, while 9 in 10 adults had heard of *trans* fat or omega-3 fatty acids, a quarter of those aware of either of the fats could not tell if the fat raises, lowers, or has no relationship with the risk of heart disease.[37]

Behavioral Risk Factor Surveillance System

The Behavioral Risk Factor Surveillance System (BRFSS) was established in 1984 by the Centers for Disease Control and Prevention and is the world's largest ongoing health surveillance system (http://www.cdc.gov/brfss/).[38] The BRFSS is a state-based telephone survey of the civilian, noninstitutionalized adult population intended to provide data on health-related risk behaviors, chronic health conditions, and use of preventive services. The BRFSS is administered by state health departments each month in all 50 states, the District of Columbia, Puerto Rico, the Virgin Islands, and Guam. Data can be analyzed by an individual state as well as by smaller geographic areas within states known as metropolitan and micropolitan statistical areas (MMSAs). A metropolitan statistical area is a group of counties that contains at least one urbanized area of 50,000 or more inhabitants, and a micropolitan statistical area is a group of counties that contains at least one urban cluster of at least 10,000 but less than 50,000 inhabitants.[38] In contrast, NHANES and other national surveys do not provide data that are specific to a particular state or region within a state.

Data from the BRFSS are used by state and local health departments to plan, initiate, and guide health promotion and disease prevention programs as well as to monitor the success of such programs over time. The questionnaire used in the BRFSS includes a core set of questions asked of respondents in all states, an optional module of questions developed by the CDC that states can elect to use if they wish, and state-added questions developed by individual states. In addition to demographic questions (e.g., sex, age, race, marital status, income, county of residence), the questionnaire asks about health status, health-care access, exercise, weight control, diabetes, oral health, tobacco use, alcohol consumption, fruit and vegetable intake, awareness of hypertension and cholesterol, and the like. Several pages from a recent BRFSS questionnaire are shown in Appendix I.

Figure 4.10 shows the increase in state-by-state prevalence of obesity based on data collected by the BRFSS. In Figure 4.10, obesity is defined as a body mass index (BMI) ≥ 30 kg/m^2, which is calculated using self-reported height and weight data collected by telephone interviews. Given the fact that overweight participants in self-reported studies tend to underestimate their weight and that all participants tend to overestimate their height, it is reasonable to assume that the data illustrated in Figure 4.10 underestimate the true prevalence of obesity. Figure 4.11 shows the percentage of U.S. adults who, during a telephone interview, reported that they had been told by a physician that they had diabetes. These data in the figure were also collected by the BRFSS and are self-reported. Despite the problems associated with self-reported data, the BRFSS is the most important source of state-based data on nutrition and health. Public health surveillance through BRFSS in the future will be much more complex and involve multiple ways of collecting public health data. Although telephone surveys will likely remain the mainstay of how BRFSS data are collected, additional modes of interviewing will also be

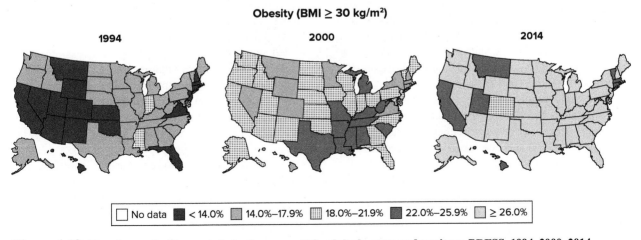

Figure 4.10 **Prevalence of self-reported obesity among U.S. adults by state and territory, BRFSS, 1994, 2000, 2014.**
The prevalence of obesity has risen sharply across the states using BRFSS data.

Source: Behavioral Risk Factor Surveillance System, Centers for Disease Control and Prevention.

Diabetes

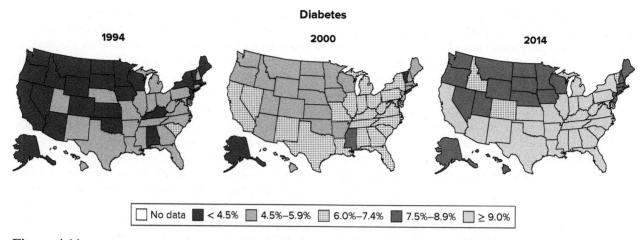

Figure 4.11 **Prevalence of diabetes among U.S. adults by state and territory, BRFSS, 1994, 2000, 2014.**
The prevalence of diabetes has risen sharply across states using BRFSS data (in parallel with the increase in obesity prevalence).
Source: Behavioral Risk Factor Surveillance System, Centers for Disease Control and Prevention.

necessary. BRFSS is developing methods for improving the quality of BRFSS data, reaching populations previously not included in the survey and expanding the utility of the surveillance data.

National Health Interview Survey

The National Health Interview Survey (NHIS) is a cross-sectional, household interview survey that has been conducted annually since its inception in 1957. It is the major source of information on the amount, distribution, and effects of illness and disability in the U.S. civilian noninstitutionalized population.[39] NHIS data are used to monitor trends in physical and mental health status; chronic conditions, including asthma and diabetes; access to and use of health-care services; health insurance coverage and type of coverage; health-related behaviors, including smoking, alcohol use, and physical activity; measures of functioning and activity limitations; and immunizations. NHIS data are collected from a nationally representative sample of approximately 35,000 to 40,000 households containing about 75,000 to 100,000 persons. The response rate is greater than 90% despite the fact that survey participation is voluntary. The confidentiality of responses is mandated by federal law.

The NHIS questionnaire has two components: a core set of questions and a set of supplemental questions. The core set of questions remains essentially unchanged from year to year and contains questions that are directed to the family unit, to one adult randomly selected from the household, and to one child, if any, randomly selected from the household. The supplemental set of questions collects data on emerging public health concerns as they arise. Data are collected through a personal household interview conducted by interviewers employed and trained by the U.S. Bureau of the Census according to procedures specified by NCHS. The interviewers are employees who are selected through an examination and testing process

and who are thoroughly trained in basic interviewing procedures. The current NHIS interview employs computer-assisted personal interviewer (CAPI) technology using a laptop computer, with interviewers entering responses directly into the computer during the interview. This procedure makes data collection faster, easier, more accurate, and more cost-effective; speeds the analysis of the data by NCHS statisticians; and makes survey results more readily available to policy analysts and epidemiologists.[39]

DIETARY TRENDS

Data on per capita food availability (also referred to as food disappearance) and consumption at the individual level have revealed a number of significant changes in the American diet.[15–17,40,41] These include changes in the sources of food energy; average amounts of energy consumed by Americans; use of specific food groups, including alcoholic and nonalcoholic beverages; and changes in eating patterns, such as snacking and eating away from home. In the following sections, some of the data presented are based on food availability, whereas other data are derived from surveys that measured actual food consumption (or at least attempted to). Food availability data are useful to nutrition policy makers, educators, researchers, and health-conscious consumers because they measure the capacity of the food supply to satisfy the nutritional needs of the population and they identify sources of nutrients and food components in the food supply. Food availability attempts to measure the flow of raw and semiprocessed commodities through the U.S. food marketing system. These data represent the amount of food that is available for consumption and, consequently, are not a direct measure of food and nutrient consumption and are not based on the quantity of food ingested, as are data from surveys such as What We Eat in America, NHANES. For this reason, food availability is a supply measure, not an intake measure.[40] As mentioned earlier in this chapter, the USDA's Economic Research Service (ERS) maintains the Food Availability (per Capita) Data System, which contains three related but separate series or sets of food availability data: Food Availability data, Loss-Adjusted Food Availability data, and Nutrient Availability data.[17] Data from the Food Availability data series, the core set of food availability data that provides estimates beginning as early as the year 1909, are not adjusted to account for food lost from spoilage, trimming, cooking, or plate waste or food fed to animals and, consequently, overstate actual food and nutrient consumption. The Loss-Adjusted Food Availability data, which provide estimates beginning from 1970 to the present, are adjusted for food losses at the primary, retail, and consumer levels and, consequently, better represent what consumers actually eat. Despite the limitations of food availability data, they are useful indicators of trends in U.S. food and nutrient availability that now span more than 100 years.[40]

Sources of Food Energy

The distribution of food energy from carbohydrate, fat, and protein has changed since the USDA's Economic Research Service first began compiling food availability data. This is shown in Figure 4.12. From 1909 to 2010, energy available from protein remained essentially unchanged at 11% to 12% of total kilocalories. Percentage of kilocalories available from carbohydrate declined from 59% in 1909 to 49% in 2010. Fat availability ranged from approximately 32% in 1909 to about 41% in 2010.

Data from NHANES 2013–2014 for percent of energy from protein, carbohydrate, total fat, and alcohol are shown in Figure 4.13. According to surveys conducted between 1965 and 2014 that measured actual food intake of individuals, the percentage of kilocalories from fat has

ranged from a high of 42.1% to a low of 32.7%, as shown in Figure 4.14. Although the percentages in Figure 4.14 seem somewhat inconsistent from one survey to the next, the figure does suggest that the mean percent of kilocalories from fat in the diets of American adults has declined slightly from several decades ago.

Factors other than changes in food consumption practices over time influence the reported percentages of kilocalories from fat in the various surveys represented in Figure 4.14. Among these are differences in how surveys collect dietary intake data, changes in the public's perceptions regarding certain "sensitive food items," ways in which foods are coded, and changes in nutrient content databases. Not all of the surveys represented in Figure 4.14 used the same methods to collect dietary intake data. Research on food intake methodology and advances in technology have led to considerable change and improvement in the way dietary intake data are collected. For example, compared with NHANES II, there was a greater percentage of 24-hour recalls collected for weekend days in NHANES III. In NHANES II, the 24-hour recalls were collected on paper forms and manually coded by dietary interviewers, whereas NHANES now uses a computer-assisted, five-step, automated multiple-pass 24-hour recall system and obtains two 24-hour recalls on virtually every respondent. In addition, the interviewers systematically probe for detailed information about all foods consumed and items added at the table. Over the years there have been improvements in the ways that food intake data have been collected and in the nutrient composition databases used. The USDA Automated Multiple Pass Method for collecting 24-hour recalls now used in NHANES has likely improved the quality of data collected in more recent surveys compared with the data collected by surveys of previous years.

As mentioned in Chapter 3, underreporting of food intake occurs, particularly in individuals with a high BMI

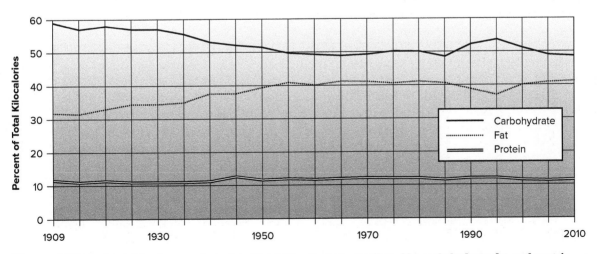

Figure 4.12 Percent of food energy (percent of total kilocalories) contributed by carbohydrate, fat, and protein from 1909 to 2010, based on food availability data from the U.S. Department of Agriculture.

The data used to develop this chart have not been adjusted for losses due to spoilage, trimming, waste, etc., and overstate actual food consumption.

Source: Data from the Economic Research Service, U.S. Department of Agriculture.

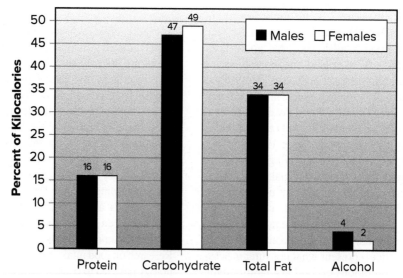

Figure 4.13 **The percent of kilocalories from protein, carbohydrate, total fat, and alcohol by sex, United States.**

Source: What We Eat in America, National Health and Nutrition Examination Survey (NHANES) 2013–2014.

and females. In NHANES, the AMPM 24-hour recall method has reduced underreporting of mean energy intake to 10% in males, 12% in females, and 3% in normal-weight individuals.[23] If given the efforts made to ensure the collection of high-quality data, recent estimates of food and nutrient intake from NHANES are the best available to date.

Percentage of energy from carbohydrate for males and females is shown in Figure 4.15. Females tend to have a greater carbohydrate intake than males, as do children and adolescents compared with older persons. Data from What We Eat in America, NHANES indicate marked discrepancies between the average intakes for Americans and several recommendations made by the Dietary Guidelines for Americans and other nutrient intake standards, such as the Dietary Reference Intakes, in terms of sources of food energy, sodium, potassium, and food groups such as whole

grains, vegetables, fruits, dairy, and seafood. Figure 4.16 shows that intakes of several food groups and key nutrients are less than the goals set by the Dietary Guidelines and other nutrient intake standards, while several exceed the recommended limits. Particularly problematic is intake of calories from solid fats and added sugars, abbreviated "SoFAS" by the Dietary Guidelines for Americans. Figure 4.16 shows that calories from solid fats and added sugars are nearly three times the recommended level.

Trends in Carbohydrates

Availability of total carbohydrates declined from about 500 g/day during 1909 to a low of about 380 g/day in the early 1960s. This decline was primarily due to decreased use of starches from grain products (flour and cereals), as

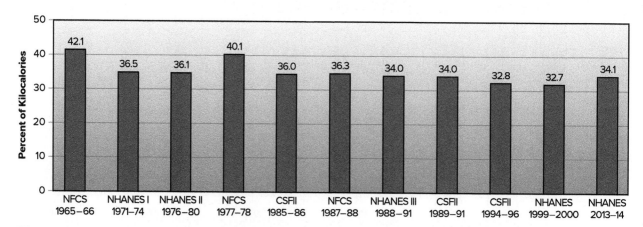

Figure 4.14 **Percent of kilocalories from fat in the diets of American adults for selected years, 1965–2014.**
Although these percentages seem somewhat inconsistent from one survey to the next, the data suggest that mean percentage of kilocalories from fat has declined slightly over the past several decades. This is particularly evident in the figure's last three surveys, which have benefited from improvements in food intake data collection methodology.

Source: Data from the USDHHS National Center for Health Statistics and the USDA Foods Survey Research Group.

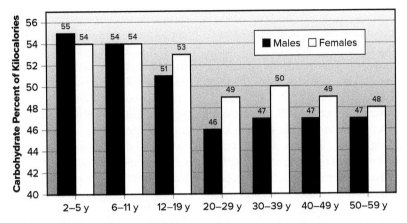

Figure 4.15 The percent of kilocalories from carbohydrate for males and females by age in years, United States, from **What We Eat in America, NHANES** Available: **www.ars.usda.gov/.**

shown in Figure 4.17. Since the mid-1960s, availability of carbohydrates increased to about 480 g/day in 2010.

Based on data from What We Eat in America, NHANES 2013–2014, mean dietary fiber intake for males and females of all ages is 18.8 g/day and 15.4 g/day, respectively. These values remain below the 20 to 35 g/day recommended by the Dietary Guidelines for Americans.

Trends in Sweeteners

Estimates of the consumption of sugar (primarily sucrose) and other caloric sweeteners come from two sources: food availability and food consumption data. Based on loss-adjusted per capita food availability data, the annual per capita availability of total caloric sweeteners peaked just before the year 2000, with corn sweeteners rising above

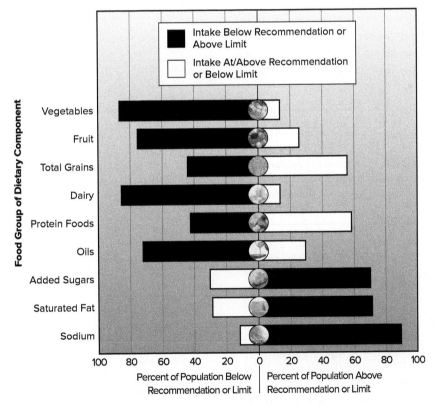

Figure 4.16 How the typical American diet compares to recommended intake levels or limits.

Dietary intakes compared to recommendations. Percent of the U.S. population ages 1 year and older who are below, at, or above each dietary goal or limit.

Source: U.S. Department of Health and Human Services and U.S. Department of Agriculture. December 2015. *2015–2020 Dietary guidelines for Americans,* 8th ed.

cane and beet sugar (Figure 4.18). Since the year 2000, availability of total caloric sweeteners and corn sweeteners has fallen, and public health officials have targeted this source of energy to reduce obesity prevalence, especially among youth.

According to the Dietary Guidelines for Americans, added sugars account on average for almost 270 calories, or more than 13% of calories per day in the U.S. population. Sugar intake is especially high among children, adolescents, and young adults. The major source of added sugars in typical U.S. diets is beverages, which include soft drinks, fruit drinks, sweetened coffee and tea, energy drinks, alcoholic beverages, and flavored waters (Figure 4.19). Beverages account for almost half (47%) of all added sugars consumed by the U.S. population. The other major source of added sugars is snacks and sweets, which include grain-based desserts such as cakes, pies, cookies, brownies, doughnuts, sweet rolls, and pastries; dairy desserts such as ice cream, other frozen desserts, and puddings; candies; sugars; jams; syrups; and sweet toppings. Together, these food categories make up more than 75% of intake of all added sugars.[42,43]

The 2015–2020 Dietary Guidelines for Americans recommend that added sugar consumption be reduced to less than 10% of calories per day.[43] Strategies include choosing beverages such as water in place of sugar-sweetened beverages and reducing portions or drinking sugar-sweetened beverages less often. Low-fat/fat-free milk or 100% fruit/vegetable juice also can be substituted in moderation in place of sugar-sweetened beverages. Additional strategies for reducing sugar intake include limiting or decreasing portion sizes of grain-based and dairy desserts and sweet snacks and choosing unsweetened or no-sugar-added versions of canned fruit, fruit sauces (e.g., applesauce), and yogurt.

Trends in Dietary Fats and Oils

The consumption of fats and oils is of considerable public health significance because of the association between saturated fatty acid intake and risk of coronary heart disease (as discussed in Chapter 9) and because all fats and oils are energy dense, providing 9 kilocalories per gram, and when consumed in excessive amounts have the potential to contribute to obesity. Figure 4.20 shows trends in the annual per capita availability (unadjusted for losses due to waste and spoilage) of the leading types of added

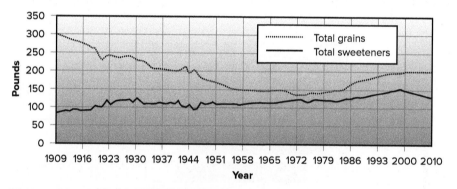

Figure 4.17 Annual per capita availability of total grain products and total sugars and caloric sweeteners from the U.S. food supply, 1909–2010.

Source: Data from the Economic Research Service, U.S. Department of Agriculture.

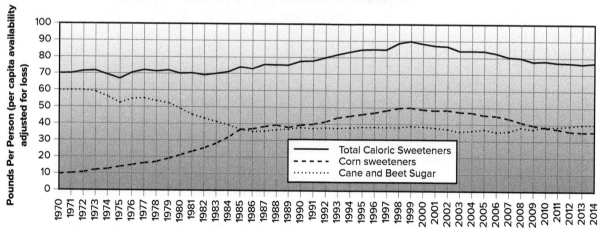

Figure 4.18 Changes in loss-adjusted per capita food availability for total caloric sweeteners, corn sweeteners, and cane and beet sugar in pounds per person from 1970 to 2014.

Source: Food Availability (Per Capita) Data System, Economic Research Service, USDA.

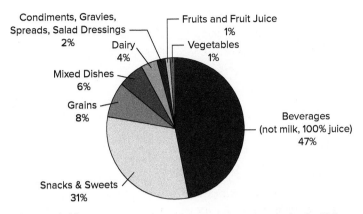

Figure 4.19 **Food Category Sources of Added Sugars in the U.S. Population Ages 2 Years and Older.**

Of any food category, sugar-sweetened beverages are the single largest source of added sweeteners in the U.S. diet.

Source: U.S. Department of Health and Human Services and U.S. Department of Agriculture. December 2015. *2015–2020 Dietary guidelines for Americans,* 8th ed. Available at http://health.gov/dietaryguidelines/2015/guidelines/.

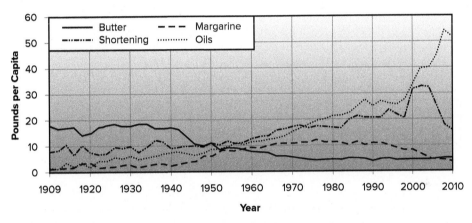

Figure 4.20 **Trends in the annual per capita availability of the leading types of added fats and oils in the United States, 1909 to 2010.**

Source: Food Availability (per Capita) Data System, Economic Research Service, USDA.

fats and oils in the United States from 1909 to 2010. In 1909, butter and vegetable shortening were the leading forms of added fats in the U.S. diet, with margarine and oils making a very small contribution. Since the early 1970s, oils have been the leading source of added fats in the U.S. diet. The per capita availability of all added fats increased from 35.5 pounds per person in 1909 to 80.3 pounds per person in 2010. This increase was in large part due to an increase in the availability of salad and cooking oils, as shown in Figure 4.20. Loss-adjusted per capita availability of added fats increased from 38.6 pounds per year in 1970 to 53.0 pounds per year in 2010. Loss-adjusted per capita availability of total fats increased from 42.6 pounds per year in 1970 to 63.5 pounds per year in 2010. Between 1909 and 2010, the per capita availability of all fats (naturally occurring in foods and added), unadjusted for losses, increased from 122 grams per day to 178 grams per day. Between 1909 and 2010, the per capita

availability of saturated fat, unadjusted for losses, remained remarkably flat at 52 to 54 grams per day. During the same interval, however, the per capita availability of monounsaturated fats increased from 47 grams per day to 77 grams per day, while polyunsaturated fats increased from 13 grams per day to 39 grams per day. Although availability data indicate a shift away from animal fats to vegetable fats, monounsaturated and saturated fatty acids remain the predominant types of fat in the American diet. Since 1909, total fat from red meat, butter, and lard have decreased, but not enough to offset the increased availability of vegetable oils used in cooking and on salads and the increased availability of fried foods produced by the fast-food industry. Data from What We Eat in America, NHANES 2013–2014 indicate that saturated fats contribute an average of 11% of total calories in the diet, a value greater than that recommended by the Dietary Guidelines for Americans, which is less than 10% of total calories from saturated fats.

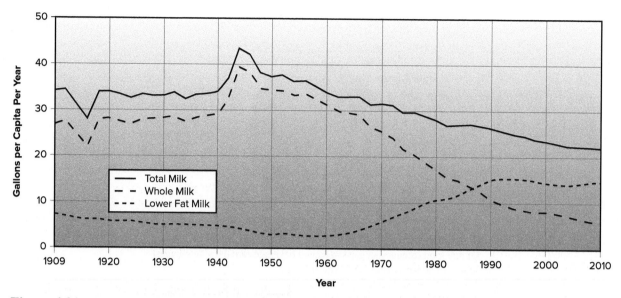

Figure 4.21 Trends in the annual per capita availability of total fluid milk, whole milk, and lower fat milk in gallons per person per year in the United States, 1909 to 2010.

Lower fat milk includes skim (fat-free) milk, 1% fat milk, and 2% fat milk combined. During the past century, per capita availability of lower fat milks has increased somewhat but not nearly enough to offset the steep decline in the availability of whole milk. Availability of total fluid milk in 2010 was one-third less than it was in 1909 and approximately one-half of what it was in 1944 when availability was at its peak.

Source: Food Availability (per Capita) Data System, Economic Research Service, USDA.

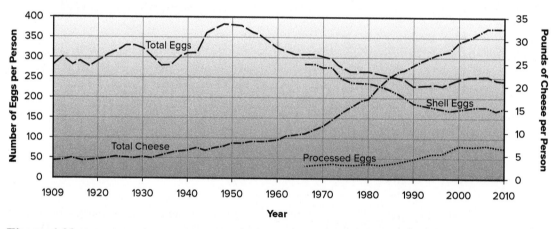

Figure 4.22 Trends in the annual per capita availability of eggs and cheese per person per year in the United States, 1909 to 2010, unadjusted for losses.

The availability of all eggs (those in the shell and those used in the processing of food) declined somewhat from 284 eggs per person per year in 1909 to 243 eggs per person per year in 2010. Between 1966 and 2010, availability of eggs in the shell declined from 284 eggs to 173 eggs per person per year while the number of eggs used in food processing increased from 30 to 73 eggs per person per year. Between 1909 and 2010, the annual per capita availability of cheese increased nearly 10-fold from 3.8 pounds per person per year to 32.8 pounds per person per year.

Source: Food Availability (per Capita) Data System, Economic Research Service, USDA.

Trends in Dairy Products

Americans have made substantial changes in the types and amount of milk they are consuming, as shown in Figure 4.21. Availability of whole milk has decreased, while the availability of low-fat and skim milk has increased markedly. Between 1909 and 2010, for example, per capita availability of whole milk (unadjusted for losses) fell from 27 to 6 gallons per person per year. During the same period, per capita availability of lower-fat milk (skim milk, 1% fat milk, and 2% fat milk), unadjusted for losses, doubled from 7 to 14 gallons per person per year. The gains in low-fat and skim milk have not offset the decline in whole milk, and overall, annual per capita availability of all fluid milk has declined from 34 gallons in 1909 to 22 gallons in 2010. Figure 4.22 illustrates changes in the annual per capita availability of eggs (left Y axis) and cheese (right Y axis) per person per year in the United States from 1909 to 2010 (unadjusted for losses). Between 1909 and 2010, the annual per capita availability of all eggs (those in the shell and those used in the processing of food) declined somewhat from 284 eggs per person per year to 243 eggs per person per year, respectively. In 1966 the USDA began collecting separate data on shell eggs and processed eggs. Between 1966 and 2010, availability of eggs in the shell declined from 284 eggs to 173 eggs per person per year while the number of eggs used in food processing increased from 30 to 73 eggs per person per year. The increased availability of processed eggs is primarily due to the greater consumption of fast foods and convenience foods prepared with processed eggs, many of which are eaten outside the home. In addition, concerns about consuming too much dietary cholesterol have led to increased popularity of commercially available cholesterol-free egg substitutes made from egg whites. Between 1909 and 2010, the annual per capita availability of cheese (unadjusted for losses) increased nearly 10-fold from 3.8 pounds per person per year to 32.8 pounds per person per year.

Trends in Beverages

A major factor in milk's drop in popularity (as shown in Figure 4.21) is competition from other beverages, especially regular carbonated soft drinks, which are now America's favorite type of beverage. As is shown in Figure 4.23, the annual per capita availability of all carbonated soft drinks combined is more than twice that of all types of fluid milk. Coffee is now the second most popular beverage, followed by beer, milk, diet carbonated soft drinks, tea, fruit juices, wine, and distilled spirits. However, as a combined group, alcoholic beverages—beer, wine, and distilled spirits—surpass coffee and milk in per capita consumption. Aggressive marketing of carbonated soft drinks and other sugar-sweetened beverages, and people's greater preference for soft drinks with meals, especially when eating away from home, also have contributed to declining milk consumption.

Between 1984 and 2008, total per capita availability of all carbonated soft drinks increased 20% from 39 gallons per person per year to 47 gallons, respectively. During the same interval, availability of diet soft drinks increased 58% from 9 gallons per person per year to 15 gallons, and the availability of regular soft drinks increased 9% from 30 to 32 gallons per person per year.[43]

Trends in Red Meat, Poultry, and Fish

Between 1909 and 2010, total per capita availability of red meat (beef, veal, pork, and lamb) and chicken (unadjusted for losses) increased 30% from 149 lb to 192 lb, respectively. During that same interval, total per capita availability of red meat decreased 16% from 133.5 lb to 111.7 lb, while availability of chicken increased 423% from 15 lb in 1909 to 80 lb in 2010, more than offsetting the decline in red meat. Between 1909 and 2010, the annual per capita availability of total fish and shellfish increased 44% from 11 lb to 16 lb, respectively. Figure 4.24 shows trends in the availability of beef, pork, chicken, and total fish and shellfish between 1909 and 2010. The primary reasons for the sharp

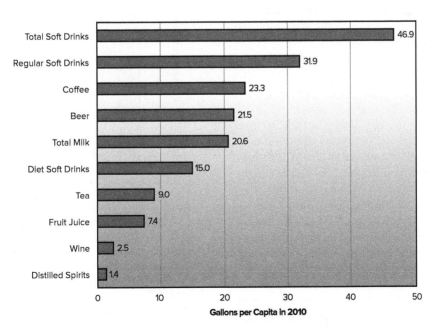

Figure 4.23 **Annual per capita availability of beverages in the United States in gallons in 2010, unadjusted for losses.**
By a wide margin, soft drinks are the most popular beverages in the United States, exceeding by more than twofold the availability of total milk. When all alcoholic beverages are combined in one group, they become the second most popular beverage in the United States.

Source: Food Availability (per Capita) Data System, Economic Research Service, USDA.

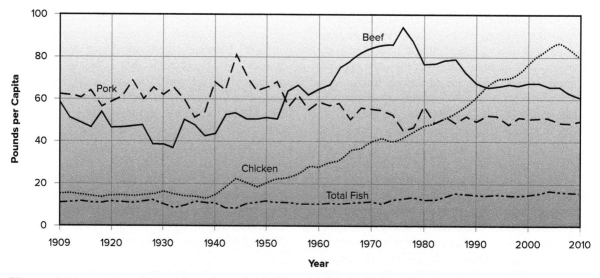

Figure 4.24 **Trends in the annual per capita availability of beef, pork, chicken, and total fish and shellfish per person per year in the United States, 1909 to 2010, unadjusted for losses.**
While the availability of beef and pork fluctuated between 1909 and 2010, overall, the availability of beef remained essentially unchanged in 2010 from what it was in 1909, while availability of pork declined slightly during this interval. Most notably, there was a more than fourfold increase in the availability of chicken during this period. Total fish and shellfish availability increased slightly.
Source: Food Availability (per Capita) Data System, Economic Research Service, USDA.

increase in chicken availability are lower prices for poultry due to technological advances and production efficiencies and aggressive marketing by the poultry industry. Greater consumer awareness of the fact that, ounce for ounce, red meat has more fat, saturated fat, and cholesterol than chicken and fish, and concerns about the link between red meat consumption and risk of coronary heart disease, have likely contributed to the overall decline in availability of red meat and the greater availability of chicken and fish.[17,40]

Trends in Fruits and Vegetables

As shown in Figure 4.25, total per capita availability of fruits and vegetables increased 21% and 11% between 1970 and 2010, respectively. Factors contributing to this increase include better quality, increased variety, and year-round availability of fresh produce. Public awareness of the health benefits of fruit and vegetable consumption may also be a factor. Much of the increase in vegetables occurred since 1982, when the U.S. National Academy of Sciences published its landmark report "Diet, Nutrition, and Cancer," which emphasized the importance of increased fruit and vegetable consumption as part of a comprehensive program to reduce cancer risk. This increased availability has been tempered by the fact that the price of fruits and vegetables has increased more than many other food items. Availability data also indicate changes in the kinds of fruits and vegetables Americans are purchasing. For example, in recent years per capita availability of iceberg lettuce has declined, while that of romaine and leaf lettuces has increased. Specialty lettuces not tracked by the USDA, such as radicchio, frisee, and arugula, have also gained in popularity. Much of the recent increase in fruits has been contributed by the greater availability of apples, bananas,

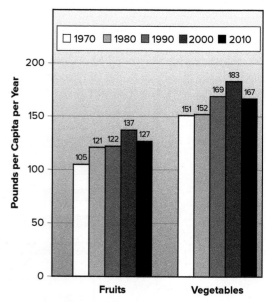

Figure 4.25 **Trends in the annual per capita availability of fruits and vegetables in pounds per person in the United States, 1970–2010, adjusted for losses.**
Between 1970 and 2010, the annual per capita availability of fruits and vegetables (adjusted for losses) increased overall.
Source: Food Availability (per Capita) Data System, Economic Research Service, USDA.

and grapes, while the increase in vegetables has been due to greater availability of tomatoes, onions, and leaf lettuces.[17,40]

Despite the increased loss-adjusted per capita availability of vegetables shown in Figure 4.25, these estimates of the amount of vegetables available for consumption remain less than what is recommended by the Dietary

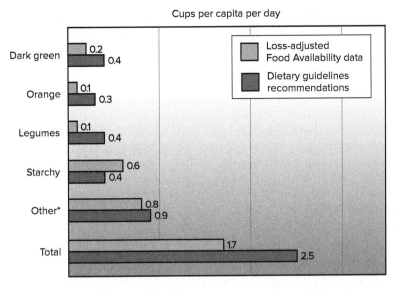

Figure 4.26 **Per capita loss adjusted food availability data for vegetables compared with the Dietary Guidelines' recommendations for vegetable consumption for someone following a 2000-calorie-per-day diet.**
Except in the case of starchy vegetables such as potatoes, the loss adjusted availability of vegetables in the United States is less than the amounts recommended by the Dietary Guidelines for Americans, especially for legumes and orange vegetables.

*Other vegetables include asparagus, broccoli, green beans, tomatoes, etc.

Source: Food Availability (per Capita) Data System, Economic Research Service, USDA.

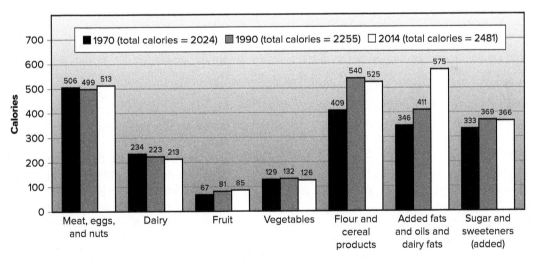

Figure 4.27 **Between 1970 and 2014, the total available calories increased 23%, with the sharpest increase in the "added fats and oils and dairy fats" category.**
Source: Food Availability (per Capita) Data System, Economic Research Service, USDA.

Guidelines for Americans, as is shown in Figure 4.26. Except in the case of starchy vegetables such as potatoes, the availability of vegetables in the United States is less than recommended by the Dietary Guidelines, especially for legumes and orange vegetables.[17]

Trends in Total Calories

As shown in Figure 4.27, the average, daily per capita number of calories available for consumption (after accounting for losses), adjusted for losses, from 2024 calories in 1970 to 2481 in 2014, a 23% increase. Calories in between 1970 and 2014, the loss-adjusted per capita number of calories availability from added fats and oils and dairy fats increased 66% from 346 calories per person per day in 1970 to 575 calories per person per day in 2014. The availability of calories from flour and cereal products increased 28%, while calories from fruit and vegetables stayed at low levels.

SUMMARY

1. National dietary and nutrition survey data are important in monitoring the nutritional status of a country's population, revealing the relationships between diet and health, identifying groups at nutritional risk and those who may benefit from food assistance programs, and evaluating the cost-effectiveness of food assistance and health education programs. These data are used to track food consumption trends and to monitor intakes of pesticides and other toxic substances.

2. Survey data provide a sound basis for agricultural policy and program development. They provide an early warning of impending food shortages and indicate how such crises may be prevented or alleviated. Food balance sheets estimate the amount of food that is available for consumption from the food distribution system.

3. Nutritional monitoring is the assessment of dietary or nutritional status at intermittent times to detect changes in the dietary or nutritional status of a population. In the United States, this has been conducted by two federal agencies: the U.S. Department of Agriculture (USDA) and the U.S. Department of Health and Human Services (HHS).

4. Passage of the National Nutrition Monitoring and Related Research Act of 1990 required the USDA and HHS to coordinate the nutritional monitoring activities of numerous federal agencies, which encompassed a wide variety of surveys and surveillance activities assessing the health and nutritional status of the U.S. population.

5. The USDA has been involved in collecting data on food availability, individual food consumption, and household food consumption. Since 1909, the USDA has used the balance sheet approach to estimate the annual per capita amount of food available for consumption. Availability (or food disappearance) is not an actual measure of food consumption. Loss-adjusted food availability data are modified to account for losses resulting from spoilage, disposal of inedible parts, trimming, cooking, food fed to pets and other animals, or wasted. It is useful for examining food trends, making international comparisons, and studying the relationships between diet and disease.

6. The USDA began assessing individual food intake with the Household Food Consumption Survey, which was later renamed the Nationwide Food Consumption Survey (NFCS) and was conducted during 1977–78 and 1987–88. The Continuing Survey of Food Intakes by Individuals replaced the NFCS. It provided timely information on U.S. diets, studied the dietary habits of persons at nutritional risk, provided data on "usual" diets by collecting several days of data over the course of a year, and demonstrated how diets varied over time.

7. Other nutritional monitoring activities of the USDA include development of food composition and nutrient databases, reporting of food and nutrient availability data, and the Supplemental Children's Survey. The Supplemental Children's Survey measured children's food consumption, so that pesticide residue exposure in children could be calculated.

8. Surveys currently conducted by the HHS include the National Health and Nutrition Examination Survey (NHANES), Total Diet Study, Health and Diet Survey, and Behavioral Risk Factor Surveillance System.

9. The NHANES monitors overall nutritional status of the U.S. population through detailed interviews (using dietary, demographic, socioeconomic, and health-related questions) and comprehensive physical examinations, including medical and dental examinations, anthropometric measurements, and diagnostic and laboratory tests.

10. The HHANES (1982–1984) was the largest and most comprehensive Hispanic health survey ever carried out in the United States. It collected health and nutritional data on the three largest subgroups of Hispanics living in the 48 continental states: Mexican Americans residing in five southwestern states, Cuban Americans living in Dade County, Florida, and Puerto Ricans residing in the New York City metropolitan area.

11. In response to the National Nutrition Monitoring and Related Research Act of 1990, NHANES became a continuous, annual survey in 1999. In 2002, the USDA's Continuing Survey of Food Intakes by Individuals and NHANES were integrated. Under the integrated framework, USDA is responsible for dietary data collection methodology, the food composition database, and the coding and processing of all dietary intake data. HHS is responsible for the sample design and data collection. Food and nutrient intake data from the integrated survey are referred to as *What We Eat in America, NHANES*.

12. Food availability data show that the percent of kilocalories from protein has held fairly steady at 11% to 12% since 1909 to the present. During the same period, the percent of kilocalories available from carbohydrate has decreased, while the percent of energy available from fat has increased.

13. Consumption of carbohydrate has declined because Americans now eat fewer grain and flour products and potatoes. Consumption of all sweeteners by Americans has increased in recent. Based on data from NHANES, dietary fiber intake is below recommended levels.

14. The availability of kilocalories from fat has increased since the early 1900s because of increased consumption of polyunsaturated and monounsaturated fats. The percent of kilocalories from saturated fat remained relatively constant throughout the 20th century.

15. Overall, Americans are drinking less milk and more sugar-sweetened beverages. Reasons for this include the popularity of soft drinks in restaurants and fast-food outlets, more meals eaten away from home, concern about saturated fat intake in dairy products, and the heavy advertising of sugar-sweetened beverages. When Americans do drink milk, they are now more likely to drink low-fat or skim milk than whole milk.

16. The annual per capita availability of red meat (beef, pork, veal, and lamb) has decreased between 1909 to the present. During the same interval, the availability of chicken has increased markedly as Americans have shown an increased preference for poultry because of its lower price and greater convenience.

17. Since 1970, the annual per capita loss-adjusted availability of added fats and oils and dairy fats has increased sharply, in contrast to low levels for fruit and vegetables.

REFERENCES

1. U.S. General Accounting Office. 1994. *Nutrition monitoring: Progress in developing a coordinated program.* Washington, DC: United States General Accounting Office. GAO/PEMD-94-23.

2. U.S. General Accounting Office. 1992. *Early intervention: Federal investments like WIC can produce savings.* Washington, DC: United States General Accounting Office. GAO/HRD-92-18.

3. National Research Council. 1989. *Diet and health: Implications for reducing chronic disease risk.* Washington, DC: National Academies Press.

4. Pao EM, Sykes KE, Cypel YS. 1989. *USDA methodological research for large-scale dietary intake surveys, 1975–88.* Washington, DC: U.S. Department of Agriculture, Human Nutrition Information Service.

5. Pelletier DL, Olson CM, Frongillo EA. 2006. Food insecurity, hunger, and undernutrition. In Bowman BA, Russell RM (eds.), *Present knowledge in nutrition,* 9th ed. Washington, DC: ILSI Press, 906–922.

6. Borrel A, Young H. 2006. Public nutrition in complex emergencies. In Bowman BA, Russell RM (eds.), *Present knowledge in nutrition,* 9th ed. Washington, DC: ILSI Press, 923–938.

7. Life Science Research Office, Federation of American Societies for Experimental Biology. 1989. *Nutrition monitoring in the United States: An update report on nutrition monitoring.* Washington, DC: U.S. Government Printing Office.

8. Moshfegh AL. 1994. The National Nutrition Monitoring and Related Research Program: Progress and activities. *Journal of Nutrition* 124:1843S–1845S.

9. Kuczmarski MF, Moshfegh A, Briefel R. 1994. Update on nutrition monitoring activities in the United States. *Journal of the American Dietetic Association* 94:753–760.

10. Woteki CE, Briefel RR, Klein CJ, Jacques PF, Kris-Etherton PM, Mares-Perlman JA, Meyers LD. 2002. Nutrition monitoring: Summary of a statement from an American Society for Nutritional Sciences working group. *Journal of Nutrition* 132:3782–3783.

11. U.S. Department of Health and Human Services, U.S. Department of Agriculture. 1993. Ten-year comprehensive plan for the national nutrition monitoring and related research program; notice. *Federal Register* 58(111):32751–32806.

12. Briefel RR. 1994. Assessment of the U.S. diet in national nutrition surveys: National collaborative efforts and NHANES. *American Journal of Clinical Nutrition* 59(suppl):164S–167S.

13. Interagency Board for Nutrition Monitoring and Related Research. Bialostosky K, ed. 2000. *Nutrition monitoring in the United States: The directory of federal and state nutrition monitoring and related research activities.* Hyattsville, MD: National Center for Health Statistics.

14. Grandjean AC. 2012. Dietary intake data collection: Challenges and limitations. *Nutrition Reviews* 70(suppl 2):S101–S104.

15. Hiza HAB, Bente L. 2011. *Nutrient content of the U.S. food supply: Developments between 2000 and 2006.* Home Economics Research Report No. 59. Washington, DC: U.S. Department of Agriculture, Center for Nutrition Policy and Promotion.

16. Muth MK, Karns SA, Nielsen SJ, Buzby JC, Wells HF. 2011.

Consumer-level food loss estimates and their use in the ERS loss-adjusted food availability data. Technical Bulletin No. 1927. Washington, DC: U.S. Department of Agriculture, Economic Research Service.

17. Wells HF, Buzby JC. 2008. *Dietary assessment of major trends in U.S. food consumption, 1970–2005*. Economic Information Bulletin, No. 33. Washington, DC: U.S. Department of Agriculture, Economic Research Service.

18. McDowell M. 2003. U.S. Department of Health and Human Services–U.S. Department of Agriculture survey integration activities. *Journal of Food Composition and Analysis* 16:343–346.

19. Coleman-Jensen A, Rabbitt MP, Gregory CA, and Singh A. September 2016. *Household food security in the United States in 2015*, ERR-215, U.S. Department of Agriculture, Economic Research Service.

20. Wunderlich GS, Norwood JL (eds.). 2006. *Food insecurity and hunger in the United States: An assessment of the measure*. Committee on National Statistics, Division of Behavioral and Social Sciences and Education, National Research Council. Washington, DC: National Academies Press.

21. Yetley E, Johnson C. 1987. Nutritional applications of the health and nutrition examination surveys (HANES). *Annual Review of Nutrition* 7:441–463.

22. Citizens Board of Inquiry into Hunger and Malnutrition. 1968. *Hunger—USA*. Washington, DC: New Community Press.

23. Ahluwalia N, Dwyer J, Terry A, Moshfegh A, Johnson C. 2016. Update on NHANES dietary data: Focus on collection, release, analytical considerations, and uses to inform public policy. *Advances in Nutrition* 7:121–134.

24. National Center for Health Statistics. 1994. *Plan and operation of the Third National Health and Examination Survey, 1988–94*. Hyattsville, MD: U.S. Department of Health and Human Services, Public Health Service, Centers for Disease Control and Prevention.

25. Delgado JL, Johnson CL, Roy I, Treviño FM. 1990. Hispanic Health and Nutrition Examination Survey: Methodological considerations. *American Journal of Public Health* 80(suppl):65–105.

26. Woteki CE. 1990. The Hispanic Health and Nutrition Examination Survey (HHANES 1982–1984): Background and introduction. *American Journal of Clinical Nutrition* 51(suppl):897S–901S.

27. Chumlea WC, Guo S, Kuczmarski RJ, Johnson CL, Leahy CK. 1990. Reliability for anthropometric measurements in the Hispanic Health and Nutrition Examination Survey (HHANES 1982–1984). *American Journal of Clinical Nutrition* 51(suppl):902S–907S.

28. Roche AF, Guo S, Baumgartner RN, Chumlea WC, Ryan AS, Kuczmarski RJ. 1990. Reference data for weight, stature, and weight/stature in Mexican Americans from the Hispanic Health and Nutrition Examination Survey (HHANES 1982–1984). *American Journal of Clinical Nutrition* 51(suppl):917S–924S.

29. Woteki CE, Briefel R, Hitchcock D, Ezzati T, Maurer K. 1990. Selection of nutrition status indicators for field surveys: The NHANES III design. *Journal of Nutrition* 120:1440–1445.

30. Kuczmarski RJ, Ogden CL, Grummer-Strawn LM, Flegal KM, Guo SS, et al. 2000. *CDC growth charts: United States. Advance data from vital and health statistics; no. 314*. Hyattsville, MD: National Center for Health Statistics.

31. Woteki CE. 2003. Integrated NHANES: Uses in national policy. *Journal of Nutrition* 133:582S–584S.

32. Pennington JAT. 2000. Total diet studies—Experiences in the United States. *Journal of Food Composition and Analysis* 13:539–544. http://www.fda.gov/Food/FoodScienceResearch/TotalDietStudy/.

33. White LL, Goldberg HI, Gilbert TJ, Ballew C, Mendlein JM, Peter DG, Percy CA, Mokdad AH. 1997. Rationale, design and methodology for the Navajo Health and Nutrition Survey.

Journal of Nutrition 127(10 suppl):2078S–2084S.

34. Byers T, Hubbard J. 1997. The Navajo Health and Nutrition Survey: Research that can make a difference. *Journal of Nutrition* 127:2075S–2077S.

35. Reinhold C, Dalenius K, Brindley P, Smith B, Grummer-Strawn L. 2011. *Pregnancy Nutrition Surveillance 2009 report*. Atlanta: U.S. Department of Health and Human Services, Centers for Disease Control and Prevention. www.cdc.gov/pednss.

36. Polhamus B, Dalenius K, Mackintosh H, Smith B, Grummer-Strawn L. 2011. *Pediatric Nutrition Surveillance 2009 report*. Atlanta: U.S. Department of Health and Human Services, Center for Disease Control and Prevention. www.cdc.gov/pednss.

37. Lin CTJ, Zhang Y, Carlton ED, Lo SC. 2016. *2014 FDA Health and Diet Survey*. www.fda.gov.

38. Behavioral Risk Factor Surveillance System, Centers for Disease Control and Prevention. www.cdc.gov/brfss/.

39. National Health Interview Survey, Centers for Disease Control and Prevention. www.cdc.gov/nchs/nhis.htm.

40. Morrison RM, Buzby JC, Wells HF. 2010. Guess who's turning 100? Tracking a century of American eating. *Amber Waves* 8(1):12–19. www.ers.usda.gov/amberwaves.

41. Hiza HAB, Bente L. 2007. *Nutrient content of the U.S. food supply, 1909–2004: A summary report*. Home Economics Research Report No. 57. Washington, DC: U.S. Department of Agriculture, Center for Nutrition Policy and Promotion.

42. Rehm CD, Peñalvo JL, Afshin A, Mozaffarian D. 2016. Dietary intake among US adults, 1999–2012. *Journal of the American Association* 315:2542–2553.

43. U.S. Department of Health and Human Services and U.S. Department of Agriculture. December 2015. *2015–2020 Dietary guidelines for Americans*, 8th ed. Available at http://health.gov/dietaryguidelines/2015/guidelines/.

ASSESSMENT ACTIVITY 4.1

Accessing Data from the Behavioral Risk Factor Surveillance System Website

As discussed earlier in this chapter, the Behavioral Risk Factor Surveillance System (BRFSS) is a state-based telephone survey of the U.S. noninstitutionalized civilian adult population established in 1984 by the U.S. Centers for Disease Control and Prevention (CDC). The BRFSS is intended to provide data on the prevalence of personal health practices identified as risk factors for one or more of the 10 leading causes of death. Data can be analyzed in several ways, including by individual state or by smaller geographic areas within states known as metropolitan and micropolitan statistical areas (MMSAs). A metropolitan statistical area is a group of counties that contains at least one urbanized area of 50,000 or more inhabitants. A micropolitan statistical area is a group of counties that contains at least one urban cluster of at least 10,000 but less than 50,000 inhabitants. Data from the BRFSS are used by state and local health departments to plan, initiate, and guide health promotion and disease prevention programs as well as to monitor the success of such programs over time.

The CDC provides several different interactive databases for accessing data from the BRFSS, including prevalence and trend data on various health risks by individual states, all states, or selected metropolitan and micropolitan statistical areas. These and other data can be accessed by going to the Behavioral Risk Factor Surveillance System's website at http://www.cdc.gov/brfss/. In this Assessment Activity, go to "Prevalence Data & Data Analysis Tools." Find your Metropolitan/Micropolitan Statistical Areas (MMSA), explore the data, and list and describe 10 interesting facts.

ASSESSMENT ACTIVITY 4.2

What's in the Foods You Eat?

The U.S. Department of Agriculture's Food Surveys Research Group has created a search tool it calls "What's in the Foods You Eat?" This search tool provides easy online access to data on the nutrient content of about 13,000 foods that Americans typically eat every day; the search tool uses the data files in the Food and Nutrient Database for Dietary Studies, which is also used in processing What We Eat in America, the dietary intake interview component of NHANES. Users can easily search the database, view and select portions and weights for a food, and then view the nutrient composition of the food. The search tool is designed to provide nutrient composition data for foods as eaten, so it contains many food mixtures, common portion sizes, and some brand names. Each result can be printed by the user.

The search tool can be found at https://www.ars. usda.gov/ (and then click on "Nutrient Data Tools"). In this Assessment Activity, go to the "What's in the Foods You East Search Tool" and enter 10 of your favorite food items. Make a table of these 10 foods and summarize at least 12 of the key nutrients for each food.

5 COMPUTERIZED DIETARY ANALYSIS SYSTEMS

STUDENT LEARNING OUTCOMES

After reading this chapter, students will be able to:

1. Understand the role of computers in nutritional assessment.

2. List criteria for selecting a quality computerized dietary analysis system.

3. Use an Internet-based dietary analysis program.

INTRODUCTION: USING COMPUTERS IN NUTRITIONAL ASSESSMENT

Prior to the development of computers and diet analysis software, the manual nutritional analysis of diets was difficult and time consuming. Consider, for example, the steps you would take to manually calculate intake of energy, protein, carbohydrate, total fat, calcium, iron, vitamin C, and other nutrients from a 24-hour recall using nutrient data from a published table. Your first step would be to find the appropriate food in the table and then compare the amount you actually ate with the portion size listed for the food. If these differed, you would have to mathematically adjust all of the nutrient values before listing them on a spreadsheet table. After doing this for each food in your 24-hour recall, you would have to add all of the values for each nutrient to calculate your final 24-hour intake. Next you would have to compare intake to a dietary standard, such as the RDA/DRI, and express this as a percentage. And you can imagine how much more difficult this process would be if you were analyzing a seven-day food record in which nutrient intake would have to be expressed as a daily average.

Clearly, computers are perfectly suited to this task of nutrient analysis, which is nothing more than number crunching, saving time, labor, and expense while reducing error (Figure 5.1).[1–5] Hundreds of software programs have been developed since the mid-1980s for all sorts of nutrition-related tasks, including analysis of food records and food frequency questionnaires, menu planning and forecasting, analysis of recipes, food service and food management tasks, nutrition education, patient interviews and counseling, and research.

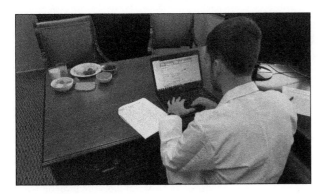

Figure 5.1
Computers are well suited to the task of nutrient analysis.
©David C. Nieman

The purpose of this chapter is to delineate important characteristics of computerized dietary analysis systems to aid you in selecting an appropriate software package for the analysis of food records, food frequency questionnaires, and recipes. Dietary analysis systems are available on the Internet, and the strengths and weaknesses of these systems will be described.

Descriptions of computer applications in nutrition and dietetics first appeared in the literature in the late 1950s. Computer hardware cost is no longer the prohibitive factor it once used to be, and most hospitals, clinics, businesses, and educational facilities provide personal computer work stations for their employees. Computerized dietary intake analysis is an important skill for dietitians and nutritionists to master.

FACTORS TO CONSIDER IN SELECTING A COMPUTERIZED DIETARY ANALYSIS SYSTEM

Hundreds of dietary analysis software packages are available, ranging from simplified programs designed for elementary school students to comprehensive programs designed for researchers. In selecting a dietary analysis program, the first step is to establish the major needs for obtaining the software, with specific tasks defined. Once this has been accomplished, choose a dietary analysis system that is suitable to these needs and tasks. For example, a research professor in a university nutrition department will probably need a completely different type of computerized dietary analysis system than a public health nutritionist working with pregnant women at nutritional risk in a county health department.

In comparing software programs, dietitians and other health professionals should consider aspects of the database, program operation, and system output.[6–9]

Nutrient Database

The most important consideration to make when selecting a computerized diet analysis system is its nutrient database.[1,2,7] The database must be accurate, well documented, and large enough to meet all intended tasks. Software vendors begin development of their databases with data from the U.S. Department of Agriculture (USDA). The USDA began publishing food composition values in 1896 and has continually revised and expanded its food composition tables ever since.[10] The USDA has also contributed to the development of food composition tables for other countries for many years and has participated in the International Network of Food Data Systems (INFOODS), organized first in 1984. INFOODS is a comprehensive effort, under the United Nations University Food and Nutrition Program and cosponsored by the Food and Agriculture Organization (FAO) of the United Nations, to improve data on the nutrient composition of foods from all parts of the world. See http://www.fao.org/infoods/ for more information on INFOODS. INFOODS maintains a list of links to software tools for dietary assessment and food composition database management systems.

USDA Nutrient Data Laboratory

The Beltsville Human Nutrition Research Center (BHNRC) is one of six human nutrition research centers within the Agricultural Research Service (ARS). The mission of BHNRC is to define, through research, the role of food and its components in optimizing human health and in reducing the risk of nutritionally related disorders in the diverse population. The Nutrient Data Laboratory (NDL) of the USDA is one of six units in the BHNRC. NDL has an interdisciplinary staff comprised of nutritionists, food technologists, and computer specialists. The mission of the Nutrient Data Laboratory is to provide leadership and to promote international cooperation in the development of authoritative nutrient databases and state-of-the-art methods to acquire, evaluate, compile, and disseminate composition data on foods available in the United States. As part of its mission, the NDL operates the National Nutrient Databank for Food Composition, a computerized information system for storing and summarizing data on the composition of foods. See Box 5.1 for a glossary of terms and acronyms used by the NDL.

The USDA NDL develops and maintains a number of databases, including the USDA Nutrient Database for Standard Reference (SR). SR nutrient data serve as the core for most commercial and many foreign databases and are the numerical foundation of essentially all public and private work in the field of human nutrition.

USDA Nutrient Databases

The primary product of the Nutrient Data Laboratory is the SR, and yearly updates are made to this database to ensure that product information is current and of the highest quality. A subset of SR is used to support the What We Eat in America component of the National Health and Nutrition Examination Survey. Data from the USDA National Nutrient Database are used for many research,

Box 5.1   **Acronyms and Documentation Terms**

The following is a list of definitions of acronyms and terms used in this chapter and in documentation for the USDA National Nutrient Database for Standard Reference.

Analytical	Data from laboratory analysis of one or more food samples
AOAC	Association of Official Analytical Chemists, independent scientific organization that published a reference of methods used in analyzing the composition of foods.
AMS	Agricultural Marketing Service, USDA
ARS	Agricultural Research Service, USDA
Atwater System	System developed by W. O. Atwater to calculate the energy contributed by protein, fat, and carbohydrates to foods.
BHNRC	Beltsville Human Nutrition Research Center
Calculated	Nutrient values computed or estimated by mathematical adjustment. Normalizing nutrients to an average moisture or fat value, use of retention factors, and substitution of similar ingredients in a formulation or recipe are examples of calculated values.
CFR	Code of Federal Regulations
CNPP	Center for Nutrition Policy and Promotion, USDA. Has information on the Dietary Guidelines, and MyPyramid.gov.
Derivation code	A 4-character, alphabetic code used to document Standard Reference nutrient data source and quality.
Discontinued item	Food product no longer sold or available commercially; item removed from Standard Reference Database.
FDA	Food and Drug Administration, U.S. Department of Health and Human Services
FNIC	Food and Nutrition Information Center. One of NAL's information centers.
Food Group	NDL categorizes foods into similar groups and assigns a Food Group Code, such as cereal grains and pasta (20), beverages (14), vegetables (11).
Food Group Code	Two-digit numeric code identifying individual Food Groups. Food Groups are further classified by subcodes, to produce a four-digit numeric code. For example, fresh pork is 1010, while cured pork is 1020. Food group codes are independent of NDB numbers.
Formulation	The estimated proportion by weight of ingredients in a multi-ingredient commercial food item when other characteristics of the food item are known or can be set. Characteristics that may be known or can be set include: order of predominance of ingredients, retention codes, target moisture level of individual ingredients and final product, and lower and upper bounds on the proportion of any individual ingredient. As a minimum, to derive a formulation, some nutrient values must be known and flagged for matching.
FSIS	Food Safety and Inspection Service, USDA
Handbook 8 (AH-8)	USDA Agriculture Handbook No. 8, *Composition of Foods*
HG-72	Home and Garden Bulletin No. 72, *Nutritive Value of Foods*
Household measure	Standard weight (sometimes with dimensions) or portion of individual food. Sometimes called serving size.
Imputed	Nutrient values developed when analytical values are unavailable. Nutrient values from another form of the same food, or another species of the same genus are examples of imputed values.
INFOODS	International Network of Food Data Systems
Item	Individual food or food product
Key Foods	Identification of foods most highly consumed and also best sources of nutrients deemed important to national dietary health. Key Foods are identified as those foods contributing up to 75% of any one nutrient. Key Foods are used by NDL to set priorities for our nutrient analysis contracts.
Label	Data printed on a food label, as supplied by its manufacturer. The values are primarily company analytical or imputed; however, the values have been rounded and/or adjusted to provide uniform serving size weights.
NAL	National Agricultural Library, USDA located in Beltsville, Maryland
NCI	National Cancer Institute, NIH

Box 5.1   *Continued*

NHANES	National Health and Nutrition Examination Survey. Conducted by the National Center for Health Statistics, U.S. Department of Health and Human Services	Refuse	Portion of food removed before consumption (meat bones, fruit pits, etc.).
NHLBI	National Heart, Lung and Blood Institute, NIH	RM	Reference Material used for evaluating the reliability of analytical methods
NNDB	USDA National Nutrient Databank	Source code	One-character numeric code to document source of nutrient data.
NDB No.	Identification number for food item in USDA Nutrient Database	SRM	Standard Reference Material from NIST used for evaluating the reliability of analytical methods
NIH	National Institutes of Health	Standard Reference (SR)	USDA National Nutrient Database for Standard Reference
NIST	National Institute of Standards and Technology, U.S. Department of Commerce	Tagname	INFOODS Tag Names identify individual nutrients for international interchange of nutrient data.
NLEA	National Labeling and Education Act of 1990. Refers to food-labeling regulations promulgated by the FDA.	UPC	Universal Product Code is a unique product identification number found on most product labels, represented by bar and number codes.
NTIS	National Technical Information Service, U.S. Department of Commerce	USDA	U.S. Department of Agriculture
PDS	Primary Data Set for USDA Nationwide Food Surveys. No longer a separate database, but part of SR.	USDA Commodity	Foods donated, or available for donation, by the Department under authorizing legislation, for use in any state in child nutrition programs, nonprofit summer camps for children, charitable institutions, nutrition programs for the elderly, the Commodity Supplemental Nutrition Program for Women, Infants, and Children (WIC), the Food Distribution Programs on Indian Reservations, and the assistance of needy people.
Recipe	The known weight or measure of ingredients in a multi-ingredient food item. Amounts of ingredients may be expressed in household volume measure units such as cups and tablespoons or may be expressed as gram weights. The term "recipe" is generally applied to a food item prepared from component ingredients in a household or institutional setting. The term may also apply to a commercial multi-ingredient food item for which the amounts of ingredients are set, rather than estimated (e.g., by Standards of Identity).	HHS	U.S. Department of Health and Human Services

Source: USDA Nutrient Data Laboratory, Agricultural Research Service.

policy, education, treatment, and nutrition monitoring programs. SR includes food composition data for nearly 9000 foods; of these, approximately 2000 are brand-name items. SR is released annually at www.ars.usda.gov/nutrientdata. Until 1992, most of this information was published in the form of *Agriculture Handbook 8* (AH-8). However, AH-8 is no longer available in printed form and SR supersedes and incorporates all of the composition data that were included in AH-8.

As information is updated, new versions of the SR database are released. Release 28 (SR28) was initially issued in September 2015 and revised in May 2016 and contained data on 8789 food items and up to 150 food components. Table 5.1 lists the 25 food groups included in SR28.

Data for SR28 were compiled from published and unpublished sources. Published sources included the scientific literature. Unpublished data were from the food industry, other government agencies, and research conducted under contracts initiated by the Agricultural Research Service (ARS). These analyses are currently conducted under the National Food and Nutrient Analysis

TABLE 5.1	USDA Nutrient Database for Standard Reference, Release 28

	Food Group
01	Dairy and Egg Products
02	Spices and Herbs
03	Baby Foods
04	Fats and Oils
05	Poultry Products
06	Soups, Sauces, and Gravies
07	Sausages and Luncheon Meats
08	Breakfast Cereals
09	Fruits and Fruit Juices
10	Pork Products
11	Vegetables and Vegetable Products
12	Nut and Seed Products
13	Beef Products
14	Beverages
15	Finfish and Shellfish Products
16	Legumes and Legume Products
17	Lamb, Veal, and Game Products
18	Baked Products
19	Sweets
20	Cereal Grains and Pasta
21	Fast Foods
22	Meals, Entrees, and Sidedishes
25	Snacks
35	American Indian/Alaska Native Foods
36	Restaurant Foods

Source: U.S. Department of Agriculture, Agricultural Research Service, Nutrient Data Laboratory. USDA National Nutrient Database for Standard Reference, Release 28 (Slightly revised).

Program (NFNAP), in cooperation with the National Cancer Institute and other offices and institutes of the National Institutes of Health, the Centers for Disease Control and Prevention (CDC), and the Food and Drug Administration (FDA). Data from the food industry represent the nutrient content of a specific food or food product at the time the data are sent to NDL. Values in the database may be based on the results of laboratory analyses or calculated by using appropriate algorithms, factors, or recipes, as indicated by the source code in the Nutrient Data file.

When nutrient data for prepared or cooked products are unavailable or incomplete, nutrient values are calculated from comparable raw items or by recipe. When values are calculated in a recipe or from the raw item, appropriate nutrient retention and food yield factors are applied. To obtain the content of nutrient per 100 g of cooked food, the nutrient content per 100 g of raw food is multiplied by the nutrient retention factor and, where appropriate, adjustments are made for fat and moisture gains and losses. Nutrient retention factors are based on data from USDA research contracts, research reported in the literature, and USDA publications.

Various checks have been built into the NDBS to ensure that, to the extent possible, all nutrient fields for each food are complete. Another check is to make sure that various calculations are completed and correct. Despite these efforts, some food items do not contain complete nutrient data. Blanks in the SR28 database are regarded as "missing data" or an indication of lack of reliable data. If a value is not present for any particular nutrient, this should not be regarded as zero or any other value—only that no value is available in SR. Table 5.2 summarizes the number of foods in the SR28 database containing selected nutrients.

Nutrient values per 100 grams and in edible portions of common measures (e.g., cup, tablespoon, or teaspoon) are contained in SR28. Other data are listed to further describe the mean value including the standard error, number of data points upon which the mean is based, the derivation code, and the source code. The derivation code documents the nutrient data source and quality. An "A," for example, means "analytical data." The source code field indicates how the data value was determined (for example, analytical, calculated, or assumed zero). Several support files that accompany SR28 provide more specific information on the source code, descriptive information about the food items, and descriptions of inedible material (for example, seeds, bone, skin).

Table 5.3 gives an example of the data that are available for each food in SR28. Analytical values represent the total amount of the nutrient present in the edible portion of the food, including any nutrients added in processing. The values do not necessarily represent the nutrient amounts available to the body.

The USDA Food and Nutrient Database for Dietary Studies (FNDDS) is a database of over 8500/beverages foods, nutrient values for 65 nutrients/food components and energy, and weights for typical food portions (formerly called Survey Nutrient Database). The FNDDS is used to process data from the survey What We Eat in America, the dietary intake component of the National Health and Nutrition Examination Survey (NHANES). The FNDDS is available for use in other dietary research studies and can be downloaded free from the website of USDA's Food Surveys Research Group (FSRG), which develops and maintains the FNDDS. The FNDDS is designed for the coding and analysis of food consumption data. Many of the foods in FNDDS are mixtures that are not available in the SR. The SR is the source of the nutrient values for foods in FNDDS, including mixed foods whose nutrient values are calculated using SR items as ingredients. The FNDDS portion descriptions include

TABLE 5.2	Number of Foods in the Database ($n = 8789$) Containing a Value for the Specified Nutrient			

Nutr. No	Nutrient	Count	Nutr. No	Nutrient	Count
255	Water* [†]	8788	321	Carotene, beta* [†]	5627
208	Energy* [†]	8789	322	Carotene, alpha* [†]	5531
268	Energy	8756	334	Cryptoxanthin, beta* [†]	5519
203	Protein* [†]	8789	337	Vitamin A, IU* [†]	8078
257	Adjusted Protein	4	318	Lycopene	5497
204	Total lipid (fat)* [†]	8789	338	Lutein + zeaxanthin	5474
207	Ash* [†]	8464	323	Vitamin E (alphatocopherol)* [†]	5900
205	Carbohydrate, by difference* [†]	8789	573	Vitamin E, added*	4777
291	Fiber, total dietary* [†]	8195	341	Tocopherol, beta	1889
269	Sugars, total* [†]	6957	342	Tocopherol, gamma	1886
210	Sucrose	1743	343	Tocopherol, delta	1870
211	Glucose (dextrose)	1752	344	Tocotrienol, alpha	1460
212	Fructose	1753	345	Tocotrienol, beta	1475
213	Lactose	1731	346	Tocotrienol gamma	1463
214	Maltose	1719	347	Tocotrienol, delta	1458
287	Galactose	1601	328	Vitamin D (D2 + D3)* [†]	5527
209	Starch	1180	325	Vitamin D2 (ergocalciferol)	139
301	Calcium, Ca* [†]	8441	326	Vitamin D3 (cholecalciferol)	1945
303	Iron, Fe* [†]	8645	324	Vitamin D [†]	5578
304	Magnesium, Mg* [†]	8050	430	Vitamin K (phylloquinone)* [†]	5226
305	Phosphorus, P* [†]	8210	429	Dihydrophylloquinone	1410
306	Potassium, K* [†]	8363	428	Menaquinone-4	588
307	Sodium, Na* [†]	8706	606	Fatty acids, total saturated* [†]	8440
309	Zinc, Zn* [†]	8083	607	4:0*	5887
312	Copper, Cu* [†]	7532	608	6:0*	5918
315	Manganese, Mn* [†]	6629	609	8:0*	6125
317	Selenium, se* [†]	7089	610	10:0*	6478
313	Fluoride, F	554	611	12:0*	6664
401	Vitamin C, total ascorbic acid* [†]	7971	696	13:0	270
404	Thiamin* [†]	8155	612	14:0*	7006
405	Riboflavin* [†]	8173	652	15:0	2399
406	Niacin* [†]	8152	613	16:0*	7213
410	Pantothenic acid	6544	653	17:0	2785
415	Vitamin B_6* [†]	7884	614	18:0*	7202
417	Folate, total* [†]	7528	615	20:0	2862
431	Folic acid* [†]	6750	624	22:0	2324
432	Folate, food* [†]	7021	654	24:0	2250
435	Folate, DFE* [†]	6732	645	Fatty acids, total monounsaturated* [†]	8123
421	Choline, total* [†]	4773	625	14:1	2755
454	Betaine	2084	697	15:1	2101
418	Vitamin B_{12}* [†]	7596	626	16:1 undifferentiated*	6999
578	Vitamin B_{12} added*	4931	673	16:1 c	1373
320	Vitamin A, RAE* [†]	7254	662	16:1 t	1243
319	Retinol* [†]	6983	687	17:1	2485

continued

| TABLE 5.2 | Number of Foods in the Database (*n* = 8789) Containing a Value for the Specified Nutrient—*continued* | | | | |

Nutr. No	Nutrient	Count	Nutr. No	Nutrient	Count
617	18:1 undifferentiated*	7229	621	22:6 n-3 (DHA)*	5955
674	18:1 c	1870	605	Fatty acids, total trans	5041
663	18:1 t	1919	693	Fatty acids, total transmonoenoic	1896
859	18:1-11 t (18:1t n-7)	168	695	Fatty acids, total transpolyenoic	1601
628	20:1	6503	601	Cholesterol* [†]	8379
630	22:1 undifferentiated*	5979	636	Phytosterols	503
676	22:1 c	1152	638	Stigmasterol	138
664	22: 1 t	866	639	Campesterol	138
671	24: 1 c	1384	641	Beta-sitosterol	139
646	Fatty acids, total polyunsaturated* [†]	8124	501	Tryptophan	5104
618	18:2 undifferentiated*	7247	502	Threonine	5153
675	18:2 n-6 c,c	1841	503	Isoleucine	5157
670	18:2 CLAs	1499	504	Leucine	5156
669	18:2 t,t	362	505	Lysine	5170
666	18:2 i	59	506	Methionine	5170
665	18:2 t not further defined	1204	507	Cystine	5004
619	18:3 undifferentiated*	7152	508	Phenylalanine	5153
851	18:3 n-3 c,c,c (ALA)	1969	509	Tyrosine	5123
685	18:3 n-6 c,c,c	1662	510	Valine	5157
856	18:3i	534	511	Arginine	5143
627	18:4	5904	512	Histidine	5150
672	20:2 n-6 c,c	2519	513	Alanine	5099
689	20:3 undifferentiated	2317	514	Aspartic acid	4946
852	20:3 n-3	1022	515	Glutamic acid	5103
853	20:3 n-6	1245	516	Glycine	5099
620	20:4 undifferentiated*	6509	517	Proline	5091
855	20:4 n-6	164	518	Serine	5099
629	20:5 n-3 (EPA)*	5998	521	Hydroxyproline	1434
857	21:5	127	221	Alcohol, ethyl*	5591
858	22:4	1068	262	Caffeine*	5396
631	22:5 n-3 (DPA)*	5954	263	Theobromine*	5356

*Indicates the 65 nutrients included in the USDA Food and Nutrient Database for Dietary Studies (FNDDS).
[†]Nutrients included in the Abbreviated file (p. 38).
Source: U.S. Department of Agriculture, Agricultural Research Service, Nutrient Data Laboratory. USDA National Nutrient Database for Standard Reference, Release 28 (Slightly revised).

common unit measures such as slice, piece, snack size, medium, teaspoon, and cup. For that reason, FNDDS includes additional weights for common food portion sizes that are not available in the SR. There are no missing values in the FNDDS, and each food has values for energy and 64 nutrients and food components. The FNDDS is updated every two years in conjunction with data released from What We Eat in America, NHANES.

Other data sets developed by the NDL are listed and described in Box 5.2. These databases include the USDA Branded Food Products Database, Dietary Supplement Ingredient Database, USDA National Nutrient Database for Standard Reference Dataset for What We Eat in America, NHANES, Cooking Yield and Nutrient Retention Factors, and specialty databases providing data for sodium, choline, flavonoids, fluoride, and oxalic acid. This website (https://ndb.nal.usda.gov/ndb/) allows users to search several USDA Food Composition Databases from one location. These include the USDA National Nutrient Database for Standard Reference, USDA Branded

TABLE 5.3	An Example of the Nutrient Data Available for Each Food in SR28

NDB No. 09003
Apples, raw, with skin (1)
Malus domestica
Includes USDA commodity food A343
Refuse: 10% Core and stem

Nutrients and Units		Amount in 100 grams or edible portion					Amount in edible portion of common measures of food		
		Mean	Std. Error	Number of Data Points	Deriv Code	Confidence Source code	Measure 1	Measure 2	Measure 3
Proximates:									
Water	g	85.56	0.241	38	A	1	106.95	93.26	190.80
Energy	kcal	52		0	NC	4	65	57	116
Energy	kj	218		0	NC	4	272	237	486
Protein (N × 6.25)	g	0.26	0.019	29	A	1	0.33	0.29	0.59
Total lipid (fat)	g	0.17	0.011	35	A	1	0.22	0.19	0.39
Ash	g	0.19	0.018	29	A	1	0.24	0.21	0.43
Carbohydrate, by difference	g	13.81		0	NC	4	17.26	15.05	30.80
Fiber, total dietary	g	2.4	0.276	29	A	1	2.9	2.6	5.2
Sugars, total	g	10.39	0.112	25	A	1	12.99	11.32	23.17
Sucrose	g	2.07	0.049	25	A	1	2.58	2.25	4.61
Glucose (dextrose)	g	2.43	0.031	25	A	1	3.03	2.65	5.41
Fructose	g	5.90	0.059	25	A	1	7.37	6.43	13.15
Lactose	g	0.00	0.000	25	A	1	0.00	0.00	0.00
Maltose	g	0.00	0.000	25	A	1	0.00	0.00	0.00
Galactose	g	0.00	0.000	25	A	1	0.00	0.00	0.00
Starch	g	0.05	0.000	10	A	1	0.07	0.06	0.12
Minerals:									
Calcium, Ca	mg	6	0.340	26	A	1	7	6	13
Iron, Fe	mg	0.12	0.009	16	A	1	0.15	0.13	0.28
Magnesium, Mg	mg	5	0.073	26	A	1	6	6	12
Phosphorus, P	mg	11	0.337	23	A	1	14	12	25
Potassium, K	mg	107	2.211	26	A	1	134	117	239
Sodium, Na	mg	1	0.071	6	A	1	2	1	3
Zinc, Zn	mg	0.04	0.004	26	A	1	0.05	0.04	0.08
Copper, Cu	mg	0.027	0.001	13	A	1	0.034	0.030	0.060
Manganese, Mn	mg	0.035	0.002	26	A	1	0.044	0.038	0.079
Selenium, Se	µg	0.0	0.000	7	A	1	0.0	0.0	0.0
Vitamins:									
Vitamin C, total ascorbic acid	mg	4.6	0.470	3	A	1	5.7	5.0	10.2
Thiamin	mg	0.017	0.002	23	A	1	0.022	0.019	0.039
Riboflavin	mg	0.026	0.004	20	A	1	0.032	0.028	0.058
Niacin	mg	0.091	0.006	13	A	1	0.114	0.099	0.203
Pantothenic acid	mg	0.061	0.012	23	A	1	0.076	0.066	0.135
Vitamin B-6	mg	0.041	0.001	23	A	1	0.051	0.045	0.092
Folate, total	µg	3	0.611	23	1	4	3	6	
Folic acid	µg	0		0	Z	7	0	0	0
Folate, food	µg	3	0.611	23		1	4	3	6

continued

TABLE 5.3	An Example of the Nutrient Data Available for Each Food in SR28—*continued*

NDB No. 09003
Apples, raw, with skin (1)
Malus domestica
Includes USDA commodity food A343
Refuse: 10% Core and stem

Nutrients and Units		Amount in 100 grams or edible portion					Amount in edible portion of common measures of food		
		Mean	Std. Error	Number of Data Points	Deriv Code	Confidence Source code	Measure 1	Measure 2	Measure 3
Folate, DFE	µg	3		0	NC	4	4	3	6
Choline, total	mg	3.4		0	AS	1	4.3	3.8	7.7
Betaine	mg	0.1		1	A	1	0.1	0.1	0.2
Vitamin B-12	µg	0.00		0	Z	7	0.00	0.00	0.00
Vitamin B-12, added	µg	0.00		0	Z	7	0.00	0.00	0.00
Vitamin A, RAE	µg	3	0.155	14	A	1	3	3	6
Retinol	µg	0		0	Z	7	0	0	0
Carotene, beta	µg	27	1.662	14	A	1	34	30	61
Carotene, alpha	µg	0	0.000	14	A	1	0	0	0
Cryptoxanthin, beta	µg	11	0.926	14	A	1	13	12	24
Vitamin A, IU	IU	54	3.108	14	A	1	68	59	121
Lycopene	µg	0	0.000	14	A	1	0	0	0
Lutein + zeaxanthin	µg	29	1.132	14	A	1	37	32	66
Vitamin E (alpha-tocopherol)	mg	0.18		10	A	1	0.23	0.20	0.41
Vitamin E, added	mg	0.00		0	Z	7	0.00	0.00	0.00
Tocopherol, beta	mg	0.00		10	A	1	0.00	0.00	0.00
Tocopherol, gamma	mg	0.00		10	A	1	0.00	0.00	0.00
Tocopherol, delta	mg	0.00		10	A	1	0.00	0.00	0.00
Tocotrienol, alpha	mg								
Tocotrienol, beta	mg								

Box 5.2	Databases Maintained by the Nutrient Data Laboratory (NDL), United States Department of Agriculture (USDA), Agricultural Research Service (ARS)

USDA NATIONAL NUTRIENT DATABASE FOR STANDARD REFERENCE

The USDA National Nutrient Database for Standard Reference (SR) is the major source of food composition data in the United States. It provides the foundation for most food composition databases in the public and private sectors. As information is updated, new versions of the database are released. Release 28 (SR28) contains data on 8789 food items and up to 150 food components.

USDA BRANDED FOOD PRODUCTS DATABASE

The submission of data to the USDA Branded Food Products Database is voluntary; however, if a manufacturer or retailer participates, a set of mandatory attributes agreed upon by the partners must be submitted. Nutrient data from the Nutrition Facts panel on each food package, as received from the manufacturer or retailer, have been included on a serving size basis (RACC) and converted to 100-gram basis. These data are publicly available and updated continuously. Uses the existing search program (http://ndb.nal.usda.gov/) that allows a user to easily find information on the nutrient content of the foods by searching on product description/name, brand, or manufacturer.

OTHER DATABASES AND REPORTS

- Monitoring Sodium Levels in Commercially Processed and Restaurant Foods
- The USDA coordinates the tracking of sodium levels of about 125 popular foods, called "Sentinel Foods," by periodically sampling them at stores and restaurants around the country, followed by laboratory analyses. Also tracks sodium levels of about 1100 other

Box 5.2   *Continued*

commercially processed and restaurant foods, called "Priority-2 Foods," every two years using information from manufacturers and restaurants. Results are shared once a year in the Sodium Monitoring Dataset and USDA National Nutrient Database for Standard Reference and once every two years in the Food and Nutrient Database for Dietary Studies.

- Dietary Supplement Ingredient Database
  - The Dietary Supplement Ingredient Database (DSID) provides estimated levels of ingredients in dietary supplement products sold in the United States. The DSID is intended primarily for research applications. The DSID was developed by the Nutrient Data Laboratory within the Agricultural Research Service, in collaboration with the Office of Dietary Supplements at NIH and other federal agencies.
- USDA National Nutrient Database for Standard Reference Dataset for What We Eat In America, NHANES (Survey-SR)
  - The dataset, Survey-SR, provides the nutrient data for assessing dietary intakes from the national survey What We Eat In America, National Health and Nutrition Examination Survey (WWEIA, NHANES). Currently, the Food and Nutrient Database for Dietary Studies (FNDDS) is used by Food Surveys Research Group, ARS, to process dietary intake data from WWEIA, NHANES. Nutrient values for FNDDS are based on Survey-SR, and this is based on the USDA National Nutrient Database for Standard Reference (SR) 28 (with 66 nutrients each for 3404 foods).
- Nutritive Value of Foods (Home and Garden Bulletin No. 72). Revised October 2002
  - Published in 2002, HG-72 contains data on over 1274 foods expressed in terms of common household units. The 19 nutrients in the table are water; calories; protein; total fat; saturated, monounsaturated, and polyunsaturated fatty acids; cholesterol; total dietary

fiber; calcium; iron; potassium; sodium; vitamin A in IU and RE units; thiamin; riboflavin; niacin; and ascorbic acid. This edition was developed using data from Release 13 of the USDA National Nutrient Database for Standard Reference.

- Cooking Yield and Nutrient Retention Factors
  - The USDA Table of Cooking Yields for Meat and Poultry are measures of changes in meat and poultry weights resulting from moisture and fat losses during cooking. The table includes percentages for cooking yield, moisture change, and fat change for specific cuts of meat and poultry prepared in USDA research studies according to specific cooking protocols. The USDA Table of Nutrient Retention Factors contains the factors for calculating retention of vitamins, minerals, alcohol, and food components during food preparation.

SPECIAL INTEREST DATABASES

- Choline, Release 2 (2008)
  - The database contains values for six choline metabolites: betaine, glycerophosphocholine, phosphocholine, phosphatidylcholine, sphingomyelin, and total choline.
- Flavonoid Databases
  - Flavonoids, Release 3.2 (November 2015)
  - Isoflavones, Release 2.1 (November 2015)
  - Proanthocyanidins, Release 2 (2015)
  - Expanded Flavonoid Database for the Assessment of Dietary Intakes
- Fluoride, Release 2 (2005)
- Oxalic Acid Content of Selected Vegetables
- Key Foods
  - Key Foods have been identified as those food items that contribute up to 75% of any one nutrient to the dietary intake of the U.S. population.
- Food Composition Classics
  - List of key publications in PDF format

Source: US Department of Agriculture, Agricultural Research Service, Nutrient Data Laboratory. USDA National Nutrient Database for Standard Reference, Release 28 (Slightly revised).

Food Products Database, and special interest databases, including Flavonoids, Isoflavones, and Proanthocyanidins. The USDA sponsors a yearly conference, the "National Nutrient Databank Conference," to facilitate cooperation among the USDA, university researchers, food companies, and others interested in nutrient data.

Criteria for Developing High-Quality Databases

Developers of commercial computerized dietary analysis systems are faced with several challenges in formulating high-quality databases.[6–9] Box 5.3 summarizes a checklist of criteria in choosing a good nutrient database.

The first challenge is to decide on how many foods and nutrients to include in the software program. Even though the USDA SR provides values on 8789 food items and up to 150 food components, relatively few recipes and name brand foods are included. As described in Box 5.2, the NDL recently developed the USDA Branded Food Products Database, and nutrient data can now be accessed using the search program found at: http://ndb. nal.usda.gov/. Users can now easily find information on the nutrient content of the foods by searching on product description/name, brand, or manufacturer. And, as emphasized in Table 5.2, a number of foods also have missing values for some nutrients, although the NDL has

Box 5.3   **Basic Checklist for Computerized Dietary Analysis Systems**

1. **The Nutrient Database**
   - How many food items are in the database? Aim for more than 15,000 to minimize food substitution decisions during data entry.
   - Does the database contain a significant number of brand name items, fast foods, baby foods, and ethnic foods? If the database contains only the foods found in the USDA SR, few brand name foods will be available, and considerable food substitution decisions will have to be made.
   - How many nutrients and nutrient factors does the software program analyze for? It should at a minimum include 12 basic components (energy sources, water, cholesterol, lipids, dietary fiber, and caffeine), 12 vitamins, and 9 minerals. Ensure that calculated nutrient factors such as percent of calories as fat, saturated fat, carbohydrate, protein, and alcohol are included. Decide if you need the large number of individual fatty acids and amino acids provided by some software programs. Look for special features, such as *trans* fatty acids, animal and vegetable protein, carbohydrate components (fructose, sucrose, starch, etc.), soluble and insoluble dietary fiber, and unique nutrients, such as beta-carotene equivalents, vitamin K, tocopherol components, lycopene, and aspartame. Also review the software for its ability to provide nutrient ratios, such as the polyunsaturated to saturated fat ratio, cholesterol to saturated fatty acid index, calcium to phosphorus ratio, and potassium to sodium ratio.
   - How many missing values are in the database? The best software companies go well beyond the USDA SR to scientific journals, food composition tables from other countries, and food manufacturers to not only add additional foods but also ensure that blanks in the nutrient database are filled in with an appropriate value.
   - Can you add new food items to the database?
   - How often are database updates provided? Aim for one update every one to two years.

2. **Program Operation**
   - What is the cost of the software package? Most of the high-quality professional computerized dietary analysis systems cost more than $500.
   - What type of computer is needed to run the program? Make sure that you have the hardware to run the software.
   - How easy is it to search for foods in the database? The best programs allow you to type in any variation of the food name and still ensure that the food will be listed during the search.
   - Can the portion size or volume and weight measure be easily adapted to conform to those listed in your food record?

   - Can you view the nutrients for a food item during data entry? Access to this information makes food substitution decisions easier.
   - How easy is it to edit the food list during entry? You are bound to make mistakes during data entry, and the best programs make it easy to correct your errors.
   - Can you easily average multiple days of dietary input to derive a daily nutrient intake average?
   - Does the software package allow you to compare dietary intake with a wide variety of standards, such as the RDA/DRI, Canadian RNI, and USDA Dietary Guidelines for Americans?
   - How fast is the overall process of entering foods, analyzing and comparing with nutrient standards, and printing results? Some programs are slow and cumbersome to use.
   - Is the program so complex that it is difficult to learn and use? The best programs are user-friendly, with a small learning curve and a good help screen system.

3. **System Output**
   - Does the software provide nutrient information in the form of tables and graphs, and does it allow you to adapt the reports as desired? The best programs provide a diversity of attractive reports, which can be adapted and shared with a variety of clients and patients. Some programs allow you to add comments via a word processor.
   - Can you print out food exchanges or a MyPlate food guide that compares food group intake with USDA standards? MyPlate values are often among the most important data to provide clients and patients during counseling.
   - Can the nutrient report be printed out as a Nutrition Facts food label? This feature can enhance communication during counseling.
   - Can you rank or sort foods in a food record from high to low for any nutrient in the database? Nutrient sorting enhances your ability to personalize comments made to clients and patients during counseling.
   - Can you export nutrient output data to a spreadsheet for additional analyses? This is an important feature for investigators and administrators.
   - Does the program give an indication of the number of missing values when calculating nutrient intake? This feature can improve the decisions made during the preparation of reports to the client or patient.

developed multiple strategies for keeping these at a minimum.

Although the USDA releases substantial amounts of new or updated information each year, the typical supermarket contains more than 40,000 brand name food products. The best software vendors attempt to provide their customers with database updates at least once a year, they use non-USDA sources to give information on brand name and ethnic foods, and they fill in missing data.

The total number of food items included in a database is important to ensure that substitution (choosing a similar food when the specific food is not in the database) is kept at a minimum.[11–13] For example, if a patient in a cardiac rehabilitation program provides a three-day food record that includes several low-fat items not found in the database, some less than ideal substitutions with other similar foods will have to be made. However, more is not necessarily better. As the database size increases, the difficulty in finding the right food and the processing time can increase.

Some software packages report having more than 100 nutrients and food components in their databases, while others contain fewer than 30. Again, more is not necessarily better, because values for certain trace minerals (e.g., chromium, selenium, molybdenum, manganese), amino acids, some fatty acids, and some vitamins (e.g., alpha-tocopherol, total tocopherol, vitamin D, vitamin K, biotin) are unknown for many foods. Thus, with an increasing number of food components, the software package developer has to cope with an expanding bank of missing values. If missing data are entered as zero and not flagged (indicated by the software as missing), nutrient totals will appear lower than they actually are. During counseling sessions with patients or clients, some confusion can develop because, for many of these nutrients, low values represent a "database deficiency," not a deficiency in the diet of the patient. The best software packages will give information on how many missing values are present for each nutrient or will warn the dietitian or user about the issue.

One way to judge the quality of a computerized dietary analysis system is to determine how the developer met the challenge of missing data in the management of its database.[7–9] Some developers go to unusual lengths to ensure that missing values are substituted with either non-USDA data or imputed values. Many food companies provide information on the nutrient content of their products on request, but usually only for a small number of nutrients. Data on the composition of foods are frequently published in the scientific literature, with several journals (e.g., *Journal of Food Science* and *Journal of Food Composition*) specializing in reporting food composition data. Following established NDL criteria, the nutrient content of mixed dishes and recipes can be estimated. Calculations are also frequently used to impute values using data for another form of food or for a similar food.

Replacing missing values with imputed values is not an easy process, and it is especially difficult when only limited information exists for a certain nutrient (e.g., trace minerals). The process requires nutritionists with expertise in data evaluation. For food items used in the FNDDS, missing data are imputed according to scientific principles. Missing values can be calculated using the recipe or formulation modules based on linear regression and are often used to generate a few missing values for some foods and complete nutrient profiles for other foods. The formulation regression program uses nutrient values and ingredients (in a specified order) from product labels. The recipe program uses known amounts from authoritative sources to generate a specific food nutrient profile.

The computerized dietary analysis system should at a minimum include the basic nutrients and nutrient factors available from the USDA SR and FNDDS (65 nutrients each for 3404 foods, Survey-SR 2013–2014, and 8536 foods in FNDDS 2013–2014) (review Box 5.3):

- Twelve basic components: energy, total fat, total carbohydrate, total protein, alcohol, water, cholesterol, total dietary fiber, caffeine, total saturated fatty acids, total monounsaturated fatty acids, and total polyunsaturated fatty acids
- Twelve vitamins (total vitamin A activity in retinol equivalents, total vitamin E activity in alpha-tocopherol equivalents, vitamin D, vitamin C, thiamin, riboflavin, niacin, vitamin B_6, folate, vitamin B_{12}, vitamin K, and choline)
- Nine minerals (calcium, iron, magnesium, phosphorus, potassium, sodium, zinc, copper, and selenium)
- Nineteen individual fatty acids
- Caffeine and theobromine
- Carotenoids

Ensure that calculated nutrient factors, such as percent of calories as fat, saturated fat, carbohydrate, protein, and alcohol, are included. Decide if you need the large number of individual fatty acids and amino acids provided by the USDA SR and FNDDS and some software programs. Look for special features, such as *trans* fatty acids, animal and vegetable protein, carbohydrate components (e.g., fructose, sucrose, starch), soluble and insoluble dietary fiber, and unique nutrients, such as beta-carotene equivalents, vitamin K, tocopherol components, lycopene, and aspartame. Also review the software for its ability to provide nutrient ratios, such as the polyunsaturated-to-saturated fat ratio, cholesterol-to-saturated fatty acid index, calcium-to-phosphorus ratio, and potassium-to-sodium ratio.

Other important measures for judging a vendor's ability to provide a high-quality database are the strength of its service policy, the number of years the vendor and the software have been in business, the frequency with which the nutrient database is updated, the credentials of the database developers, and the cost of upgrades and technical support.

In summary, the content quality of nutrient databases from different software vendors may vary widely, depending on the number of food items and nutrients included, whether the most recent USDA releases have been incorporated, and the degree to which non-USDA sources (e.g., food industry, scientific literature) or estimating calculations are used to fill in the missing values. Three questions to ask when evaluating a nutrient database for personal or professional use are

- Does the database contain all of the foods and nutrients of interest?
- Is the database complete for the nutrients of interest (i.e., few missing values)?
- Is the nutrient database kept up-to-date with the changing marketplace and the availability of new nutrient data?[2]

Program Operation

General operating features of the computerized dietary analysis system are extremely important, determining whether a software package is easy to use while generating the desired information.[6–9] (Review Box 5.3 for a checklist of features to look for in the program operation of computerized dietary analysis systems.)

Important operating features include computer hardware requirements, cost of the software package, quality of help screens and user's manual, methods of searching for and entering foods to be analyzed (e.g., food codes, food names, and/or food groups), ability to preview single food nutrients while entering foods, ability to assign a variety of volume or weight measures for each food item, ease of editing the food list, food entry number limit, ease of averaging multiple days of dietary input, ability to compare results with a variety of dietary standards, and quality and variety of printed reports. The ability to modify the database (e.g., adding new foods, deleting old ones, or altering the nutrient values) is another important concern.

Software package prices are typically more than $500 for high-quality programs used by nutrition professionals and researchers. However, some research-based systems can cost much more than this.

The method for searching and entering foods to be analyzed by the microcomputer is one of the most important program operation features. Most software programs allow users to search and enter foods by full name, partial name, or code numbers. However, dietary analysis systems have different ways of accomplishing this task, with some requiring more effort and keystrokes than others. For example, some programs require the user to choose a food group prior to selecting the specific food, a step that can slow down the food entry process. Users tend to prefer searching for the appropriate foods using food names rather than code numbers (which requires use of a food code manual) or food groups. Most of the best programs have nearly instantaneous listing of foods after the user enters the food name. Some programs have a search capability, which allows the user to find the food quickly and directly using only a few appropriate keystrokes (e.g., the first few letters of each word of the food description in any order).

While searching the database for the appropriate food from a patient or client diet record, substitutions (using a food that is as similar as possible) often have to be made, even with databases containing more than 10,000 food items. Finding appropriate substitutes is much easier when the user is allowed to preview the nutrient breakdown of a certain food. Most of the top-quality programs provide a pop-up window during food search and entry, summarizing the nutrient components for the specific amount of the food chosen.

Once the appropriate food has been located in the database, the user must assign a volume or weight measure for each food item. In comparison with earlier software programs, many current dietary analysis programs allow users to assign a wide variety of such measures in an easy and accurate manner.

Often there is the need to edit the food list either during or following food search and entry. Ease of editing the food list is an important feature to evaluate when deciding on a software program. The best programs allow users to easily delete or insert foods or allow the volume or weight measure to be changed with little additional effort.

Software packages often include a wide variety of dietary standards against which individual nutrient intake can be compared. These dietary standards typically include the Dietary Reference Intakes (DRIs), the Canadian Recommended Nutrient Intakes (RNIs), and the MyPlate food group standards (see Chapter 2). Additionally, most programs compare basic food component intake (e.g., total fat, saturated fat, cholesterol, dietary fiber) with the USDA Dietary Guidelines for Americans. This comparison allows the tables and graphs to look complete and professional.

Food composition data are continually being updated. Users need to ensure that they are using the most current data available. There are times when a user may want to add foods, delete old ones, or add nutrients to the database. Nearly all dietary analysis systems allow users to modify the database in this fashion.

System Output

Once the data have been entered into the computerized dietary analysis system, two important features are the software program's ability to print out a variety of reports and its ability to export data to electronic files for further analysis. (Review Box 5.3.)

Most software packages allow users to preview the output in both tabular and graphic form on the monitor prior to storage on a disk and/or printing. A variety of output formats are desirable to present the nutrient analysis data, including graphic and tabular comparisons with the DRI, RNI, or other nutrient standards, and a spreadsheet table that outlines the nutrient values for each food in the analysis. While some software programs print a spreadsheet table with all of the nutrients for each food after one or two keystrokes, others will print only two to five nutrients for each food at a time, requiring the user to print out a series of repeated reports.

A few computerized dietary analysis systems have unique features that greatly improve the value of printed information. Few nutrient databases have no missing values. To aid in the interpretation of results, some software programs list missing nutrient values. For example, if a nutritionist is analyzing a three-day food record with 70 foods, the number of missing values for zinc, vitamin E, copper, and so on is listed separately beside each nutrient. Some software packages allow users to sort and print the analyzed diet for nutrients that may be of concern. For example, if a patient's diet is low in iron, the iron values for each food within the diet can be printed in descending order, allowing the nutritionist to make individualized recommendations. A few software packages also allow personal messages from the nutritionist to the client or patient to be included with each printed report through use of a text editor. Another feature that is extremely useful is the automatic calculation of food choices or MyPlate food groups contained within the analyzed diet. This allows the nutritionist to counsel the client or patient about potential deficiencies from a food group perspective. The scope, content, and presentation of the information generated vary greatly from one program to another, and users should ensure that printouts are appropriate, meaningful, and useful for specific needs.

Another system output feature that is useful to some nutritionists and most researchers is the ability of the software package to export the nutrient data to electronic files in a format that is useful for further statistical analysis. For example, if a researcher is analyzing the seven-day food records of 100 cancer patients, being able to electronically transport the nutrient summaries of each individual patient to a spreadsheet software program prior to statistical analysis can save a tremendous amount of effort.

Computerized Dietary Analysis Systems

Some comparative reviews of computerized dietary analysis systems are available, but most of these were published during the 1980s and 1990s when these systems were being developed. Some websites compare available dietary analysis systems, but these are generally biased in favor of the company providing the review (e.g., see www.nutribase.com).[6–8]

ESHA Research (www.esha.com) released the first version of Food Processor in 1984. Multiple versions have been released since then, and this program is the most popular and critically acclaimed computerized dietary analysis system among dietitians, nutritionists, nutrition professors, and allied health personnel. The Food Processor Nutrition Analysis software combines an extensive database with an easy-to-use interface for comprehensive nutrition, recipe, and menu analysis. Multiple reports in several formats (CSV, RTF, PDF) can be generated, including the MyPlate, data spreadsheet, single nutrient, and food label reports. The food and nutrition database includes more than 72,000 foods and food items, including popular foods, restaurant items, ingredients, and recipes, and analyzes for up to 163 nutritional components, diabetic exchanges, and MyPlate food groups. The exercise database contains about 1000 individual activities and reports METs. The ESHA port utility allows databases to be imported. Another widely used dietary analysis system, Nutritionist Pro, was terminated by First DataBank in 2004, but then restarted and revised in 2005 by Axxya Systems (www.nutritionistpro. com). The original Nutritionist Pro software was developed in 1982 and has remained popular despite sifting through three separate companies. The Nutritionist Pro Diet Analysis software package has an extensive database with over 80,000 foods, recipes, and ingredients and analyzes for over 120 nutrients. Nutritionist Pro can be used to analyze diet recalls, food frequency questionnaires, recipes, and menus, with data extracted in multiple formats (CSV, PDF, RTF). Nutrient data can be organized into multiple reports, including MyPlate food groups, menus, recipes, food labels, food lists, and graphs. Nutrients for a particular food can be viewed instantly while adding foods.

NutritionCalc Plus is available to students using this textbook and was jointly developed by The McGraw-Hill Education and ESHA Research, Inc. NutritionCalc is a powerful dietary self assessment tool that allows users to analyze and monitor personal diet goals. The program is easy to use and includes an abridged ESHA database with more than 30,000 foods and 27 nutrients. Dietary intake can be printed out using 11 different report options. Users can add unique foods and recipes to the database.

In 1988, the Nutrition Coordinating Center (NCC) at the University of Minnesota released the Nutrition Data System, a microcomputer-based version of the mainframe computer system that had been developed beginning in 1974 in collaboration with the National Heart, Lung, and Blood Institute (NHLBI) and outside experts in nutrition, statistics, computer science, and education. In 1998, NCC released the Nutrition Data System for Research (NDSR), a Windows-based software package incorporating an up-to-date interface with its highly accurate database. The strength of the NDSR is its extensive database, which contains more than 18,000 foods, 8000 brand name products, and many ethnic foods, with values for up to 165 nutrients and nutrient ratios, with virtually no missing nutrient values. There is a price, however, for this comprehensive database ($5700 and $3800/year support), and most users include medical and nutrition researchers, epidemiologists, and food and restaurant industries.

DIETARY ANALYSIS ON THE INTERNET

Use of the Internet through work and home personal computers became widespread during the late 1990s and

Box 5.4   Internet Sources for Sound Nutrition Information

- USDA Choose MyPlate
  www.choosemyplate.gov and **www.usda.gov**
  Access point for learning how to build a healthy plate
- President's Council on Fitness, Sports & Nutrition
  www.fitness.gov
  Information on promoting health through fitness, sports, and nutrition
- Mayo Clinic
  www.mayoclinic.com
  Provides consumers with good nutrition information in a fun, user-friendly format
- Federal Citizen Information Center
  publications.USA.gov
  Provides access to hundreds of educational materials
- FDA Center for Food Safety and Applied Nutrition
  www.fda.gov/Food
  Provides government updates on food and nutrition issues and basic nutrition guidelines
- Meals for You (My Menus)
  www.MealsForYou.com
  Provides thousands of recipes with menu plans, shopping lists, and nutritional analysis
- USDA Food and Nutrition Information Center
  fnic.nal.usda.gov or **www.nutrition.gov** or **teamnutrition.usda.gov**
  Connects readers to the vast nutrition-related resources of the National Agricultural Library

- Healthfinder
  www.healthfinder.gov and **www.health.gov**
  Organizes the health and nutrition information from federal and state agencies
- Vegetarian Resource Group
  www.vrg.org
  Provides nutrition information and recipes for those interested in the vegetarian diet
- American Dietetic Association
  www.eatright.org
  Provides nutrition information for both consumers and dietitians
- International Food Information Council
  www.foodinsight.org
  Provides guidelines on nutrition and food safety for consumers and professionals
- National Heart, Lung, and Blood Institute
  www.nhlbi.nih.gov
  Provides science-based, plain-language information related to heart, lung, and blood diseases and conditions, with prevention information for health professionals

commonplace early in the 21st century. Thousands of websites provide nutrition-based information, and the quality of this information ranges from excellent to very poor. Box 5.4 lists several websites providing sound nutrition information.

Free dietary analysis on the Internet first became available during the mid-1990s. Box 5.5 summarizes several of the best Internet sites for dietary assessment. The top-rated online dietary assessment tool is the SuperTracker by the USDA's Center for Nutrition Policy and Promotion (CNPP). The application is based on the Dietary Guidelines for Americans and designed to help individuals identify how their personal dietary and physical activity choices compare to recommended amounts customized for each user. This free application helps individuals determine what and how much to eat and track foods, physical activities, and weight (Figure 5.2). Users at this site can enter food intake over several days and tabular reports on average nutrient intake and a comparison with MyPlate food group standards.

Multiple 24-hour dietary recalls, when conducted properly, provide the highest-quality, least biased dietary data. To allow the use of 24-hour recalls in a wider range

of research, investigators at the National Cancer Institute (NCI) created the Automated Self-Administered 24-hour (ASA24)® dietary recall system, a Web-based tool that enables multiple, automatically coded, self-administered 24-hour recalls. The latest release, ASA24-2016, also permits researchers to collect data using single or multi-day food records, also known as food diaries. The ASA24 system is freely available for use by researchers, clinicians, and teachers. The ASA24 system consists of a respondent website used to collect dietary intake data and a researcher website used to manage study logistics and obtain nutrient and food group data files. This website provides details on the ASA24 system and how to access and use it in your research: https://epi.grants.cancer.gov/asa24/.

The Diet History Questionnaire (DHQ) is a freely available food frequency questionnaire (FFQ) developed by staff at the Risk Factor Assessment Branch (RFAB), National Cancer Institute. It can be used by researchers, clinicians, or teachers without permission. The DHQ II has an updated food list with 134 food items and 8 dietary supplement questions. See this website for more information: https://epi.grants.cancer.gov/dhq2/.

Box 5.5 **Dietary Assessment on the Internet**

SuperTracker (www.supertracker.usda.gov)

The SuperTracker is a comprehensive diet and physical activity analysis resource available at www.supertracker.usda.gov. SuperTracker offers consumers the ability to (1) personalize recommendations for what and how much to eat and amount of physical activity; (2) track foods and physical activity from a database of foods and physical activities; (3) customize features such as goal setting, virtual coaching, weight tracking, and journaling; (4) measure progress with comprehensive reports ranging from a simple meal summary to in-depth analysis of food groups and nutrient intake over time; and (5) operationalize the 2008 Physical Activity Guidelines. The "Food-A-Pedia" option allows a nutrient comparison between two different foods. The "Food Tracker" option allows the user to enter food intake from multiple days and find the average intake of energy and 33 nutrients, and then compare to nutrition targets.

NutritionQuest Food Screeners for Adults (www.nutritionquest.com)

NutritionQuest was founded by Dr. Gladys Block in 1993, initially to provide services to health researchers. NutritionQuest provides a full range of reliable, validated, up-to-date diet and physical activity assessment tools, in a variety of formats, including food frequency questionnaires and short screening questionnaires.

Agricultural Research Service Nutrient Data Laboratory (https://ndb.nal.usda.gov/ndb/)

This website (https://ndb.nal.usda.gov/ndb/) allows users to search several USDA Food Composition Databases from one location. These include the USDA National Nutrient Database for Standard Reference, USDA Branded Food Products Database, and special interest databases, including Flavonoids, Isoflavones, and Proanthocyandidins. Over 77,000 foods can be searched at this website, and it provides information on up to 150 food components.

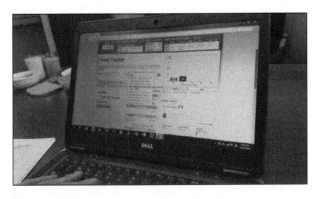

Figure 5.2 **The top-rated online dietary assessment tool is the SuperTracker by the USDA's Center for Nutrition Policy and Promotion (CNPP).**
©David C. Nieman

As discussed in Chapter 3, there are both strengths and limitations in assessing dietary intake using 24-hour recalls, food records or food diaries, and food frequency questionnaires. The National Cancer Institute (NCI) has developed dietary analysis software for the analysis of food frequency questionnaires. The Block-NCI Health Habits and History Questionnaires (HHHQ) are food frequency questionnaires developed by Dr. Gladys Block and her colleagues at the NCI and have been repeatedly validated and used in epidemiologic studies.[14,15] Dr. Block is now associated with NutritionQuest (Berkeley, CA). Software was originally developed in the early 1980s as an analysis tool for the first Block-NCI HHHQ and then updated as the HHHQ was adapted. (See www.nutritionquest.com/ for more information.)

NCI investigators have developed a self-administered, scannable food frequency questionnaire, the Diet History Questionnaire (DHQ). The DHQ and the Diet*Calc analysis software can be downloaded from the NCI Internet site: http://riskfactor.cancer.gov/DHQ/. The DHQ is recommended by the NCI for epidemiologic research and for nutrition professionals who prefer food frequency questionnaires over food records for estimation of nutrient intake. A Web-based DHQ is now available.

SUMMARY

1. Computers are perfectly suited to the task of nutrient analysis, which is one of the most widespread applications of computer technology in dietetics. Computerized nutrient analysis tasks include clinical, educational, administrative, epidemiologic, and metabolic/experimental applications.

2. There are many factors to consider in selecting computerized dietary analysis systems. The first step is to establish the major needs for obtaining the software, with specific tasks defined. Once this has been accomplished, the next step is to choose a dietary analysis system that is suitable to these needs and tasks. There are three characteristics of software programs that dietitians and other health professionals can use to compare programs: (a) aspects of the database, (b) software program operation, and (c) system output.

3. The most important consideration to make when selecting a computerized diet analysis system is the nutrient database. The database must be accurate, verified, and large enough to meet all intended tasks.

4. The USDA Nutrient Data Laboratory develops and maintains a number of databases, including the USDA Nutrient Database for Standard Reference (SR) and the Food and Nutrient Database for Dietary Studies (FNDDS). SR and FNDDS nutrient data serve as the core for most commercial and many foreign databases and are the numerical foundation of essentially all public and private work on the field of human nutrition. These USDA nutrient databases can be downloaded from the Internet.

5. Developers of commercial computerized dietary analysis systems are faced with several challenges in formulating a high-quality database. These include deciding on how many foods and nutrients to include in the software program and use of non-USDA sources to give information on certain brand name foods and to fill in the missing data. The contents of nutrient databases from different software vendors may vary widely, depending on the number of food items and nutrients included, whether or not the most recent USDA releases have been incorporated, and the degree to which non-USDA sources (e.g., food industry, scientific literature) or estimating calculations are used to fill in the missing values.

6. The general operating features of the computerized dietary analysis system are extremely important, determining whether a software package is easy to use while generating the desired information. These features include everything from search and entry of food items to the comparison of results with a variety of dietary standards.

7. Once the data have been entered into the computerized dietary analysis system, two important features are the software program's ability to print out a variety of printed reports, and export the data to a variety of electronic files for further analysis.

8. Use of the Internet through work and home personal computers became widespread during the late 1990s and commonplace early in the 21st century. Free dietary analysis on the Internet first became available during the mid-1990s. The top-rated online dietary assessment program is SuperTracker, which is maintained by the USDA: www.supertracker. usda.gov.

REFERENCES

1. Dwyer J, Picciano MF, Raiten DJ, National Health and Nutrition Examination Survey. 2003. Food and dietary supplement databases for What We Eat in America, NHANES. *Journal of Nutrition* 133:624S–634S.

2. Forster H, Walsh MC, Gibney MJ, Brennan L, Gibney ER. 2016. Personalized nutrition: The role of new dietary assessment methods. *The Proceedings of the Nutrition Society* 75:96–105.

3. Ahluwalia N, Dwyer J, Terry A, Moshfegh A, Johnson C. 2016. Update on NHANES dietary data: Focus on collection, release, analytical considerations, and uses to inform public policy. *Advances in Nutrition* 7:121–134.

4. Falomir Z, Arregui M, Madueño F, Corella D, Coltell Ó. 2012. Automation of food questionnaires in medical studies: A state-of-the-art review and future prospects. *Computers in Biology and Medicine* 42:964–974.

5. Kirkpatrick SI, Subar AF, Douglass D, Zimmerman TP, Thompson FE, Kahle LL, George SM, Dodd KW, Potischman N. 2014. Performance of the Automated Self-Administered 24-hour Recall relative to a measure of true intakes and to an interviewer-administered 24-h recall. *American Journal of Clinical Nutrition* 100:233–240.

6. Seaman C. 2008. Review of some computer software packages for dietary analysis. *Journal of Human Nutrition and Dietetics* 5:263–264.

7. Lee RD, Nieman DC, Rainwater M. 1995. Comparison of eight microcomputer dietary analysis programs with the USDA Nutrient Data Base for Standard Reference. *Journal of the American Dietetic Association* 95:858–867.

8. Nieman DC, Butterworth DE, Nieman CN, Lee KE, Lee RD. 1992. Comparison of six microcomputer dietary analysis systems with the USDA Nutrient

Database for Standard Reference. *Journal of the American Dietetic Association* 92:48–56.

9. Nieman DC, Nieman CN. 1987. A comparative study of two microcomputer nutrient databases with the USDA Nutrient Database for Standard Reference. *Journal of the American Dietetic Association* 87:930–932.

10. Pao EM, Sykes KE, Cypel YS. 1990. Dietary intake—Large scale survey methods. *Nutrition Today* 25(6):11–17.

11. Lentjes MA, Bhaniani A, Mulligan AA, Khaw KT, Welch AA. 2010. Developing a database of vitamin and mineral supplements (ViMiS) for the Norfolk arm of the European Prospective Investigation into Cancer (EPIC-Norfolk). *Public Health Nutrition* 17:1–13.

12. Phillips KM, Patterson KY, Rasor AS, Exier J, Haytowitz DB, Holden JM, Pehrsson PR. 2006. Quality-control materials in the USDA National Food and Nutrient Analysis Program (NFNAP). *Analytical and Bioanalytical Chemistry* 384:1341–1355.

13. Yamini S, Juan W, Marcoe K, Britten P. 2006. Impact of using updated food consumption and composition data on selected MyPyramid food group nutrient profiles. *Journal of Nutrition Education and Behavior* 38(6 suppl):S136–S142.

14. Potischman N, Carroll RJ, Iturria SJ, Mittl B, Curtin J, Thompson FE, Brinton LA. 1999. Comparison of the 60- and 100-item NCI-Block questionnaires with validation data. *Nutrition and Cancer* 34:70–75.

15. Velie E, Kulldorff M, Schairer C, Block G, Albanes D, Schatzkin A. 2000. Dietary fat, fat subtypes, and breast cancer in postmenopausal women: A prospective cohort study. *Journal of the National Cancer Institute* 92:833–839.

ASSESSMENT ACTIVITY 5.1

Analysis of Your 24-Hour Recall on the Internet

Fill out a 24-hour recall (see Chapter 3) and analyze your nutrient intake using the SuperTracker as described in Box 5.5 (https://www.supertracker.usda.gov/). Print out results and fill in the table. Also print out the food groups and calories report. Bring it to class. Discuss in class your experience in using the SuperTracker.

Nutrient	SuperTracker
Energy (kcal)	_____
Protein (gm)	_____
Carbohydrate (gm)	_____
Dietary fiber (gm)	_____
Total fat (gm)	_____
Cholesterol (mg)	_____
Vitamin A (RE)	_____
Vitamin C (mg)	_____
Calcium (mg)	_____
Iron (mg)	_____
Zinc (mg)	_____
Sodium (mg)	_____

1. What food groups were you "under" for? Discuss strategies to improve.

_____

_____

_____

2. Do you feel that this 24-hour food record nutrient and food group analysis from SuperTracker adequately represented your normal intake? If not, explain why.

_____

_____

_____

_____

ASSESSMENT ACTIVITY 5.2

Internet Sources for Sound Nutrition Information

Box 5.4 summarized Internet sites that provide sound nutrition information. Go to three of these sites and describe at least one topic that increased your understanding of nutrition.

Three Internet sites that contain some aspect of dietary analysis and are highly rated:

1. Name of Internet site: _____

New topic description: _____

_____

_____

2. Name of Internet site: _____

New topic description: _____

_____

_____

3. Name of Internet site: _____

New topic description: _____

_____

_____

_____

_____

STUDENT LEARNING OUTCOMES

After studying this chapter, the student will be able to:

1. Demonstrate the ability to accurately measure length, stature, and body weight.

2. Differentiate between the measurement of standing height or stature and the measurement of recumbent length.

3. Demonstrate the ability to calculate and interpret body mass index.

4. Demonstrate the ability to accurately measure waist circumference.

5. Discuss trends in the prevalence of overweight among American adults from the early 1960s to the present.

6. Discuss trends in the prevalence of obesity among American children and adolescents.

7. Distinguish between overweight and obesity.

8. Explain the difference between the two-compartment model and the four-compartment model of assessing body composition.

9. Compare different methods of assessing body composition.

INTRODUCTION

Anthropometry is of considerable interest to scientists and the public and is a valuable adjunct in assessing nutritional status. Concerns about the social and health implications of overweight and obesity have led many people to question the appropriateness of their weight, body composition, and body image. This has resulted in debate and confusion about which methods and standards should be used in assessing body weight and composition. Unfortunately, in some people it has led to such a preoccupation with body weight that their eating habits and body image have become disordered.

The effect of nutrition on human growth and development has made accurate measurement of the body's dimensions and weight indispensable to the practice of nutritional assessment. Properly assessing growth and development requires that standardized methods be followed for measuring the body. Assessment of the body's protein and muscle stores is fundamental to the diagnosis and treatment of malnutrition and to the evaluation of a patient's response to medical nutrition therapy. Nutritional research often depends on methods of accurately assessing changes in body growth and composition.

This chapter describes the available techniques for measuring the body's dimensions and composition. Some of these techniques are used daily by practitioners, and others are limited to nutritional research. This chapter establishes an essential foundation for applying the principles for assessing growth and development, nutritional status, and response to nutrition and other therapy.

Mastering and intelligently applying the techniques and information in this chapter will provide you with skills that will be invaluable to your work in the field of nutrition.

WHAT IS ANTHROPOMETRY?

Anthropometry is the measurement of body size, weight, and proportions.[1-3] The word "anthropometry" is derived from the Greek word "anthropo," meaning "human," and the Greek word "metron," meaning "measure."[2] Measures obtained from anthropometry can be sensitive indicators of health, development, and growth in infants and children.[2] Anthropometric measurements include weight, stature (standing height), recumbent length, skinfold thicknesses, circumferences (head, waist limb), limb lengths, diameters (sagittal abdominal diameter, or SAD), and breadths (shoulder, elbow, wrist). Several indices and ratios can be calculated from anthropometric measurements, including the body mass index (BMI) and the waist-hip ratio.[2] Anthropometric measures can be used to evaluate nutritional status, whether it be obesity caused by overnutrition or emaciation resulting from protein-energy malnutrition. They are valuable in monitoring the effects of nutritional intervention for disease, trauma,

surgery, or malnutrition.[1,4] Anthropometry also is considered the method of choice for estimating body composition in a clinical setting.[5] NHANES is the only study that collects and publishes national anthropometric measurement estimates for the U.S. population—all ages and all sizes.[2] (See http://www.cdc.gov/nchs/nhanes/.)

MEASURING LENGTH, STATURE, AND HEAD CIRCUMFERENCE

Measurements of length, stature (or height), weight, and head circumference are among the most fundamental and easily obtained anthropometric measurements. Among infants and children, these measurements are the most sensitive and commonly used indicators of health. A child's growth and development can be assessed by comparing stature for age, weight for age, weight for stature, and BMI for age with standards obtained from studies of large numbers of healthy, normal children. The measurement of stature is important for calculating certain indices such as weight for stature, weight divided by stature, and the creatinine height index and for estimating basal energy expenditure.[2,5,6]

In measurements of length and stature, reference will be made to positioning the head in the **Frankfort horizontal plane.** As shown in Figure 6.1, this plane is represented by a line between the lowest point on the margin of the orbit (the bony socket of the eye) and the *tragion* (the notch above the tragus, the cartilaginous projection just anterior to the external opening of the ear). With the head in line with the spine, this plane should be horizontal.[7] Many people will assume this position naturally.[2]

In all anthropometric measurements, consistency in technique and units of measurement (feet/inches, centimeter/millimeter, and so on) will help eliminate potential sources of error.[2,5]

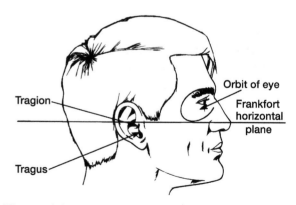

Figure 6.1

Length and stature are measured with the head in the Frankfort horizontal plane. This plane is represented by a line between the lowest point on the margin of the orbit (the bony socket of the eye) and the tragion (the notch above the tragus, the cartilaginous projection just anterior to the external opening of the ear).

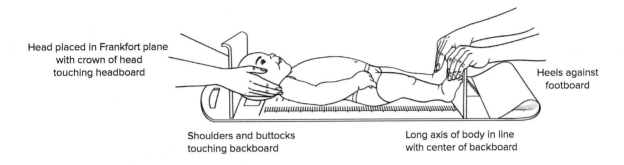

Head placed in Frankfort plane with crown of head touching headboard

Heels against footboard

Shoulders and buttocks touching backboard

Long axis of body in line with center of backboard

Figure 6.2 Special device (infantometer) for measuring the length of children who cannot stand erectly without assistance; the device has a stationary headboard and a movable footboard.

Length

Length (also referred to as recumbent length) is obtained with the subject lying down, in a supine or face-up position, and generally is reserved for children up to 24 months of age or for children who cannot stand erectly without assistance.[2,7] The growth charts used for persons birth to 24 months of age are based on recumbent length, whereas the growth charts for those age 2 to 20 years are based on stature.[8,9] Measurement of recumbent length requires a special measuring device called an infantometer (Figure 6.2) with a stationary headboard and movable footboard that are perpendicular to the backboard. The device's measuring scale (in millimeters or inches) should have its zero end at the edge of the headboard and allow the child's length to be read from the footboard.[2]

Two persons are required to measure recumbent length, as shown in Figure 6.2. With the child in the supine position (lying on his or her back), one person holds the child's head against the backboard, with the crown securely against the headboard and with the Frankfort plane perpendicular to the backboard. This person also keeps the long axis of the child's body aligned with the center line of the backboard, the child's shoulders and buttocks securely touching the backboard, and the shoulders and hips at right angles to the long axis of the body. The other person keeps the child's legs straight and against the backboard, slides the footboard against the bottom of the feet (without shoes or socks) with the toes pointing upward, and reads the measurement. The footboard should be pressed firmly enough to compress the soft tissues of the soles but without diminishing the vertebral column length. Length should be recorded to the nearest 0.1 cm or $\frac{1}{8}$ in., using a consistent unit over repeated measurements.[2,7] Gentle restraint is often required to keep a squirming infant properly positioned during measuring. When this is not possible, the best estimate should be recorded with a notation of the circumstances.[2]

Stature

Stature, or standing height, can be measured for subjects 2 to 3 years of age and older who are cooperative and able to stand without assistance.[2,7] Stature can be measured in

several ways. The simplest is to fasten a measuring stick or nonstretchable tape measure to a flat, vertical surface (for example, a wall) and use a right-angle headboard for reading the measurement. If a wall is used, it should not have a thick baseboard, and the subject should not stand on carpet, which could affect the accuracy of measurements.[7] Using the movable rod on a platform scale is not recommended because it often lacks rigidity, the headboard is not always correctly aligned, there is no rigid surface against which to position the body, and the platform height will vary depending on the subject's weight.[9]

Another approach is to use a **stadiometer,** a medical device for measuring height that is typically constructed with a ruler and a sliding horizontal headpiece. Some high-end stadiometers provide a digital measurement of height that can be transferred to a computer through the wireless network and include a movable Frankfurt Line for precise positioning of the head. When being measured with the stadiometer, the subject should be barefoot and wear minimal clothing to facilitate correct positioning of the body. The subject should stand with heels together, arms to the side, legs straight, shoulders relaxed, and head in the Frankfort horizontal plane ("look straight ahead"). Heels, buttocks, scapulae (shoulder blades), and back of the head should, if possible, be against the vertical surface of the stadiometer, as shown in Figure 6.3. Some people may not be able to touch all four points against the stadiometer because of obesity, protruding buttocks, or curvature of the spine. Rather than creating an embarrassing situation by trying to force a subject into a physically impossible position, have the subject touch two or three of the four points to the vertical surface of the stadiometer or estimate height from knee height, as is discussed in Chapter 7.

Just before the measurement is taken, the subject should inhale deeply, hold the breath, and maintain an erect posture ("stand up tall") while the headboard is lowered on the highest point of the head with enough pressure to compress the hair.[1,2,7] The measurement should be read to the nearest 0.1 cm or $\frac{1}{8}$ in. and with the eye level with the headboard to avoid errors caused by **parallax,** which is a difference in the apparent reading of a measurement scale (for example, a skinfold caliper's needle) when viewed from various points not in a straight line

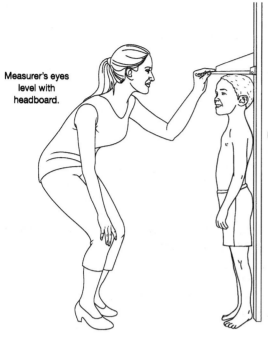

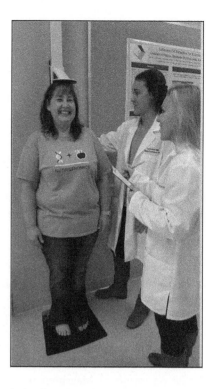

Headboard flat against the wall and resting on crown of head. Head in the Frankfort plane.

Measurer's eyes level with headboard.

Head, shoulder blades, and buttocks against the wall.

Shoulders relaxed, arms at sides.

Feet bare, flat on floor. Heels close together and against the wall.

Figure 6.3 **Body position when measuring stature.**
When measuring height, the individual should have heels together, with the back of the head, shoulder blades, buttocks, and heels making contact with the backboard. The head should be in the Frankfort horizontal plane. Lower the stadiometer piece and tell the individual to stand as tall as possible, take a deep breath, and hold this position.
©David C. Nieman

with the eye.[1,2,7] Hair ornamentation may have to be removed if this interferes with the measurement.

Nonambulatory Persons

In nonambulatory persons (those unable to walk) or those who have such severe spinal curvature that measurement of height would be inaccurate, stature can be estimated from knee height.[1,6] This and other recumbent measures and their application in nutritional assessment of older persons are discussed in Chapter 7.

Head Circumference

Head circumference measurement is an important screening procedure to detect abnormalities of head and brain growth, especially in the first year of life. Although these conditions may or may not be related to nutritional factors, discussion of head circumference measurement is included here for convenience.[2] Head circumference increases rapidly during the first 12 months of life but, by 36 months, growth is much slower. Head circumference-for-age can be evaluated using a suitable pediatric growth chart, as discussed later in this chapter.[9] Appendix H has U.S. reference data for head circumference.

Head circumference is most easily measured when the infant or child is sitting on the lap of the caregiver, although older children can be measured when they are standing.[2,7] A flexible, nonstretchable measuring tape is required. Objects such as pins should be removed from the hair. As

shown in Figure 6.4, the lower edge of the tape should be positioned just above the eyebrows, above (not over) the ears, and around the back of the head, so that the maximum circumference is measured. The tape should be in the same plane on both sides of the head and pulled snug to compress the hair. The measurement is read to the nearest 0.1 cm or ⅛ in. and written in the infant's file. Reliability of the measurement should be verified with a second reading.[2,7]

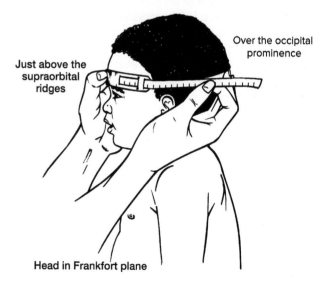

Over the occipital prominence

Just above the supraorbital ridges

Head in Frankfort plane

Figure 6.4
When measuring head circumference, the lower edge of the tape should be just above the eyebrows and ears, around the occipital prominence of the head, tight enough to compress the hair.

MEASURING WEIGHT

One of the most important measurements in nutritional assessment is body weight. Weight is an important variable in equations predicting caloric expenditure and in indices of body composition.[11]

Body weights can be obtained using an electronic scale or a balance-beam scale (Figure 6.5). Electronic scales tend to be lighter in weight, more portable, and faster and easier to use than balance-beam scales. They provide easy-to-read digital output in either metric or English units and, when properly calibrated, are highly accurate. Compared to most balance-beam scales, they have a much greater weight capacity, which can be as high as 1000 lb (450 kg). Most models can be connected to a computer network so that data on weight, height, and body mass index can be automatically entered into the patient's electronic medical record. They can record a subject's weight quickly, which is advantageous when weighing infants, who tend to resist lying still for very long. When treated with care and operated according to the manufacturer's instructions, electronic scales are quite durable and long-lasting. Like any scale, they should be periodically checked for calibration by qualified instrument technicians and/or state inspectors.

Infants

Infants should be weighed on a pan-type pediatric electronic scale that is accurate to within at least 10 g (0.01 kg) or 0.5 oz, as shown in Figure 6.5.[2,7] Any cushion (for example, either a towel or diaper) used in the pan should be in place when the zero adjustments are made on the scale or its weight should be subtracted from the infant's weight. Whatever practice is used, it must be uniformly followed and noted in the infant's file. Infants can be weighed nude, or the weight of the infant's diaper can be subtracted from the infant's weight. The infant should be set lying down in the middle of the pan. The average of two or three weighings is recorded numerically in the infant's file to the nearest 10 g (0.01 kg) or 0.5 oz and then is plotted on the growth chart in the presence of the subject's caregiver. If, on comparison with previous data, the current values appear unusual, the measurements should be repeated.[2,7]

Excessive infant movement can make it difficult to obtain an accurate weight, in which case the weighing can be deferred until later in the examination. When too active to weigh on a baby scale, an infant can be weighed on a platform scale while being held by an adult with the weight derived by difference. Because this weight will be less accurate than desired (but still better than no weight), the method should be noted in the infant's chart.

Children and Adults

Children and adults who can stand without assistance are weighed on a platform electronic scale that is accurate to 100 g (0.1 kg) or 0.2 lb, as shown in Figure 6.5.[1,2,7] The subject should stand still in the middle of the scale's platform without touching anything and with the body weight equally distributed on both feet. The weight should be read to the nearest 100 g (0.1 kg) or 0.2 lb and recorded. Two measurements taken in immediate succession should agree to within 100 g (0.1 kg) or 0.2 lb.[2] The weight of children then can be plotted on their growth charts. As with infants, if there seems to be any discrepancy between the current and past values, the measurement should be repeated for verification. Diurnal variations (cyclical changes occurring throughout the day) in weight of about 1 kg in children and 2 kg in adults are known to occur.[7,11] For this reason, it is a good practice to also record the time weight was measured.

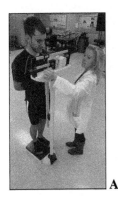
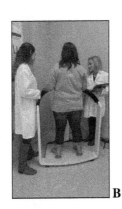
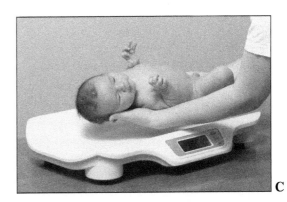

Figure 6.5 Measurement of body weight.
The scale on the left (A) is a standard physician's balance-beam scale. The scale in the center (B) is a bariatric scale with the digital display at waist level, a hand rail attached to the platform on which the patient stands, and a weight capacity of 660 pounds. This electronic scale also measures body composition using bioelectrical impedance. When height is measured along with weight, this unit is capable of calculating the patient's body mass index and displaying it on the digital read-out. The digital scale on the right (C) has a tray that is used for weighing infants and a weight capacity of 40 lb (20 kg).

(a, b) ©David C. Nieman; (c) ©Miroslav Beneda/123RF

Ideally, children and adults should be weighed after voiding and dressed in an examination gown of known weight or in light underclothing with the scales placed where adequate privacy is provided.[2,7] NHANES procedures require that participants wear a lightweight examination gown, which consists of a disposable shirt, pants, and slippers. Infants are measured wearing only diapers.[2] Should the weight of clothing be subtracted from the subject's weight? It depends on the purpose for which measurements are obtained and how accurate they need to be. In settings requiring a high degree of accuracy, subjects can be clothed in an examination gown of known weight for which consideration can be easily made. In situations having somewhat less stringent requirements, a reasonable estimate of clothing weight can be subtracted from a subject's weight.[7]

Nonambulatory Persons

Persons who cannot stand unassisted on a scale can be weighed in a bed scale or wheelchair scale.[2,7] The subject to be weighed in the bed scale (shown in Figure 6.6) is comfortably positioned in the weighing sling, which then is gently raised until the subject is suspended off the bed. In a chair scale, the subject sits upright in the center of the chair while leaning against the backrest. Using either method, once the subject is still, weight can be read and recorded to the nearest 100 g (0.1 kg) or 0.2 lb. Reliability of the measurement can be verified with a second reading, which should agree to within 100 g or 0.2 lb.[2]

Body weight also can be computed from knee height, calf circumference, midarm circumference, and subscapular skinfold thickness.[2,10] Descriptions of these anthropometric measurements and computational formulas for computing body weight are given in Chapter 7.

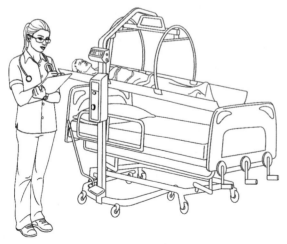

Figure 6.6
A bed scale can be used to weigh bedridden patients.

CDC Growth Charts

The physical growth and development of infants and children are important indicators of the value a society places on the health and wellness of its most vulnerable members. Growth charts are a fundamental tool for evaluating physical growth and development and for assessing the nutritional status and general well-being of infants, children, and adolescents.[8–11] For at least a century they have been used to determine whether a child is adequately nourished and to screen for inadequate growth that might indicate some medical, nutritional, or developmental condition having an adverse effect on the child's health.[9] Growth charts also can be used for monitoring the growth of infants and children undergoing medical treatment so that dietary intake, including enteral or parenteral nutrition support, can be evaluated and adjusted to best meet the infant's or child's needs.[10] As valuable as they are, growth charts are intended to be used not as a sole diagnostic instrument but, rather, as tools contributing to the formation of an overall clinical impression for the child being measured. Traditionally, they have primarily been used for detecting malnutrition, but in the past few decades concerns about the rising prevalence of overweight and obesity among children and adolescents have led to the increased use of growth charts to screen for unhealthy weight gain, overweight, and obesity in the pediatric population.[9]

Figure 6.7 shows a CDC growth chart developed for assessing length-for-age and weight-for-age in females from birth to 24 months of age. The CDC has developed growth charts for females and males for two age intervals: birth to 24 months, and 2 to 20 years. The charts for the age interval birth to 24 months give **percentile** curves for length-for-age, weight-for-age, weight-for-length, and head circumference-for-age. For the age interval 2 to 20 years, the charts give percentile curves for stature-for-age, weight-for-age, body mass index-for-age, and weight-for-stature. Figure 6.8 shows the body mass index-for-age chart for females ages 2 to 20 years. All of the growth charts developed by the CDC and recommended for use in assessing the growth and development of children from birth up to 20 years of age are shown in Appendix G. When using the birth-to-24-months charts, length is measured in the recumbent position (lying down). When using the charts for persons 2 to 20 years old, stature (height) should be measured with the person standing. The median difference between length and stature at 2 years of age is 0.3 in. or 0.7–0.8 cm.[9] Head circumference, a variable included in the birth-to-24-months age charts, is omitted in the charts for those 2 to 20 years old.

Many users of growth charts assume that they represent an ideal or desirable norm, enabling clinicians to evaluate children for inadequate or excessive growth. But this may not be the case, depending on how the chart was developed. There are two different conceptual approaches to developing pediatric growth charts. One is to create a

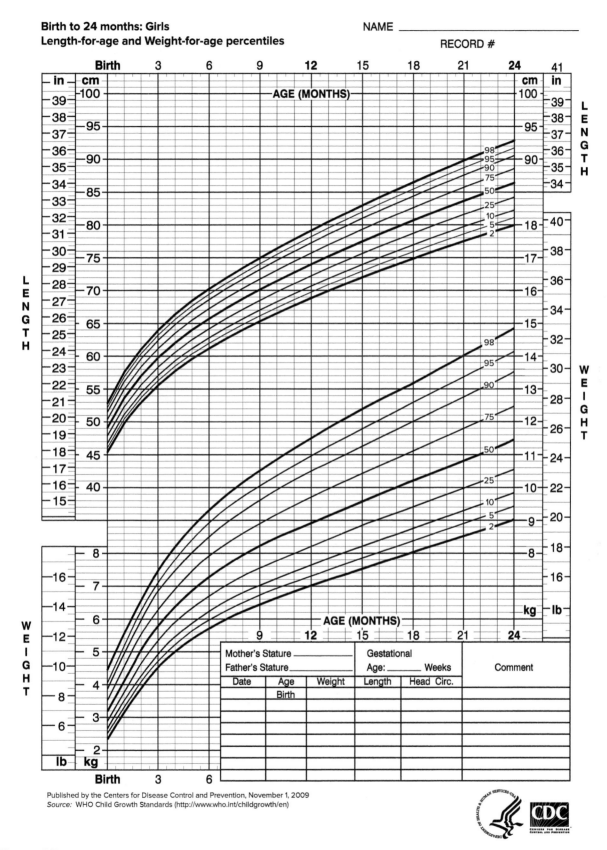

Birth to 24 months: Girls
Length-for-age and Weight-for-age percentiles

NAME _____

RECORD # _____

Published by the Centers for Disease Control and Prevention, November 1, 2009
Source: WHO Child Growth Standards (http://www.who.int/childgrowth/en)

Figure 6.7

An example of a growth chart developed by the U.S. Centers for Disease Control and Prevention (CDC). This one assesses both length-for-age and weight-for-age in U.S. females from birth to 24 months. All of the growth charts recommended for use by the CDC are shown in Appendix G.

Source: U.S. Centers for Disease Control and Prevention. http://www.cdc.gov/growthcharts/.

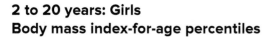

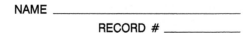

2 to 20 years: Girls
Body mass index-for-age percentiles

NAME _____

RECORD # _____

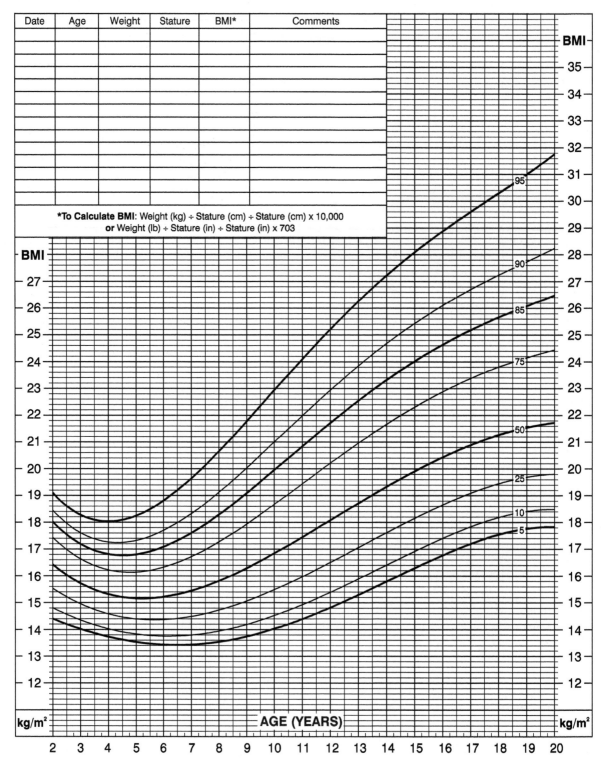

*To Calculate BMI: Weight (kg) ÷ Stature (cm) ÷ Stature (cm) x 10,000
or Weight (lb) ÷ Stature (in) ÷ Stature (in) x 703

SOURCE: Developed by the National Center for Health Statistics in collaboration with
the National Center for Chronic Disease Prevention and Health Promotion (2000).
http://www.cdc.gov/growthcharts

Figure 6.8

The body mass index-for-age growth charts developed by the CDC are an important advancement over the 1977 NCHS charts, which did not include BMI as an assessment variable. This chart is for females ages 2 to 20 years. The one for males is included in Appendix G.

Source: U.S. Centers for Disease Control and Prevention. http://www.cdc.gov/growthcharts/.

chart based on anthropometric measures (length, stature, weight, and head circumference) performed on a large group of infants and children in a particular place and time. This is known as a **growth reference** and describes *what is* or *what exists*, and does not necessarily represent what is ideal. The children whose anthropometric data are used in developing a growth reference may not all be healthy, especially in terms of weight or body mass index, or may not have been breast-fed as infants. The other approach is to create a chart using anthropometric data collected from a large group of infants and children who are growing under optimal health and environmental conditions. This is known as a **growth standard** and describes *what should be*, and represents how healthy children should grow under optimal conditions. The growth standard is developed by collecting the anthropometric data from a large number of children from selected communities who meet specific inclusion and exclusion criteria.[9,10] Of the two types of growth charts, those based on a growth standard are preferred, because in practice, clinicians use growth charts as a standard of what is optimal rather than as a reference that only describes what exists at a given time and place.

Charts for Birth up to 24 Months

The growth charts now recommended by the CDC and the American Academy of Pediatrics for assessing the growth of children from birth up to 24 months were developed by the CDC using growth standard data collected by the World Health Organization (WHO) in its Multicentre Growth Reference Study (MGRS).[9] An example of one of these charts is shown in Figure 6.7, while the other charts for use with this age category are shown in Appendix G and are available from the CDC's website (http://www.cdc.gov/growthcharts). These charts are a *growth standard* developed using high-quality data collected from infants and young children participating in the MGRS, an international study of the growth of infants and young children living under optimal environmental and health conditions. The study was conducted between 1997 and 2003 in six sites: Pelotas, Brazil; Accra, Ghana; Delhi, India; Oslo, Norway; Muscat, Oman; and Davis, California. Mothers, infants, and young children participating in the study had to meet strict inclusion and exclusion criteria. For example, mothers who smoked during pregnancy or lactation or who had a low socioeconomic status were excluded from the study. Infants born < 37 weeks of gestation or ≥ 42 weeks of gestation or who were part of a multiple delivery (when more than one fetus is carried to term in a single pregnancy) were excluded from the study.[9] The most important stipulation was that all infants participating in the MGRS were to be breast-fed for 12 months and predominantly breast-fed for at least 4 months (but preferably for 6 months) with complementary foods introduced

by at least 6 months but not before 4 months of age. This is important because breast-feeding is the recommended standard for infant feeding and healthy breast-fed infants should be the standard against which all other infants are compared. These charts are superior to previous charts developed by the CDC because they represent how infants and young children up to age 24 months should grow under ideal environmental and health conditions and in accordance to internationally recommended infant feeding practices, which emphasize exclusive breast-feeding for at least 4 months and continued breast-feeding for at least 12 months with the introduction of complementary foods not occurring before 4 months of age.[9] They were developed using high-quality data from a prospective study specifically designed to establish a standard of infant and young child growth under ideal conditions. They supersede the previous CDC charts for this age range, which were based on reference data collected from infants and children, 50% of which were not breast-fed and who may not have been growing under ideal circumstances.[9–10]

To use the charts properly, be sure to select the chart that correctly matches the child's age and sex. Measurements for length, head circumference, and weight must be carefully taken following the standardized methods originally used in collecting the data from which the charts were developed. The approaches outlined in this book conform to those standardized methods and therefore are appropriate. Because chronological age is the most influential variable in rapidly growing children, it is essential that the subject's exact age be known before plotting age-dependent variables (for example, weight for age).[2] Age should be calculated to the nearest month.[2] These data, along with the mother's and father's stature and the child's gestational age in weeks, should first be recorded in the appropriate row and column in the table in the lower right-hand corner of the chart. To plot the data, locate the subject's age on the chart's horizontal axis (see Figure 6.7). Then locate the subject's length, weight, or head circumference on the vertical axis. Draw a small circle on the chart where the lines representing these two values intersect. Check to make sure that the circle you have drawn is at the correct point in reference to the two variables. A complete growth chart should include data that are both recorded numerically and plotted on the chart. If you plot the data while the subject is still present, you may repeat the measurements if unusual or changed values appear.[2] Variables on the chart, shown in Figure 6.7, are presented as nine percentile curves: 2, 5, 10, 25, 50, 75, 90, 95, and 98. A child's length for age, for example, would be considered average when, once it is plotted, it is on or near the 50th percentile curve. In other words, the 50th percentile is considered the average, or **median,** value for the specific population of interest. If the plotted length for age were on the 75th percentile curve, 75% of girls her age would be shorter than she is. If a child's height for age were at the 10th percentile, only 10% of children of the same age and sex would be shorter. Ranking persons this way is appropriate if they are part of the population from which the data were obtained. Values less than the 2nd percentile and greater than the 98th percentile warrant evaluation. If, over time, a subject's plotted values change markedly (i.e., cross two percentile lines), the reasons for that change should be investigated.

Charts for Ages 2 to 20 Years

The charts recommended for assessing growth in children and adolescents from age 2 up to 20 years were published in 2000 and developed by the CDC using *growth reference* data because high-quality growth standard data for this age range do not exist.[9] An example of one of these charts is shown in Figure 6.8, while the other charts for use with this age range are shown in Appendix G. These charts are based primarily on anthropometric measurements performed on nationally representative samples of infants, children, and adolescents during a series of national health examination surveys conducted by the CDC between 1963 and 1994. These include cycle II of the National Health Examination Survey (NHES) (1963–1965), cycle III of the NHES (1966–1970), the first National Health and Nutrition Examination Survey

(NHANES I) (1971–1974), NHANES II (1976–1980), and NHANES III (1988–1994).[8]

There are some minor differences in how these charts are used, compared to the charts for children from birth up to 24 months of age. Stature (or standing height) is used instead of length, and head circumference is not used as a variable. The tables for recording this subject's anthropometric data and, when appropriate, the mother's and father's stature, are located in the upper left-hand corner of the charts. Another difference is in the number of percentile curves. In the stature-for-age and weight-for-age charts for both sexes, there are seven percentile curves: 5, 10, 25, 50, 75, 90, and 95. In the weight-for-stature charts for both sexes, there is an 85th percentile curve in addition to the other seven percentile curves. Values less than the 5th percentile and greater than the 95th percentile warrant evaluation, and if, over time, a subject's plotted values change markedly (i.e., cross two percentile lines), the reasons for that change should be investigated. The body mass index-for-age charts, an example of which is shown in Figure 6.8, also have an additional 85th percentile curve. As shown in Box 6.1, children and adolescents having a BMI-for-age ≥ 85th percentile but > 95th percentile are classified as "overweight" and those having a BMI-for-age that is ≥ 95th percentile are classified as "obese."[12–14]

  Box 6.1   **Defining Overweight and Obesity in the Pediatric Population**

The body mass index-for-age percentile charts developed by the CDC and published in 2000 should be used for classifying body mass index (BMI) in children and adolescents age 2 years of age and older, as shown below.[12–14] An example of the chart for females is shown in Figure 6.8 and the chart for males is in Appendix G. The charts are also available from the CDC's website (http://www.cdc.gov/growthcharts). Weight and stature should be carefully measured following the standardized methods outlined in this book, and recorded in the appropriate location in the table in the upper left-hand corner of the chart, along with the date and the subject's age to the nearest month. BMI should be accurately calculated to the nearest one-tenth (carried out one decimal point) and recorded in the appropriate line of

the table. Age should be plotted along the horizontal axis of the chart, and BMI should be plotted along the vertical axis of the chart. Draw a small circle on the chart where the lines representing these two values intersect. Check to make sure that the circle is at the correct point in reference to the two variables. A child or adolescent age 2 to 20 years having a BMI-for-age ≥ 85th percentile but < 95th percentile is classified as "overweight," and a child or adolescent is classified as "obese" when the BMI-for-age is ≥ 95th percentile. Notice in Figure 6.8 that the 95th percentile curve exceeds a BMI of 30 kg/m^2 beginning at approximately 18 years of age for boys and 17 years of age for girls. If a child or teen has a BMI of 30 kg/m^2 or higher, a diagnosis of obesity is certain.[12–14]

Percentile Cut-Off Value	Classification of BMI
< 5th percentile	Underweight
≥ 5th and < 85th percentile	Normal or healthy weight
≥ 85th and < 95th percentile	Overweight
≥ 95th percentile *or* ≥ 30 kg/m^2 (whichever is smaller)	Obese

WEIGHT STANDARDS

Technically speaking, **overweight** is defined as a body weight greater than some reference point of acceptable weight that usually is defined in relation to height. While it is possible for a highly muscular person to be overweight because of his or her muscle mass, in the vast majority of cases, particularly in developed countries such as the United States and Canada, people are overweight because their bodies contain an excess amount of body fat. **Obesity,** on the other hand, is technically defined as an excess amount of body fat in relation to lean body mass.[15] As will be discussed later in this chapter, determining the relative amounts of fat and lean tissue (i.e., body composition analysis) requires certain techniques. Body composition cannot be determined by simply measuring weight and height, for example, to calculate body mass index, or BMI (discussed later in this chapter), which is weight in kilograms divided by height in meters squared (BMI = kg ÷ m^2). However, because of the technical difficulties of body composition analysis and the ease by which weight and height can be measured and BMI can be calculated, clinicians often define overweight as a BMI ≥ 25 kg/m^2 but < 30 kg/m^2 and define obesity as a BMI ≥ 30 kg/m^2. Again, the assumption is that most people are overweight and obese because of excess body fat.

There is overwhelming scientific evidence that overweight and obese individuals, as a group, tend to die at a younger age compared to persons who are not overweight or obese.[16–20] Excess body fat is an important risk factor for type 2 diabetes, hypertension, coronary heart disease, certain types of cancer, osteoarthritis, and other health conditions. However, because excess body fat is only one of many factors influencing disease risk, it is difficult to estimate the extent to which excess body fat increases disease risk. Because disease risk is affected by factors other than excess body fat, such as cigarette smoking and physical inactivity, it is difficult to estimate the extent to which excess body fat increases disease risk. A recent study that pooled data from 57 different prospective studies with nearly 900,000 participants mostly from western Europe and North America showed that risk of death was lowest when BMI was approximately 22.5 kg/m^2 to 25.0 kg/m^2, which, according to this study, appears to be the optimal BMI range for adults.[16] Every additional 5 kg/m^2 of BMI greater than 25.0 kg/m^2 was associated with a 30% greater risk of death from all causes, a 40% greater risk of death from cardiovascular diseases, a 60% to 120% greater risk of death from diabetic, renal, and hepatic diseases, and a 10% increased risk of death from neoplastic diseases. Compared to those in the optimal BMI range, those whose BMI was in the 30.0 to 35.0 kg/m^2 range died 2 to 4 years earlier and those whose BMI was in the 40.0 to 45.0 kg/m^2 died 8 to 10 years earlier (which is comparable to the effects of cigarette smoking). Those having a BMI less than this optimal range of 22.5 to 25.0 kg/m^2 are also at increased risk of death compared to

those whose BMI is in the optimal range, but much of the excess mortality seen in this group is primarily due to cigarette smoking.[16] This relationship between BMI and risk of death is illustrated in Figure 6.9.

A variety of approaches exist for determining a person's recommended (or "ideal") body weight range. Among these are the **Hamwi equations,** which were first published in 1964 by George J. Hamwi, MD (1915–1967), who, at the time of his death, was Chief of the Division of Endocrinology and Metabolism, College of Medicine, The Ohio State University. For men, 106 lb are allowed for the first 5 ft of stature and 6 lb are added for each additional inch over 5 ft. If the man is less than 5 ft tall, 6 lb are subtracted from the 106 lb for each inch under 5 ft. For women, 100 lb are allowed for the first 5 ft of stature and 5 lb are added for each additional inch over 5 ft. If the woman is less than 5 ft tall, 5 lb are subtracted from the 100 lb for each inch under 5 ft. This is then expressed as a range of plus or minus 10% to provide an allowance for the effects of frame size.

Men:

106 lb for the first 5 ft + 6 lb for each inch over 5 ft ± 10%

106 lb for the first 5 ft − 6 lb for each inch under 5 ft ± 10%

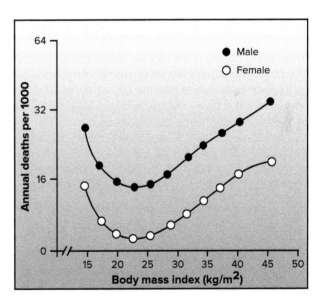

Figure 6.9 The relationship between body mass index (kg/m^2) and risk of death from all causes in males and females.

Risk of death is lowest when body mass index (BMI) is approximately 22.5 kg/m^2 to 25.0 kg/m^2 and for every 5 kg/m^2 greater BMI risk of death increases by 30%. Below 22.5 kg/m^2 risk of death increases, especially for smoking-related diseases such as respiratory diseases and lung cancer. The relationship between BMI and risk of death is referred to as a "J-shaped" curve, as illustrated in the figure.

Source: Prospective Studies Collaboration. 2009. Body-mass index and cause-specific mortality in 900,000 adults: Collaborative analyses of 57 prospective studies. *Lancet* 373:1083–1096.

Women:

>   100 lb for the first 5 ft + 5 lb for each inch over
>   5 ft ± 10%
>   100 lb for the first 5 ft − 5 lb for each inch under
>   5 ft ± 10%

Consider, for example, a woman who is 68 inches tall. Based on the Hamwi equation, her recommended body weight range would be 126 to 154 lb, which is 140 lb ± 10%.

Height-Weight Tables

Body weight can be assessed through the use of height-weight tables and the use of **relative weight** and **height-weight indices.** Height-weight tables are convenient, quick, easy to use, and understood by practically every adult. However, because of their limitations, they are obsolete and have been supplanted by better approaches, such as body mass index (kg/m^2).

The life insurance industry has been in the forefront of developing height-weight tables because of its access to the data necessary for generating them. The tables were developed by comparing the heights and weights of life insurance policyholders with statistical data (known as actuarial data) on mortality rates and/or longevity of policyholders. Actuarial data were compiled on literally millions of insured persons in the United States and Canada in an attempt to define weights associated with the greatest longevity and lowest mortality rates.[15,19,21] The insurance industry has used data from the tables to help screen applicants to avoid insuring persons who are poor risks. Good reviews of the topic have been published by Weigley[21] and Manson and coworkers.[22]

The Metropolitan Life Insurance Company published the Ideal Weight Tables in 1942 and 1943,[23,24] the Desirable Weight Tables in 1959,[25] and the Height-Weight Tables in 1983.[26] Table 6.1 is the 1983 Metropolitan Life table.

Appendix H shows NHANES 2011–2014 data for the distribution of weight, height, and body mass index in the U.S. population.[1]

Limitations of Height-Weight Tables

Height-weight tables have several limitations, which are summarized in Box 6.2.[19,22,27] Because tables are formulated from data drawn from specific groups or populations, they may not be applicable to other groups or populations. This is especially true of tables based on insurance industry data, which are derived from people who apply for life insurance—predominantly white, middle-class adults. African Americans, Asians, Native Americans, Hispanics, and low-income persons are not proportionally represented.[10]

The quality of the data on height and weight is variable. The same care in obtaining the NHANES data was not used in collecting data for the Metropolitan tables, where approximately 10% of the heights and weights were self-reported. Self-reporting of height and weight has been shown to be inaccurate, and the error is influenced by such factors as sex, actual height, and actual weight.[28–30] Rowland,[29] for example, showed that errors in self-reported weight were directly related to a person's overweight status and increased directly with the magnitude of overweight. The frequency of overreporting height increases with increasing height and is more common in males than females.[31]

There is often inadequate documentation and control of certain variables known to confound the relationships between weight and mortality.[22] Most important among these confounding variables is cigarette smoking. Smokers tend to weigh less than nonsmokers but have higher mortality rates because of smoking-related diseases. Including data on smokers in height-weight tables tends to make lower weights appear less healthy and higher weights appear more healthy.[32]

 Box 6.2   **Strengths and Limitations of Height-Weight Tables**

STRENGTHS

Weight is an important distinguishing feature of identification.

Weight and height can be accurately measured.

Height-weight tables are easily understood by many.

Height-weight tables are a part of our culture.

LIMITATIONS

The data on which height-weight tables are based are not representative of the entire population.

Quality of the data is variable.

Some of the data are cross-sectional and do not allow associations between weight and mortality to be drawn.

There is inadequate control of potentially confounding variables, especially smoking.

It is not always clear how frame size was determined.

Tables do not provide information on body composition.

| TABLE 6.1 | Height-Weight Table for Persons Ages 25 to 59 Years (Height Without Shoes, Weight Without Clothing)* |

Height		Small Frame		Medium Frame		Large Frame	
in.	cm	lb	kg	lb	kg	lb	kg
Men							
61	155	123–129	56–59	126–136	57–62	133–145	60–66
62	157	125–131	57–60	128–138	58–63	135–148	61–67
63	160	127–133	58–60	130–140	59–64	137–151	62–69
64	163	129–135	59–61	132–143	60–65	139–155	63–70
65	165	131–137	60–62	134–146	61–66	141–159	64–72
66	168	133–140	60–64	137–149	62–68	144–163	65–74
67	170	135–143	61–65	140–152	64–69	147–167	67–76
68	173	137–146	62–66	143–155	65–70	150–171	68–78
69	175	139–149	63–68	146–158	66–72	153–175	70–80
70	178	141–152	64–69	149–161	68–73	156–179	71–81
71	180	144–155	65–70	152–165	69–75	159–183	72–83
72	183	147–159	67–72	155–169	70–77	163–187	74–85
73	185	150–163	68–74	159–173	72–79	167–192	76–87
74	188	153–167	70–76	162–177	74–80	171–197	78–90
75	191	157–171	71–78	166–182	75–83	176–202	80–92
Women							
57	145	99–108	45–49	106–118	48–54	115–128	52–58
58	147	100–110	45–50	108–120	49–55	117–131	53–60
59	150	101–112	46–51	110–123	50–56	119–134	54–61
60	152	103–115	47–52	112–126	51–57	122–137	55–62
61	155	105–118	48–54	115–129	52–59	125–140	57–64
62	157	108–121	49–55	118–132	54–60	128–144	58–65
63	160	111–124	50–56	121–135	55–61	131–148	60–67
64	163	114–127	52–58	124–138	56–63	134–152	61–69
65	165	117–130	53–59	127–141	58–64	137–156	62–71
66	168	120–133	55–60	130–144	59–65	140–160	64–73
67	170	123–136	56–62	133–147	60–67	143–164	65–75
68	173	126–139	57–63	136–150	62–68	146–167	66–76
69	175	129–142	59–65	139–153	63–70	149–170	68–77
70	178	132–145	60–66	142–156	65–71	152–173	69–79
71	180	135–148	61–67	145–159	66–72	155–176	70–80

Source: 1983 Metropolitan Height and Weight Tables. 1983. *Statistical Bulletin of the Metropolitan Life Insurance Company* 64 (Jan.–June):3.

*Height without shoes obtained by subtracting 1 in. from heights with shoes for males and females. Weight without clothes obtained by subtracting 5 lb and 3 lb from weight with clothes for males and females, respectively.

There have been problems associated with frame measurements.[27] The 1959 Metropolitan tables never defined how frame size was determined. The frame size measurements used in the 1983 Metropolitan tables are based on NHANES I and NHANES II data and are so devised that 25% of the population is classified as having a small frame, 50% as having a medium frame, and 25% as having a large frame. Within the range of body weights considered acceptable for a given height and sex, the lower end of the weight range was assumed to be for small-framed persons, the middle of the range for medium-framed persons, and the upper end of the range for large-framed persons. This practice may not be appropriate because data on height/weight and frame size were obtained from two distinct population groups.

The weight measurements used in compiling the data were only those taken when the subjects initially applied for life insurance.[27] If weight changed between issuance of the policy and death, this was not taken into account. Age also was not taken into account.

Finally, weight tables fail to provide information on actual body composition—the proportions of fat and lean tissue—or on the distribution of body fat. This is a critical weakness because the quantity of weight (a person's actual weight) is considerably less important than the quality of weight (how much of that weight is fat and how much is lean tissue). An unusually muscular person with a low body fat content (for example, a football player or weight lifter) may be overweight according to a height-weight table but not obese. Body composition can be estimated from measurements of skinfolds, densitometry (hydrostatic or underwater weighing), and other methods.

Strengths of Height-Weight Tables

Height-weight tables have some strengths. Body weight is an important concept, and next to age, sex, and race it is regarded as the most distinguishing feature of identification. Height and weight are easily measured, and most adults and many adolescents and children are able to understand and use height-weight tables.

Despite these strengths, height-weight tables are essentially obsolete. They have been replaced by body mass index (BMI), which is regarded as a better measure of adiposity.[19]

MEASURING FRAME SIZE

Several approaches to determining frame size have been proposed,[33,34] including biacromial breadth (distance between the tips of the biacromial processes at the top of the shoulders) and bitrochanteric breadth (distance between the most lateral projections of the greater trochanter of the two femurs),[33,35–37] the ratio of stature to wrist circumference;[38] breadth of the chest based on chest X rays,[39] knee and wrist breadth,[40] and elbow breadth.[41] The accessibility of the elbow and the ease by which elbow breadth can be measured makes it one of the most practical ways of determining frame size. The other methods are limited by such factors as lack of population norms, difficulty in obtaining measurements, and the influence of adiposity.[27,33]

When measuring elbow breadth, the subject stands erectly, with the right upper arm extended forward perpendicular to the body, as shown in Figure 6.10. The forearm is then flexed until the elbow forms a 90-degree angle, with fingers up, palm facing the subject. The measurer then should feel for the widest bony width of the elbow and place the heads of a flat-blade sliding caliper at those points. Pressure should be firm enough to compress soft tissues. The measurement should be read to the nearest 0.1 cm or 1/8 in.[35] Elbow breadth percentiles for males and females are given in Table 6.2. Some data suggest that frame measurements do not materially improve the ability to predict body fat from body weight.[40,42] Other researchers suggest avoiding frame-adjusted tables because of the lack of data on the relationship of frame size to body weight.

The following formula can be used to determine frame size from the ratio of body height to wrist circumference,[38]

$$r = \frac{H}{C}$$

where r = the ratio of body height to wrist circumference; H = body height in centimeters; and C = circumference of the right wrist in centimeters.[38] A small frame size is defined as ratios greater than 10.5 for males and 11.0 for females, with a large frame size linked to ratios below 9.6 for males and 10.1 for females, and a medium frame size determined when ratios intermediate to these values are measured.

To measure the right wrist circumference, the arm should be flexed at the elbow with the palm facing upward and the hand muscles relaxed. Place the measuring tape around the wrist crease just distal to (beyond) the styloid processes of the radius and ulna (the two bony prominences at the wrist). The measuring tape must be no wider than 0.7 cm, so that it can fit into the depressions between the styloid processes and the bones of the hand. The tape should be perpendicular to the long axis of the forearm. The tape should be touching the skin but not compressing the soft tissues. Record the measurement to the nearest 0.1 cm.[43]

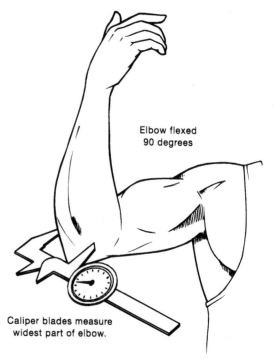

Elbow flexed
90 degrees

Caliper blades measure
widest part of elbow.

Upper arm parallel to floor

Figure 6.10
Elbow breadth is sometimes used for determining frame size. With the arm and hand in this position, a sliding caliper can be used to measure the widest point at the elbow.

TABLE 6.2	Elbow Breadth in Centimeters for Males and Females 20 Years and Older	
Percentile	**Males**	**Females**
5th	6.6	5.7
10th	6.8	5.9
15th	6.9	6
25th	7	6.1
50th	7.4	6.4
75th	7.7	6.8
85th	7.9	7
90th	8	7.2
95th	8.2	7.4

Source: McDowell MA, Fryar CD, Ogden CL. 2009. *Anthropometric reference data for children and adults: United States, 1988–1994.* National Center for Health Statistics. Vital Health Statistics 11(249).

HEIGHT-WEIGHT INDICES

In view of the shortcomings of height-weight tables, particularly their inability to provide information on actual body composition, investigators have sought better approaches to assessing body weight and fatness (or adiposity) that can be derived from easily obtainable anthropometric measures, such as weight and stature. This has led to the development of various height-weight indices or body mass indices, which are shown in Table 6.3. An index is simply a ratio of one dimension (e.g., weight) to another dimension (e.g., height). The height-weight indices are of two types: relative weight and power-type indices.

Relative Weight

Relative weight is a person's *actual weight* divided by some *reference weight* for that person's height and

TABLE 6.3	Height-Weight Indices*
Relative weight:	$\frac{\text{Actual weight}}{\text{Reference weight}} \times 100$
Weight/height ratio:	$\frac{\text{Weight}}{\text{Height}}$
Quetelet's index:	$\frac{\text{Weight}}{\text{Height}^2}$
Khosla-Lowe index:	$\frac{\text{Weight}}{\text{Height}^3}$
Ponderal index:	$\frac{\text{Height}}{\text{Weight}^{1/3}}$
Benn's index:[†]	$\frac{\text{Weight}}{\text{Height}^p}$

Source: Lee J, Kolonel LN, Hinds MW. 1981. Relative merits of the weight-corrected-for-height indices. *American Journal of Clinical Nutrition* 34:2521–2529.

*The numerical values of the indices depend on the values used (for example, kilograms and meters or pounds and inches).

[†]"p" is a population-specific exponent derived from height-weight data of the population sample. Consequently, its value changes from sample to sample.

multiplied by 100, so that it can be expressed as a percentage. Several approaches could be taken to arrive at a person's reference weight: the Hamwi equation, one of the height-weight tables discussed previously (e.g., the midpoint of the weight range for a person of medium frame from Table 6.1), the median weight for a given height and sex, the body weight for a given height and BMI, or the 50th percentile of weight-for-age or weight-for-stature using the CDC growth charts.

To calculate relative weight, take as an example a 19-year-old male who weighs 183 lb. Using the appropriate CDC growth chart in Appendix G (2 to 20 years: boys, stature-for-age and weight-for-age), the 50th percentile weight-for-age of a 19-year-old male would be 152 lb. The relative weight (RW) would be calculated as follows:

$$\frac{183 \text{ lb (actual weight)}}{152 \text{ lb (reference weight)}} \times 100 = 12\% \text{ RW}$$

Thus, this adolescent's relative weight (RW) is 120%, or his weight is 20% greater than the reference weight. Depending as it does on some approach for determining reference weight, relative weight is subject to the same limitations as the approach used to determine reference weight. A relative weight within the range of 90% to 120% is generally considered acceptable.

Power-Type Indices

As shown in Table 6.3, several power-type indices are available for assessing body weight relative to height.[44–47] The preferred index should be maximally correlated with body mass (weight) and should be minimally correlated with stature. In other words, it should be equally good at indicating body mass, no matter how tall or short a person is. Of those indices shown in Table 6.3, there is general agreement among researchers and expert panels that Quetelet's index is preferred for assessing the body weight of children, adolescents, and adults.[19,48–50]

The most widely used height-weight index is the **Quetelet's index** (W/H^2), which is more commonly known as **body mass index (BMI)**.[19,48–51] Because all the power-type indices are body mass indices, the more technically correct name for W/H^2 is Quetelet's index. Quetelet's index is obtained by dividing weight in kilograms by height in meters squared. Consider a male weighing 70 kg (154 lb) and standing 178 cm, or 1.78 m, (70 in.) tall. His body mass index would be

$$\frac{70 \text{ kg (weight in kilograms)}}{1.78 \text{ m}^2 \text{(height in meters squared)}} = 22.1 \text{ kg/m}^2$$

Body mass index has a relatively high correlation with estimates of body fatness and a low correlation with stature.[48] Garrow and Webster,[47] for example, showed that Quetelet's index correlated well with estimates of body composition from three methods—body density, total body water, and total body potassium—and concluded that Quetelet's index "is both a convenient and reliable indicator of obesity." The American College of Cardiology with the American Heart Association and Obesity Society recommend that the BMI be calculated for each patient on a yearly basis by physicians.[19] Many scientists consider Quetelet's index to be an appropriate way to assess body weight in children and adolescents.[52–55] Roche and coworkers[56] have found Quetelet's index to be the best single indicator of total body fat in girls and adults and the best single indicator of percent body fat in men. Of the other height-weight indices shown in Table 6.3, Quetelet's index has shown the closest correlation with estimates of body fatness by skinfold measurements and densitometry.[57,58]

Frisancho and Flegel[59] have shown Quetelet's index to correlate well with estimates of body fatness based on skinfold measurements, and they recommend combining Quetelet's index with skinfold measurements whenever possible. Investigators have suggested combining Quetelet's index with the rather easily obtained waist circumference as an improved means of assessing increased risk in adults for heart disease, stroke, type 2 diabetes, and premature death.[19,48,60,61]

A **nomogram** for determining Quetelet's index is shown in Figure 6.11. To use the nomogram, place a

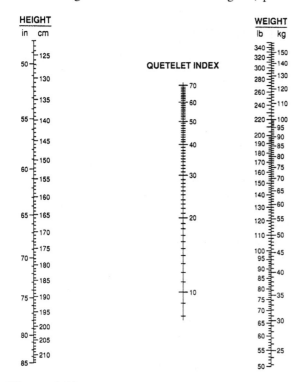

Figure 6.11

Quetelet's index (kg/m^2), or body mass index (BMI), is calculated from this nomogram by placing a straightedge on the measurements for height and body weight and reading the point at which the straightedge intersects the central scale.

Source: Nieman DC. 2011. *Exercise testing and prescription: A health-related approach,* 7th ed. Boston: McGraw-Hill Higher Education.

straightedge on the point of the height scale that corresponds to height in centimeters or inches and on the point of the weight scale that corresponds to weight in kilograms or pounds. Then read Quetelet's index on the center scale. Use nomograms with caution. In some publications, nomograms may be inadvertently modified and thus rendered inaccurate.[62] This occurred in two highly respected reports: *The Surgeon General's Report on Nutrition and Health* and the National Research Council's *Diet and Health.* BMI can also be determined using Table 6.4.

Table 6.5 shows classifications of overweight and obesity and associated disease risk based on Quetelet's index (BMI) and waist circumference in adults. In Table 6.5, it should be noted that even in persons with a "normal" BMI, increased waist circumference can be a marker for increased risk of type 2 diabetes, hypertension, and cardiovascular disease.[60] There is no standard approach for using anthropometric measures to assess regional fat distribution in children. Consequently, use of waist circumference in conjunction with BMI is not recommended for children.[49] The recommended approach for use of BMI for evaluating body weight in children and adolescents is use of the BMI-for-age growth charts developed by the CDC, discussed in the section "CDC Growth Charts" and in Box 6.1.

As BMI increases above approximately 25.0 kg/m^2, there is a gradual increase in risk of morbidity from such conditions as type 2 diabetes, hypertension, coronary heart disease, stroke, gallbladder disease, osteoarthritis, sleep apnea and other respiratory problems, and some types of cancer (prostate, colon, endometrial, and breast).[48,60] However, risk of morbidity and mortality from these conditions increases precipitously when BMI is greater than 30.0 kg/m^2. This observation resulted in *overweight* being defined as having a BMI of 25.0 to 29.9 kg/m^2 and in *obesity* being defined as a BMI of 30.0 kg/m^2 or greater.

Based on data from NHANES III, for example, the prevalence of hypertension in adults with a BMI < 25 kg/m^2 is 18.2% and 16.5% for males and females, respectively. At a BMI ≥ 30 kg/m^2, the prevalence of hypertension is 38.4% and 32.2% in males and females, respectively.[60] Data from the Nurses' Health Study show that risk for colon cancer is twice as high in women with a BMI > 29 kg/m^2 than in women with a BMI < 21 kg/m^2.[63] Data from the Women's Health Study showed that risk of type 2 diabetes in women increases as BMI increases.[18] This ongoing cohort study of nearly 40,000 female health professionals aged 45 years and older began in 1992 and relies on self-reported data on height, weight, sociodemographics, health habits, and medical history, all obtained using a questionnaire periodically completed by participants. Compared with women with a self-reported BMI of less than 25 kg/m^2, risk of type 2 diabetes is increased threefold in women having a BMI of 25 kg/m^2 to less than 30 kg/m^2 and is increased ninefold among women having a BMI of 30 kg/m^2 or greater.[18] This observed increase in morbidity and mortality with increased BMI is seen across all population groups. However, the

TABLE 6.4 | Body Mass Index Table

To determine your BMI, first find your height (in inches without shoes) in the column at the far left of the table. Then, moving to the right along the row that represents your height, locate your weight in pounds. The number at the top of that column is the BMI for your height and weight.

Height (in)	Healthy Weight						Overweight					Obese											Very Obese													
BMI	19	20	21	22	23	24	25	26	27	28	29	30	31	32	33	34	35	36	37	38	39	40	41	42	43	44	45	46	47	48	49	50	51	52	53	54
												Body Weight (lb)																								
58	91	96	100	105	110	115	119	124	129	134	138	143	148	153	158	162	167	172	177	181	186	191	196	201	205	210	215	220	224	229	234	239	244	248	253	258
59	94	99	104	109	114	119	124	128	133	138	143	148	153	158	163	168	173	178	183	188	193	198	203	208	212	217	222	227	232	237	242	247	252	257	262	267
60	97	102	107	112	118	123	128	133	138	143	148	153	158	163	168	174	179	184	189	194	199	204	209	215	220	225	230	235	240	245	250	255	261	266	271	276
61	100	106	111	116	122	127	132	137	143	148	153	158	164	169	174	180	185	190	195	201	206	211	217	222	227	232	238	243	248	254	259	264	269	275	280	285
62	104	109	115	120	126	131	136	142	147	153	158	164	169	175	180	186	191	196	202	207	213	218	224	229	235	240	246	251	256	262	267	273	278	284	289	295
63	107	113	118	124	130	135	141	146	152	158	163	169	175	180	186	191	197	203	208	214	220	225	231	237	242	248	254	259	265	270	278	282	287	293	299	304
64	110	116	122	128	134	140	145	151	157	163	169	174	180	186	192	197	204	209	215	221	227	232	238	244	250	256	262	267	273	279	285	291	296	302	308	314
65	114	120	126	132	138	144	150	156	162	168	174	180	186	192	198	204	210	216	222	228	234	240	246	252	258	264	270	276	282	288	294	300	306	312	318	324
66	118	124	130	136	142	148	155	161	167	173	179	186	192	198	204	210	216	223	229	235	241	247	253	260	266	272	278	284	291	297	303	309	315	322	328	334
67	121	127	134	140	146	153	159	166	172	178	185	191	198	204	211	217	223	230	236	242	249	255	261	268	274	280	287	293	299	306	312	319	325	331	338	344
68	125	131	138	144	151	158	164	171	177	184	190	197	203	210	216	223	230	236	243	249	256	262	269	276	282	289	295	302	308	315	322	328	335	341	348	354
69	128	135	142	149	155	162	169	176	182	189	196	203	209	216	223	230	236	243	250	257	263	270	277	284	291	297	304	311	318	324	331	338	345	351	358	365
70	132	139	146	153	160	167	174	181	188	195	202	209	216	222	229	236	243	250	257	264	271	278	285	292	299	306	313	320	327	334	341	348	355	362	369	376
71	136	143	150	157	165	172	179	186	193	200	208	215	222	229	236	243	250	257	265	272	279	286	293	301	308	315	322	329	338	343	351	358	365	372	379	386
72	140	147	154	162	169	177	184	191	199	206	213	221	228	235	242	250	258	265	272	279	287	294	302	309	316	324	331	338	346	353	361	368	375	383	390	397
73	144	151	159	166	174	182	189	197	204	212	219	227	235	242	250	257	265	272	280	288	295	302	310	318	325	333	340	348	355	363	371	378	386	393	401	408
74	148	155	163	171	179	186	194	202	210	218	225	233	241	249	256	264	272	280	287	295	303	311	319	326	334	342	350	358	365	373	381	389	396	404	412	420
75	152	160	168	176	184	192	200	208	216	224	232	240	248	256	264	272	279	287	295	303	311	319	327	335	343	351	359	367	375	383	391	399	407	415	423	431
76	156	164	172	180	189	197	205	213	221	230	238	246	254	263	271	279	287	295	304	312	320	328	336	344	353	361	369	377	385	394	402	410	418	426	435	443

TABLE 6.5	Classification of Overweight and Obesity by Body Mass Index (BMI), Waist Circumference, and Associated Disease Risk[*] in Adults

| | BMI (kg/m²) | Obesity Class | Disease Risk[*] Relative to Normal Weight and Waist Circumference | |
			Men ≤ 40 in. (≤ 102 cm); Women ≤ 35 in. (≤ 88 cm)	Men > 40 in. (> 102 cm); Women > 35 in. (> 88 cm)
Underweight	< 18.5		——	——
Normal[†]	18.5–24.9		——	——
Overweight	25.0–29.9		Increased	High
Obesity	30.0–34.9	I	High	Very high
	35.0–39.9	II	Very high	Very high
Extreme obesity	≥ 40.0	III	Extremely high	Extremely high

Source: Center for Disease Control and Prevention, https://www.cdc.gov/healthyweight/assessing/

*Disease risk for type 2 diabetes, hypertension, and cardiovascular disease.

[†]Increased waist circumference can also be a marker for increased risk even in persons of normal weight.

specific degree of increased risk associated with any given level of overweight varies with race/ethnicity, age, gender, societal condition, physical activity, and family history of disease or presence of other disease risk factors. Consequently, the classifications of overweight and obesity and associated disease risks shown in Table 6.5 are approximations based on the best available data and are influenced by a variety of factors, which must be carefully considered by the clinician.[60]

How do the BMIs of American adults compare with these standards and how have they changed since the early 1960s? Figure 6.12 shows how the percent of American adults with a BMI ≥ 25.0 kg/m² (includes both overweight and obese adults) and those with a BMI ≥ 30 kg/m² (obese adults) have changed since 1960, based on measured weight and height collected by nationally representative surveys: the first National Health Examination Survey (NHES I), the first National Health and Nutrition Examination Survey (NHANES I), NHANES II, NHANES III, NHANES 2003–2006, and NHANES 2011–2014. As shown in Figure 6.12, between 1960 and 1980 the percent of American men and women classified as obese (having a BMI ≥ 30.0 kg/m²) remained relatively stable but then increased dramatically.

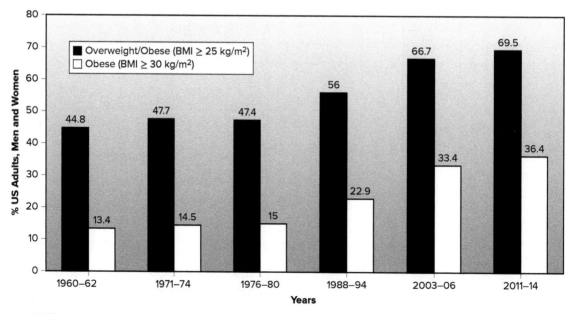

Figure 6.12 Change in the percent of American adults (20 years of age and older) with a BMI ≥ 25 kg/m² (includes both overweight and obese individuals) and those with BMI ≥ 30 kg/m² (obese individuals) between 1960 and 2011–2014.

Source: National Center for Health Statistics. http://www.cdc.gov/nchs/hus.htm.

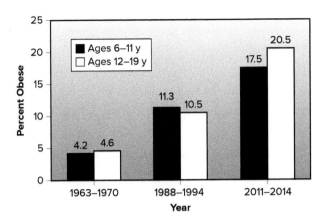

Figure 6.13 Change in the percent of American children (6 to 11 years of age) and adolescents (12 to 19 years of age) classified as obese starting in 1963.
Obese is defined as a BMI-for-age ≥ 95th percentile of BMI-for-age and sex using the CDC growth charts.
Source: National Center for Health Statistics. http://www.cdc.gov/nchs/hus.htm.

Figure 6.13 shows how the percent of obese American children and adolescents ages 6 to 11 years and 12 to 19 years changed between 1963–1970 and 2011–2014. These percentages are based on data from nationally representative surveys, NHES cycles II and III, NHANES III, and NHANES 2011–2014. As outlined in Box 6.1, a BMI-for-age ≥ 95th percentile is used to define obesity in children and adolescents, which is associated with a significant likelihood of persistence of obesity into adulthood.[8,13,14,49] A BMI-for-age ≥ 95th percentile is associated with elevated blood pressure and lipid and lipoprotein profiles that increase the risk for obesity-related disease and mortality. Pediatric obesity experts recommend that these children and adolescents have an in-depth medical assessment and possibly undergo treatment for weight loss.[14,49]

In most situations, people having a high BMI have a large amount of total body fat. However, BMI has limitations and in some instances is not a reliable indicator of total body fat.[60] For example, BMI overestimates total body fat in persons who are very muscular or who have clinically evident edema, and it underestimates body fat in persons who have lost muscle mass such as the frail and elderly. However, because of the ease of measuring weight and height and the ready availability of weight and height data, BMI is frequently used as a surrogate approach and is recommended as a practical approach for assessing body fat in the clinical setting.

Definitive measurement of body fat content requires using techniques that are expensive and/or often not readily available to most clinicians, such as skinfold measurements, underwater weighing, air displacement plethysmography, and bioelectrical impedance analysis. These measurement techniques and the concept of body composition are discussed in the next sections.

BODY FAT DISTRIBUTION

Body fat distribution is an important concept when considering the health implications of obesity.[15,19,60] Where fat is placed, or distributed, within the body may actually be more important than quantity of body fat. Body fat distribution can be classified into two types: (1) upper body, android, or male type, and (2) lower body, gynoid, or female type.[19] Obese persons having a greater proportion of fat within the upper body, especially within the abdomen, compared with that within the hips and thighs, have **android obesity.** Obese persons with most of their fat within the hips and thighs have **gynoid obesity.** Android obesity is generally (but not always) seen in obese males, whereas females generally carry a greater proportion of their body fat on the hips and thighs.[19]

Numerous studies have shown that risk for insulin resistance, hyperinsulinemia (elevated blood insulin levels), prediabetes (impaired glucose tolerance), type 2 diabetes mellitus, hypertension, hyperlipidemia (elevated blood cholesterol and triglyceride levels), and stroke, as well as risk for death are increased in persons with android obesity.[60,65,66] Although the approaches used to assess fat distribution varied somewhat among these studies, they consistently showed that disease risk is associated with upper-body placement of body fat.[19,60,65–67] They also showed that fat distribution is a more important risk factor for morbidity and mortality than is obesity per se.[19,68] In obese adolescent females, android obesity tends to be associated with elevated levels of triglyceride, serum cholesterol, and low-density lipoprotein (LDL) cholesterol. Android obesity in adolescent males tends to be associated with lower levels of high-density lipoprotein (HDL) cholesterol, a higher ratio of total cholesterol to HDL cholesterol, and higher levels of LDL cholesterol.[69]

Total abdominal fat has been described as the sum of the fat, or adipose tissue, present in three compartments of the body's abdominal region: subcutaneous (just under the skin), visceral (surrounding the organs within the peritoneal cavity), and retroperitoneal (outside of and posterior to the peritoneal cavity). Research suggests that excessive fat in the visceral compartment is most strongly correlated with increased risk for morbidity and mortality; however, this is a matter of debate and remains to be determined. What is certain is that the presence of increased total abdominal fat is an independent risk predictor, even when BMI is not markedly increased.[60,70] Total abdominal fat can be most accurately measured using magnetic resonance imaging or computed tomography. However, these approaches are expensive and not readily available in the clinical setting. Two other approaches for assessing total abdominal fat that are relatively easy to perform in the clinical setting are the waist-to-hip ratio and waist circumference. The waist-to-hip ratio (WHR) is calculated by dividing the waist circumference by the hip (or gluteal) circumference. Because of the increased risk for hypertension, prediabetes, type 2 diabetes, and hyperlipidemia associated with increased abdominal fat and the lower risks associated with fat placement in the hips and thighs, it is preferred that the waist circumference be less than the hip circumference, and consequently the WHR be somewhat less than 1. Some authorities recommend that the WHR be < 0.9 and < 0.8 for adult males and females, respectively, and that when WHR is greater than these cutpoints the risk for disease rises steeply.[15] In recent years, researchers have shown that waist circumference is actually a better predictor of total abdominal fat content than the WHR and a better predictor of disease risk.[60,65,71–73] For example, a team of Canadian researchers used computed tomography to measure abdominal fat content in nearly 800 adult males and females.[71] When they compared these measurements with estimates of abdominal fat content derived from WHR and waist circumference measurements, they found that waist circumference was the best overall predictor of abdominal visceral obesity and that, in women, WHR was a poor predictor and its use should be avoided. Because of this and other research, the National Institutes of Health (NIH) recommends using waist circumference to assess abdominal fat content.[60,70] The NIH has concluded that waist circumference is an easy and practical method for assessing regional body fat distribution. It is a valuable guide in assessing health risk in persons categorized as normal or overweight (in terms of BMI) and provides an independent prediction of risk over and above that of BMI.[60,70] Waist circumference has been shown to be positively correlated with the amount of fat within the abdomen and to serve as a good indicator of abdominal visceral obesity.[71]

Figure 6.14 illustrates how waist circumference is measured in adults.[60,70] Ask the subject to remove any outer clothing restricting easy access to the abdomen and waist or interfering with placement of the measuring tape against the bare skin or interfering with measurement accuracy (by compressing the abdomen or distorting the natural shape of the subject's abdomen and waist). The subject should be undressed to light underclothing and wearing a gown or smock to maintain his or her modesty. Locate the right iliac crest by using the fingertips to gently feel for the highest point of the hip bone on the subject's right side. Using a soft-tipped, washable pen, draw a short horizontal mark just above the uppermost lateral border of the right iliac crest. Then cross this with a vertical mark along the midaxillary line. Place an inelastic, flexible tape measure in a horizontal plane (parallel to the floor) around the abdomen at the level of this marked point on the right side of the subject. The subject should stand erectly, abdominal muscles relaxed, arms at the side, and feet together. The tape should be snug against the skin but not so tight as to compress the skin. Take the reading at the end of a normal expiration. Repeat the measurement once or twice to ensure that an

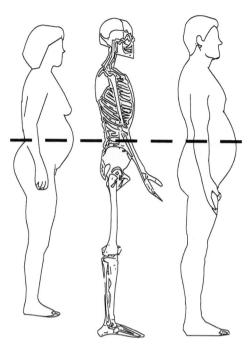

Figure 6.14

To measure waist circumference in adults, locate the top of the right iliac crest, the highest point of the hip bone on the right side. Place a measuring tape in a horizontal plane (parallel to the floor) around the abdomen at the level of the iliac crest. The tape should be snug but should not compress the skin. Take the reading at the end of a normal expiration. Repeat the measurement to ensure accuracy.

Source: National Health and Nutrition Examination Survey (NHANES). 2016. *Anthropometry procedures manual.* http://www.cdc.gov/nchs/nhanes/nhanes2015-2016/manuals15_16.htm.

accurate measurement has been obtained and record the measurement to the nearest 0.1 cm. NHANES 2011–2014 waist circumference data for ages 2 years and older across various demographic groups is included in Appendix H.

As shown in Table 6.6, a "high-risk" waist circumference in adults is defined as > 40 in. (> 102 cm) in males and > 35 in. (> 88 cm) in females.[60,70] In addition to being used in the initial assessment of body weight and risk for disease, waist circumference is also useful for evaluating the success of weight loss treatment. Note that waist circumference has little predictive value in subjects having a BMI ≥ 35 kg/m² and that, in these persons, waist circumference does not need to be measured. Also, the cutpoints in Table 6.6 may not be applicable to

TABLE 6.6	High-Risk Waist Circumferences for Adult Males and Females
Males	> 40 in. (> 102 cm)
Females	> 35 in. (> 88 cm)

Source: https://www.cdc.gov/healthyweight/assessing/.

persons whose height is < 60 in. (< 152 cm). The waist circumference cutpoints shown in Table 6.6 generally apply to all adult racial and ethnic groups in North America, although there are ethnic and age-related differences in regional body fat distribution that may influence the accuracy of waist circumference as a surrogate measure of abdominal fat content. For example, waist circumference is a better predictor of disease risk than is BMI for persons of Asian descent. In older persons, waist circumference is more valuable at estimating obesity-related disease risk.[60,70]

Sagittal Abdominal Diameter (SAD) Measurement

The sagittal abdominal diameter (SAD) measurement is a simple anthropometric index of visceral adiposity.[2,5] SAD is well correlated with obesity-related metabolic disturbances, and limited data support that SAD is a better predictor of cardiovascular disease than other anthropometric measurements, including BMI, waist circumference, and waist-hip ratio.[2,5] The use of SAD in clinical environments has been impeded by a lack of normative data, but recent NHANES cycles have included SAD measurements on participants 8 years of age and older across various demographic groups for the first time (see Appendix H).[1] Pregnant females and persons over 600 pounds were excluded from SAD measurements in NHANES 2011–2014. NHANES SAD data will allow epidemiologic investigators to better examine the relationship between SAD and chronic disease risk, prevalence, incidence, and mortality.[2] Cut-off SAD values for predicting elevated cardiovascular risk have been proposed (≥ 23 cm for males and ≥ 20 cm for females), but additional research is needed to establish clinically useful values.

SAD is measured with the participant in a supine position with the knees bent and feet flat on an examination table (Figure 6.15).[2,5] An abdominal caliper is used to establish the external distance between the front of the

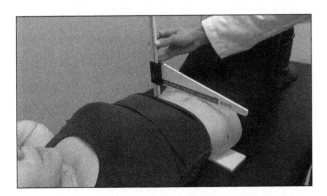

Figure 6.15
The sagittal abdominal diameter (SAD) is measured at the height of the iliac crest with the participant in a supine position, knees bent and feet flat on an examination table.
©David C. Nieman

abdomen and the small of the back at the iliac level line. The measurement site should first be marked. Locate the right iliac crest at the point where it intersects the midaxillary line. With a cosmetic pencil, draw a line perpendicular to the table on the uppermost lateral border of the right ilium. Locate the left iliac crest where it also intersects the midaxillary line and extend the measuring tape over the abdomen without compressing the skin from the left iliac crest to the mark on the right iliac crest. The arc of this extended tape should be aligned perpendicular to the table. Draw a horizontal line, around 5 cm long, on the abdomen along the iliac level line. The line should be drawn on the top left edge of the tape. Take at least two SAD measurements. Ask the participant to briefly raise his or her hips and insert the caliper's lower arm under the small of the back, making sure the caliper's upper arm exceeds the participant's abdominal diameter. Check that the caliper's lower arm is in contact with the participant's back. Grasp the shaft of the caliper with one hand and adjust it in a vertical position (confirmed by the bubble in the spirit level). Using the other hand, slide the caliper's upper arm down to about 2 cm above the abdomen with the edge aligned with the iliac level line mark but without touching the abdomen. Instruct the participant to slowly take in a gentle breath, slowly let the air out, and then pause (rest, relax). Promptly slide down the caliper's upper arm, letting it lightly touch the abdomen but without compressing it, and take the measurement. Read the measurement (to the nearest 0.1 cm) on the shaft of the caliper. Repeat, and if the difference between the first and second measurements is greater than 0.5 cm, third and fourth measurements should be conducted until there is consistency.

BODY COMPOSITION

Interest in human body composition has increased over the past several decades, primarily because obesity has been associated with such diseases as diabetes mellitus, hypertension, and coronary heart disease.[16–18,74–76] Overweight is one of the most prevalent diet-related problems in the United States. As shown in Figures 6.12 and 6.13, the prevalence of obesity in the United States has markedly increased. Globally, the prevalence of obesity varies widely, from less than 5% in India, China, Japan, and Korea to more than 25% in the United States, Mexico, New Zealand, and Canada.[77] Globally, the prevalence of obesity is increasing, as is the prevalence of obesity-linked diseases, such as type 2 diabetes, hypertension, and coronary heart disease.

Measurement of body fat is important in studying the nature of obesity and the obese person's response to treatment. As previously mentioned, the percent of body fat, as well as its placement, can have profound effects on health.

Estimating fat and protein reserves is a common practice in assessing a patient's nutritional status. During nutritional deprivation, these stores are depleted, leading to increased morbidity and mortality, caused at least in part by nutrition-related impairment of the body's immune system.[78,79] Simple techniques to screen fat and protein reserves of patients are critical in the light of reports that malnutrition is seen in as many as half of all hospitalized patients in the United States, Canada, and other industrialized countries.[80–82]

Body composition can be an important factor in certain athletic events. For example, carrying excess fat can be detrimental to the performance of runners and gymnasts. Body composition measurements can help these athletes maintain body fat at levels that are neither too high nor too low.[27] Too low a percent body fat can adversely affect metabolism and health. Female athletes will experience oligomenorrhea (abnormally infrequent menstruation) and amenorrhea (absence or abnormal cessation of menstruation) when their percent body fat is too low. This, in turn, can result in bone demineralization and increased risk of osteoporosis and bone fractures. Inadequate body fat may indicate disease, starvation, or an eating disorder, such as anorexia nervosa.

The perspective that the body consists of two chemically distinct compartments forms the model on which most body composition methods are based.[83,84] In the two-compartment model, the body can be divided into fat mass and fat-free mass or, according to an alternative approach, into adipose tissue and lean body mass. In the former view, developed by Keys and Brozek,[85] the fat mass includes all the solvent-extractable lipids contained in both adipose tissue and other tissues, and the residual is the fat-free mass. The fat-free mass is composed of muscle, water, bone, and other tissues devoid of fat and lipid. For example, the solvent ether could be used to extract all the fat and lipid from a minced animal carcass. That remaining after all the fat and lipid were extracted would be the fat-free mass. The lean body mass of the latter approach is similar to the fat-free mass except that lean body mass includes a small amount of lipid that our bodies must have—for example, lipid that serves as a structural component of cell membranes or lipid contained in the nervous system.[86] This essential lipid constitutes about 1.5% to 3% of the weight of the lean body.

Body composition often is defined as the *ratio of fat to fat-free mass* and frequently is expressed as a percentage of body fat. Adipose tissue contains about 14% water, is nearly 100% free of the electrolyte potassium, and is assumed to have a density of 0.90 g/cm^3.[27,83] The less homogenous *fat-free compartment* is primarily composed of bone, muscle, other fat-free tissue, and body water. Its chemical composition is assumed to be relatively constant, with a water content of 72% to 74%, a potassium content of 60 to 70 mmol/kg in males and 50 to 60 mmol/kg in females, and a density of 1.10 g/cm^3 at normal body temperature.[83] However, several factors can affect the density of the fat-free compartment. Among these are age (the fat-free compartment in children is less dense than

that of middle-aged persons, and bone density is decreased in elderly persons, especially those with osteoporosis), the degree of fitness (athletes have denser bone and muscle), and the body's state of hydration.[27] The use of anthropometry (measures of skinfold thicknesses, bone dimensions, and limb circumferences), determination of whole-body density (most commonly by underwater weighing), electrical conductance and impedance, and other methods to estimate body composition are based on the two-compartment model.[83]

An alternative approach to the two-compartment model is the four-compartment model, which views the human body as composed of four chemical groups: water, protein, mineral, and fat.[83] Methods for estimating body composition based on the four-compartment model include neutron activation analysis, isotope dilution techniques, bioelectrical impedance, total body electrical conductivity, and absorptiometry.[83]

A variety of methods exist for estimating body composition, and each has its strengths and limitations. Except for cadaveric studies, all of the following techniques are *indirect* measures.

CADAVERIC STUDIES

Only by analyzing cadavers can direct measurement of human body composition be made.[4] The most comprehensive direct study of body composition was the Brussels Cadaver Analysis Study (CAS), in which more than 30 cadavers were studied from 1979 to 1983.[87] The CAS helped validate various in vivo methods for estimating body composition and collected data for developing new anthropometric models for determining body composition.[87] Recumbent length, hydrostatic (underwater) weight, numerous girths and breadths, and skin surface area were measured. Skinfolds were measured at 14 standard sites. The skin and subcutaneous tissue then were cut open and carefully measured, so that skinfold measurements could be directly compared with measurements of skin and subcutaneous adipose tissue thickness. The skin, adipose tissue, skeletal muscle, bone, and viscera were dissected out and weighed in air and under water to determine density of the organs and tissues. The CAS allowed examination of several assumptions underlying the use of skinfold measurements and hydrostatic weighing to determine body composition. A major assumption of the CAS was that anthropometric measures and body composition in cadavers are similar to those of living subjects.[87,88]

SKINFOLD MEASUREMENTS

The most widely used method of indirectly estimating percent body fat in clinical settings is to measure skinfolds—the thickness of a double fold of skin and compressed subcutaneous adipose tissue (Figure 6.16).[5,88] Although more accurate methods for assessing percent body fat

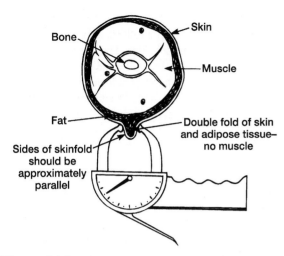

Bone

Skin

Muscle

Fat

Double fold of skin
and adipose tissue–
no muscle

Sides of skinfold
should be
approximately
parallel

Figure 6.16

The double fold of skin and adipose tissue between the tips of
the skinfold caliper should be large enough to form
approximately parallel sides. Care should be taken to elevate
only skin and adipose tissue, not muscle.

exist, skinfold measurement has these advantages: the
equipment needed is inexpensive and requires little space;
measurements are easily and quickly obtained; and, when
correctly done, skinfold measurement provides estimates
of body composition that correlate well with those derived
from hydrostatic weighing, the most widely used laboratory method for determining body composition.

Assumptions in Using Skinfold Measurements

Estimating body fat from skinfold thickness measurements
involves several assumptions, outlined in Box 6.3, that may
not always hold true.[88] When a caliper is initially applied to a
skinfold, the caliper reading decreases as its tips compress the
fold of skin and subcutaneous adipose tissue. Thus, it is recommended to read the caliper dial about 4 seconds after the
caliper tips have been applied to the skinfold.[89] Research has
shown significant differences in skinfold compressibility at a
particular site among individuals (interindividual variation)

and at different sites on one individual (intraindividual variation).[88,90] Even after the timing of caliper readings has been
standardized, similar thicknesses of adipose tissue may yield
different caliper readings because of differences in
compressibility.[88] Alternatively, compressibility differences
may result in skinfolds of different thicknesses yielding similar caliper readings.[33] Of all the assumptions considered in
this section, this probably has the greatest potential for being
a significant source of error in estimating body composition
from skinfold measurements.[88]

The CAS showed that skin thickness as a percent of
total caliper reading varies at different sites and that
"while the contribution of skin to total skinfold thickness
is generally not large, it may lead to significant error
especially in lean subjects."[88]

Thickness of subcutaneous adipose tissue varies
widely among different skinfold sites within individuals
and for the same skinfold site between individuals.[87,88,91]
Consequently, overall subcutaneous adipose tissue is best
assessed by measuring multiple skinfold sites. A minimum of three is recommended. Proper site selection is
critical because subcutaneous fat layer thickness can vary
significantly within a 2- to 3-cm proximity of certain
sites.[83,92] Research has shown that certain skinfold sites
are highly correlated to total subcutaneous adipose tissue
and that sites from the lower limbs should be included in
body composition prediction formulas.[88,93]

Adipose tissue can be divided into external, or subcutaneous (what lies directly under the skin), and internal
portions (that within and around muscles and surrounding organs).[92] The only direct data on the relationship of
external-to-internal adipose tissue come from the CAS.
These data show that each kilogram of subcutaneous adipose tissue is associated with approximately 200 g of
internal adipose tissue and that skinfolds are significantly
correlated with total adiposity.[87]

Although estimating body composition by skinfold
measurements fails to meet all the assumptions of Box 6.3,
it is preferred over use of other anthropometric variables
and is certainly better than height-weight indices.[94] Thus,
skinfold measurement is the most widely used method of
indirectly estimating percent body fat in clinical settings.

 Box 6.3   **Assumptions Involved in Using Skinfold Thickness Measurements to Predict Body Fat**

1. The double thickness of skin and subcutaneous adipose
   tissue has a constant compressibility.
2. Thickness of the skin is negligible or a constant
   fraction of the skinfold.
3. The thickness of subcutaneous adipose tissue is
   constant or predictable within and between individuals.

4. The fat content of adipose tissue is constant.
5. The proportion of internal to external fat is constant.
6. Body fat is normally distributed.

Source: Martin AD, Ross WD, Drinkwater DT, Clarys JP. 1985. Prediction of body fat by skinfold caliper: Assumptions and cadaver evidence. *International Journal of Obesity* 9(suppl 1):31–39.

Measurement Technique

Proper measurement of skinfolds requires careful attention to site selection and strict adherence to the following protocol, which is standard among researchers who have developed the prediction equations for determining body fatness from skinfold measurements.

1. Most North American investigators (including those conducting large national surveys from which reference data are derived) take skinfold measurements on the right side of the body. European investigators typically perform measurements on the left side.[95] From a practical standpoint, it matters little on which side measurements are taken. However, the authors of this textbook suggest that North American students be taught to take all measurements on the right side (except where indicated otherwise) to coincide with the efforts of most U.S. and Canadian researchers.

2. As a general rule, those with little experience in skinfold measurement should mark the site to be measured once it has been carefully identified. A flexible, nonstretchable tape measure can be used to locate midpoints on the body.[89]

3. The skinfold should be firmly grasped by the thumb and index finger of the left hand about 1 cm or ½ in. **proximal** to the skinfold site and pulled away from the body. This is usually easy with thin people, but it may be difficult with the obese and may be somewhat uncomfortable. The amount of tissue grasped must be enough to form a fold with approximately parallel sides. The thicker the fat layer under the skin, the wider the necessary fold.

4. The caliper is held in the right hand, perpendicular to the long axis of the skinfold and with the caliper's dial facing up and easily readable. The caliper tips should be placed on the site and should be about 1 cm or ½ in. **distal** to the fingers holding the skinfold, so that pressure from the fingers will not affect the measured value, as shown in Figure 6.17.

5. The caliper should not be placed too deeply into the skinfold or too close to the tip of the skinfold. The measurer should try to visualize where a true double fold of skin thickness is and place the caliper tips there. It is a good practice to position the caliper arms one at a time on the skinfold.

6. The dial is read approximately 4 seconds after the pressure from the measurer's hand has been released on the lever arm of the caliper. If caliper tips exert force for longer than 4 seconds, the reading will gradually become smaller as fluids are forced from the compressed tissues. The measurer's eyes and caliper dial should be positioned to avoid errors caused by parallax. Readings should be recorded to the nearest 1 mm.

7. A minimum of two measurements should be taken at each site. Measurements should be at least 15 seconds apart to allow the skinfold site to return to normal. If consecutive measurements vary by more than 1 mm, more should be taken until there is consistency.

8. The measurer should maintain pressure with the thumb and index finger throughout each measurement.

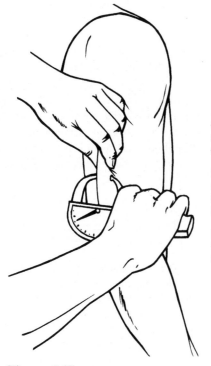

Grasp a double fold of skin and subcutaneous adipose tissue with the thumb and index finger of the left hand.

Place the caliper tips on the site where the sides of the skinfold are approximately parallel and 1 cm distal to where the skinfold is grasped.

Position the caliper dial so that it can be read easily. Obtain the measurement about 4 sec after placing the caliper tips on the skinfold.

Figure 6.17
Accurate skinfold measurements require careful site selection and proper technique in placing and reading the caliper.

9. When measuring the obese, it may be impossible to elevate a skinfold with parallel sides, particularly over the abdomen. In this situation, the measurer should use both hands to pull the skinfold away while a partner attempts to measure the width. If the skinfold is too wide for the calipers, underwater weighing or another technique will have to be used.

10. Measurements should not be taken immediately after exercise or when the person being measured is overheated because the shift in body fluid to the skin will inflate normal skinfold size.

11. It takes practice to consistently grasp skinfolds at the same location every time. Accuracy can be tested by having several technicians take the same measurements and comparing results. It may take up to 50 practice sessions to become proficient in measuring skinfolds.

Two types of skinfold calipers are depicted in Figure 6.18 The Lange skinfold caliper is most popular among U.S. researchers and clinicians. The Harpenden and Holtain are two other types of skinfold calipers, and are commonly used in Europe. Several less expensive plastic calipers are available, such as the Slim Guide and the Fat-Control Caliper. Some of the plastic calipers have been shown to give results comparable to the more expensive calipers.[96,97] The Slim Guide may be an acceptable caliper for those who cannot afford a more expensive instrument. The Holtain, Lange, and Harpenden calipers are highly recommended because these were used in developing prediction equations and reference values. Whatever the type of skinfold caliper used, the jaw tips should exert a pressure of 10 g/mm^2 throughout the caliper's full measurement range. The calipers should be calibrated periodically (for

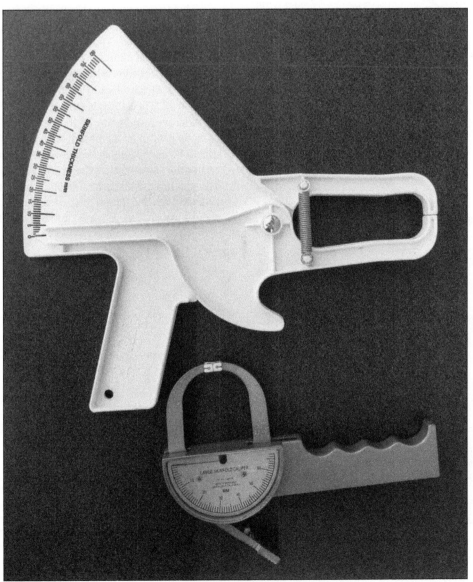

Figure 6.18 "Two types of commercially available skinfold calipers that are accurate include the inexpensive Slim Guide and more expensive Lange models."

©David C. Nieman

example, before measuring skinfolds on groups of subjects) by checking the dial reading against a graduated calibration block. Caliper readings should be within at least $\pm$ 1 mm at each 5-mm interval from 5 to 50 mm.[2]

Site Selection

This section describes eight of the most commonly used skinfold sites following the Airlie Consensus Conference protocol as outlined in the *Anthropometric Standardization Reference Manual.*[93]

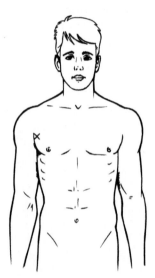

Figure 6.19
The location of the pectoral or chest skinfold site is the same for males and females.

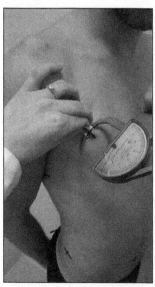

Figure 6.20   Measurement of the pectoral or chest skinfold.
Note that the caliper is held perpendicular to the long axis of the skinfold. The blade tips are approximately 1 cm distal to the fingers grasping the skinfold.
©David C. Nieman

Chest

The chest, or pectoral skinfold site, is measured using a skinfold with its long axis running from the top of the anterior axillary fold to the nipple. The skinfold is grasped as high as possible on the anterior axillary fold, and the thickness of the fat fold is measured 1 cm or $\frac{1}{2}$ in. below the fingers along the axis, as shown in Figures 6.19 and 6.20. The skinfold site is the same for males and females. Other than to help determine the long axis of the skinfold, the nipple is not used as a landmark for either males or females. This site can be measured on a female wearing a brassiere or two-piece bathing suit.

Triceps

Because of its accessibility, the triceps is the most commonly measured site. The triceps skinfold site is on the posterior aspect of the right arm, over the triceps muscle, midway between the lateral projection of the acromion process of the scapula and the inferior margin of the olecranon process of the ulna. These bony landmarks are shown in Figure 6.21. The midpoint between the acromion and olecranon processes should be marked along the *lateral* side of the arm with the elbow flexed 90 degrees, as shown in Figure 6.22. The subject's arm should now hang loosely at the side, with the palm of the hand facing *anteriorly* to properly determine the posterior midline. The skinfold site should be marked along the posterior midline of the upper arm at the same level as the previously marked midpoint. The measurer should stand behind the subject, grasp the skinfold with the thumb and index finger of the left hand about 1 cm or $\frac{1}{2}$ in. proximal to the skinfold site, as shown

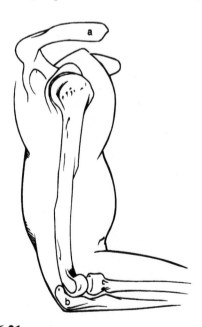

Figure 6.21
The triceps skinfold site is located midway between the lateral projection of the acromion process of the scapula, **a,** and the olecranon process of the ulna, **b,** with the elbow flexed 90 degrees.

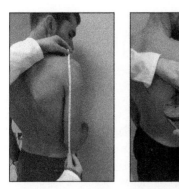

Figure 6.22 **Measurement of the triceps skinfold.**
©David C. Nieman

in Figure 6.22. Again, notice in Figure 6.22 that the caliper tips are about 1 cm or $\frac{1}{2}$ in. from the thumb and finger, the caliper is perpendicular to the long axis of the skinfold, and the dial can be easily read.

Subscapular

The subscapular site is 1 cm below the lowest, or inferior, angle of the scapula, as shown in Figure 6.23. The long axis of the skinfold is on a 45-degree angle directed down and to the right side. The site can be located by gently feeling for the inferior angle of the scapula or by having the subject place his or her right arm behind the back.

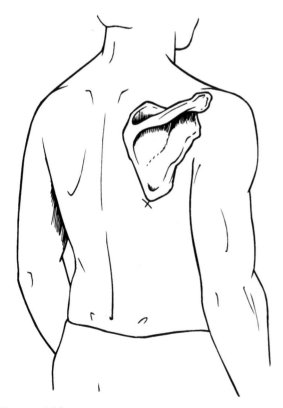

Figure 6.23
The subscapular skinfold site is just below the inferior border of the scapula. The long axis of the site runs at 45 degrees of horizontal.

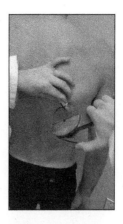

Figure 6.24 **Measurement of the subscapular skinfold site.**
©David C. Nieman

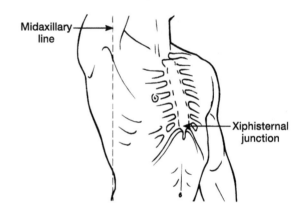

Figure 6.25
The midaxillary site is a horizontal skinfold along the midaxillary line at the level of the xiphisternal junction.

It is measured with the subject standing with arms relaxed to the sides. The skin is grasped 1 cm above and medial to the site along the axis (see Figure 6.24).

Midaxillary

As shown in Figure 6.25, this site is at the right midaxillary line (a vertical line extending from the middle of the axilla) level with the xiphisternal junction (at the bottom of the sternum where the xiphoid process begins). It is measured with the subject standing erectly and with the right arm slightly abducted (moved away from center of the body) and flexed (bent posteriorly), as in Figure 6.26.

Suprailiac

This skinfold is measured just above the iliac crest at the midaxillary line (see Figures 6.27 and 6.28). The long axis follows the natural cleavage lines of the skin and runs diagonally. The subject should stand erectly with feet together and arms hanging at the sides, although the right arm can be abducted and flexed slightly to improve access to the site. The measurer should grasp the skinfold about 1 cm posterior to the midaxillary line and measure the skinfold at the midaxillary line.

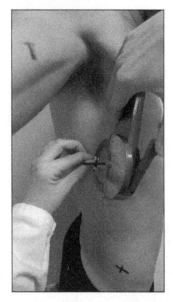

Figure 6.26 Measurement of the midaxillary skinfold.
©David C. Nieman

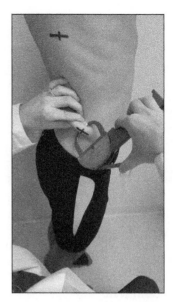

Figure 6.28 Measurement of the suprailiac skinfold.
©David C. Nieman

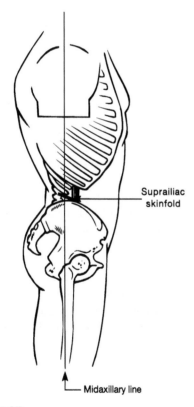

Suprailiac
skinfold

Midaxillary line

Figure 6.27
The suprailiac skinfold is measured just above the iliac crest at the midaxillary line. The long axis of the skinfold follows the natural cleavage lines of the skin.

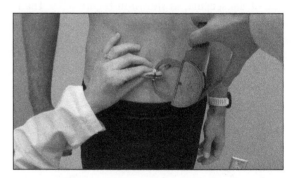

Figure 6.29 Measurement of the abdominal skinfold.
©David C. Nieman

of and 1 cm below the midpoint of the umbilicus is measured (Figure 6.29).

Thigh

This site is a vertical skinfold along the midline of the anterior aspect of the thigh midway between the junction of the midline and the inguinal crease and the proximal (upper) border of the patella, or kneecap (Figure 6.30). Flexing the subject's hip helps locate the inguinal crease. The subject shifts the weight to the left foot and relaxes the leg being measured by slightly flexing the knee with the foot flat on the floor. The skinfold is measured as shown in Figure 6.31.

Medial Calf

With the subject sitting, the right leg is flexed about 90 degrees at the knee with the sole of the foot flat on the floor. The measurement also may be taken with the subject standing with the foot resting on a platform, so that

Abdomen

The subject stands erectly with the body weight evenly distributed on both feet, abdominal muscles relaxed, and breathing quietly. A horizontal skinfold 3 cm to the right

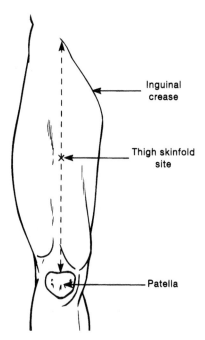

Figure 6.30
The thigh skinfold lies along the anterior midline of the thigh halfway between the inguinal crease and the proximal border of the patella.

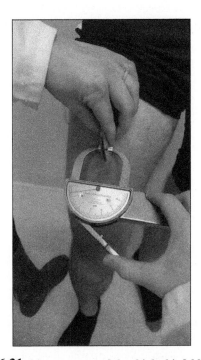

Figure 6.31 Measurement of the thigh skinfold.
©David C. Nieman

the knee and hip are flexed about 90 degrees. The point of maximum calf circumference is marked at the medial (inner) aspect of the calf. A vertical skinfold is grasped about 1 cm proximal to the marked site and measured at the site (Figure 6.32).

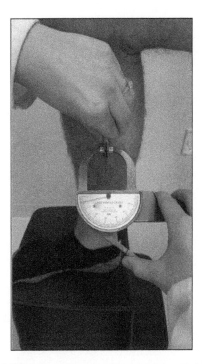

Figure 6.32 Measurement of the medial calf skinfold.
©David C. Nieman

Triceps and Subscapular Skinfold Measurements

The triceps and subscapular skinfolds are accessible and easy to measure and have been included in large population studies such as the NHANES. Reference data for triceps and subscapular skinfolds derived from NHANES 2007–2010 are shown in Appendix I. Using the tables, the 50th percentile represents the median value for each age/sex group. If a subject had a skinfold thickness at the 85th percentile for his or her age/sex group, 85% of the subjects studied in that group would have smaller measurements, and only 15% would have larger measurements. Thus, the triceps and subscapular skinfold measurements allow comparisons to be made with national reference data starting at age 2 months.

Various attempts have been made to calculate percent body fat from triceps and subscapular skinfold measurements, especially when combined with additional information.[98,99]

The American Body Composition Calculator (ABCC) (http://uncbodycalc.sph.unc.edu/) uses sex, ethnicity, age, height, and weight to determine body fat percent.[99] Additional factors improve the accuracy of the calculated results, and these include two skinfolds (triceps, subscapular), four circumferences (waist, arm, thigh, calf), and two lengths (upper arm, upper leg). Measurement methods are based on the *NHANES Anthropometry and Physical Activity Monitor Procedures Manual* (https://www.cdc.gov/nchs/data/nhanes/nhanes_05_06/BM.pdf).[100] Review Box 6.4 for a full description of the ABCC, and how two skinfold measurements (triceps and subscapular) can be combined with other information to accurately estimate percent body fat.

Box 6.4   The American Body Composition Calculator (ABCC)

The American Body Composition Calculator (ABCC) (http://uncbodycalc.sph.unc.edu/) uses sex, ethnicity, age, height, and weight to determine body fat percent.[99] Additional factors improve the accuracy of the calculated results, and these include two skinfolds (triceps, subscapular), four circumferences (waist, arm, thigh, calf), and two lengths (upper arm, upper leg). Measurement methods are based on the *NHANES Anthropometry and Physical Activity Monitor Procedures Manual* (https://www.cdc.gov/nchs/data/nhanes/nhanes_05_06/BM.pdf).[100]

Step 1: Select Your Preferred Measurement System.

Preference
- U.S./Imperial
- Metric

Step 2: Enter Your Information for the Required Fields Below.

Sex
- Male
- Female

Ethnicity
- White
- Black
- Latina/Latino
- Other

Age	**30 years**

Age range is from 8 years to 85 years.

Height	**5' 5"**

Height range is from 3' 6" to 6' 5."

Weight	**140 lb**

Weight range is from 41 lb to 300 lb.

Step 3: Enter Additional Measurements for Improved Accuracy.

Waist Circumference	**25"**

Waist Circumference range is from 18" to 59."

Dual-emission X-ray absorptiometry (DXA) assessed during the 1999–2006 NHANES was used as the reference standard. These are the first equations that have been shown to be valid and unbiased for both youth and adults in estimating percent body fat from DXA. Here is the website display and calculation for a 30-year-old white female with a height of 5 feet 5 inches, weight of 140 pounds, triceps skinfold of 23 mm, subscapular skinfold of 20 mm, and waist circumference of 25 inches.

Arm Circumference	**None**

Arm Circumference range is from 4.0" to 22.0."

Thigh Circumference	**None**

Thigh Circumference range is from 10.0" to 33.0."

Calf Circumference	**None**

Calf Circumference range is from 6.0" to 22.0."

Upper Arm Length	**None**

Upper Arm Length range is from 8.0" to 20.0."

Upper Leg Length	**None**

Upper Leg Length range is from 8.0" to 22.0."

Triceps Skinfold Thickness	**23 mm**

Triceps Skinfold Thickness range is from 2 mm to 45 mm.

Subscapular Skinfold Thickness	**20 mm**

Subscapular Skinfold Thickness range is from 2 mm to 45 mm.

Your calculated body composition is **33.03%.** Congratulations. Your percent body fat is within the healthy range of 27.5% to 37.4% for white American females 30 to 49 years of age.

NOTE: The Body Composition Calculator is not accurate for individuals who are less than 8 years of age, are less than 3'6" or more than 6'5" tall, weigh less than 42 or more than 300 pounds, are pregnant, have had sex reassignment hormone therapy, or have had an amputation other than fingers or toes. The ABCC calculations are based on this source: Stevens J, Ou F-S, Cai J, Heymsfield SB, Truesdale KP. 2016. Prediction of percent body fat measurements in Americans 8 years and older. *International Journal of Obesity* 40:587–594.[99]

The "healthy range" of percent body fat for children is based on this source: Taylor RW, Jones IE, Williams SM, Goulding A. 2002. Body fat percentages measured by dual-energy X-ray absorptiometry corresponding to recently recommended body mass index cutoffs for overweight and obesity in children and adolescents aged 3–18 y. *American Journal of Clinical Nutrition* 76:1416–1421.

The "healthy range" of percent body fat for adults is based on this source: Heo M, Faith MS, Pietrobelli A, Heymsfield SB. 2012. Percentage of body fat cutoffs by sex, age, and race-ethnicity in the US adult population from NHANES 1999–2004. *American Journal of Clinical Nutrition* 95:594–602.

ADDITIONAL GUIDELINES FOR CIRCUMFERENCE AND LENGTH MEASUREMENTS (FIRST MARK, THEN MEASURE):

Arm circumference: Circumference at mid-arm (halfway between uppermost edge of the posterior border of the acromion process to the olecranon process, same as triceps skinfold), while standing with the right arm hanging loosely

Thigh circumference: Circumference at mid-thigh (halfway between proximal patalla and inguinal crease, same as thigh skinfold) with most of the weight on the left leg with the right leg forward, knee slightly flexed, and soles of both feet flat on the floor

Calf circumference: Maximal calf circumference while in the seated position

Upper arm length: Measured with a tape measure down the back of the arm from the posterior border of the acromion process to the tip of the olecranon process, arm flexed 90 degrees at the elbow with the palm facing up

Upper leg length: Measured with a tape measure down the front of the thight from the inguinal crease to the proximal border of the patella, while in the seated position

Multiple-Site Skinfold Measurements

Predicting body density and then percent of body fat from skinfold measurements requires estimating equations. These formulas have been developed by comparing a variety of skinfold and other anthropometric measures with measurements of body density or body fat percentage (usually by hydrostatic weighing and dual-energy X-ray absorptiometry (DXA)) to see which anthropometric measures fit best. Various statistical approaches are used to develop gender-specific percent body fat equations.[4,94,101–103]

Many estimating equations have been developed and can be classified as either population-specific equations or generalized equations.[92,94,98] Population-specific equations are derived from data on groups of people sharing certain characteristics, such as age and gender. The first valid equations, for example, were developed in 1951 for young and middle-aged men.[104] Numerous other population-specific equations have been developed since then, but their use is limited. Equations developed from data on middle-aged females, for example, may not be valid for females of other ages.

More recently, generalized equations have been developed that are applicable to persons varying greatly in age and body fatness. The primary advantage of this approach is that one generalized equation can replace several population-specific equations with no loss in prediction accuracy.[5,94,98,99] Table 6.7 shows several generalized prediction equations for calculating body density or percent body fat using skinfolds. Because fat placement differs between males and females, separate equations are given for each sex.

The equations in Table 6.7 predict either body fat percent or body density. Body density formulas require an additional calculation to estimate percent body fat. Two formulas are available for this step: the Brozek and the Siri equations:

Brozek: Percent body fat = (457 ÷ body density) − 414

Siri: Percent body fat = (495 ÷ body density) − 450

The recent trend in development of equations to calculate percent body fat has been to use DXA measurements from NHANES as the criterion measure.[99–107] Associations between various anthropometric measurements and percent body fat can differ based on gender, age, and race/ethnicity. As described earlier, 28 equations have been developed for the prediction of percent body fat in children and adults using NHANES DXA data combined with 2 and 10 anthropometric measurements (height, weight, skinfolds, circumferences, lengths).[99] These are currently the best generalized equations available for calculating percent body fat and can be applied at the excellent website maintained by the University of North Carolina at Chapel Hill (http://ABCC.sph.unc.edu).

What Is a Desirable Level of Fatness?

Various attempts have been made to develop norms for percent body fat. This has proven to be a challenging task due to the lack of long-term studies linking body fat levels and disease mortality, difficulties in accurately and repeatedly measuring body composition in large population groups, and the lack of consensus on optimal body fat percentage levels (especially within the United States, where 70% of adults are overweight or obese). Tables 6.8 and 6.9 and Figure 6.33 show DXA-derived body fat percentage data for males and females, ages 8 and older.[103,105,106,107] These data are percent body fat values obtained from whole-body dual-energy x-ray absorptiometry (DXA)

TABLE 6.7	**Generalized Body Composition Equations for Male and Female Adults***

Males

Body density = $1.11200000 - 0.00043499(X_1) + 0.00000055 (X_1)^2 - 0.00028826 (X_8)$

Percent body fat = $0.29288 (X_2) - 0.00050 (X_2)^2 + 0.15845 (X_8) - 5.76377$

Body density = $1.1093800 - 0.0008267 (X_3) + 0.0000016 (X_3)^2 - 0.0002574 (X_8)$

Body density = $1.1125025 - 0.0013125 (X_4) + 0.00000055 (X_4)^2 - 0.0002440 (X_8)$

Percent body fat = $0.39287 (X_5) - 0.00105 (X_5)^2 + 0.15772 (X_8) - 5.18845$

Females

Body density = $1.0970 - 0.00046971 (X_1) + 0.00000056 (X_1)^2 - 0.00012828 (X_8)$

Percent body fat = $0.29699 (X_2) - 0.00043 (X_2)^2 + 0.02963 (X_8) + 1.4072$

Percent body fat = $0.41563 (X_6) - 0.00112 (X_6)^2 + 0.03661 (X_8) + 4.03653$

Body density = $1.0994921 - 0.0009929 (X_7) + 0.0000023 (X_7)^2 - 0.0001392 (X_8)$

Source: Jackson AS, Pollock ML. 1985. Practical assessment of body composition. *Physician and Sportsmedicine* 13(5):76–90; Golding LA, Myers CR, Sinning WE. 1989. *The Y's way to physical fitness,* 3rd ed. Champaign, IL: Human Kinetics Books.

*X_1 = sum of chest, midaxillary, triceps, subscapular, abdomen, suprailiac, and thigh skinfolds; X_2 = sum of abdomen, suprailiac, triceps, and thigh skinfolds; X_3 = sum of chest, abdomen, and subscapular skinfolds; X_4 = sum of chest, triceps, and subscapular skinfolds; X_5 = sum of abdomen, suprailiac, and triceps skinfolds; X_6 = sum of triceps, abdomen, and suprailiac skinfolds; X_7 = sum of triceps, suprailiac, and thigh skinfolds; X_8 = age in years.

TABLE 6.8	Percent Body Fat Distribution by Age Group for Males Males, Percentile Distribution for Total Body Fat (all race and ethnicity)								
Age	5th	10th	15th	25th	50th	75th	85th	90th	95th
8–11 y	18.2	19.6	20.6	22.1	25.9	33.2	37.5	39.6	42.9
12–15 y	15.1	16.1	16.9	18.6	23.0	31.1	34.3	37.7	40.6
16–19 y	14.0	14.9	15.6	17.0	20.7	27.5	31.3	33.6	37.3
20–39 y	15.5	17.4	18.9	21.2	26.1	30.4	32.8	34.6	37.2
40–59 y	19.3	21.5	23.0	24.2	28.5	32.2	34.1	35.5	37.7
60–79 y	22.0	24.2	25.3	27.3	30.7	34.4	36.4	37.7	39.6
≥ 80 y	21.9	24.2	25.4	27.3	30.8	33.9	36.1	37.3	38.8

Source: Borrud LG, Flegal KM, Looker AC, Everhart JE, et al. 2010. Body composition data for individuals 8 years of age and older: U.S. population, 1999–2004. National Center for Health Statistics. *Vital Health Statistics* 11(250).

TABLE 6.9	Percent Body Fat Distribution by Age Group for Females Females, Percentile Distribution for Total Body Fat (all race and ethnicity)								
Age	5th	10th	15th	25th	50th	75th	85th	90th	95th
8–11 y	21.7	22.9	24.3	26.3	31.2	37.1	40.3	41.9	43.9
12–15 y	21.7	23.4	24.9	27.4	31.9	37.3	40.1	42.0	44.9
16–19 y	24.2	26.3	27.6	30.0	34.0	39.2	42.9	44.8	47.7
20–39 y	25.8	28.4	29.9	32.5	37.8	42.9	45.6	47.4	49.8
40–59 y	28.5	31.8	33.6	36.4	41.0	45.1	47.1	48.6	50.7
60–79 y	32.3	34.9	36.4	38.9	42.8	46.2	48.0	49.1	50.7
≤ 80 y	29.8	32.7	34.3	36.9	41.0	44.4	46.3	47.5	48.9

Source: Borrud LG, Flegal KM, Looker AC, Everhart JE, et al. 2010. Body composition data for individuals 8 years of age and older: U.S. population, 1999–2004. National Center for Health Statistics. *Vital Health Statistics* 11(250).

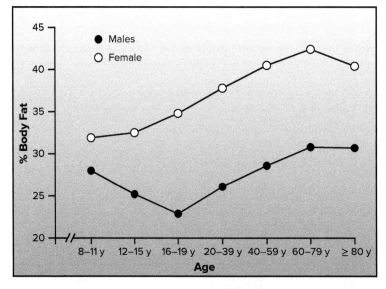

Figure 6.33 **Percent body fat for males and females 8 years of age and older.**

Source: Borrud LG, Flegal KM, Looker AC, Everhart JE, et al. 2010. Body composition data for individuals 8 years of age and older: U.S. population, 1999–2004. National Center for Health Statistics. *Vital and Health Statistics* 11(250).

scans for persons 8 years of age and older who participated in the National Health and Nutrition Examination Survey (NHANES) 1999–2004 (see Appendix J).[107] Valid total body measurements were obtained on 16,973 individuals. Through the use of multiple imputation, a usable sample of 22,010 individuals was achieved for analysis. Although these are interesting data, they represent a cross-sectional snapshot of the body fat percentage levels of children, adolescents, and adults. In other words, these percentile distributions do not allow "optimal" body fat percentage values to be defined. The recent focus in developing body fat percentage norms has been to establish equivalent levels with BMI for which there is abundant disease prevention data. Table 6.10 summarizes percentage of body fat cutoffs by sex and age on the basis of the relation between DXA and BMI using NHANES data. Cutoffs of percentage of body fat varied depending on age and sex, with slight differences for different race-ethnicity groups (not included in Table 6.10).[103,105] The data in Table 6.10 will continue to be updated as long-term studies on the relationship between body composition and mortality are published. It should be noted that a wide range of percent body fat levels are compatible with athletic endeavor, but in general, athletes have low levels of body fat, typically less than 15% and 25% in males and females, respectively.[27]

TABLE 6.10	Percent Body Fat and BMI Classifications for Males and Females by Age Group		
Gender and Age	Normal *Equal to BMI < 24.9 kg/m²*	Overweight/Fat *Equal to BMI 25 to 29.9 kg/m²*	Obese *Equal to BMI ≥ 30 kg/m²*
Males	% Body Fat	% Body Fat	% Body Fat
3–10 y	< 20	20–29.9	≥ 30
11–17 y	< 22	22–31.9	≥ 32
18–49 y	< 24.9	25–29.9	≥ 30
50–84 y	< 27.9	28–31.9	≥ 32
Females			
3–6 y	< 21	21–25.9	≥ 26
7–10 y	< 25	25–34.9	≥ 35
11–17 y	< 34	34–44.9	≥ 45
18–49 y	< 36.9	37–41.9	≥ 42
50–84 y	< 39.9	40–43.9	≥ 44

Note: Data are based on percentages of body fat measured from dual-energy x-ray absorptiometry (DXA).

Sources:

Heo M, Faith MS, Pietrobelli A, Heymsfield SB. 2012. Percentage of body fat cutoffs by sex, age, and race-ethnicity in the US adult population from NHANES 1999–2004. *American Journal of Clinical Nutrition* 95:594–602.

Taylor RW, Jones EI, Williams SM, Goulding A. 2002. Body fat percentages measured by dual-energy X-ray absorptiometry corresponding to recently recommended body mass index cutoffs for overweight and obesity in children and adolescents aged 3–18 y. *American Journal of Clinical Nutrition* 76:1416–1421.

Using the values in Table 6.10, the form shown in Figure 6.34, and the following formulas, a person can calculate a target weight necessary to achieve a certain percent body fat.[27]

Weight of fat = Total body weight × Percent body fat
Fat-free weight = Total body weight-Fat weight
Target weight = Present fat-free weight ÷ (100% − desired percent body fat)

For example, take a subject who weighs 200 lb, has 25% body fat, and desires to have a 15% body fat (for athletic reasons):

Weight of fat = 200 lb × 0.25 = 50 lb
Fat-free weight = 200 lb − 50 lb = 150 lb
Target weight = 150 lb ÷ 0.85 = 176 lb

DENSITOMETRY

Densitometry is assessing body composition by measuring the density of the entire body.[83,84] Density is expressed as mass per unit volume and usually is obtained through **hydrostatic,** or underwater weighing, DXA, and air displacement plethysmography.[108]

Underwater Weighing

A common research technique of determining whole-body density is hydrostatic, or underwater, weighing.[83,84]

Figure 6.34 Skinfold recording and calculation form.

The technique is based on **Archimedes' principle,** which states that the volume of an object submerged in water equals the volume of water the object displaces. Thus, if the mass and the volume of a body are known, the density of that body can be calculated. Using another formula, percent body fat can be calculated from body density.

This approach is based on the two-compartment model of body composition: the fat and fat-free mass. The fat-free mass is assumed to have a constant level of hydration and a constant proportion of bone mineral to muscle. The approach also assumes a constant fat mass density of 0.90 g/cm^3 and a density of the fat-free mass of 1.10 g/cm^3.[83,84] The densities of bone and muscle tissue are greater than the density of water (density of distilled water = 1.00 g/cm^3), whereas fat is less dense than water. Thus, muscular subjects having a low percentage of body fat tend to weigh more submerged in water than do subjects having a higher percentage of body fat.

Body density can be calculated from the following formula,[4]

$$Body\ density = \frac{WA}{\dfrac{(WA - WW)}{DW} - (RV + VGI)}$$

where WA = body weight in air; WW = body weight submerged in water; DW = density of water; RV = residual lung volume; VGI = volume of gas in the gastrointestinal tract.

Equipment

The necessary equipment for underwater weighing includes a tank, tub, or pool of water of sufficient size for total body submersion; a scale or another method of determining the subject's underwater weight; and, attached to the scale, a chair or frame lowered into the water on which the subject sits (Figure 6.35).

The water should be comfortably warm, filtered, chlorinated, and undisturbed by wind or other activity in the water during testing.[27] A method of underwater weighing in a swimming pool using a wooden shell placed within the pool to reduce water movement, which can adversely affect weighing, has been described by Katch.[108]

The chair should be constructed so that the subject can sit under the water with legs slightly bent and the water at neck level, as shown in Figure 6.35. Weights should be attached to the chair, so that its empty or tare weight while under water is at least 3 kg for subjects of moderate body fatness and at least 4 to 6 kg for obese subjects.[27] Some researchers use a frame on which the subject lies submerged in the prone (face down) position while breathing through a snorkel.[27,108] This causes less up-and-down movement of the body in the water, thus resulting in fewer fluctuations of the scale.

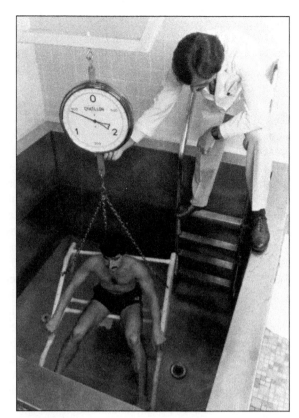

Figure 6.35
Equipment for underwater weighing includes a tank of sufficient size and shape for total human submersion, an accurate scale for measuring weight with 10-gram divisions, a method of measuring water temperature, and a chair that is weighted to prevent flotation.
©David C. Nieman

Typically, an autopsy scale (such as the 9-kg capacity Chatillon autopsy scale shown in Figure 6.35) is used in underwater weighing. A strain gauge, or force cell, gives more precise measurements.[27,83,109] These instruments can be interfaced with a computer, which, with the appropriate software, can easily determine the midpoint of fluctuations and can use that as the basis for further calculations.[27]

Procedure[27]

1. Basic data—name, date, age, sex, stature, and weight (in kilograms) in air—should be collected and recorded on a form such as the one shown in Figure 6.36. The tester should record the tare weight—the underwater weight of the chair (and any attached weights)—before the subject sits in it. The subject should be several hours **postprandial,** clean, wearing only a swimsuit. The subject should have urinated and defecated immediately before weighing. Carbonated beverages and flatus-causing foods should be avoided before the procedure because gastrointestinal tract gas will decrease the subject's underwater weight, resulting in erroneously low measurements of body density.

Body Composition Worksheet

Name _____ Date _____

Age _____ Sex _____ Height _____

Skinfolds (mm)

_____ Chest   _____ Suprailiac

_____ Triceps   _____ Abdominal

_____ Subscapular   _____ Thigh

_____ Midaxillary   _____ Medial calf

Hydrostatic Measurements

_____ Weight in air (Wa)

_____ Tare weight

_____ Average gross weight (average of best two trials)

Underwater weighing trials

1 ____ 2 ____ 3 ____ 4 ____ 5 ____

6 ____ 7 ____ 8 ____ 9 ____ 10 ____

_____ Weight in water (Ww) (average gross weight—tare weight)

_____ Density of water (Dw)

_____ Residual volume (RV)

Calculations

$$\text{Density} = \frac{Wa}{\dfrac{(Wa - Ww)}{Dw} - (RV + 100\ ml)}$$

_____ Percent body fat = (495 ÷ density) − 450

_____ Fat weight (weight in the air × fat%)

_____ Lean body weight (weight in the air − fat weight)

_____ Classification

Figure 6.36 Body composition worksheet.

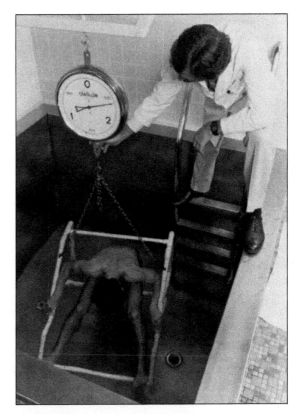

Figure 6.37 Subject's body position while submerged during underwater weighing.
The water should be kept as calm as possible to get a good reading on the scale. Note how the tester is steadying the scale with his hand. Once the scale is relatively steady, the tester should remove the hand and take the reading.
©David C. Nieman

2. Measuring skinfolds: skinfold measurements can help verify results from underwater weighing. These can be recorded on the form shown in Figure 6.36.

3. Submerging: while comfortably seated in the chair, the subject exhales as fully as possible and slowly leans forward until the head is completely under the water, as shown in Figure 6.37. The subject continues to press as much air from the lungs as possible. After exhaling fully, the subject remains motionless and counts for 5 to 7 seconds before coming up for air. This allows the tester time to read the scale. While in the water, the subject should move slowly and deliberately to prevent water turbulence, which can make the subject bob up and down and make scale reading difficult. When the subject submerges, the tester can keep one hand on the scale to steady it, as shown in Figure 6.37.

4. Recording underwater weight: several trials usually are necessary before the subject becomes accustomed to the procedure and consistent readings are obtained. Katch and coworkers[108] weighed subjects 9 or 10 times and took the average of the last 3 underwater readings as the "true" underwater weight. Underwater weight should be recorded on the Body Composition Worksheet (Figure 6.36) as the gross weight in water. The net body weight in water is the gross weight in water minus the tare weight. The temperature of the water should be measured, and water density should be determined from standard tables.

5. Determining residual volume: residual volume (RV) is the amount of air remaining in the lungs after a maximal exhalation. All other things being equal, a subject with a large RV will be more buoyant (have a lower underwater weight) than one with a smaller RV. Although RV often is estimated, whenever possible it should be measured directly. When RV is estimated, hydrostatically determined percent body

fat is no more accurate than when derived from skinfold measurements.[27] Techniques for measuring RV include nitrogen washout, helium dilution, and oxygen dilution. The choice of technique is generally a matter of which is available to the investigator.

If equipment for measuring RV is not available, it can be estimated from vital lung capacity.[110] RV is approximately 24% of vital lung capacity, provided the vital capacity is measured while the subject is in water. Another approach is to use the following sex-specific formulas,[111]

$$\text{Male RV} = 0.017 \text{ A} + 0.06858 \text{ S} - 3.477$$

$$\text{Female RV} = 0.009 \text{ A} + 0.08128 \text{ S} - 3.900$$

where A = age in years and S = stature in inches. Because measuring gastrointestinal tract gas is impossible using conventional methods, it is nearly always estimated to be 100 mL in adults.[83] The value is likely smaller in children and larger in subjects who consumed flatus-producing foods or carbonated beverages before being measured. The volume of gastrointestinal gas can range from 50 to 300 ml.[83]

6. Calculate estimates of body density and percent body fat using the worksheet (Figure 6.36). The remainder of the calculations on the Body Composition Worksheet are the same as those discussed in the section "What Is a Desirable Level of Fatness?"

Weaknesses of Underwater Weighing

Underwater weighing has several weaknesses. It is not practical for testing large numbers of people. Subjects must be willing and able to remain submerged and motionless long enough for an accurate measurement of weight to be made. This requires considerable subject cooperation and training.[83,112,113] Consequently, about 10% to 20% of subjects find it difficult to be weighed under water. The technique requires some special equipment, experience, and financial investment. In many situations, skinfold measurements may be more practical.[27]

Densitometry is based on several assumptions. Perhaps the most tenuous of these is a constant density of the fat-free compartment.[27,83,87] A number of factors can affect the density of the fat-free mass, and these can influence the accuracy of body density measurement by 3% to 4%.[27] Athletes, for example, tend to have denser bone and muscle tissue, which may result in underestimation of body fat (possibly even *negative* body fat values), whereas the tendency of older persons to have less dense bones will likely result in overestimation of body fat.[4] Fat-free tissue density values for adults are probably not appropriate for use with children. Another concern is gas trapped in the gut, the amount of which can only be estimated. Other factors affecting the accuracy of body density measurements include the consumption of food and carbonated beverages shortly before underwater weighing, fluid loss during intensive training, fluid retention before menstruation, and the degree of forcible exhalation while submerged.[27] Air displacement plethysmography, 8-electrode, segmental multifrequency bioelectrical impedance, and DXA have largely replaced underwater weighing for determination of body composition in many research and clinical laboratories.

Air Displacement Plethysmography

As an alternative to underwater weighing, body volume (and, consequently, body density and percent body fat) can be measured using a technique known as air displacement plethysmography. Air displacement plethysmography originated in Germany over 100 years ago with the first viable operating system becoming commercially available in 1995. Air displacement plethysmography determines total body volume (volume of empty chamber minus volume of chamber with subject). Body volume varies inversely with pressure so long as temperature remains constant (Boyle's law). Cosmed (Concord, CA) has several types of air displacement plethysmographic devices, including the BOD POD for children, adolescents, and adults (Figure 6.38), and the PEA POD

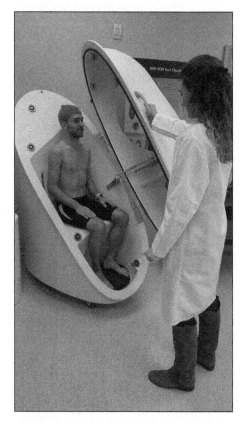

Figure 6.38
The BOD POD Gold Standard Body Composition Tracking System is an air displacement plethysmograph that uses whole-body densitometry to determine body composition (fat and fat-free mass) in adults and children, and it can accommodate a wide range of populations. A full test requires only about five minutes and provides highly accurate, safe, comfortable, and fast results.
©David C. Nieman

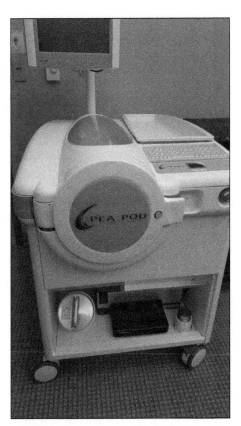

Figure 6.39
The PEA POD is an air displacement plethysmography (ADP)
system using whole-body densitometry to determine body
composition (fat and fat-free mass) in infants weighing between
1 and 8 kg. The PEA POD is accurate, easy to operate, and
takes about seven minutes. See http://www.cosmedusa.com/.
©David C. Nieman

(Figure 6.39) for infants (up to 6 months of age). The BOD
POD with the pediatric option accessory allows the assessment of body composition of young children 2 to 6 years of
age using a customized seat insert. The unit is constructed
of fiberglass and consists of two chambers (front and rear),
which are separated by a wall, which also serves as a
molded seat on which the subject sits during testing. The
subject enters and exits the front chamber of the unit
through a hinged door containing a large acrylic window,
giving the subject a comfortable sense of openness when
the door is closed. The rear chamber houses electronic
instruments, an air circulation system, valves, pressure
transducers, and a breathing circuit. Attached to the wall
separating the two chambers is a diaphragm, which, when
moved during calibration and subject measurement,
slightly alters the volume of the two chambers. These volume alterations during calibration and subject measurement are used, along with other values, to calculate the
subject's volume. Connected to but outside the unit are a
scale for weighing the subject and a computer for controlling the system and for collecting, analyzing, and out-
putting data.[112,114] In order to accurately measure body

volume, it is necessary to minimize or account for the
effects of clothing, hair, body surface area, and thoracic
(lung and airway) gas volume. The effects of clothing and
hair are minimized by having the subject dress in a tight-
fitting swimsuit and wear a swimcap to compress the hair.
Body surface area is calculated using a formula and accurate measurement of height and weight. Thoracic gas volume can be measured or estimated using an equation
during the final step of the measurement process.[114,116]

After voiding, the subject is weighed on the system's
scale, and height is measured using a stadiometer. A two-
step calibration process is performed, first with the front
chamber empty and the door closed and then with a 50-liter
calibration cylinder in the front chamber with the door
closed. During each step of the calibration process, the
electronically controlled diaphragm oscillates back and
forth to alter the volume in the two chambers.[114] The subject then enters the front chamber, the door is closed, and
the subject relaxes and breathes normally while the diaphragm oscillates back and forth. At the end of this 20-sec-
ond measurement, the door is momentarily opened and
then closed and the measurement process is repeated. If
these two volume measurements are within 150 ml of each
other, the measurements are accepted and the mean value
is used for calculations. If they are not within 150 ml, a
third measurement is taken. Any two of the three measurements that are within 150 ml of each other are averaged,
and that value is used in calculations of body volume.
Pressure differences within the front chamber when it is
empty and when the subject is present are used in calculating the subject's body volume.[114–116]

In research environments, the final step is measurement of the subject's thoracic gas volume, which includes
all air in the lungs and airways. The door is opened and
the subject is given a single-use, disposable breathing
tube, which is connected to a breathing circuit housed in
the unit's rear chamber. The subject's nostrils are sealed
with a nose clip and the subject is instructed to breathe
quietly through the mouth. The door is then closed. After
several normal breaths, a valve in the breathing circuit
momentarily closes at the midpoint of an exhalation. As
previously instructed, the subject compresses and then
relaxes the diaphragm muscle. This produces small pressure fluctuations within the subject's airway and in the
chamber, which are used to calculate thoracic gas volume. The final body volume is calculated based on the
initial volume measurement, corrected for thoracic gas
volume and the subject's body surface area. This is then
used to calculate percent body fat mass and percent body
lean mass.[115,116]

Measurements of body composition derived from air
displacement plethysmography among different groups of
subjects have been compared with those derived from
other criterion methods, such as underwater weighing and
dual-energy X-ray absorptiometry.[115–124] In general, these
validation studies show good agreement between

measurements of body composition based on air displacement plethysmography and these two other criterion methods when group means are compared. Overall, air displacement plethysmography is an accurate and practical technique for body composition analysis in the clinical setting. Most noteworthy is the fact that plethysmography overcomes some of the methodological and technical constraints of underwater weighing. It is fairly quick and easy and is much more suitable for use with children, the elderly, and the disabled than is underwater weighing.[116–119,122,124] Like underwater weighing, calculations of body density from volume measurements derived from air displacement plethysmography are dependent on the assumption that fat-free tissue has a constant density.[112,117]

BIOELECTRICAL IMPEDANCE

Bioelectrical impedance analysis (BIA) was developed in the 1960s and has emerged as one of the most popular methods for measuring body composition.[125] A harmless current is generated and passed through the individual being measured. The electrical current primarily passes through fat-free mass body compartments with high amounts of electrolyte-rich water where resistance is lowest. Impedance to the electrical current is greatest in fat tissue (only 14–22% water content). BIA measures the electrical impedance of body tissues and can be used to assess fluid volumes, total body water, and fat-free body mass, and through estimation, percent body fat. NHANES included BIA measurements in several NHANES cycles, first with a tetrapolar, single-frequency (50 kHz) BIA method (years 1988–1994), and then more recently (years 1999–2004) with a multi-frequency analyzer that measured impedance at 50 frequencies logarithmically spaced from 5 kHz to 1000 kHz.[126,127]

In practice, BIA is performed by measuring shifts in impedance between electrodes that are positioned on various parts of the body. Figure 6.40 shows a scale that measures leg-to-leg BIA through electrodes that contact the bare feet. Other BIA devices use electrodes in a tetrapolar arrangement on the wrists and ankles. A wide variety of equations have been developed to estimate fat-free mass and percent body fat from single-frequency (50 kHz) BIA devices, and in general, most studies show that when compared to various reference techniques (e.g., DXA, underwater weighing), BIA (when conducted appropriately) has about the same accuracy as skinfold methods.[128–130] There are several potential sources of measurement error with BIA that center around the hydration status of the individual being tested. Every attempt should be made to ensure that the individual is in a state of normal hydration.

BIA devices have become more sophisticated, with a focus on multiple frequencies and a higher number of electrodes to improve accuracy and precision. Segmental multi-frequency BIA uses multiple broadband frequencies

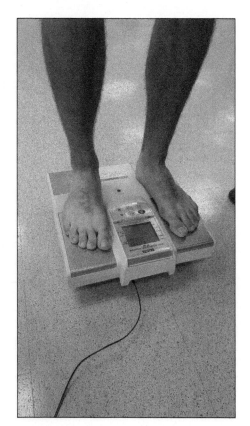

Figure 6.40
Bioelectrical impedance offers a convenient, rapid, noninvasive, and safe approach for assessing body composition. In this unit, four electrodes are built into the top of a digital scale, and a harmless current is passed leg to leg, with impedance measured. The electrical impedance can be used to assess fluid volumes, total body water, and fat-free body mass.
©David C. Nieman

in the range of 1 kHz to 1000 kHz with eight electrodes (i.e., 8-polar BIA), two for each hand and foot (Figure 6.41). This BIA method improves the accuracy of measuring total body water, fat-free mass, and percent body fat, especially for the assessment of healthy, nonobese individuals. Eight-polar BIA correlates closely with DXA and other reference methods, and in-day precision of multiple tests on the same individual is high.[131–133] However, both single- and multiple-frequency bioimpedance techniques can be erroneous for whole-body estimates in clinical populations when fluid abnormalities and extreme adiposity are present.[127] Eight-polar BIA is very practical because of the tactile electrodes, the development of devices that allow an individual to stand on a scale while grasping side rails that have in-built electrodes, and the rapidity of measurement. Body composition values for the whole body, trunk, and each limb are measured and included in test results. Fat-free mass is accurately assessed with 8-polar BIA, allowing the resting metabolic rate to be estimated.

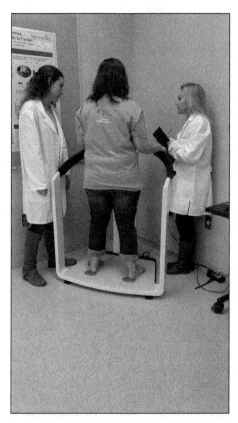

Figure 6.41 **Segmental multi-frequency BIA uses multiple broadband frequencies in the range of 1 kHz to 1000 kHz with eight electrodes (i.e., 8-polar BIA), two for each hand and foot. Eight-polar BIA is very practical because of the tactile electrodes, the development of devices that allow an individual to stand on a scale while grasping side rails that have in-built electrodes, and the rapidity of measurement.**
©David C. Nieman

DUAL-ENERGY X-RAY ABSORPTIOMETRY

Several imaging methods can be used to distinguish and quantify types of tissue (adipose, lean, bone). These include dual-energy X-ray absorptiometry (DXA), computed axial tomography (CT), magnetic resonance (MR), and positron emission tomographic (PET) scanners. Each technique has its own strengths and limitations, and they vary in accuracy, precision or reproducibility, accessibility, and costs.

DXA was originally designed for determining bone mineral density, but it can also be used to assess fat and fat-free soft tissue. The fundamental principle of DXA is the measurement of the transmission of X-rays through the body at high and low energies.[134,135] The X-ray source generates a beam of X-rays, which consists of photon particles carried through electromagnetic energy. As photons pass through the tissues, physical interactions take place that reduce beam intensity depending on the energy of the photons and the density and thickness of the human tissues. DXA measures the absorption (attenuation) of two X-ray photon energies, typically near 40 and 70 keV, which allows for the distinguishing of bone from soft tissue. After excluding pixels that represent bone tissue, DXA estimates fat from the proportion of fat to lean soft tissue in each pixel of a whole-body image based on X-ray attenuation. DXA assumes that the attenuation coefficients of fat and lean soft tissue remain constant among individuals, and that DXA measurements are not affected by the anteroposterior thickness of a body.

DXA technology and software have improved over time. Major technological advances have taken place with the progressive transition from pencil-beam densitometers to narrow fan-beam densitometers with multiple detectors that allow quick, high-resolution scans of the whole body. The enhanced resolution allows for better bone edge detection and body composition assessment.[134–138]

In general, DXA body composition assessment is highly accessible, convenient, quick (5- to 13-minute scan time), accurate, precise, and safe (Figure 6.42). DXA has a very low ionizing radiation exposure (~0.001 mSv per scan or about the same as three hours of natural "background" radiation exposure). DXA has been evaluated against the "gold standard" 4-compartment (4-C) model that divides the body into four compartments—fat mass, bone mineral, total body water, and other (i.e., protein, non-bone minerals, and glycogen). Most

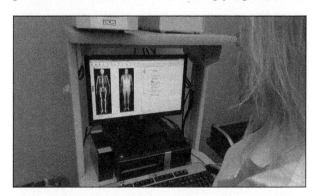

Figure 6.42 **DXA can be used for measurement of body composition and bone mineral density, and is convenient, quick, accurate, precise, and safe.**
©David C. Nieman

studies show that the mean difference in percent body fat between DXA and 4-C is within plus or minus 4%, and that repeat testing on individuals is precise (generally less than 3% variance).[134,135] DXA has been included in NHANES for the development of body composition reference values.[105]

Precision of DXA testing for body composition changes over time can be improved by ensuring consistent positioning and preparation (e.g., fasting state, clothing, time of day, physical activity, empty bladder).[136,137] Positioning of the arms, hands, legs, and feet whenever possible should be according to the NHANES method (palms down isolated from the body, feet neutral, ankles strapped, arms straight or slightly angled, face up with neutral chin). Discrepancies in body composition outcomes have also been reported between DXA machines, both within the same manufacturer and across manufacturers. So repeat tests on individuals should be made with the same DXA machine.

Due to its good precision, widespread availability, and low radiation dose, DXA is a convenient and useful diagnostic tool for body composition assessment in a wide variety of individuals, and future improvements in technology and software will strengthen this consensus.[134,138] Box 6.5 summarizes the use of DXA in screening for osteoporosis. NHANES reference data for spinal lumbar and femur bone mineral density are provided in Appendixes K and L.

 Box 6.5 — **Osteoporosis Screening Using DXA**

Osteoporosis, the most common bone disorder in humans, is characterized by the loss of bone mass and deterioration of bone microarchitecture, compromised bone strength, and an increased susceptibility to fracture and painful morbidity.[139]

Osteoporosis can be classified as either primary (not related to other disease) or secondary (when an identifiable cause other than age or menopause is present). Osteoporosis can be secondary to such conditions as Cushing's syndrome, malignancies of the bone (myeloma), hyperthyroidism, hyperparathyroidism, male hypogonadism, and amenorrhea. Certain inherited diseases, such as osteogenesis imperfecta, can also result in osteoporosis, as can long-term use of such medications as thiazide diuretics and heparin. The most common form is primary osteoporosis, in which no other disease is apparent, and is most frequently seen in middle-aged and older adults. Primary Type I osteoporosis is seen in postmenopausal females between 51 and 75 years of age and is a consequence of reduced estrogen levels. Primary Type II osteoporosis is seen in both sexes after age 70 years.

Building strong bones, especially before the age of 35, and then reducing bone loss in later years are the best strategies for preventing osteoporosis. There are many risk factors for osteoporosis, including personal and family history of low bone mass and fracture; being a thin, older female; early estrogen deficiency and amenorrhea; anorexia nervosa; low lifetime calcium intake and vitamin D deficiency; use of certain medications; a physically inactive lifestyle; and current cigarette smoking and excessive use of alcohol.[139] Osteoporosis prevention is centered around consuming a balanced diet rich in calcium and vitamin D, regular weight-bearing exercise, a healthy lifestyle with no smoking or excessive alcohol intake, and bone density testing and medication when appropriate.

DXA is the preferred approach for measuring bone mineral density (BMD) because of its capacity to measure bone mineral content at axial and appendicular sites, the rapid scan time and low radiation exposure, and superior quality-control procedures and accuracy.

Osteoporosis is generally diagnosed by comparing a patient's BMD (determined by DXA) with the mean normal BMD in a population of healthy young adults of the same sex and assigning what is referred to as a T-score.[139] The comparison group serves as the reference population and is considered the standard for peak bone mass. The T-score is the number of standard deviations above or below the mean BMD of the reference population. The most widely accepted diagnostic criterion for osteoporosis is that developed by the World Health Organization (WHO), which defines osteoporosis as a T-score at or below –2.5, as shown in Table 6.11. When the T-score is between –1.0 and –2.5 standard deviations, a condition known as osteopenia is present. Osteopenia is not considered a diagnosis but, rather, is a term used to describe a bone mineral density that is somewhat low but not so low as to warrant a diagnosis of osteoporosis. A normal T-score is -1.0 or greater.

Figure 6.43 summarizes the Surgeon General's guidelines for assessing bone health and preventing bone disease.[139] In general, all women aged 65 and older regardless of risk factors should be tested for BMD with DXA. Women under the age of 65 years can be considered for BMD DXA

TABLE 6.11	World Health Organization T-Score Criteria for Classifying Normal Bone Mineral Density (BMD), Osteoporois
Classification	**T-score**
Normal BMD	–1.0 or greater
Osteopenia	Between –1.0 and –2.5
Osteoporosis	–2.5 or less
Severe osteoporosis	22.5 or less and fragility fracture

Source: World Health Organization and the International Society for Clinical Densitometry.

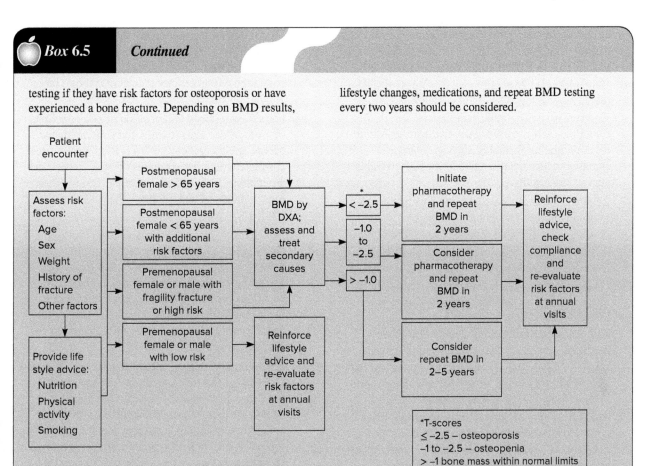

Box 6.5   *Continued*

testing if they have risk factors for osteoporosis or have experienced a bone fracture. Depending on BMD results,

lifestyle changes, medications, and repeat BMD testing every two years should be considered.

Figure 6.43 **The Surgeon General's guidelines for assessing bone health and preventing bone disease.**

Source: U.S. Department of Health and Human Services. 2004. Bone health and osteoporosis: A report of the surgeon general. Rockville, MD: U.S. Department of Health and Human Services, Office of the Surgeon General.

Summary

1. Anthropometry is the measurement of body size, weight, and proportions. Adherence to proper technique is critical to obtaining accurate and precise measurements. Among children, length, stature, weight, and head circumference are the most sensitive and commonly used anthropometric indicators of health.

2. Body weight, one of the most important measurements in nutritional assessment, should be obtained using an electronic or balance-beam scale with nondetachable weights that is appropriate for the subject.

3. Standards for assessing physical growth of persons from birth to age 20 years have been developed by the Centers for Disease Control and Prevention.

These growth charts allow a child's development to be easily categorized relative to the development of other children of similar age and sex.

4. Overweight is a body weight above some reference weight, which usually is defined in relation to stature. Obesity is an excess of body fat in relation to lean body mass. Overweight persons tend to die sooner than average-weight persons, especially those who are overweight at younger ages. The lowest mortality in the United States is associated with body weights that are somewhat below average for a given group based on sex and stature.

5. Approaches to assessing body weight include height-weight tables, relative weight, and height-weight indices. The life insurance industry, a leader in the

development of height-weight tables, has attempted to define body weights for a given sex and stature that are associated with the lowest mortality.

6. Height-weight tables fail to provide information on body composition. Their data are not drawn from representative population samples and are sometimes self-reported. They inadequately control for confounding variables, such as cigarette smoking, which tend to make lower body weights appear less healthy.

7. Relative weight is a person's actual weight divided by some reference weight for that person's height, multiplied by 100, and expressed as a percentage of reference weight. Relative weights between 90% and 120% are considered within normal limits.

8. Of the various body mass indices available, the most common is Quetelet's index—weight in kilograms divided by height in meters squared. Although body mass indices tend to be better predictors of obesity than height-weight tables or relative weight, they still do not distinguish between overweight resulting from obesity and that resulting from unusual muscular development.

9. The distribution of body fat may be as important a consideration as total quantity of fat. Body fat distribution can be classified into two types: upper body (android, or male, type) and lower body (gynoid, or female, type). Android obesity is associated with increased risk of insulin resistance, hyperinsulinemia, impaired glucose tolerance (prediabetes), type 2 diabetes mellitus, hypertension, hyperlipidemia, stroke, and death. The waist-to-hip ratio and waist circumference are valuable indices of regional body fat distribution.

10. Body composition analysis can provide estimates of the body's reserves of fat, protein, water, and several minerals. The two-compartment model divides the body into fat and fat-free masses. The four-compartment model views the human body as composed of four chemical groups: water, protein, mineral, and fat. Most approaches to determining body composition are indirect measures.

11. Measurement of skinfolds is the most widely used method of indirectly estimating percent body fat. What is actually measured is the thickness of a double fold of skin and compressed subcutaneous adipose tissue.

12. Skinfold measures have several advantages. The equipment is inexpensive and portable. Measurements can be easily and quickly obtained, and they correlate well with body density measurements. Proper measurement of skinfolds requires careful site selection and strict adherence to the standardized techniques outlined in this chapter.

13. The triceps is the most commonly used single skinfold site. Single-site skinfold measurements must be interpreted with caution. Results should be compared with reference data derived from large population surveys, such as NHANES.

14. For assessing body composition of young people, the sum of two sites (triceps and subscapular or triceps and medial calf) often is used. These sites correlate with other measures of body fatness and are more reliably and objectively measured than most other sites, and reference data are available.

15. Regression equations allow body density and percent body fat to be estimated from multiple skinfold measures. These equations were developed by seeing which combination of anthropometric measures best predict body density. Generalized equations can be applied to groups varying greatly in age and body fatness and can replace several population-specific equations with little loss in prediction accuracy.

16. Densitometry involves measuring the density of the entire body, usually by hydrostatic (underwater) weighing. If mass and volume of the body are known, its density can be calculated. However, hydrostatic weighing is not practical for testing large groups. It requires considerable subject cooperation, special equipment, experience, and financial investment.

17. Air displacement plethysmography involves using a specially designed two-chambered unit for measuring the body's volume, which is then used to calculate body density and composition. Subjects better tolerate this method than underwater weighing. It requires less subject cooperation, and residual lung volume measurements are not needed. It appears as accurate and precise as underwater weighing, but the equipment is considerably more complex and costly.

18. The marked difference in electrolyte content between fat and fat-free tissues is a basic principle behind body composition estimates from bioelectrical impedance analysis (BIA) and total body electrical conductivity (TOBEC). In BIA, the body's resistance to a minute electrical current is used to calculate total body water, from which the percentages of body fat and fat-free mass are calculated using various formulas.

19. Body composition estimates derived from dual-energy X-ray absorptiometry (DXA) compare favorably with those from underwater weighing. DXA has the advantage of requiring little subject cooperation, being relatively quick, and having a low radiation dose.

REFERENCES

1. Fryar CD, Gu Q, Ogden CL, Flegal KM. 2016. Anthropometric reference data for children and adults: United States, 2011–2014. National Center for Health Statistics. *Vital Health Statistics* 3(39).

2. National Health and Nutrition Examination Survey (NHANES). 2016. *Anthropometry Procedures Manual.* http://www.cdc.gov/nchs/nhanes/nhanes2015-2016/manuals15_16.htm.

3. Fryar CD, Gu Q, Ogden CL. 2012. Anthropometric reference data for children and adults: United States, 2007–2010. National Center for Health Statistics. *Vital Health Statistics* 11(252).

4. Lohman TG, Roche AF, Martorell R, eds. 1988. *Anthropometric standardization reference manual.* Champaign, IL: Human Kinetics Books.

5. Madden AM, Smith S. 2016. Body composition and morphological assessment of nutritional status in adults: A review of anthropometric variables. *Journal of Human Nutrition and Dietetics* 29:7–25.

6. Chumlea WC, Roche AF, Steinbaugh ML. 1985. Estimating stature from knee height for persons 60 to 90 years of age. *Journal of the American Geriatrics Society* 33:116–120.

7. Gordon CC, Chumlea WC, Roche AF. 1988. Stature, recumbent length, and weight. In Lohman TG, Roche AF, Martorell R (eds.), *Anthropometric standardization reference manual.* Champaign, IL: Human Kinetics Books.

8. Kuczmarski RJ, Ogden CL, Guo SS, et al. 2002. *2000 CDC growth charts for the United States: Methods and development.* National Center for Health Statistics. Vital and Health Statistics, Series 11, Number 246.

9. Centers for Disease Control and Prevention. 2010. Use of World Health Organization and CDC growth charts for children aged 0–59 months in the United States.

Morbidity and Mortality Weekly Report 59(No. RR-9):1–15.

10. Parsons HG, George MA, Innis SM. 2011. Growth assessment in clinical practice: Whose growth curve? *Current Gastroenterology Reports* 13:286–292.

11. Mei Z, Grummer-Strawn LM. 2011. Comparison of changes in growth percentiles of US children on CDC 2000 growth charts with corresponding changes on WHO 2006 growth charts. *Clinical Pediatrics* 50:402–407.

12. Ogden CL, Flegel KM. 2010. Changes in terminology for childhood overweight and obesity. National Health Statistics Reports No. 25, National Center for Health Statistics, U.S. Centers for Disease Control and Prevention, U.S. Department of Health and Human Services.

13. Krebs NS, Himes JH, Jacobson D, Nicklas TA, Guilday P. 2007. Assessment of child and adolescent overweight and obesity. *Pediatrics* 120(suppl 4):S193–S228.

14. Barlow SE. 2007. Expert committee recommendations regarding the prevention, assessment, and treatment of child and adolescent overweight and obesity: Summary report. *Pediatrics* 120(suppl 4):S164–S192.

15. Food and Nutrition Board, National Research Council. 1989. *Diet and health: Implications for reducing chronic disease risk.* Washington, DC: National Academies Press.

16. Prospective Studies Collaboration. 2009. Body-mass index and cause-specific mortality in 900,000 adults: Collaborative analyses of 57 prospective studies. *Lancet* 373:1083–1096.

17. Manson JE, Skerrett PJ, Greenland P, VanItallie TB. 2004. The escalating pandemics of obesity and sedentary lifestyle: A call to action for clinicians. *Archives of Internal Medicine* 164:249–258.

18. Weinstein AR, Sesso HD, Lee IM, Cook NR, Manson JE, Buring JE, Gaziano JM. 2004. Relationship of physical activity vs. body mass index with type 2 diabetes in women. *Journal of the American Medical Association* 292:1188–1194.

19. Jensen MD, Rya DH, Apovian CM, et al. 2014. 2013 AHA/ACC/TOS guideline for the management of overweight and obesity in adults: A report of the American College of Cardiology/American Heart Association Task Force on Practice Guidelines and The Obesity Society. *Circulation* 129(25 Suppl 2):S102–S138.

20. May AL, Kuklina EV, Yoon PW. 2012. Prevalence of cardiovascular disease risk factors among US adolescents, 1999–2008. *Pediatrics* 129:1035–1041.

21. Weigley ES. 1984. Average? Ideal? Desirable? A brief overview of height-weight tables in the United States. *Journal of the American Dietetic Association* 84:417–423.

22. Manson JE, Stampfer MJ, Hennekens CH, Willett WC. 1987. Body weight and longevity: A reassessment. *Journal of the American Medical Association* 257:353–358.

23. Ideal weights for women. 1942. *Statistical Bulletin of the Metropolitan Life Insurance Company* 23(October):6–8.

24. Ideal weights for men. 1943. *Statistical Bulletin of the Metropolitan Life Insurance Company* 24(June):6–8.

25. New weight standards for men and women. 1959. *Statistical Bulletin of the Metropolitan Life Insurance Company* 40(November–December):1–3.

26. Metropolitan height and weight tables. 1983. *Statistical Bulletin of the Metropolitan Life Insurance Company* 64(January–June):2.

27. Nieman DC. 2011. *Exercise testing and prescription: A health-related approach,* 7th ed. Boston: McGraw-Hill.

28. Pirie P, Jacobs D, Jeffery R, Hannan P. 1981. Distortion in self-reported height and weight data. *Journal of the American Dietetic Association* 78:601–606.

29. Rowland ML. 1991. Self-reported weight and height. *American Journal of Clinical Nutrition* 52:1125–1133.

30. Schlichting PF, Hoilund-Carlsen PF, Quaade F, Lauritzen SL. 1981. Comparison of self-reported height and weight with controlled height and weight in women and men. *International Journal of Obesity* 5:67–76.

31. DelPrete LR, Caldwell M, English C, Banspach SW, Lefebvre C. 1992. Self-reported and measured weights and heights of participants in community-based weight loss programs. *Journal of the American Dietetic Association* 92:1483–1486.

32. Willett WC, Stampfer M, Manson J, VanItallie T. 1991. New weight guidelines for Americans: Justified or injudicious? *American Journal of Clinical Nutrition* 53:1102–1103.

33. Frisancho AR. 1990. *Anthropometric standards for the assessment of growth and nutritional status.* Ann Arbor: University of Michigan Press.

34. Novascone MA, Smith EP. 1989. Frame size estimation: A comparative analysis of methods based on height, wrist circumference, and elbow breadth. *Journal of the American Dietetic Association* 89:964–966.

35. Wilmore JH, Frisancho RA, Gordon CC, Himes JH, Martin AD, Martorell R, Seefeldt VD. 1988. Body breadth equipment and measurement techniques. In Lohman TG, Roche AF, Martorell R, eds. *Anthropometric standardization reference manual.* Champaign, IL: Human Kinetics Books.

36. Katch VL, Freedson PS. 1982. Body size and shape: Derivation of the HAT frame size model. *American Journal of Clinical Nutrition* 36:669–675.

37. Katch VL, Freedson PS, Katch FI, Smith L. 1982. Body frame size: Validity of self-appraisal. *American Journal of Clinical Nutrition* 36:676–679.

38. Grant JP, Custer PB, Thurlow J. 1981. Current techniques of nutritional assessment. *Surgical Clinics of North America* 61:437–463.

39. Garn SM, Pesick SD, Hawthorne VM. 1983. The bony chest breadth as a frame size standard in nutritional assessment. *American Journal of Clinical Nutrition* 37:315–318.

40. Baecke JAH, Burema J, Deurenberg P. 1982. Body fatness, relative weight and frame size in young adults. *British Journal of Nutrition* 48:1–6.

41. Frisancho AR, Flegel PN. 1983. Elbow breadth as a measure of frame size for U.S. males and females. *American Journal of Clinical Nutrition* 37:311–314.

42. Garrow JS. 1983. Indices of adiposity. *Nutrition Abstracts and Reviews* 53:697–708.

43. Callaway CW, Chumlea WC, Bouchard C, Himes JH, Lohman GT, Martin AD, Mitchell CD, Mueller WH, Roche AF, Seefeldt VD. 1988. Circumferences. In Lohman TG, Roche AF, Martorell R, eds. *Anthropometric standardization reference manual.* Champaign, IL: Human Kinetics Books.

44. Lee J, Kolonel LN, Hinds MW. 1981. Relative merits of the weight-corrected-for-height indices. *American Journal of Clinical Nutrition* 34:2521–2529.

45. Lee J, Kolonel LN, Hinds MW. 1982. Relative merits of old and new indices of body mass: A commentary. *American Journal of Clinical Nutrition* 36:727–728.

46. Lee J, Kolonel LN. 1983. Body mass indices: A further commentary. *American Journal of Clinical Nutrition* 38:660–661.

47. Garrow JS, Webster J. 1985. Quetelet's index (W/H^2) as a measure of fatness. *International Journal of Obesity* 9:147–153.

48. Willett WC, Dietz WH, Colditz GA. 1999. Guidelines for healthy weight. *New England Journal of Medicine* 341:427–434.

49. Barlow SE, Dietz WH. 1998. Obesity evaluation and treatment: Expert committee recommendations. *Pediatrics* 102(3). http://www.pediatrics.org/cgi/content/full/102/3/e29.

50. Flegal KM. 1999. The obesity epidemic in children and adults: Current evidence and research issues. *Medicine and Science in Sports and Exercise* 31(suppl):S509–S514.

51. Smalley KJ, Knerr AN, Kendrick ZV, Colliver JA, Owen OE. 1990. Reassessment of body mass indices. *American Journal of Clinical Nutrition* 52:405–408.

52. Dietz WH, Robinson TN. 1998. Uses of the body mass index as a measure of overweight in children and adolescents. *Journal of Pediatrics* 132:191–193.

53. Killeen J, Vanderburg D, Harlan W. 1978. Application of weight-height ratios and body mass indices to juvenile populations—The National Health Examination Survey data. *Journal of Chronic Diseases* 31:529–537.

54. Dietz WH, Bellizzi MC. 1999. Introduction: The use of body mass index to assess obesity in children. *American Journal of Clinical Nutrition* 70(suppl):S123–S125.

55. Bellizzi MC, Dietz WC. 1999. Workshop on childhood obesity: Summary of the discussion. *American Journal of Clinical Nutrition* 70(suppl):S173–S175.

56. Roche AF, Siervogel RM, Chumlea WC, Webb P. 1981. Grading body fatness from limited anthropometric data. *American Journal of Clinical Nutrition* 34:2831–2838.

57. Keys A, Fidanza F, Karvonen MJ, Kimura N, Taylor HL. 1972. Indices of relative weight and obesity. *Journal of Chronic Diseases* 25:329–343.

58. Norgan NG, Ferro-Luzzi A. 1982. Weight-height indices as estimators of fatness in men. *Human Nutrition: Clinical Nutrition* 36C:363–372.

59. Frisancho AR, Flegel PN. 1982. Relative merits of old and new indices of body mass with reference to skinfold thickness. *American Journal of Clinical Nutrition* 36:697–699.

60. National Institutes of Health. 1998. *Clinical guidelines on the identification, evaluation, and treatment of overweight and obesity in adults.* National Heart, Lung, and Blood Institute. NIH publication number 98-4083.

61. U.S. Department of Health and Human Services and U.S. Department of Agriculture. 2010. *Dietary guidelines for Americans, 2010.* Washington, DC: U.S. Government Printing Office. www.dietaryguidelines.gov.

62. Kahn HS. 1991. A major error in nomograms for estimating body mass index. *American Journal of Clinical Nutrition* 54:435–437.

63. Giovannucci E, Colditz GA, Stampfer MJ, Willett WC. 1996. Physical activity, obesity, and risk of colorectal adenoma in women (United States). *Cancer Causes and Control* 7:253–263.

64. Troiano RP, Flegal KM. 1999. Overweight prevalence among youth in the United States: Why so many different numbers? *International Journal of Obesity* 23(suppl 2):S22–S27.

65. Wang Y, Rimm EB, Stampfer MJ, Willett WC, Hu FB. 2005. Comparison of abdominal adiposity and overall obesity in predicting risk of type 2 diabetes among men. *American Journal of Clinical Nutrition* 81:555–563.

66. Bray GA, Champagne CM. 2004. Obesity and the metabolic syndrome: Implications for dietetics practitioners. *Journal of the American Dietetic Association* 104:86–89.

67. Kaye SA, Folsom AR, Prineas RJ, Potter JD, Gapstur SM. 1990. The association of body fat distribution with lifestyle and reproductive factors in a population study of postmenopausal women. *International Journal of Obesity* 14:583–591.

68. Troisi RJ, Weiss ST, Segal MR, Cassano PA, Vokonas PS, Landsberg L. 1990. The relationship of body fat distribution to blood pressure in normotensive men: The normative aging study. *International Journal of Obesity* 14:515–525.

69. Zwiauer K, Widhalm K, Kerbl B. 1990. Relationship between body fat distribution and blood lipids in obese adolescents. *International Journal of Obesity* 14:271–277.

70. National Institutes of Health. 2000. *The practical guide; identification, evaluation, and treatment of overweight and obesity in adults.* National Heart, Lung, and Blood Institute. NIH publication number 00-4084.

71. Rankinen T, Kim SY, Perusse L, Despres JP, Bouchard C. 1999. The prediction of abdominal visceral fat level from body composition and anthropometry: ROC analysis. *International Journal of Obesity and Related Metabolic Research* 23:801–809.

72. Turcato E, Bosello O, Francesco VD, Harris TB, Zoico E, et al. 2000. Waist circumference and abdominal sagittal diameter as surrogates of body fat distribution in the elderly: Their relation with cardiovascular risk factors. *International Journal of Obesity and Related Metabolic Research* 24:1005–1010.

73. Clasey JL, Bouchard C, Teates CD, Riblett JE, Thorner MO, et al. 1999. The use of anthropometric and dual-energy x-ray absorptiometry (DXA) measures to estimate total abdominal and abdominal visceral fat in men and women. *Obesity Research* 7:256–264.

74. Must A, Strauss RS. 1999. Risk and consequences of childhood and adolescent obesity. *International Journal of Obesity and Related Metabolic Disorders* 23(suppl 2): S2–S11.

75. Flegal KM. 1999. The obesity epidemic in children and adults: Current evidence and research issues. *Medicine and Science in Sports and Exercise* 31(suppl):S509–S514.

76. Colditz GA. 1999. Economic costs of obesity and overweight. *Medicine and Science in Sports and Exercise* 31(suppl):S663–S667.

77. OECD. 2014. *OECD health statistics 2014*, forthcoming, www.oecd.org/health/healthdata.

78. Chandra RK. 1981. Immunodeficiency in undernutrition and overnutrition. *Nutrition Reviews* 39:225–231.

79. Chandra RK. 1991. 1990 McCollum Award lecture. Nutrition and immunity: Lessons from the past and new insights into the future. *American Journal of Clinical Nutrition* 53:1087–1101.

80. Bistrian BR, Blackburn GL, Hallowel E, Heddle R. 1974. Protein status of general surgical patients. *Journal of the American Medical Association* 230:858–860.

81. Bistrian BR, Blackburn GL, Vitale J, Cochran D, Naylor J. 1976. Prevalence of malnutrition in general medical patients. *Journal of the American Medical Association* 235:1567–1570.

82. Coats KG, Morgan SL, Bartolucci AA, Weinsier RL. 1993. Hospital-associated malnutrition: A reevaluation 12 years later. *Journal of the American Dietetic Association* 93:27–33.

83. Lukaski HC. 1987. Methods for the assessment of human body composition: Traditional and new. *American Journal of Clinical Nutrition* 46:537–556.

84. Wang J, Thornton JC, Kolesnik S, Pierson RN. 2000. Anthropometry in body composition. An overview. *Annals of the New York Academy of Sciences* 904:317–326.

85. Keys A, Brozek J. 1953. Body fat in adult man. *Physiological Reviews* 33:245–325.

86. Wilmore JH, Buskirk ER, DiGirolamo M, Lohman TG. 1986. Body composition: A round table. *Physician and Sportsmedicine* 14:144–162.

87. Clarys JP, Martin AD, Drinkwater DT, Marfell-Jones MJ. 1987. The skinfold: Myth and reality. *Journal of Sports Sciences* 5:3–33.

88. Martin AD, Ross WD, Drinkwater DT, Clarys JP. 1985. Prediction of body fat by skinfold caliper: Assumptions and cadaver evidence. *International Journal of Obesity* 9:31–39.

89. Harrison GG, Buskirk EB, Carter JEL, Johnston JE, Lohman TG, Pollock ML, Roche AF, Wilmore J. 1988. Skinfold thicknesses and measurement technique. In Lohman TG, Roche AF, Martorell R (eds.), *Anthropometric standardization reference manual.* Champaign, IL: Human Kinetics Books.

90. Himes JH, Roche AF, Siervogel RM. 1979. Compressibility of skinfolds and the measurement of subcutaneous fatness. *American Journal of Clinical Nutrition* 32:1734–1740.

91. Siervogel RM, Roche AF, Himes JH, Chumlea WC, McCammon R. 1982. Subcutaneous fat distribution

in males and females from 1 to 39 years of age. *American Journal of Clinical Nutrition* 36:162–171.

92. Lohman TG. 1981. Skinfolds and body density and their relation of body fatness: A review. *Human Biology* 53:181–225.

93. Lohman TG. 1988. Anthropometry and body composition. In Lohman TG, Roche AF, Martorell R (eds.), *Anthropometric standardization reference manual*. Champaign, IL: Human Kinetics Books.

94. Jackson AS, Pollock ML. 1985. Practical assessment of body composition. *Physician and Sportsmedicine* 13(5):76–90.

95. Martorell R, Mendoza F, Mueller WH, Pawson IG. 1988. Which side to measure: Right or left? In Lohman TG, Roche AF, Martorell R (eds.), *Anthropometric standardization reference manual*. Champaign, IL: Human Kinetics Books.

96. Leger LA, Lambert J, Martin P. 1982. Validity of plastic skinfold caliper measurements. *Human Biology* 54:667–675.

97. Burgert SL, Anderson CF. 1979. A comparison of triceps skinfold values as measured by the plastic McGaw caliper and Lange caliper. *American Journal of Clinical Nutrition* 32:1531–1533.

98. Cui Z, Truesdale KP, Cai J, Stevens J. 2014. Evaluation of anthropometric equations to assess body fat in adults: NHANES 1999–2004. *Medicine and Science in Sports and Exercise* 46:1147–1158.

99. Stevens J, Ou F-S, Cai J, Heymsfield SB, Truesdale KP. 2016. Prediction of percent body fat measurements in Americans 8 years and older. *International Journal of Obesity* 40:587–594.

100. National Health and Nutrition Examination Survey. NHANES Anthropometry and Physical Activity Monitor Procedures Manual. https://www.cdc.gov/nchs/data/nhanes/nhanes_05_06/BM.pdf.

101. Jackson AS, Pollock ML, Ward A. 1980. Generalized equations for predicting body density of women. *Medicine and Science in Sports and Exercise* 12:175–182.

102. Stevens J, Cai J, Truesdale KP, Cuttler L, Robinson TN, Roberts AL. 2013. Percent body fat prediction equations for 8- to 17-year-old American children. *Pediatric Obesity* 9:260–271.

103. Taylor RW, Jones IE, Williams SM, Goulding A. 2002. Body fat percentages measured by dual-energy X-ray absorptiometry corresponding to recently recommended body mass index cutoffs for overweight and obesity in children and adolescents aged 3–18 y. *American Journal of Clinical Nutrition* 76:1416–1421.

104. Brozek J, Keys A. 1951. The evaluation of leanness-fatness in man: Norms and intercorrelations. *British Journal of Nutrition* 5:194–205.

105. Heo M, Faith MS, Pietrobelli A, Heymsfield SB. 2012. Percentage of body fat cutoffs by sex, age, and race-ethnicity in the US adult population from NHANES 1999–2004. *American Journal of Clinical Nutrition* 95:594–602.

106. Ogden CL, Li Y, Freedman DS, Borrud LG, Flegal KM. 2011. Smoothed percentage body fat percentiles for U.S. children and adolescents, 1999–2004. *National Health Statistics Report* (43):1–7.

107. Borrud LG, Flegal KM, Looker AC, Everhart JE, et al. 2010. Body composition data for individuals 8 years of age and older: U.S. population, 1999–2004. National Center for Health Statistics. *Vital and Health Statistics* 11(250).

108. Katch F, Michael ED, Horvath SM. 1967. Estimation of body volume by underwater weighing: Description of a simple method. *Journal of Applied Physiology* 23:811–813.

109. Akers R, Buskirk ER. 1969. An underwater weighing system utilizing "force cube" transducers. *Journal of Applied Physiology* 26:649–652.

110. Wilmore JH. 1969. A simplified method for determination of residual volumes. *Journal of Applied Physiology* 27:96–100.

111. Goldman HI, Becklake MR. 1959. Respiratory function tests: Normal values at median altitudes and the prediction of normal results. *American Review of Tuberculosis and Pulmonary Diseases* 79:457–467.

112. Ellis KJ. 2000. Human body composition: In vivo methods. *Physiological Reviews* 80:649–680.

113. Wagner DR, Heyward VH. 1999. Techniques of body composition assessment: A review of laboratory and field methods. *Research Quarterly for Exercise and Sport* 70:135–149.

114. Dempster P, Aitkens S. 1995. A new air displacement method for the determination of human body composition. *Medicine and Science in Sports and Exercise* 27:1692–1697.

115. Fields DA, Gunatilake R, Kalaitzoglou E. 2015. Air displacement plethysmography: Cradle to grave. *Nutrition in Clinical Practice* 30:219–226.

116. Wingfield HL, Smith-Ryan AE, Woessner MN, Melvin MN, Fultz SN, Graff RM. 2014. Body composition assessment in overweight women: Validation of air displacement plethysmography. *Clinical Physiology and Function Imaging* 34:72–76.

117. Fields DA, Goran MJ, McCrory MA. 2002. Body-composition assessment via air-displacement plethysmography in adults and children: A review. *American Journal of Clinical Nutrition* 75:453–467.

118. Radley D, Gately PJ, Cooke CB, Carroll S, Oldroyd B, Truscott JG. 2005. Percentage fat in overweight and obese children: Comparison of DXA and air displacement plethysmography. *Obesity Research* 13:75–85.

119. Demerath EW, Guo SS, Chumlea WC, Towne B, Roche AF, Siervogel RM. 2002. Comparison

of percent body fat estimates using air displacement plethysmography and hydrodensitometry in adults and children. *International Journal of Obesity and Related Metabolic Disorders* 26:389–397.

120. Fields DA, Hunter GR, Goran MI. 2000. Validation of the Bod Pod with hydrostatic weighing: Influence of body clothing. *International Journal of Obesity* 24:200–205.

121. Collins MA, Millard-Stafford ML, Sparling PB, Snow TK, Rosskopf LB, Webb SA, Omar J. 1999. Evaluation of the Bod Pod for assessing body fat in collegiate football players. *Medicine and Science in Sports and Exercise* 31:1350–1356.

122. Dewit O, Fuller NJ, Fewtrell MS, Wells JCK. 2000. Whole body air displacement plethysmography compared with hydrodensitometry for body composition analysis. *Archives of Disease in Childhood* 82:159–164.

123. Biaggi RR, Vollman MW, Nies MA, Brener CE, Flakoll PJ, et al. 1999. Comparison of air-displacement plethysmography with hydrostatic weighing and bioelectrical impedance analysis for the assessment of body composition in healthy adults. *American Journal of Clinical Nutrition* 69:898–903.

124. Nunez C, Kovera AJ, Pietrobelli A, Heshka S, Horlick M, Kehayias JJ, et al. 1999. Body composition in children and adults by air displacement plethysmography. *European Journal of Clinical Nutrition* 53:382–387.

125. Fosbøl MØ, Zerahn B. 2015. Contemporary methods of body composition measurement. *Clinical Physiology and Functional Imaging* 35:81–97.

126. Kuczmarski RJ. 1996. Bioelectrical impedance analysis measurements as part of a national nutrition survey. *American Journal of Clinical Nutrition* 64(3 Suppl):453S–458S.

127. Kuchnia AJ, Teigen LM, Cole AJ, Mulasi U, Gonzalez MC, Heymsfield SB, Vock DM, Earthman CP. Phase angle and impedance ratio: Reference cut-points from the United States National Health and Nutrition Examination Survey 1999–2004 from bioimpedance spectroscopy data. *JPEN Journal of Parenteral and Enteral Nutrition* (in press) pii: 0148607116670378.

128. Mulasi U, Kuchnia AJ, Cole AJ, Earthman CP. 2015. Bioimpedance at the bedside: Current applications, limitations, and opportunities. *Nutrition in Clinical Practice* 30:180–193.

129. Jaffrin MY. Body composition determination by bioimpedance: An update. 2009. *Current Opinion in Clinical Nutrition and Metabolic Care* 12:482–486.

130. Dehghan M, Merchant AT. 2008. Is bioelectrical impedance accurate for use in large epidemiological studies? *Nutrition Journal* 7:26.

131. Bosy-Westphal A, Schautz B, Later W, Kehayias JJ, Gallagher D. 2013. What makes a BIA equation unique? Validity of eight-electrode multifrequency BIA to estimate body composition in a healthy adult population. *European Journal of Clinical Nutrition* 67:14–21

132. Medici G, Mussi C, Fantuzzi AL, Malavolti M, Albertazzi A, Bedogni G. 2005. Accuracy of eight-polar bioelectrical impedance analysis for the assessment of total and appendicular body composition in peritoneal dialysis patients. *European Journal of Clinical Nutrition* 59:932–937.

133. Kriemler S, Puder J, Zahner L, Roth R, Braun-Fahrländer C, Bedogni G. 2009. Cross-validation of bioelectrical impedance analysis for the assessment of body composition in a representative sample of 6- to 13-year-old children. *European Journal of Clinical Nutrition* 63:619–626.

134. Seabolt LA, Welch EB, Silver HJ. 2015. Imaging methods for analyzing body composition in human obesity and cardiometabolic disease. *Annals of the New York Academy of Science* 1353:41–59.

135. Toombs RJ, Ducher G, Shepherd JA, De Souza MJ. 2012. The impact of recent technological advances on the trueness and precision of DXA to assess body composition. *Obesity (Silver Spring)* 20:30–39.

136. Shepherd JA, Baim S, Bilezikian JP, Schousboe JT. 2013. Executive summary of the 2013 International Society for Clinical Densitometry Position Development Conference on Body Composition. *Journal of Clinical Densitometry* 16:489–495.

137. Hangartner TN, Warner S, Braillon P, Jankowski L, Shepherd J. 2013. The official positions of the International Society for Clinical Densitometry: Acquisition of dual-energy X-ray absorptiometry body composition and considerations regarding analysis and repeatability of measures. *Journal of Clinical Densitometry* 16:520–536.

138. Shepherd JA, Sommer MJ, Fan B, Powers C, Stranix-Chibanda L, Zadzilka A, Basar M, George K, Mukwasi-Kahari C, Siberry G. (2017). Advanced analysis techniques improve infant bone and body composition measures by dual-energy X-ray absorptiometry. Journal of Pediatrics 181:248–253.

139. U.S. Department of Health and Human Services. 2004. *Bone health and osteoporosis: A report of the surgeon general*. Rockville, MD: U.S. Department of Health and Human Services, Office of the Surgeon General.

ASSESSMENT ACTIVITY 6.1

Assessment and Classification of Body Weight

Successful treatment of overweight begins with the assessment and classification of body weight. This assessment activity explains how to assess and classify body weight, waist circumference, and risk status using the approaches recommended by the U.S. National Institutes of Health in its publication *The Practical Guide; Identification, Evaluation, and Treatment of Overweight and Obesity in Adults.*[70] Although several accurate methods exist for measuring body fat, most of these methods are not readily available in the clinical setting. Body mass index (BMI) is recommended as the most practical approach for assessing body weight in the clinical setting and can be used as a surrogate method for assessing body fat content. Table 6.5 gave classifications of overweight and obesity, based on BMI (also see Figure 6.44). It should be noted that BMI overestimates body fat in very muscular persons and in patients with edema. It can underestimate body fat in persons who have lost muscle mass (such as the elderly). Waist circumference is recommended

as the most practical tool for assessing a person's abdominal fat content. The cutpoints for high-risk waist circumference were given in Table 6.6. BMI and waist circumference also can be used to monitor response to weight management treatment in persons whose BMI is < 35 kg/m^2.

Begin this assessment activity by accurately measuring your stature, body weight, and waist circumference and then calculating your body mass index (BMI), following the instructions in this chapter. Classify your BMI and waist circumference (high-risk or low-risk) using Tables 6.5 and 6.6; if applicable, classify your disease risk ("increased," "high," "very high," or "extremely high") using Table 6.5. Record your results in the following spaces:

Body weight:
_____ lb _____ kg (pounds ÷ 2.2 = kg)

Body stature:
_____ in. _____ m (inches × 0.0254 = m)

Waist circumference:
_____ in. _____ cm (inches × 2.54 = cm)

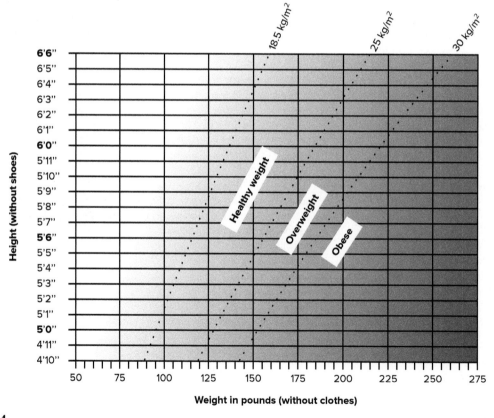

Figure 6.44
Using body mass index (BMI), body weight can be grouped into three categories. Healthy weight is defined as a BMI of 18.5 kg/m^2 up to 25 kg/m^2, overweight is a BMI of 25 kg/m^2 up to 30 kg/m^2, and obese is a BMI of 30 kg/m^2 or greater.

TABLE 6.12	Diseases and Risk Factors That Place Patients at Increased Risk for Mortality

Diseases Placing Patients at Very High Risk for Mortality

- Established coronary heart disease
- Atherosclerotic diseases other than coronary heart disease (e.g., peripheral arterial disease, abdominal aortic aneurysm, symptomatic carotid artery disease)
- Type 2 diabetes (fasting plasma glucose $\geq$ 126 mg/dL or 2-hour postprandial plasma glucose $\geq$ 200 mg/dL)
- Sleep apnea

Cardiovascular Disease Risk Factors

- Cigarette smoking
- Hypertension (systolic blood pressure $\geq$ 140 mm Hg or diastolic blood pressure $\geq$ 90 mm Hg) or current use of antihypertensive medication
- High-risk low-density lipoprotein cholesterol ($\geq$ 160 mg/dL) or borderline high-risk (130 to 159 mg/dL), along with two or more other risk factors
- Low high-density lipoprotein cholesterol (< 35 mg/dL)
- Impaired fasting glucose (between 110 and 125 mg/dL)
- Family history of premature coronary heart disease
- Age (if male, $\geq$ 45 years; if female, $\geq$ 55 years or postmenopausal)
- Physical inactivity

Body mass index:

_____ kg/m^2

BMI classification:

_____

Waist circumference classification:

_____

Disease risk classification:

_____

Elevated BMI, high-risk waist circumference, or both suggest the need for weight loss but do not indicate the required intensity of intervention. Patients who have certain obesity-related diseases (*comorbidities*) or who have cardiovascular disease risk factors (Table 6.12) are at a higher risk for mortality than those who do not have these diseases or risk factors. Consequently, patients need to be screened for these diseases and risk factors and, when present, placed on a program of intense risk-factor modification and weight management intervention.

ASSESSMENT ACTIVITY 6.2

Body Composition Evaluation Using Skinfold Measurements

This assessment activity gives you an opportunity to use skinfold measurements to estimate percent body fat and to evaluate body composition.

Step 1

Photocopy the "Skinfold Measurements" form in Figure 6.34. Using the information described in this chapter, have your instructor or a classmate measure the thickness of three of your skinfolds (chest, abdomen, and thigh for men; triceps, suprailiac, and thigh for women), and record the values on the "Skinfold Measurements" form.

Step 2

Total the values of the three skinfold measurements and enter this number on the appropriate line in the "Skinfold Measurements" form.

Step 3

Estimate percent body fat using the appropriate formula from Table 6.7 and the Siri equation. Enter this percentage on the appropriate line in the "Skinfold Measurements" form. Using Table 6.10, classify your percent body fat and write that classification on the appropriate line in the "Skinfold Measurements" form.

Step 4

Calculate your fat weight, lean body weight, and desired body weight, as indicated in the "Skinfold Measurements" form and the text.

ASSESSMENT ACTIVITY 6.3

The American Body Composition Calculator (ABCC)

As described in Box 6.4, The American Body Composition Calculator (ABCC) (http://uncbodycalc.sph.unc.edu/) uses sex, ethnicity, age, height, weight, skinfolds, circumferences, and lengths to determine body fat percent using newly developed equations from NHANES data. In this Assessment Activity, you will first make several measurements with the assistance of your instructor and classmate, and then enter the data at the ABCC website to calculate your percent body fat.

ENTER YOUR DATA HERE (closely adhere to measurement guidelines described in this chapter):

1. Age (years):   _____
2. Height in feet, inches: _____
3. Weight, lbs: _____
4. Triceps skinfold, mm: _____
5. Subscapular skinfold, mm: _____
6. Waist circumference, in: _____
7. % body fat from ABCC: _____
8. Classification of % body fat: _____ (use Table 6.10)

NOTE: you can add additional circumference and lengths to refine your percent body fat estimate.

ASSESSMENT OF THE HOSPITALIZED PATIENT

STUDENT LEARNING OUTCOMES

After studying this chapter, the student will be able to:

1. Identify characteristics for diagnosing malnutrition.

2. Describe the four components of comprehensive geriatric assessment.

3. Use the Mini Nutritional Assessment short form for assessing malnutrition.

4. Know how to conduct anthropometric measurements used in diagnosing malnutrition, including mid-upper arm circumference, mid-upper arm muscle circumference, mid-upper arm muscle area, calf circumference, and height estimates from ulna length, demispan, and knee height.

5. Compare and contrast the Harris-Benedict equations, the World Health Organization equations, and the equations used to calculate EER in terms of the variables they require, how they were developed, how they are applied, and their accuracy.

6. Differentiate between resting energy expenditure and basal metabolic rate.

7. Describe how various stresses (diseases or traumatic events) affect resting energy expenditure and energy requirement in humans.

8. Describe how various stresses (diseases or traumatic events) affect nitrogen excretion and protein requirement in humans.

INTRODUCTION

The Nutrition Care Process was described in Chapter 1. The four steps of the Nutrition Care Process include nutritional assessment, nutrition diagnosis, nutrition intervention, and nutritional monitoring and evaluation. This process applies to the nutrition care provided by the dietetic practitioner to all patients, clients, and groups, including the hospitalized patient. This chapter will not repeat the information provided in Chapter 1 on the Nutrition Care Process but, instead, will focus on the specific challenge of identifying and documenting adult malnutrition.

Malnutrition and undernutrition are experienced when there is a deficiency of energy (kilocalories), protein, or other nutrients, causing measurable and adverse effects on body composition, function, and health.[1-4] Although specific criteria for the identification of malnutrition differ between organizations, an unintentional weight loss of more than 10% in the past six months or more than 5% in the last month is often used.[4]

Malnutrition is common in hospitalized patients and has been linked to muscle wasting (sarcopenia), immune suppression and increased infections, prolonged length of hospital stay and higher treatment costs, a greater likelihood of hospital readmission, higher mortality rates, increased risk of pressure ulcers and impaired wound healing, anemia, lower quality of life and risk of social isolation, decreased mental health and cognition, and increased risk of falling and bone fractures[1-3] (Figure 7.1). A comprehensive review of published studies showed that malnutrition ranges from 13% to 78% among acute care patients.[1] This wide range is due to the type of patient studied, different methods of detecting malnutrition, and hospital resources. Malnutrition continues to be underdiagnosed in many hospitals, and approximately one-third of patients who are not malnourished on admission may become malnourished while hospitalized.[3]

Simple measures, such as documenting height and weight on admission and assessing patients' nutritional intake, weight status, and medications that alter nutritional intake, can assist in early detection of malnutrition in the acute care patient. Validated nutritional screening instruments have been designed to identify individuals who are malnourished or at risk of malnutrition, and these will be described and compared in this chapter.

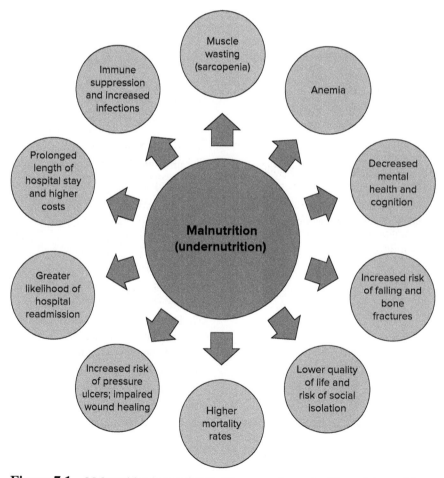

Figure 7.1   **Malnutrition is associated with many adverse health, social, mental, and financial outcomes.**

Unfortunately, survey data from hospital-based clinicians indicate that nutrition screening is conducted only half the time on admission, with only one-fourth using a validated nutrition assessment tool.[3] Reported barriers to completion of nutrition assessment are insufficient personnel, inadequate resources, and insufficient expertise.[3]

The goal in many hospitals and clinical care sites is the early detection of malnutrition with appropriate nutrition support and follow-up. Until 2016, nutrition screening had been mandated by the Joint Commission on Accreditation of Healthcare Organizations (JCAHO) for all hospital patients within 24 hours of admission. JCAHO now recommends that nutrition screening be a part of the clinical care process and that identification of components of the assessment should be defined by each organization.[3,4]

A comprehensive systematic review showed that nutritional interventions increase daily caloric and protein intake, leading to increased body weight.[2] Readmission rates decrease, with a trend for shorter length of hospital stay. Although researchers debate the overall clinical benefits, most studies support that nutrition intervention is an effective strategy for prevention of health care–acquired malnutrition and associated complications.[1–4]

ASSESSING MALNUTRITION

All hospitalized patients should be screened shortly after admission, with those at risk of malnutrition going through additional assessment and appropriate intervention. The average length of stay of hospitalized patients is 4.5 days, underscoring the need to move as rapidly as possible.[3] In addition, nutrition must be addressed early in discharge planning so that needs are met in the transition from hospital to home or alternate care setting.

Health-care organizations should take specific actions to address prevention or treatment of acute or chronic disease-related malnutrition in hospitalized patients to improve the quality of patient care, improve clinical outcomes, and reduce costs. The top three priority actions to take are as follows:[3]

1. **Each clinician on the interdisciplinary care team should participate in the execution of the nutrition care plan.** Clinicians should create an institutionalized culture in which everyone involved values clinical nutrition care. Nutrition support teams should include physicians, dietitians, nurses, and pharmacists.[3,5] The nurse is often the first health-care professional to assess the patient upon admission to the hospital and plays a vital role in the implementation of nutritional assessment and intervention.[5]
2. **Develop systems to quickly diagnose all malnourished patients and those at risk.** If malnutrition is present, it should be included as one of the patient's coded diagnoses.
3. **Develop nutrition care plans in a timely fashion and implement comprehensive nutrition interventions (optimally within 48 hours of identification of the malnourished patient).** Hospitals should support development of dedicated teams for protocol development and management of enteral or parenteral nutrition as appropriate to facilitate timely initiation of the prescribed nutrition support therapy.

The Academy of Nutrition and Dietetics (Academy) and the American Society for Parenteral and Enteral Nutrition (A.S.P.E.N.) recommend that a standardized set of diagnostic characteristics be used to identify and document adult malnutrition in routine clinical practice. The identification of two or more of the following six characteristics is recommended for diagnosing malnutrition, and it should be assessed on admission and at frequent intervals throughout the patient's stay in an acute, chronic, or transitional care setting:

1. Insufficient energy intake
2. Weight loss
3. Loss of muscle mass
4. Loss of subcutaneous fat
5. Localized or generalized fluid accumulation that may sometimes mask weight loss
6. Diminished functional status as measured by handgrip strength

COMPREHENSIVE GERIATRIC ASSESSMENT

The United States is experiencing considerable growth in its older population, according to the U.S. Census Bureau (www.census.gov). In 2050, the population aged 65 and over (i.e., the elderly) is projected to be 83.7 million, almost double its current level (Figure 7.2). The elderly will represent 21% of the 400 million individuals living in the year 2050. The number of people in the oldest-old age group, which refers to those aged 85 and over, is projected to grow to 18 million in 2050 (4.5% of the U.S. population).

Aging is accompanied by numerous physiologic changes that negatively impact nutritional status and increase the risk of malnutrition. These changes include a decreased sense of taste and smell; poor oral health and dental problems that make chewing difficult; inflammation; a monotonous, low-quality diet; and limited mobility due to osteoarthritis that affects the ability to shop for food and prepare meals. The elderly experience loss of muscle mass (sarcopenia), further limiting functional ability. Nutritional status is also impacted as the elderly experience profound psychosocial and environmental changes, such as isolation, loneliness, depression, and inadequate finances.[5,6] A systematic review of the scientific literature established these risk factors for malnutrition in the older

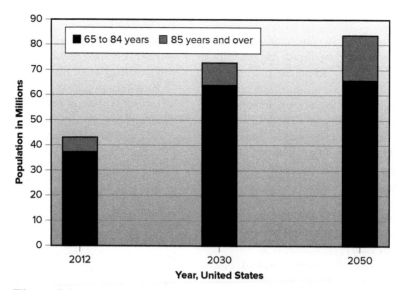

Figure 7.2   In 2050, the population aged 65 and over is projected to be 83.7 million, almost double its current level.

Source: Ortman JM, Velkoff VA, Hogan H. 2014. An aging nation: The older population in the United States. *Current Population Reports, P25-1140.* Washington, DC: U.S. Census Bureau.

population: frailty in institutionalized persons; excessive polypharmacy; general health decline, including physical function; Parkinson disease; constipation; poor or moderate self-reported health status; cognitive decline; dementia; eating dependences; loss of interest in life; poor appetite; basal oral dysphagia; signs of impaired efficacy of swallowing; and institutionalization.[6]

The net effect of these aging-related changes is progressive undernutrition, which often goes undiagnosed. Early detection of malnutrition is important, and it is an important component of comprehensive geriatric assessment (CGA). There are at least four components in CGA:

1. **Physical health:** Evaluate medication use, the risk for malnutrition, falling, incontinence, immobility, specific disease and conditions, and visual or hearing impairment.
2. **Mental health:** Assess dementia, depression, cognition, stress, and emotional status.
3. **Social and economic status:** Examine the social support network, competence of caregivers, quality of life, economic resources, and cultural, ethnic, and spiritual resources.
4. **Functional status:** Evaluate the physical environment and access to essential services, such as shopping, pharmacy, and transportation.

These four CGA components are discussed below, with a focus on commonly used assessment tools. The dietitian is not responsible for collecting all of the CGA data. Members of the nutrition support team, including physicians, dietitians, nurses, and pharmacists, work together to ensure that each elderly patient is assessed comprehensively, with the goal of providing appropriate nutrition support.

1. Physical health: Evaluate medication use, the risk for malnutrition, falling, incontinence, immobility, specific disease and conditions, and visual or hearing impairment.

The central issue raised by increasing longevity is that of net gain in active functional years versus total years of disability and dysfunction (www.healthypeople/gov). Aging adults experience a higher risk of chronic disease, with 60% of the elderly managing two or more chronic conditions. Falls are the leading cause of injury among older adults, and 3 in 10 experience moderate to severe functional limitations. Older individuals often complain of a decreased ability to taste and enjoy food as taste buds decrease in number and size. Visual function worsens gradually with age, and after age 80, less than 15% have normal vision. Gradual hearing loss affects about 66% of people reaching age 80. Up to 20% of elderly adults living at home and 75% of those in long-term care facilities cannot control the muscle that controls urination, a condition called urinary incontinence. Physical health information can be gleaned from the physical examination and medical history reports, with contributions from nurses, physicians, pharmacists, and dietitians.

Malnutrition can be assessed with several assessment tools, including the six-component Mini Nutritional Assessment Short Form (MNA-SF)® (http://www.mna-elderly.com) (see Figure 7.3 and Table 7.1 for a comparison of different methods). The MNA-SF is quick (less than five minutes) and easy to administer with six questions, including an option to substitute calf circumference when BMI is not available. The MNA incorporates three

TABLE 7.1	Identification and Documentation of Adult Malnutrition (Undernutrition)				
Malnutrition Indicator	Mini Nutritional Assessment (MNA-SF)	Subjective Global Assessment (SGA)	Nutritional Risk Screening (NRS 2002)	Malnutrition Universal Screening Tool (MUST)	Simplified Nutritional Appetite Questionnaire (SNAQ) 65+
Insufficient energy intake	Has food intake declined over past 3 months	Change in dietary intake	Reduced dietary intake in last week		Poor appetite past week
Weight loss	Weight loss during last 3 months (> 3 kg = malnourished)	Weight change in past 2 weeks and 6 months	Weight loss during last 3 months	% unplanned weight loss past 3–6 months	Unintentional weight loss of ≥ 4 kg past 6 months
Body mass index (from height and weight)	< 19 kg/m^2* (malnourished)		< 20.5 kg/m^2 (malnourished)	< 18.5 kg/m^2** (malnourished)***	
Loss of muscle mass	Calf circumference in cm	Muscle wasting (temple, clavicle, shoulder, ribs, quadriceps, calf, knee, hand)			Mid-upper arm circumference (MUAC) < 25 cm
Loss of subcutaneous fat		Fat under eyes, triceps, biceps			
Fluid accumulation		Edema and ascites (fluid in peritoneal cavity)			
Gastrointestinal symptoms; illness		Frequency and duration of nausea, vomiting, diarrhea, anorexia	Severe illness or in intensive therapy	Acute illness, > 5 d no nutritional intake	
Diminished functional capacity	Mobility (bed or chair bound)	Dysfunction, difficulty ambulation and normal activities; bed/chair ridden			Poor functioning; ability to walk up and down a staircase of 15 steps without resting
Psychological stress	Stress or acute disease in past 3 months				
Neuro-psychological problems	Dementia or depression				

*If BMI not available, measure calf circumference in cm (less than 31 cm is malnourished).

**Estimate BMI category from mid-upper arm circumference (MUAC). If MUAC < 23.5 cm, BMI likely to be < 20 kg/m^2; if > 32.0 cm, BMI likely to be > 30 kg/m^2.

***Use height estimate from ulna length if height cannot be obtained (length from olecranon process to styloid process on wrist, left side while arm is bent and placed across the chest with the fingers pointing to the opposite shoulder). Use these equations:

Men: Predicted height (cm) = 79.2 + [3.60 · ulna length (cm)]; Women: Predicted height (cm) = 95.6 + [2.77 · ulna length (cm)]

Sources: MNA-SF: http://www.mna-elderly.com/; SGA: http://subjectiveglobalassessment.com/; NRS 2002: http://espen.info/documents/screening.pdf; MUST: http://www.bapen.org.uk/screening-and-must/must-calculator; SNAQ: http://www.fightmalnutrition.eu/fight-malnutrition/screening-tools/snaq-tools-in-english/.

cut-off points for nutritional status (Figure 7.3). The six components of the MNA-SF are weight loss, appetite, mobility, psychological stress, neuro-psychological problems, and BMI. All components are scored from 0 to 2 or 3, with a total score of 0–4, thus classifying patients into three nutritional groups: well-nourished, at risk of malnutrition, and malnourished if scores of 12–14, 8–11, and 0–7 points, respectively, are tallied. Multiple studies show that the MNA-SF is highly sensitive in identifying malnourished patients.[7–12] The original MNA was developed in the 1990s and had 18 items, but the current version consists of 6 questions to streamline the screen process and has 99% diagnostic accuracy for predicting undernutrition (www.mna-elderly.com). The MNA-SF is the most widely used and investigated screening tool for malnutrition and undernutrition.

If height cannot be measured with a stadiometer, MNA-SF guidelines recommend estimating height using the half arm-span, demispan, or knee height. The half arm-span is the distance from the midline at the sternal notch to the tip of the middle finger while the nondominant arm is stretched out in a horizontal position

Mini Nutritional Assessment MNA®

Last name:			First name:	
Sex:	Age:	Weight, kg:	Height, cm:	Date:

Complete the screen by filling in the boxes with the appropriate numbers. Total the numbers for the final screening score.

Screening

A Has food intake declined over the past 3 months due to loss of appetite, digestive problems, chewing or swallowing difficulties?
0 = severe decrease in food intake
1 = moderate decrease in food intake
2 = no decrease in food intake   ◯

B Weight loss during the last 3 months
0 = weight loss greater than 3 kg (6.6 lbs)
1 = does not know
2 = weight loss between 1 and 3 kg (2.2 and 6.6 lbs)
3 = no weight loss   ◯

C Mobility
0 = bed or chair bound
1 = able to get out of bed / chair but does not go out
2 = goes out   ◯

D Has suffered psychological stress or acute disease in the past 3 months?
0 = yes   2 = no   ◯

E Neuropsychological problems
0 = severe dementia or depression
1 = mild dementia
2 = no psychological problems   ◯

F1 Body Mass Index (BMI) (weight in kg) / (height in m)^2
0 = BMI less than 19
1 = BMI 19 to less than 21
2 = BMI 21 to less than 23
3 = BMI 23 or greater   ◯

IF BMI IS NOT AVAILABLE, REPLACE QUESTION F1 WITH QUESTION F2.
DO NOT ANSWER QUESTION F2 IF QUESTION F1 IS ALREADY COMPLETED.

F2 Calf circumference (CC) in cm
0 = CC less than 31
3 = CC 31 or greater   ◯

Screening score   ◯ ◯
(max. 14 points)

12–14 points: ◯   Normal nutritional status | Save |
8–11 points: ◯   At risk of malnutrition | Print |
0–7 points: ◯   Malnourished | Reset |

Figure 7.3   The six-component Mini Nutritional Assessment short form (MNA-SF).

(Figure 7.4). Height is then simply calculated by doubling the half arm-span measurement. Particular care should be made to ensure the arm is kept in line with the shoulder and the patient is able to stretch it out straight. The measurement should be made to the nearest 0.1 cm, and at least two measurements should be taken until they are within 0.5 cm of each other. Patients with contractions or deformities of the shoulder, elbow, or wrist joints should be excluded. Demispan is the distance from the midline at the sternal notch to the web between the middle and ring

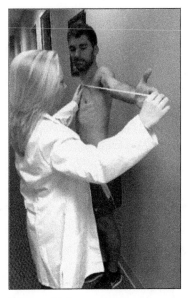
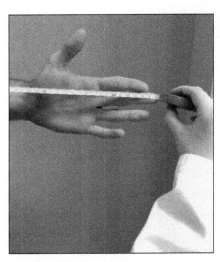
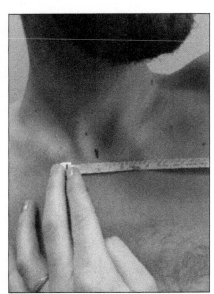

Figure 7.4   The half arm-span is the distance from the midline at the sternal notch to the tip of the middle finger while the nondominant arm is stretched out in a horizontal position. Height is then simply calculated by doubling the half arm-span measurement.
©David C. Nieman

fingers along the outstretched nondominant arm (Figure 7.5). Height is calculated from these formulas:

- Females: Height in cm = (1.35 × demispan cm) + 60.1
- Males: Height in cm = (1.40 × demispan cm) + 57.8

Knee height is one method for estimating height with bed- or chair-bound patients and is best measured using a sliding knee height caliper (Figure 7.6). The patient should bend the knee of one leg at a 90°angle while lying supine or sitting on a table with legs hanging off the table. Measure from the heel of the foot to the anterior surface of the thigh about 3 cm above the patella. The fixed blade of the caliper

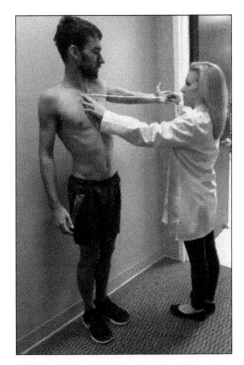
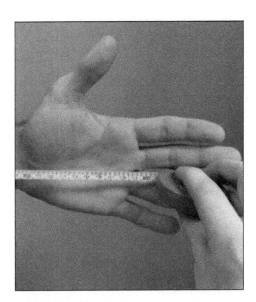

Figure 7.5   Demispan is the distance from the midline at the sternal notch to the web between the middle and ring fingers along the outstretched nondominant arm. Height can be calculated by two simple gender-specific formulas.
©David C. Nieman

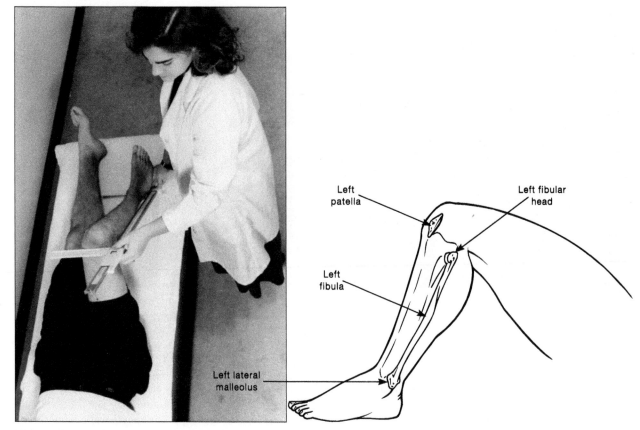

Figure 7.6   Knee height is best measured using a sliding knee height caliper with the patient's knee at a 90°angle while lying supine or sitting on a table with legs hanging off the table. Measure from the heel of the foot to the anterior surface of the thigh about 3 cm above the patella, and use an appropriate population-specific formula to calculate height (see Table 7.2).
©David C. Nieman

is placed under the heel of the foot, and the movable blade is placed above the patella. The caliper shaft is positioned parallel to the fibula and over the lateral malleolus. Take two or more measurements until there is agreement within 0.5 cm, and then use the appropriate population-specific formula to calculate height (Table 7.2).

During MNA-SF screening, if the BMI cannot be calculated for various reasons, measure the calf circumference in cm (Figure 7.7). The calf circumference is easy to measure, is used as a surrogate measure of muscle and subcutaneous adipose tissue, and is correlated with lean body mass. If the calf circumference is less than 31 cm, the patient gets 0 points, indicating that he or she is malnourished. To obtain the calf circumference, the patient should be sitting with the left leg hanging loosely or lying supine with the leg bent at a 90° angle. Wrap the tape around the calf at the widest circumference and take the measurement. A limitation of calf circumference measurement is peripheral edema, which is prevalent in approximately 25% of older adults.

The MNA-SF screening process also provides procedures for determining BMI for amputees. To determine the BMI for amputees, first calculate the patient's estimated weight, including the weight of the missing body

TABLE 7.2	**Population-Specific Formulas for Estimating Total Body Height from Knee Height**
Population	**Formula (Height cm =)**
Non-Hispanic white men	$78.31 + (1.94 \times \text{knee height cm}) - (0.14 \times \text{age})$
Non-Hispanic black men	$79.69 + (1.85 \times \text{knee height cm}) - (0.14 \times \text{age})$
Mexican-American men	$82.77 + (1.83 \times \text{knee height cm}) - (0.16 \times \text{age})$
Non-Hispanic white women	$82.21 + (1.85 \times \text{knee height cm}) - (0.21 \times \text{age})$
Non-Hispanic black women	$89.58 + (1.61 \times \text{knee height cm}) - (0.17 \times \text{age})$
Mexican-American women	$84.25 + (1.82 \times \text{knee height cm}) - (0.26 \times \text{age})$

Source: Chumlea WC, Guo SS, Wholihan K, Cockram D, Kuczmarski RJ, Johnson CL. 1998. Stature prediction equations for elderly non-Hispanic white, non-Hispanic black, and Mexican-American persons developed from NHANES III data. *Journal of the American Dietetic Association* 98:137–142.

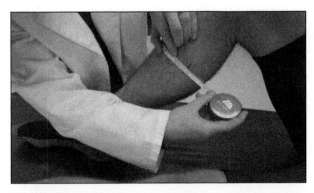

Figure 7.7   **Wrap the tape around the calf at the widest circumference and take the measurement while the patient is sitting with the left leg hanging loosely or lying supine with the leg bent at a 90° angle.**
©David C. Nieman

part. Use the information in Table 7.3 to determine the percentage of body weight contributed by a body part, subtract (in decimal form) from 1.0, and divide the current weight by the difference. For example, if a 75-year-old man weighing 70 kg at a height of 1.778 m (70 inches) had his entire arm amputated (5.0%), estimated body weight and BMI would be

- 70 kg / (1 − 0.05) = 73.7 kg
- BMI = 73.7 / $(1.778)^2$ = 23.3 kg/m^2

Table 7.1 compares the MNA-SF with four other tools used for assessing nutritional status and malnutrition. The Subjective Global Assessment (SGA) method encompasses a clinical history and physical exam.[13] The SGA is composed of the following components: diet and weight change history, gastrointestinal symptoms (nausea, vomiting, diarrhea, anorexia), functional capacity (difficulty with ambulation and normal activities, bed/chair-ridden), and evidence from the physical examination showing loss of muscle mass and subcutaneous fat as well as fluid

TABLE 7.3	Percentage of Total Body Weight for Selected Body Components
Missing Body Part	**Percentage**
Hand	0.7%
Foot	1.5%
Forearm and hand	2.3%
Entire arm	5.0%
Lower leg and foot	5.9%
Entire leg	16%

Source: Osterkamp LK. 1995. Current perspective on assessment of human body proportions of relevance to amputees. *Journal of the American Dietetic Association* 95:215–218.

accumulation (edema and ascites). Patients are given "A", "B", and "C" ratings for the SGA components. Studies support the use of the SGA for detecting malnutrition in clinical settings, but its accuracy depends on the experience of the clinician due to the subjectivity of the grading system.

The Nutrition Risk Screening tool (NRS-2002) was developed and promoted by the European Society for Clinical Nutrition and Metabolism (ESPEN).[14] The NRS-2002 tool encompasses three domains: nutritional parameters (BMI < 20.5 kg/m^2, weight loss in the past three months, reduced food intake), severity of disease, and age (> 70 years). The total NRS-2002 score can range from 0 to 7, with values > 3 indicating an increased risk of malnutrition and a likelihood of benefit from nutritional intervention. The NRS-2002 has received mixed support in validation and comparative studies.[7–9]

The Malnutrition University Screening Tool (MUST) was developed by the Malnutrition Advisory Group, a standing committee of BAPEN in the United Kingdom. MUST can be used by all care workers in hospitals, community settings, and other care institutions. MUST is a screening tool to identify adults who are at risk of malnutrition, and it is composed of three clinical parameters rated as 0, 1, or 2, as follows: BMI ≥ 20.0 kg/m^2 = 0 points, 18.5–20.0 kg/m^2 = 1 point; < 18.5 kg/m^2 = 2 points; weight loss within the last three to six months less than 5% = 0 points; 5%–10% = 1 point; > 10% = 2 points; presence of acute disease, with 2 points added in the case of acutely ill patients with no nutritional intake or likelihood of no nutritional intake for more than five days. MUST has received mixed support in validation and comparative studies.[7,8,15,16] In one systematic review, MUST performed well in detecting malnutrition in about half the studies reviewed in adults, but not in older patients.[15] Among nursing home residents, MUST screening estimated a prevalence of malnutrition significantly below the MNA.[16]

During MUST screening, height can be estimated in special circumstances from measuring ulna (forearm) length. Ulna length should be measured in centimeters from the elbow olecranon process to the midpoint of the styloid process at the wrist, with the left arm crossed over the chest and fingers at the right shoulder (Figure 7.8). These equations can be used to predict height in men and women 65 years of age and older:[17]

- Men: Predicted height (cm) = 79.2 + [3.60 · ulna length (cm)]

- Women: Predicted height (cm) = 95.6 + [2.77 · ulna length (cm)]

The MUAC is the circumference of the upper arm at the triceps skinfold site, and it is used to identify undernutrition. During MUST screening, BMI can be estimated from the mid-upper arm circumference (MUAC) if weight

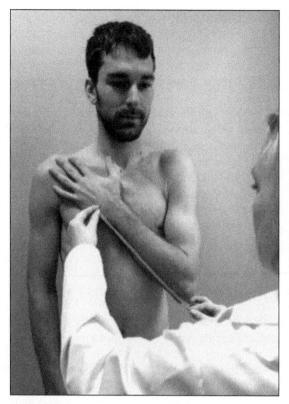
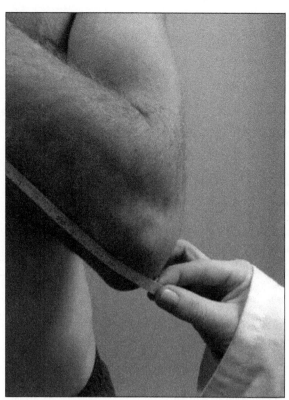

Figure 7.8   Height can be estimated with a gender-specific formula using ulna length, which is the centimeter distance from the olecranon process at the elbow to the midpoint of the styloid process at the wrist, with the left arm crossed over the chest and fingers at the right shoulder.
©David C. Nieman

or height cannot be obtained using these equations (with MUAC measured in centimeters):

- Male: $BMI = 1.01 \times MUAC - 4.7$

- Female: $BMI = 1.10 \times MUAC - 6.7$

From these equations, MUAC measurement of less than 23.5 cm approximately equates to BMI of < 18.5 kg/m², raising the potential concern about nutritional status and indicating the need for more detailed assessment.

To obtain the MUAC measurement in the ambulatory patient, the triceps skinfold site is measured and marked as described in Chapter 6. The arm is relaxed to the side with the palm of the hand facing the thigh. A nonstretchable measuring tape is placed around the arm, perpendicular to the long axis of the arm and at the level of the triceps skinfold site. The tape should be placed in contact with the arm but without compressing the soft tissues. The measurement should be recorded to the nearest 0.1 cm (Figure 7.9).

In the nonambulatory patient, MUAC is measured while the patient is in the supine position. With the upper arm approximately parallel to the body, the forearm is placed palm down across the middle of the body with the elbow bent 90°. Using a nonstretchable tape measure, the

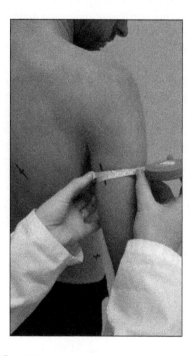

Figure 7.9   The mid-upper arm circumference (MUAC) is measured in the ambulatory patient while the patient is standing. The tape is placed around the arm, perpendicular to the long axis, at the level of the triceps skinfold site.
©David C. Nieman

midpoint of the upper arm is located between the tip of the acromion process and the olecranon process and marked, as shown in Figure 7.10. Once the midpoint of the upper arm is properly marked, the arm is returned to the patient's side with the palm facing upward. The arm is then raised slightly off the surface of the examination table by placing a folded towel under the patient's elbow. A nonstretchable tape measure is placed around the upper arm at the level of the marked midpoint and perpendicular to the long axis of the arm, and the circumference is measured as described for an ambulatory patient (Figure 7.11).

The Simplified Nutritional Appetite Questionaire (SNAQ) was developed in 2005 by various organizations in The Netherlands to assess the loss of appetite.[11,19,20] The SNAQ[65+] was targeted for the elderly who are living at home and who may or may not receive home care, and other versions are targeted for adults under the age of 65 years, SNAQ[65-], and for those in nursing and care homes, SNAQ[RC]. With the SNAQ[65+], the first step is to assess whether the patient has unintentionally lost 4 kg or more within the past six months. If the patient does not know, probe for whether or not clothes have become too big or the belt has had to be tightened recently. Step 2 involves measuring the MUAC, with a measurement less than

25 cm used as one indicator of malnutrition. Step 3 assesses appetite (e.g., "Did you have a poor appetite in the past week?") and functional status ("Can you walk up and down a staircase of 15 steps without resting?"). If the patient doesn't climb stairs, ask, "Are you able to walk outside for five minutes without resting?" If the patient is in a wheelchair, ask, "Are you able to move your own wheelchair for five minutes without resting?" In general, the SNAQ[65+] has moderate predictive validity for determining risk of undernutrition in community-dwelling older persons.[20] The SNAQ[65+] and other versions are very easy and quick to use, but one study found this tool to be less sensitive in detecting malnutrition in older people compared to the MNA tool.[11]

2. Mental health: Assess dementia, depression, cognition, stress, and emotional status.

According to *Healthy People 2020* (www.healthypeople.gov), mental health is a state of successful performance of mental function, resulting in productive activities, fulfilling relationships with other people, and the ability to adapt to change and to cope with challenges. Mental disorders are characterized by alterations in thinking, mood,

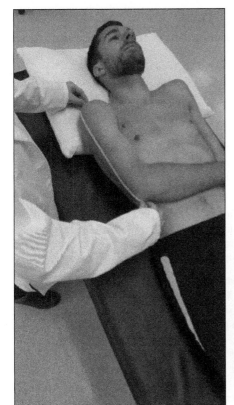

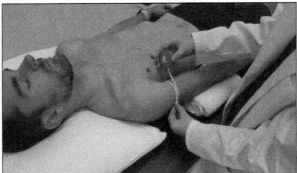

Figures 7.10 and 7.11　**Measurement of MUAC in the nonambulatory patient.**
When the patient cannot stand, MUAC is measured by first locating and marking the midpoint of the upper arm between the tip of the acromion process and the olecranon process (i.e., the triceps skinfold site). A folded towel under the elbow raises the arm off the surface of the table. The arm circumference is measured without compressing soft tissues.
©David C. Nieman

and/or behavior that are associated with distress and/or impaired functioning. Mental disorders contribute to a host of problems, which may include depression, anxiety, disability, pain, or death. Among nursing home residents, 18.7% of people age 65 to 74, and 23.5% of people age 85 and older, have reported mental illness. Senility or organic brain syndrome is common among the elderly and is associated with impairment of memory, judgment, feelings, personality, and ability to speak. Alzheimer's disease is the fifth leading cause of death among the elderly.

The Mini Mental State Examination (MMSE) is a tool that can be used to assess mental status, and it includes 11 questions that test five areas of cognitive function: orientation (e.g., what is the year, season, date, day, month), registration (ability to repeat names of three objects), attention and calculation (e.g., serial 7's or spell *world* backward), recall (rename the three objects), and language (e.g., repeat "no ifs, ands, or buts" or write a sentence). A score of 23 or lower out of 30 indicates cognitive impairment (http://www4.parinc.com).

The Geriatric Depression Scale (GDS) is a brief (15 items), valid questionnaire for assessing depression in older adults in community, acute care, and long-term care settings. A score of 5 and higher should prompt an in-depth psychological assessment and evaluation for suicidality (see Figure 7.12).[21]

3. Social and economic status: Examine the social support network, competence of caregivers, quality of life, economic resources, and cultural, ethnic, and spiritual resources.

Mental and physical health are linked to many social and economic factors, including income level; education level; sexual orientation; geographic location; interpersonal, family, and community dynamics; housing quality; and social support (www.healthypeople.gov).

Social and economic data can be gleaned from the physical examination and medical reports, as well as follow-up questions with the patient. Quality of life, an important measure that is intimately linked with social and economic status, can be assessed with the brief Older People's Quality of Life questionnaire (OPQOL-brief).[22] The OPQOL-brief has 13 items with 5-point response scales (Figure 7.13). Scores of 33 and lower indicate poor quality of life.

4. Functional status: Evaluate the physical environment and access to essential services, such as shopping, pharmacy, and transportation.

These data can be gleaned from the physical examination and medical reports, as well as follow-up questions with the patient. Most importantly, focus on assessment of the

Geriatric Depression Scale (GDS): Short Form

Choose the best answer for how you have felt **over the past week**:

1.	Are you basically satisfied with your life?	YES / **NO**
2.	Have you dropped many of your activities and interests?	**YES** / NO
3.	Do you feel that your life is empty?	**YES** / NO
4.	Do you often get bored?	**YES** / NO
5.	Are you in good spirits most of the time?	YES / **NO**
6.	Are you afraid that something bad is going to happen to you?	**YES** / NO
7.	Do you feel happy most of the time?	YES / **NO**
8.	Do you often feel helpless?	**YES** / NO
9.	Do you prefer to stay at home, rather than going out and doing new things?	**YES** / NO
10.	Do you feel you have more problems with memory than most?	**YES** / NO
11.	Do you think it is wonderful to be alive now?	YES / **NO**
12.	Do you feel pretty worthless the way you are now?	**YES** / NO
13.	Do you feel full of energy?	YES / **NO**
14.	Do you feel that your situation is hopeless?	**YES** / NO
15.	Do you think that most people are better off than you are?	**YES** / NO

Figure 7.12 **The Geriatric Depression Scale (GDS) assesses depression in older adults in community, acute care, and long-term care settings.**

Answers in **bold indicate depression**. Score 1 point for each bolded answer.

Interpretation:
A score > 5 points is suggestive of depression.
A score ≥ 10 points is almost always indicative of depression.
A score > 5 points should warrant a follow-up comprehensive assessment.

Target Population: The GDS may be used with healthy, medically ill and mild to moderately cognitively impaired older adults. It has been extensively used in community, acute and long-term care settings.

Validity And Reliability: The GDS has a 92% sensitivity and a 89% specificity when evaluated against diagnostic criteria. The validity and reliability of the tool have been supported through both clinical practice and research.

Source: http://www.stanford.edu/~yesavage/GDS.html. This scale is in the public domain.

patient's ability to accomplish basic activities of daily living (ADLs) and to participate in behavioral and social activities (instrumental activities of daily living, or IADLs).[23]

ADLs include bathing, dressing, toileting, transferring, continence, and feeding. IADLs require a higher level of cognition and judgment than ADLs and include preparation of meals, shopping, light housework, financial management,

Brief OLDER PEOPLE'S QUALITY OF LIFE QUESTIONNAIRE (opqol-brief)

The OPQOL-brief questionnaire has 13 items, with a preliminary single item on global QoL, shown below. This single item is not scored with the OPQOL; it is coded as Very good (1) to Very bad (5).

We would like to ask you about your quality of life: Single item–global QoL: *Thinking about both the good and bad things that make up your quality of life, how would you rate the quality of your life as a whole?* (Put an "X" in the box that matches your rating).

	Very good	Good	Alright	Bad	Very bad
Your quality of life AS A WHOLE IS:					

OLQOL-BRIEF: Please tick one box in each row. Please select the response that best describes you/your views. There are no right or wrong answers.

Question	Strongly agree	Agree	Neither agree nor disagree	Disagree	Strongly disagree
1. I enjoy my life overall					
2. I look forward to things					
3. I am healthy enough to get out and about					
4. My family, friends, or neighbors would help me if needed					
5. I have social or leisure activities/hobbies that I enjoy doing					
6. I try to stay involved with things					
7. I am healthy enough to have my independence					
8. I can please myself with what I do					
9. I feel safe where I live					
10. I get pleasure from my home					
11. I take life as it comes and make the best of things					
12. I feel lucky compared to most people					
13. I have enough money to pay for household bills					

OPQOL-Brief scoring:

Each of the 13 items is scored: Strongly agree = 5, Agree = 4, Neither = 3, Disagree = 2, Strongly disagree = 1.

The theoretical range for the summed OPQOL-brief is 13–65 (13 items by their 5-point response scales, coded 1 to 5).

Tentative Norms:

Low QOL:	33 to 50
Borderline low QOL:	51–55
Good QOL:	56–59
High QOL:	60–65

Figure 7.13   Quality of life can be assessed with the brief Older People's Quality of Life questionnaire (OPQOL-brief).

Source: Bowling A, Hankins M, Windle G, Bilotta C, Grant R. 2013. A short measure of quality of life in older age: The performance of the brief Older People's Quality of Life questionnaire (OPQOL-brief). *Archives of Geriatrics and Gerontology*, 56:181–187.

Note: This questionnaire is free to use and no permission is needed.

medication management, use of transportation, and use of the phone. Many eldercare financial assistance programs use the inability to perform a specific number of the activities of daily living as eligibility criteria.

ADLs are basic activities performed by individuals on a daily basis necessary for independent living at home or in the community. A common ADL assessment tool is the Katz Index of Independence in Activities of Daily Living (https://consultgeri.org/try-this/general-assessment/issue-2.pdf). There are many variations on the definition of the activities of daily living, but most organizations agree there are five basic categories:

1. Personal hygiene—bathing, grooming, and oral care
2. Dressing—the ability to make appropriate clothing decisions and physically dress oneself
3. Eating—the ability to feed oneself, though not necessarily to prepare food
4. Toileting and continence—both the mental and physical abilities to use a restroom

5. Transferring—moving oneself from seated to standing and getting into and out of bed

IADLs are actions that are important to being able to live independently but are not necessarily required activities on a daily basis. They can help determine with greater detail the level of assistance required by an elderly or disabled person. A common IADL assessment tool is the Lawton Instrumental Activities of Daily Living (IADL) scale (http://micmrc.org/system/files/IADL.pdf). The IADLs typically include

1. Basic communication skills—such as using a regular phone, mobile phone, email, or the Internet
2. Transportation—either by driving oneself, arranging rides, or using public transportation
3. Meal preparation—meal planning, preparation, and storage and the ability to safely use kitchen equipment
4. Shopping—the ability to make appropriate food and clothing purchase decisions
5. Housework—doing laundry, cleaning dishes, and maintaining a hygienic place of residence
6. Managing medications—taking accurate dosages at the appropriate times, managing refills and avoiding conflicts
7. Managing personal finances—operating within a budget, writing checks, paying bills, and avoiding scams

There are other measures of function that can be utilized during geriatric comprehensive assessment. Low muscle mass and weakness are potentially disabling in older adults, and the Foundation for the National Institutes of Health Sarcopenia Project recommends the use of hand-grip strength testing to determine weakness.[24] The final recommended cutpoints for weakness are grip strength values of less than 26 kg for men and less than 16 kg for women (the maximum value of any of six grip strength tests, three with each hand separately).[25] For men and women, grip strengths of 26–32 kg and 16–20 kg, respectively, are classified as "intermediate." Using these criteria, 5% of persons aged 60 and over had weak muscle strength, 13% had intermediate strength, and 82% had normal strength during the 2011–2012 NHANES cycle.[26] Among those aged 80 and over, 19% had weak strength, 34% had intermediate strength, and 47% had normal strength. Fifty-five percent of those with weak strength reported difficulty rising from an armless chair, compared with 26% of those with intermediate strength and 13% of those with normal strength. In general, these data will draw more attention to weak muscle strength, an important predictor of slow gait speed and impaired mobility.

The muscle strength/grip test measures the isometric grip strength using a hand-grip dynamometer. NHANES used the Takei Digital Grip Strength Dynamometer (Model T.K.K.5401).[27] There are many different models of hand-grip dynamometers, and the Jamar dynamometer is widely used and recommended (http://www.topendsports.com/testing/products/grip-dynamometer/index.htm).

To perform the hand-grip strength test, NHANES recommends these procedures:[27]

1. The test should first be explained and demonstrated to the patient. Have the patient loosen up the hand and fingers by shaking them and bending and stretching all fingers several times.
2. Adjust the grip size of the dynamometer to the patient's hand size. The second joint of the hand should fit snugly under the handle, which should be gripped between the fingers and the palm at the base of the thumb (Figure 7.14).
3. After the practice, the patient should be asked to stand straight up with feet hip width apart (Figure 7.15a). The dynamometer is gripped in line with the forearm at the thigh level, elbow straight, so that the dynamometer is not touching the body (Figure 7.15b). If the patient cannot stand, the test can be performed in the seated position, with the arm hanging straight down to the side of the chair or wheelchair (Figure 7.15c).
4. The test involves an all-out gripping effort for two to three seconds, without leaning forward. The hand should shake because of the quickness and hardness of the squeezing motion. The head is straight and the eyes are looking forward. The patient should exhale during the test to avoid buildup of intra-thoracic pressure. No swinging or pumping of the arm is allowed. A suggested verbal command of encouragement is *When I say "squeeze," squeeze as hard as you can until you can't squeeze any harder. Remember to blow out when you squeeze. ready, take a breath in, let it out, squeeze! squeeze as hard as you can until you can't squeeze any harder.*
5. Each hand should be tested three times, alternating hands between trials with a 60-second rest between measurements on the same hand. The top grip strength score in kilograms from each hand is recorded.

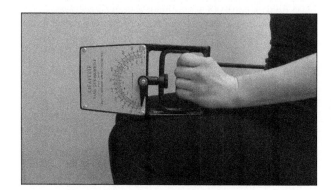

Figure 7.14 Adjust the dynamometer to the patient's hand size, with the second joint of the hand fitting snugly under the handle.
©David C. Nieman

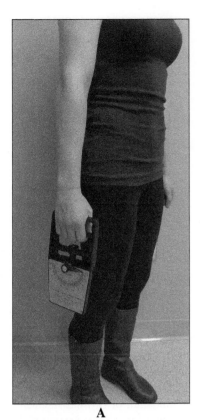
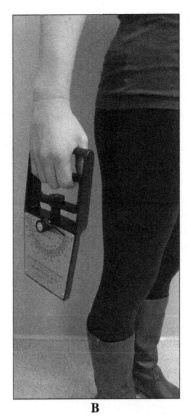
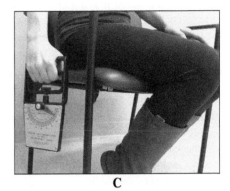

A   B   C

Figure 7.15   **The hand-grip test should be assessed with the patient standing or sitting straight up, with the arm hanging straight down.**
©David C. Nieman

NUTRITION SCREENING TOOL FOR PEDIATRIC PATIENTS

Nutrition screening of hospitalized elderly adults has received much attention in comparison to that of pediatric patients. Several validated pediatric nutrition risk screening tools are available, but most of them are complex and do not have the simplicity of similar tools used with adults.[28,29] Examples include the pediatric Subjective Global Nutrition Assessment (SGNA), Screening Tool for the Assessment of Malnutrition in Pediatrics (STAMP), Screening Tool Risk on Nutritional Status and Growth (STRONGkids), and Paediatric Yorkhill Malnutrition Score (PYMS). The SGNA involves a nutrition-focused medical history (height and weight percentiles for age, unintentional changes in body weight, adequacy of dietary intake, gastrointestinal symptoms, functional capacity, and metabolic stress of disease) and a physical examination for loss of subcutaneous fat, muscle wasting, and edema.[28]

In 2016, a quick, simple, and valid pediatric nutrition screening tool (PNST) was developed.[29] Weight and height measures were not included because nurses expressed a reluctance to compare children's weights and heights with any form of growth standard, including BMI cutoff tables. Questions had to be brief to be included in the admission forms. The PNST consists of four simple questions that require a yes or no response, and two affirmative responses are used as a cutoff for identifying pediatric patients at nutrition risk (prior to being referred to a health professional for an in-depth nutritional assessment):

1. Has the child unintentionally lost weight lately?
2. Has the child had poor weight gain over the last few months?
3. Has the child been eating/feeding less in the last few weeks?
4. Is the child obviously underweight/significantly overweight?

These four questions from the PNST were nearly as sensitive as the SGNA in detecting pediatric malnutrition, thus providing a valid and simple alternative to complex pediatric-specific nutrition screening tools.[29] This simple tool should advance the early and cost-effective identification of children who will benefit from targeted nutrition intervention.

ADDITIONAL ANTHROPOMETRIC MEASUREMENTS FOR THE HOSPITALIZED PATIENT

Several additional anthropometric measurements can be taken from hospitalized patients, depending on decisions made by the hospital nutrition support team. These include skinfold measurements, estimates of body weight, and arm muscle area. Measurement of subcutaneous fat using skinfold calipers allows body fat to be estimated and can be used in equations to estimate muscle stores.

Recumbent Skinfold Measurements

In the recumbent patient, the triceps and subscapular skinfolds can be measured with the patient lying on the left side.[18] Apart from differences in body positioning, the techniques for measuring skinfolds in the recumbent patient are essentially the same as those described in Chapter 6.

The subject is positioned as shown in Figure 7.16. The bottom arm is in front of the body at a 45-degree angle, the trunk is in a straight line, the shoulders are perpendicular to the spine and examination table, and the arm to be measured is lying on the trunk with the palm down. The legs are slightly flexed at the hips and knees.[18]

As in the standing ambulatory patient, the triceps skinfold is measured at the back of the upper arm at the level of the marked midpoint. With the thumb and index finger of the left hand, the measurer grasps a double fold of skin and adipose tissue about 1 cm (½ in.) above the marked midpoint of the upper arm. The long axes of the skinfold and arm must be parallel. Holding the skinfold, the measurer places the caliper tips on the skinfold and reads the dial after about four seconds (Figure 7.17). The measurer's eyes should be in line with the needle and dial of the caliper to avoid errors caused by parallax.[18]

For measuring the subscapular skinfold, the body is positioned as shown in Figure 7.16. The same site is used as when the subject is standing, and the skinfold is grasped

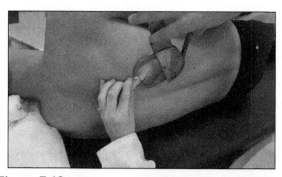

Figure 7.18   Measurement of subscapular skinfold of the recumbent subject.
©David C. Nieman

and measured along the same axis (see Chapter 6). As shown in Figure 7.18, the measurer grasps the double layer of skin and adipose tissue along the axis of the skinfold, so that the thumb and index finger of the left hand are about 1 cm (½ in.) from the actual measurement site. Note that the left hand is distal and lateral to the skinfold site. Holding the skinfold, the measurer places the caliper tips at the site and reads the dial after about 4 seconds. The measurer should look directly at the dial of the caliper to avoid errors caused by parallax.[18] A minimum of two measurements should be taken at each site. Successive measurements should be at least 15 seconds apart from each other to allow the skinfold site to return to normal. If consecutive measurements vary by more than 1 mm, additional measurements should be taken until the readings are consistent.

The sum of the triceps and subscapular skinfold thicknesses can be used as an indicator of the body's energy reserves. Appendix K provides percentiles for triceps and subscapular skinfold thicknesses for males and females ages 2 to 90 years.

Estimating Body Weight

Most patients can be weighed on scales, but sometimes it is difficult or impossible to obtain a patient's weight. This may be because of the patient's medical condition, equipment attached to the patient (for example, life support devices, traction equipment, casts, or braces), or lack of a suitable bed or wheelchair scale.[4]

When it is difficult or impossible to obtain a patient's body weight directly, it can be estimated from various anthropometric measures (that is, knee height, midarm circumference, calf circumference, and subscapular skinfold thickness) using the equations given in Tables 7.4 and 7.5. The decision of which equation to use will depend on the patient's age and the anthropometric measures that can be obtained or are available.

From Tables 7.4 and 7.5, it can be noted that a certain amount of error is inherent in the process of estimating body weight from anthropometric measures. This error can be minimized by using an equation requiring a larger number of variables (four as opposed to two) and by paying strict attention to measurement technique. Although

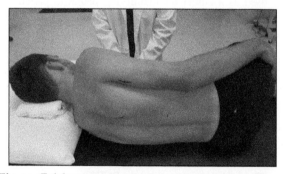

Figure 7.16   Body position for measurement of triceps and subscapular skinfolds of the recumbent subject.
©David C. Nieman

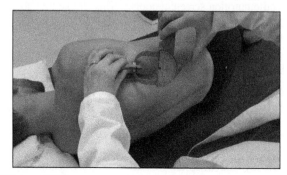

Figure 7.17   Measurement of triceps skinfold of the recumbent subject.
©David C. Nieman

TABLE 7.4	Equations for Estimating Body Weight in Persons 65 Years of Age and Older from Anthropometric Measures

Females*	SEE†
Weight = (MUAC × 1.63) + (CC × 1.43) − 37.46	± 4.96 kg
Weight = (MUAC × 0.92) + (CC × 1.50) + (SSF × 0.42) − 26.19	± 4.21 kg
Weight = (MUAC × 0.98) + (CC × 1.27) + (SSF × 0.40) + (KH × 0.87) − 62.35	± 3.80 kg
Males*	
Weight = (MUAC × 2.31) + (CC × 1.50) − 50.10	± 5.37 kg
Weight = (MUAC × 1.92) + (CC × 1.44) + (SSF × 0.26) − 39.97	± 5.34 kg
Weight = (MUAC × 1.73) + (CC × 0.98) + (SSF × 0.37) + (KH × 1.16) − 81.69	± 4.48 kg

Source: Chumlea WC, Guo S, Roche AF, Steinbaugh ML. 1988. Prediction of body weight for the nonambulatory elderly from anthropometry. *Journal of the American Dietetic Association* 88:564–568.

*Weight is in kg; MUAC = midarm circumference, in cm; CC = calf circumference, in cm; SSF = subscapular skinfold thickness, in mm; KH = knee height, in cm.

†SEE = standard error of the estimate.

TABLE 7.5	Equations for Estimating Body Weight from Knee Height (KH) and Midarm Circumference (MUAC) for Various Groups

Age*	Race	Equation†	Accuracy‡
Females			
6–18	Black	Weight = (KH × 0.71) + (MUAC × 2.59) − 50.43	± 7.65 kg
6–18	White	Weight = (KH × 0.77) + (MUAC × 2.47) − 50.16	± 7.20 kg
19–59	Black	Weight = (KH × 1.24) + (MUAC × 2.97) − 82.48	± 11.98 kg
19–59	White	Weight = (KH × 1.01) + (MUAC × 2.81) − 66.04	± 10.60 kg
60–80	Black	Weight = (KH × 1.50) + (MUAC × 2.58) − 84.22	± 14.52 kg
60–80	White	Weight = (KH × 1.09) + (MUAC × 2.68) − 65.51	± 11.42 kg
Males			
6–18	Black	Weight = (KH × 0.59) + (MUAC × 2.73) − 48.32	± 7.50 kg
6–18	White	Weight = (KH × 0.68) + (MUAC × 2.64) − 50.08	± 7.82 kg
19–59	Black	Weight = (KH × 1.09) + (MUAC × 3.14) − 83.72	± 11.30 kg
19–59	White	Weight = (KH × 1.19) + (MUAC × 3.21) − 86.82	± 11.42 kg
60–80	Black	Weight = (KH × 0.44) + (MUAC × 2.86) − 39.21	± 7.04 kg
60–80	White	Weight = (KH × 1.10) + (MUAC × 3.07) − 75.81	± 11.46 kg

*Age (in years) is rounded to the nearest year.

†Weight is in kg: lb ÷ 2.2 = kg; kg × 2.2 = lb. Knee height is in cm; in. × 2.54 = cm; cm ÷ 2.54 = in.

‡For persons within each group, estimated body weight should be within the stated value for 95% of the subjects.

Source: Brunnstrom S. 1983. *Clinical Kinesiology,* 4th ed. Philadelphia: Davis.

estimates of body weight may be as much as 14 kg greater than or less than actual body weight, an estimate of body weight recorded on a patient's chart is better than no weight recorded. The use of estimated weights should be reserved for patients who cannot be weighed or for whom weights would be inaccurate, and every reasonable effort should be made to obtain direct measurements of body weights on patients.

Arm Anthropometry: Muscle Circumference and Muscle Area

Mid-upper arm muscle circumference (MAMC) is calculated from MUAC and the triceps skinfold and can be used to evaluate fat-free mass.[30] The formula is

MAMC (cm) = MUAC (cm) − [triceps skinfold (mm) × 0.3142]

For example, if the MUAC is 30.5 cm, and the triceps skinfold is 29.2 mm, MAMC = 30.5 − [29.2 × 0.3142] = 21.3 cm.

The MAMC is relatively easy to assess and calculate, and low values have been associated with adverse outcomes.[31,32] In one study of older adults, the well-nourished group had an average MAMC of 21.3 cm compared to averages of 18.8 cm for moderately malnourished and 17.2 cm for severely malnourished older adults.[31]

The mid-upper arm muscle area (MAMA) can be used to evaluate fat-free mass and, similar to MAMC, is calculated from MUAC and the triceps skinfold:[30,33]

$$MAMA\ (cm^2) = \frac{(MUAC\ cm - [triceps\ skinfold\ mm \times 0.3142])^2}{12.57}$$

For example, is the MUAC is 30.5 cm, and the triceps skinfold is 29.2,

$$MAMA = (30.5 - [29.2 \times 0.3142])^2/12.57 = 36.2 \text{ cm}^2$$

Revised equations were proposed by Heymsfield et al.[33] to address some incorrect assumptions and the area occupied by bone. The revised equations are the same as described here except that the estimated MAMA is corrected by subtracting 10 for male patients, 6.5 for female patients. Low values for both MAMA and corrected MAMA are linked to adverse outcomes.[30]

Low values for MAMC or MAMA predict health risk in adults, and MAMC may be preferable for use in nutrition support screening because it is marginally easier to calculate. Population and ethnic-specific standards have not been established.[30] Reference values for MAMC from adults were collected in the 1971–1974 and 1988–1994 NHANES.

MAMA reference values from persons aged 2 months to 90 years collected in NHANES III (1988–94) are available and expressed as 5th to 95th percentiles.[34,35] If the 15th and 5th percentiles are used as a cutoff for mild and severe malnutrition, respectively, then Table 7.6 can be used for MAMA measurements. As with all anthropometric measurements, other factors and assessments should be combined until malnutrition is diagnosed.

Reference percentile ranges for MUAC and MAMA have been developed for children and adolescents ages 1 to 20 years, and provide a useful nutritional assessment

TABLE 7.6	MAMA Cutoffs for Mild (15th percentile) and Severe (5th percentile) Malnutrition	
Gender and Age Group	MAMA (cm²) 15th Percentile, Mild Malnutrition	MAMA (cm²) 5th Percentile, Severe Malnutrition
Males, Age Range (years)		
30–59.9	55	49
60–69.9	53	47
70–79.9	49	44
80–90	43	38
Females, Age Range (years)		
30–59.9	33	28
60–69.9	33	28
70–79.9	32	27
80–90	31	26

Sources: Based on data from two papers using NHANES reference and percentile data.

Bishop CW. 1984. Reference values for arm muscle area, arm fat area, subscapular skinfold thickness, and sum of skinfold thicknesses for American adults. *Journal of Parenteral and Enteral Nutrition* 8:515–522.

Frisancho AR. 2008. *Anthropometric standards: An interactive nutritional reference of body size and body composition for children and adults*, 2nd ed. Ann Arbor: University of Michigan Press.

tool in a wide variety of settings.[36,37] Figure 7.19 depicts the 5th, 50th, and 95th percentile MUAC and MAMA values for children and adolescents using NHANES data. The Academy of Nutrition and Dietetics consensus report on the nutritional assessment of critically ill children recommends the use of MUAC to assess nutritional status in bedbound children when measurements of weight and length or height are not feasible.

DETERMINING ENERGY REQUIREMENTS

Twenty-four-hour energy expenditure is primarily determined by resting energy expenditure, the thermic effect of food, the thermic effect of exercise, and whether disease or injury is present.[38] As Sims and Danforth[38] pointed out, these "components of energy expenditure are not entirely discrete but are useful divisions when attempting to investigate factors that might regulate or control them."

Twenty-four-hour energy expenditure can be represented by the following equation:

$$24\text{-EE} = REE + TEF + TEE + TED$$

where 24-EE = 24-hour energy expenditure; REE = resting energy expenditure; TEF = thermic effect of food; TEE = thermic effect of exercise; and TED = thermic effect of disease and injury.

Basal metabolic rate (BMR) is defined as the lowest rate of energy expenditure of an individual. It is calculated from oxygen consumption measured over a 6- to 12-minute period when the subject is in a postabsorptive state (no food consumed during the previous 12 hours) and has rested quietly during the previous 30 minutes in a thermally neutral environment (room temperature is perceived as neither hot nor cold). Obtaining a truly basal metabolic measurement is impractical in most instances. Therefore, a more appropriate term for metabolic rate or energy expenditure in the awake, resting, postabsorptive subject is *resting energy expenditure (REE)*.

In the clinical setting, achieving optimal conditions for determining REE can be difficult sometimes because of the continuous care patients undergo. In these situations, the term *REE* is used in the scientific literature to represent energy expenditure measured by indirect calorimetry under conditions that are as controlled as the clinical situation allows.[39] As shown in Figure 7.20, REE is the largest component of 24-hour energy expenditure, accounting for roughly 65% to 75% of 24-hour energy expenditure in healthy persons.

The second largest contributor to 24-hour energy expenditure is the energy expended for muscular work, or the thermic effect of exercise (TEE).[40] Of all the components of a healthy person's 24-hour energy expenditure, it is the most variable. For most North Americans, it accounts for about 15% to 20% of 24-hour energy expenditure but can increase by a factor of two or more with

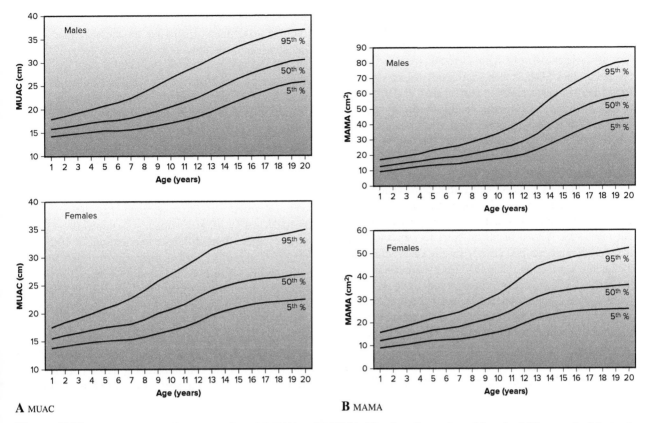

A MUAC   **B** MAMA

Figure 7.19   **5th, 50th, and 95th percentile MUAC (A) and MAMA (B) values for male and female children and adolescents using NHANES data.**

Source: Addo OY, Himes JH, Zemel BS. Reference ranges for midupper arm circumference, upper arm muscle area, and upper arm fat area in US children and adolescents aged 1–20 y. *American Journal of Clinical Nutrition* (in press).

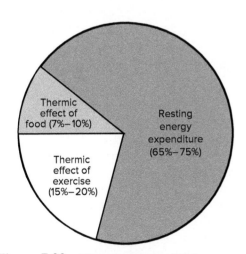

Figure 7.20   **The components of 24-hour energy expenditure in healthy persons.**

regular, high-intensity, long-duration physical activity.[40] Energy expended in exercise can exceed the REE in some athletes who train several hours daily.

The thermic effect of food (TEF), also known as diet-induced thermogenesis or the specific dynamic action of food, is the increased energy expenditure following food consumption or administration of parenteral or enteral nutrition. The TEF is the energy cost of nutrient absorption, transport, storage, and metabolism. It accounts for about 7% to 10% of 24-hour energy expenditure.[38,40]

The energy needs of patients can be determined in two ways: measuring energy expenditure or estimating these needs using a variety of guidelines.[39–44]

Measuring Energy Expenditure

Calorimetry is the measurement of the body's energy expenditure. Direct calorimetry measures the body's heat output, whereas indirect calorimetry determines energy expenditure by measuring the body's oxygen consumption and carbon dioxide production. Because energy expenditure measurements using direct and indirect calorimetry are performed in a laboratory, they may not accurately represent energy expenditure of free-living subjects (i.e., persons living at home and engaged in typical work and leisure-time activities). To more accurately measure the energy expenditure of free-living subjects, researchers can use two other methods: doubly labeled water and the bicarbonate-urea method.

Direct Calorimetry

Direct calorimetry uses a specially designed chamber to measure the amount of heat given off by the body through radiation, convection, and evaporation.[45] Direct calorimeters range in size from just large enough to comfortably accommodate an adult human lying in the recumbent position to those the size of a small room, such as the one located at the USDA Human Nutrition Research Center at Beltsville, Maryland, and shown in Figure 7.21.[46] The walls of the USDA direct calorimeter contain a layer of water that is warmed by the subject's body heat. Changes in the water temperature are recorded, and the amount of energy expended by the subject is calculated. The composition of air entering and exiting the chamber is analyzed to determine the subject's production of carbon dioxide and methane and consumption of oxygen. Temperature, pressure, and humidity within the chamber and the subject's motion are measured. A total of 30 different measurements are monitored, recorded, and analyzed using electronic instrumentation. The interior of the chamber measures 8 ft by 9 ft by 10 ft and is comfortably furnished with a bed, table, toilet, sink, video monitor, telephone, and exercise equipment, as shown in Figure 7.21. The calorimeter provides highly accurate measurements of human energy expenditure for periods as long as 24 hours. However, the expense of building and maintaining the chamber and instrumentation is prohibitive, and thus, this approach is rarely used.[45,46]

Indirect Calorimetry

Indirect calorimetry is based on the fact that energy metabolism ultimately depends on oxygen utilization (VO_2) and carbon dioxide production (VCO_2).[39] Thus, expired air contains less oxygen and more carbon dioxide than inspired air. When the volume of expired air is known and the differences in oxygen and carbon dioxide concentrations in inspired and expired air are known, the body's energy expenditure can be calculated. Estimations of energy expenditure by indirect calorimetry are the same as those derived from direct calorimetry.

Several techniques can be used in indirect calorimetry. In *closed circuit calorimetry*, the subject is connected via a mouthpiece, mask, or endotracheal tube to a spirometer filled with a known amount of 100% oxygen.[45,47] The subject rebreathes only the gas within the spirometer—a closed system. Carbon dioxide is removed from the system by a canister of soda lime (potassium hydroxide) placed in the breathing circuit. The subject's VO_2 is determined either from the amount of oxygen consumed from the spirometer or from the amount of added oxygen needed to maintain a constant volume within the spirometer. The closed circuit technique is neither portable nor suitable to use on

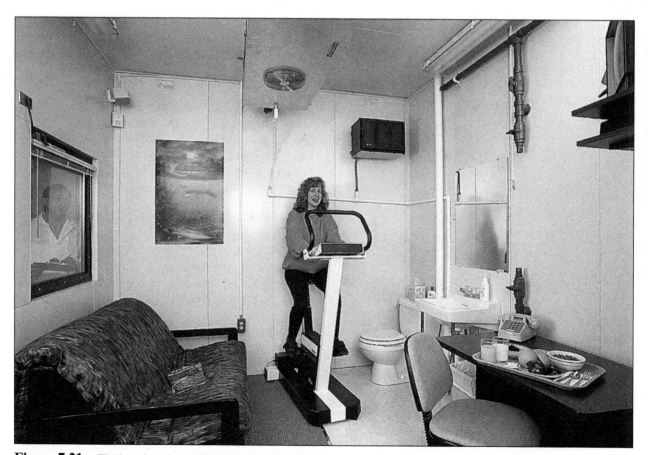

Figure 7.21   The interior of the USDA Human Nutrition Research Center's direct calorimeter provides a small but comfortable living space to subjects undergoing energy expenditure measurements lasting as long as 24 hours.

Source: U.S. Department of Agriculture, Agriculture Research Service, Beltsville Human Nutrition Research Center.

exercising subjects. During exercise, the apparatus offers excessive resistance to gas flow, and the removal of carbon dioxide is inadequate.

In *open circuit calorimetry,* the subject breathes through a two-way valve in which room air is inspired from one side of the valve, and expired air passes through the opposite side to where it is either analyzed immediately or collected for later analysis. In the *Douglas bag method* of open circuit calorimetry, the expired air is collected in large vinyl bags or latex rubber meteorologic balloons for later analysis.

A more common approach to open circuit indirect calorimetry in clinical settings is use of a *computerized metabolic monitor,* which can be taken to the bedside for measuring energy expenditure of patients who are either spontaneously breathing or breathing with the assistance of a mechanical ventilator.[38] The portable computerized metabolic monitor shown in Figure 7.22 has a ventilated hood, which can be placed over the face of a patient while in bed and can be made air-tight with a snugly fitting collar. The volume of inspired and expired air (known as minute ventilation) can be measured with a bidirectional digital turbine device. Gas analyzers in the unit determine the oxygen and carbon dioxide content of both inspired and expired air, and they determine the caloric requirements and substrate utilization. Data can be displayed on the unit's video screen, recorded on an optional printer, or downloaded to a computer for storage and/or further analysis.

The Academy of Nutrition and Dietetics recommends several guidelines when performing indirect calorimetry in healthy and noncritically ill individuals (see Figure 7.23 for a summary):[39]

1. Patients should be fasted for at least 7 hours, avoid moderate to vigorous physical activity for 12 to 48 hours, and rest for 30 minutes in a thermoneutral, quiet, and dimly lit room in the supine position before the test, without doing any activities, including fidgeting, reading, or listening to music. A blanket can be provided as desired. If a 7-hour fast is not clinically feasible, the practitioner should instruct the individual that a small meal (≤ 300 kcal) may be consumed 4 hours before the measurement.

2. RMR can be measured at any time of the day as long as resting conditions are met.

3. When measuring RMR, discard the data for the first five minutes, and then use four minutes of measurements taken during steady state (i.e., 10% or less coefficient of variation in VO_2 and CO_2).

4. The practitioner may select any gas collection device (ventilated hood/canopy, mouthpiece and nose clip, or face mask) for the RMR measurement (see Figure 7.20).

5. The practitioner should ensure that the patient refrains from ingesting caffeine or other stimulants for at least four hours before the RMR measurement. If the individual uses nicotine products, the practitioner should ask the individual to abstain for more than 140 minutes before the RMR measurement.

6. If the respiratory quotient (RQ or VCO_2/VO_2) falls outside the physiologic range (<0.67 or >1.3), the practitioner should suspect an error and repeat the RMR measurement. If the RQ is between 0.91 and 1.3 in an individual who has fasted, the practitioner should suspect a problem and consider repeating the measurement.

Doubly Labeled Water

Another approach to measuring energy expenditure is the doubly labeled water (DLW) method. Using this approach, a subject drinks a known amount of two different stable isotopic forms of water: $H_2^{18}O$ and ^2H_2O. Ordinary water is a molecule composed of two atoms of hydrogen, each having an atomic mass of 1 (^1H), and one atom of oxygen having an atomic mass of 16 (^{16}O). Although hydrogen atoms with an atomic mass of 2 (^2H, or deuterium) and oxygen atoms with an atomic mass of 18 (^{18}O) are naturally present in nature, they are found only in extremely minute quantities. Consequently, it is reasonable to assume that essentially all the ^2H and ^{18}O present in the body came from the doubly labeled water. After the subject drinks the two different isotopic forms of water, they mix with the body's water and are gradually eliminated from the body. The ^2H_2O is lost from the body only as water and reflects water flux, whereas the $H_2^{18}O$ is lost from the body in water and as $C^{18}O_2$ and reflects both water flux and CO_2 produced by the body.[41,47] Over the next one to three weeks the subject provides a series of urine samples that are used to measure the rate at which the two isotopes disappear from the body. The rate of disappearance is then used to calculate energy

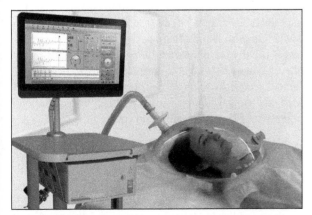

Figure 7.22 **An example of a computerized metabolic monitor in operation.**
This unit uses indirect calorimetry with a ventilated hood to determine a patient's resting energy.
Courtesy of COSMED USA, Inc.

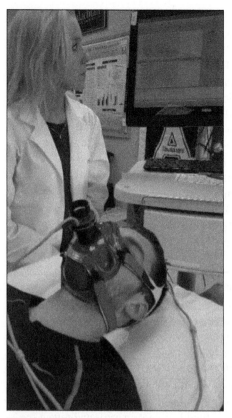

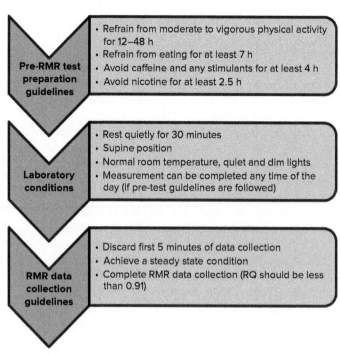

| Pre-RMR test preparation guidelines | • Refrain from moderate to vigorous physical activity for 12–48 h
• Refrain from eating for at least 7 h
• Avoid caffeine and any stimulants for at least 4 h
• Avoid nicotine for at least 2.5 h |

| Laboratory conditions | • Rest quietly for 30 minutes
• Supine position
• Normal room temperature, quiet and dim lights
• Measurement can be completed any time of the day (if pre-test guidelines are followed) |

| RMR data collection guidelines | • Discard first 5 minutes of data collection
• Achieve a steady state condition
• Complete RMR data collection (RQ should be less than 0.91) |

Figure 7.23   **The face mask is an appropriate type of gas-collection device for RMR measurement.**
©David C. Nieman

expenditure. The method is noninvasive and provides an accurate measurement of energy expenditure over a period of one to three weeks, and because the two isotopes are stable (nonradioactive), the procedure is considered safe to use even on infants and females who are pregnant or lactating.

The method has been validated in humans by use of carefully performed energy balance studies and by direct and indirect calorimetry.[41,47] In laboratory testing, DLW has demonstrated an accuracy of 1% and a coefficient of variation of 3% to 6%.[47,48] The DLW technique is considered the best available method for providing average estimates of the 24-hour energy expenditure of free-living subjects (those outside a controlled setting) over an extended period of time of one to three weeks. Although it does not provide a direct measurement of energy expended in physical activity (thermic effect of exercise), this can be calculated by subtracting estimates of resting metabolic rate and the thermic effect of food from measured 24-hour energy expenditure. Use of DLW is limited by the expense of the isotopes and its dependence on isotope ratio mass spectrometry for analysis of urine samples, and consequently it is not ideally suited for use in large, epidemiologic studies.[47,48] As mentioned in Chapter 3, comparisons of energy expenditure determined by DLW with reported energy intake from 24-hour recalls and food records have raised serious questions

about the accuracy of reported energy intakes in dietary studies.

Estimating Energy Needs

Indirect calorimetry is the gold standard for measuring resting energy expenditure and should be utilized whenever possible. The use of predictive equations can be problematic in the critical care setting because of the unpredictable effects of disease, injury, and stress on RMR.[49] In most clinical settings, however, energy expenditure is usually not measured. Instead, it is estimated using one of numerous available formulas such as the Harris-Benedict equations, those developed by the Institute of Medicine for calculating Estimated Energy Requirement, or the World Health Organization equations.

Commonly Used Equations

There are many equations that have been developed for estimating the nonprotein energy requirements of hospitalized patients.[40–43] Commonly used equations for predicting REE are those published in 1919 by Harris and Benedict[43] and those developed by an expert panel of the World Health Organization, which are shown in Table 7.7. Harris and Benedict used indirect calorimetry to determine the REE of 239 healthy young adults (136 males and 103 females with a mean age of 27 and 31 years, respectively). From these

TABLE 7.7	Examples of Equations for Estimating Resting Energy Expenditure in Healthy Persons

Harris-Benedict

Females   REE = 655.096 + 9.563 W + 1.850 S − 4.676 A

Males   REE = 66.473 + 13.752 W + 5.003 S − 6.755 A

Harris-Benedict (Values Rounded for Simplicity)

Females   REE = 655.1 + 9.6 W + 1.9 S − 4.7 A

Males   REE = 66.5 + 13.8 W + 5.0 S − 6.8 A

World Health Organization (WHO)

			SD*
Females	3–9 years old	22.5 W + 499	± 63
	10–17 years old	12.2 W + 746	± 117
	18–29 years old	14.7 W + 496	± 121
	30–60 years old	8.7 W + 829	± 108
	> 60 years old	10.5 W + 596	± 108
Males	3–9 years old	22.7 W + 495	± 62
	10–17 years old	17.5 W + 651	± 100
	18–29 years old	15.3 W + 679	± 151
	30–60 years old	11.6 W + 879	± 164
	> 60 years old	13.5 W + 487	± 148

National Institutes of Health

REE = 638 + (15.9 × FFM)

University of Vermont

REE = 418 + (20.3 × FFM)

Abbreviations: W = weight in kilograms; A = age in years; S = stature in cm; FFM = fat-free mass in kilograms.

*SD = standard deviation of the differences between actual and computed values—68% of the time the actual REE will be within ± 1 standard deviation of the predicted REE.

Sources: Harris JA, Benedict FG. 1919. *A biometric study of basal metabolism in man.* Publication 279. Washington, DC: Carnegie Institution of Washington; World Health Organization. 1985. *Energy and protein requirements. Report of a joint FAO/WHO/UNU expert consultation.* Technical Report Series 724. Geneva, Switzerland: World Health Organization; Nieman DC. 2011. *Exercise testing and prescription: A health-related approach,* 7th ed. Boston: McGraw-Hill.

data, they derived regression equations (Table 7.7) that best predicted REE using the variables weight, stature, age, and sex.[43] Research has shown the Harris-Benedict equations' accuracy of prediction among healthy, adequately nourished persons to be within ± 14% of REE measured by indirect calorimetry.[43] In malnourished, ill patients, however, the Harris-Benedict equations tend to underestimate REE by as much as 22%.[43] Despite these shortcomings, the Harris-Benedict equations are often widely used in estimating the energy needs of patients in clinical settings.

A major decision in developing prediction equations is which variables to include. The major determinant of REE is fat-free mass—what some researchers call the active protoplasmic tissue, or the body cell mass.[44] These cells are the body's metabolically active, energy-consuming cells, and they determine about 70% to 80% of the variance in REE. The remaining 20% to 30% of variance in REE is primarily determined by genetics.[41] As discussed in Chapter 6, fat-free mass can be determined using a variety of approaches such as skinfold measurement, underwater weighing, air displacement plethysmography, or dual-energy X-ray absorptiometry. If known, an individual's fat-free mass in kilograms can be used to accurately estimate resting energy expenditure using equations shown in Table 7.7.

Numerous other equations for predicting REE in healthy populations are available.[41] The WHO equations (shown in Table 7.7) were developed by a group of experts.[42] Because stature was not found to significantly improve the predictive ability of the equations, it was omitted. Using measured energy expenditure based on the doubly labeled water technique, the Institute of Medicine developed a set of equations for estimating REE in healthy people. These are shown in Table 7.8.

TABLE 7.8	Institute of Medicine Equations for Calculating Resting Energy Expenditure (REE) in Kilocalories per Day

REE for males ages 3–18 years, healthy weight (BMI < 85th percentile for age and sex)

REE = 68 − (43.3 × age) + (712 × height) + (19.2 × weight)

REE for males ages 3–18, at risk of overweight or overweight (BMI ≥ 85th percentile for age and sex)

REE = 419.9 − (33.5 × age) + (418.9 × height) + (16.7 × weight)

REE for females ages 3–18 years, healthy weight (BMI < 85th percentile for age and sex)

REE = 189 − (17.6 × age) + (625 × height) + (7.9 × weight)

REE for females ages 3–18, at risk of overweight or overweight (BMI ≥ 85th percentile for age and sex)

REE = 515.8 − (26.8 × age) + (347 × height) + (12.4 × weight)

REE for males ages 19 and older

REE = 293 − (3.8 × age) + (456.4 × height) + (10.12 × weight)

REE for females ages 19 and older

REE = 247 − (2.67 × age) + (401.5 × height) + (8.6 × weight)

Abbreviations: REE = resting energy expenditure; age is in years; height is in meters; weight is in kilograms.

Source: Panel on Macronutrients, Panel on the Definition of Dietary Fiber, Subcommittee on Upper Reference Levels of Nutrients, Subcommittee on Interpretation and Uses of Dietary Reference Intakes, Standing Committee on the Scientific Evaluation of Dietary Reference Intakes. 2002. *Dietary reference intakes for energy, carbohydrate, fiber, fat, fatty acids, cholesterol, protein, and amino acids.* Washington, DC: National Academies Press.

The equations in Table 7.7 and Table 7.8 predict REE in kilocalories, and to arrive at estimates of 24-hour energy expenditure, the REE must be increased to account for TEE. This is done by multiplying REE by one of the activity factors shown in Table 7.9 to arrive at TEE. Use of an additional factor to account for increased metabolism caused by disease, injury, and surgery is often necessary to estimate the 24-hour energy expenditure of patients.

When using these equations, keep in mind that there is a large interindividual variability in energy requirements. Even though a particular equation may be able to

TABLE **7.9**	**Equations for Calculating Estimated Energy Requirement (EER) in Kilocalories per Day**

EER for Infants and Young Children

EER = TEE + tissue deposition[a]

0–3 months	$(89 \times \text{weight} - 100) + 175$
4–6 months	$(89 \times \text{weight} - 100) + 56$
7–12 months	$(89 \times \text{weight} - 100) + 22$
13–35 months	$(89 \times \text{weight} - 100) + 20$

EER for Males 3–8 years

EER = TEE + tissue deposition

EER = $88.5 - 61.9 \times \text{age} + \text{PA} \times (26.7 \times \text{weight} + 903 \times \text{height}) + 20$

where PA is the physical activity coefficient:

PA = 1.00 for sedentary

PA = 1.13 for low active

PA = 1.26 for active

PA = 1.42 for very active

EER for Females 3–8 years

EER = TEE + tissue deposition

EER = $135.3 - 30.8 \times \text{age} + \text{PA} \times (10.0 \times \text{weight} + 934 \times \text{height}) + 20$

where PA is the physical activity coefficient:

PA = 1.00 for sedentary

PA = 1.16 for low active

PA = 1.31 for active

PA = 1.56 for very active

EER for Males 9–18 years

EER = TEE + tissue deposition

EER = $88.5 - 61.9 \times \text{age} + \text{PA} \times (26.7 \times \text{weight} + 903 \times \text{height}) + 25$

where PA is the physical activity coefficient:

PA = 1.00 for sedentary

PA = 1.13 for low active

PA = 1.26 for active

PA = 1.42 for very active

EER for Females 9–18 years

EER = TEE + tissue deposition

EER = $135.3 - 30.8 \times \text{age} + \text{PA} \times (10.0 \times \text{weight} + 934 \times \text{height}) + 25$

where PA is the physical activity coefficient:

PA = 1.00 for sedentary

PA = 1.16 for low active

PA = 1.31 for active

PA = 1.56 for very active

EER for Males 19 years of age and older

EER = TEE

EER = $662 - 9.53 \times \text{age} + \text{PA} \times (15.91 \times \text{weight} + 539.6 \times \text{height})$

where PA is the physical activity coefficient:

PA = 1.00 for sedentary

PA = 1.11 for low active

PA = 1.25 for active

PA = 1.48 for very active

EER for Females 19 years of age and older

EER = TEE

EER = $354 - 6.91 \times \text{age} + \text{PA} \times (9.36 \times \text{weight} + 726 \times \text{height})$

where PA is the physical activity coefficient:

PA = 1.00 for sedentary

PA = 1.12 for low active

PA = 1.27 for active

PA = 1.45 for very active

EER for Pregnancy

EER = EER for age + pregnancy energy needs[b] + tissue deposition

1st trimester = EER for age + 0

2nd trimester = EER for age + 160 + 180

3rd trimester = EER for age + 272 + 180

EER for Lactation

EER = EER for age + milk energy output[c] − weight loss[d]

1st 6 months = EER for age + 500 − 170

2nd 6 months = EER for age + 400 − 0

Abbreviations: EER = Estimated Energy Requirement; TEE = Total Energy Expenditure; PA = physical activity coefficient; age is in years; height is in meters; weight is in kilograms.

[a]Tissue deposition represents the energy cost of growth during infancy, childhood, adolescence, and pregnancy as measured in kilocalories.

[b]Pregnancy energy needs represents the additional energy required to support the metabolic demands of pregnancy.

[c]Milk energy output represents the energy needed to produce the milk during lactation. Milk output is somewhat greater in the first 6 months than in the second 6 months of breastfeeding.

[d]Weight loss represents an average decline in EER of 170 kcal/day that well-nourished lactating women experience during the first 6 months postpartum, resulting in an average weight loss of 0.8 kg/month.

Source: Panel on Macronutrients, Panel on the Definition of Dietary Fiber, Subcommittee on Upper Reference Levels of Nutrients, Subcommittee on Interpretation and Uses of Dietary Reference Intakes, Standing Committee on the Scientific Evaluation of Dietary Reference Intakes. 2002. *Dietary reference intakes for energy, carbohydrate, fiber, fat, fatty acids, cholesterol, protein, and amino acids.* Washington, DC: National Academies Press.

predict the mean REE for a given group of people with a rather high degree of accuracy, the accuracy of that same equation in predicting one individual's value may be quite low. Thus, remember that even the best prediction equation provides only an approximation of an individual's energy requirement.

Estimated Energy Requirement Equations

The National Academy of Sciences, as part of its ongoing work in developing the Dietary Reference Intakes (DRIs) (discussed in Chapter 2), has developed a set of prediction equations to calculate the Estimated Energy Requirement (EER).[41] These equations are shown in Table 7.9. The EER is defined as the average dietary energy intake that is predicted to maintain energy balance in a healthy person of a defined age, gender, weight, height, and level of physical activity consistent with good health.[41] For infants, children, and adolescents the EER includes the energy needed for a desirable level of physical activity and optimal growth, maturation, and development at an age- and gender-appropriate rate that is consistent with good health, including maintenance of a healthy body weight and appropriate body composition. For females who are pregnant or lactating, the EER includes the energy needed for physical activity, maternal and fetal development, and lactation at a rate consistent with good health.[41]

The EER is calculated using a series of prediction equations developed by the DRI Committee for healthy-weight individuals age 0 to 100 years based on the 24-hour total energy expenditures of more than 1200 subjects measured using the doubly labeled water technique.[41] Using measured 24-hour total energy expenditure data obtained from these healthy-weight subjects, the DRI Committee developed a series of regression equations that best predict the energy requirement of healthy-weight individuals using such variables as age, gender, life stage (pregnant or lactating), body weight, height, and physical activity level. As shown in Table 7.9, EER equations have been developed for infants and young children of both sexes age 0 to 35 months, males and females age 3 to 8 years, males and females age 9 to 18 years, males and females age 19 years and older, and females who are pregnant or lactating. Except for those for infants and young children age 0 to 35 months, the equations contain a physical activity coefficient (PA) that represents one of four different categories of physical activity level: sedentary, low active, active, and very active. Energy expenditure at the sedentary level includes basal energy expenditure, the thermic effect of food, and physical activities required for independent living. A low active lifestyle would be roughly equivalent to the energy expended by a 70 kg (154 lb) adult walking 2.2 miles per day at a rate of 3 to 4 miles per hour (or an equivalent amount of energy expended in other activities) in addition to the activities necessary for independent living. An active lifestyle would be roughly equivalent to the energy expended by a 70 kg (154 lb) adult walking 7 miles per day at a rate of 3 to 4

miles per hour in addition to the activities related to independent living. Energy expenditure by a very active lifestyle would be equivalent to walking 17 miles per day in addition to the activities of independent living. The extra energy needed for growth during infancy, childhood, adolescence, and pregnancy is included in an allowance referred to as tissue deposition. During pregnancy, metabolic rate is also increased because of the energy requirements of the uterus and fetus and the increased work of the heart and lungs. During lactation, extra energy is needed to support milk production, which is somewhat greater in the first six months of breastfeeding than in the second six months. Because most women lose an average of 0.8 kg per month in the first six months postpartum (i.e., after delivery), EER is, on average, 170 kcal per day less.[41]

EER equations apply only to persons having a healthy weight, and EER values have not been established for persons who are overweight or obese.[41] Instead, the DRI Committee has developed a separate set of equations for calculating total energy expenditure (TEE) for the maintenance of weight for adults age 19 years and older who are overweight (BMI between 25.0 kg/m² and 29.9 kg/m²) and or obese (BMI ≥ 30.0 kg/m²), and an additional set was developed for children and adolescents age 3 to 18 years who are overweight (a BMI for age and sex ≥ 95th percentile).[41] These equations are shown in Table 7.10. The DRI Committee adopted the definition of healthy weight for adults (age 19 years and older) used by the Dietary Guidelines for Americans, which is a BMI ≥ 18.5 kg/m² but ≤ 24.9 kg/m². Healthy weight for persons age 2 to 18 years is defined as a BMI that is > 5th percentile but < 85th percentile of BMI for age and sex, a concept discussed at length in Chapter 6. The equations developed for overweight or obese persons shown in Table 7.10 allow calculation of the TEE necessary for weight maintenance using the variables of gender, age, weight, height, and physical activity level. If weight loss is desired, a recommended approach is to reduce energy intake by 500 to 1000 kilocalories less than that needed for maintenance and to increase energy expenditure by engaging in moderate physical activity for approximately 60 minutes per day on most days of the week.

Energy Expenditure in Disease and Injury

Surgery, trauma, infection, burns, and various diseases can cause 24-hour energy expenditure and urinary nitrogen excretion to increase markedly.[50,51] The effect of various stresses on REE in hospitalized patients is shown in Figure 7.24.[50] The normal range of resting energy expenditure is represented by the light horizontal bar across the middle of the figure. Starvation in the unstressed person results in a hypometabolic state (below average metabolic rate) as the body attempts to conserve its energy reserves. The time when peak energy expenditure occurs in

TABLE 7.10	**Equations for Calculating Total Energy Expenditure (TEE) for Weight Maintenance in Kilocalories per Day for Overweight and Obese Adults and for Overweight Children and Adolescents**

TEE for Overweight and Obese Males Age 19 Years and Older

TEE = 1086 − 10.1 × age + PA × (13.7 × weight + 416 × height)

where PA is the physical activity coefficient:

    PA = 1.00 for sedentary

    PA = 1.12 for low active

    PA = 1.29 for active

    PA = 1.59 for very active

TEE for Overweight and Obese Females Age 19 Years and Older

TEE = 448 − 7.95 × age + PA × (11.4 × weight + 619 × height)

where PA is the physical activity coefficient:

    PA = 1.00 for sedentary

    PA = 1.16 for low active

    PA = 1.27 for active

    PA = 1.44 for very active

TEE for Overweight Males Age 3–18 Years

TEE = 114 − 50.9 × age + PA × (19.5 × weight + 1161.4 × height)

where PA is the physical activity coefficient:

    PA = 1.00 for sedentary

    PA = 1.12 for low active

    PA = 1.24 for active

    PA = 1.45 for very active

TEE for Overweight Females Age 3–18 Years

TEE = 389 − 41.2 × age + PA × (15.0 × weight + 701.6 × height)

where PA is the physical activity coefficient:

    PA = 1.00 for sedentary

    PA = 1.18 for low active

    PA = 1.35 for active

    PA = 1.60 for very active

Abbreviations: TEE = Total Energy Expenditure; PA = physical activity coefficient; age is in years; height is in meters; weight is in kilograms. In persons age 19 years and older overweight is defined as a BMI between 25.0 kg/m² and 29.9 kg/m² and obese is defined as a BMI ≥ 30.0 kg/m². In persons age 3–18 years, overweight is defined as a BMI for age and sex ≥ 95th percentile.[54]

Source: Panel on Macronutrients, Panel on the Definition of Dietary Fiber, Subcommittee on Upper Reference Levels of Nutrients, Subcommittee on Interpretation and Uses of Dietary Reference Intakes, Standing Committee on the Scientific Evaluation of Dietary Reference Intakes. 2002. *Dietary reference intakes for energy, carbohydrate, fiber, fat, fatty acids, cholesterol, protein, and amino acids.* Washington, DC: National Academies Press.

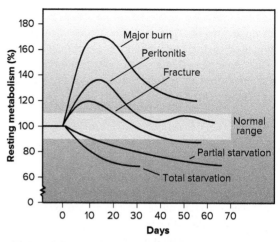

Figure 7.24   **Effect of various stresses on resting energy expenditure in hospitalized patients.**

Source: Long CL, Schaffel N, et al. 1979. Metabolic response to injury and illness: Estimation of energy and protein needs from indirect calorimetry and nitrogen balance. *Journal of Parenteral and Enteral Nutrition* 3:452–456.

A common approach to estimating a patient's energy needs is to calculate the 24-hour energy expenditure, as outlined in Box 7.1, and then to increase this value by the appropriate injury factors shown in Table 7.11. This second step is necessary because the equations developed by Harris-Benedict, the DRI equations for calculating EER, and the World Health Organization equations are all based on data collected from healthy subjects.

Of all the conditions in Table 7.11, burns have the greatest potential for increasing energy expenditure.[52–56] When caloric intake fails to adequately meet energy

TABLE 7.11	**Injury Factors Used to Account for the Thermic Effect of Disease and Injury**

Condition	Injury Factor*
Minor surgery	1.0–1.1
Major surgery	1.1–1.3
Mild infection	1.0–1.2
Moderate infection	1.2–1.4
Severe infection	1.4–1.8
Skeletal or blunt trauma	1.2–1.4
Skeletal or head trauma (steroid treated)	1.6–1.8
Burns involving ≤ 20% BSA†	1.2–1.5
Burns involving 20% to 40% BSA	1.5–1.8
Burns involving > 40% BSA	1.8–2.0

Source: Long CL. 1984. The energy and protein requirements of the critically ill patient. In Wright RA, Heymsfield SB, eds. *Nutritional assessment.* Boston: Blackwell Scientific Publications.

*Multiply the predicted resting energy expenditure adjusted for the thermic effect of food and the thermic effect of exercise by the appropriate injury factor to arrive at an estimate of the patient's 24-hour energy expenditure. The range in values allows adjustment depending on the severity of the disease or injury.

†BSA = body surface area.

response to stress varies, depending on the severity of the illness or injury, and energy needs gradually return to normal during recovery. Figure 7.24 represents average values for both males and females of varying ages and body sizes and assumes no secondary complications, which can prolong periods of increased energy needs. The clinical course of individual patients can be expected to vary somewhat from these average values.

Box 7.1 **Estimating Resting Energy Expenditure (REE) and 24-Hour Energy Expenditure Using the World Health Organization (WHO) Equations**

Using the WHO equations in Table 7.7, the Harris-Benedict equations in Table 7.7, or the DRI equations for calculating REE in Table 7.8 is quite easy. As an example, take a 23-year-old female with a body weight of 64 kg (141 lb). Begin by selecting the proper equation for the subject's sex and age. Then calculate the predicted REE using the appropriate WHO equation.

$$REE = 14.7\,W + 496$$
$$REE = (14.7 \times 64) + 496$$
$$REE = 941 + 496$$
$$REE = 1437\ kcal$$

To arrive at an estimate of 24-hour energy expenditure, the value for REE (1437 kcal) is then multiplied by an activity factor (Table 7.9) that accounts for the thermic effect of exercise—the calories expended during physical activity. Assuming this person has an activity level at the low end of the average activity category, the activity factor of 1.2 will be used.

$$1437\ kcal \times 1.2 = 1724\ kcal$$

This gives an estimated 24-hour energy expenditure of 1724 kcal. Assuming that the subject is 168 cm (66 in.) tall, how do these values compare with those obtained by using the DRI equations for calculating EER?

expenditure in burn patients, weight loss, delayed wound healing, and poor clinical outcome will result. A number of equations or approaches have been proposed for estimating the energy and protein needs of burn patients.[53–56] Several of these are shown in Table 7.12. An approach to estimating the energy requirements of a burn patient is to simply calculate his or her REE using the WHO RMR equation and then increase this value by an injury factor (1.6 to 2.2) and possibly an activity factor to account for energy the patient expends while in therapy.[57] A very simple approach, shown in Table 7.12, is merely to double the REE derived from the Harris-Benedict equation.[52]

The equations developed by Curreri and coworkers, shown in Table 7.12, have been frequently used for calculating the energy needs of burned patients.[55,58] In these equations, energy requirements for patients of different ages are estimated by adding resting energy expenditure (REE) as predicted by the Harris-Benedict equation to the product of the percent of body surface area burned (%BSAB) and an age-dependent constant. In the originally published equation for adults, resting or basal energy requirement was estimated by multiplying the patient's body weight in kilograms by 25.[55] This is based on the observation that REE is approximately 25 kcal/kg of body weight. The Curreri

TABLE 7.12	**Equations for Estimating the Energy Requirements of Patients with Burns***
Age	**Equation**
Allard[56]	
Adults	kcal = –4343 + (10.5 × %BSAB) + (0.23 CI) + (0.84 REE) + (114 T) – (4.5 PBD)
Cunningham[52]	
0–3 yr	kcal = 2 × REE
Curreri[55]	
0–1 yr	kcal = REE + (15 × %BSAB)
1–3 yr	kcal = REE + (25 × %BSAB)
4–15 yr	kcal = REE + (40 × %BSAB)
16–59 yr	kcal = REE + (40 × %BSAB)
≥ 60 yr	kcal = REE + (65 × %BSAB)
Hildreth[54]	
Child	kcal = (1800 × m² BSA) + (2200 × m² BSAB)
Adolescent	kcal = (1500 × m² BSA) + (1500 × m² BSAB)
Long[50]	
Any age	kcal = REE × injury factor × activity factor

*kcal = estimated daily energy requirement in kilocalories; REE = resting energy expenditure as predicted by the Harris-Benedict equation; BSA = body surface area in m²; BSAB = body surface area burned in m²; %BSAB = percent of body surface area burned; CI = the number of kilocalories the patient received in the previous 24 hours; T = average rectal temperature of the previous 24 hours in degrees Celsius; PBD = the number of postburn days prior to the day the energy requirements are calculated; see Table 7.7 for activity factors and Table 7.6 for injury factors.

equations have the advantage of linking energy estimates with percent of body surface area burned. However, studies comparing the energy needs of severely burned patients as measured by indirect calorimetry and as estimated by the Curreri equations show that the equations tend to overestimate energy needs, resulting in overfeeding.[59] One explanation for this may be that recent advances in the management of severe burns result in less of a hypermetabolic response to the thermal injury as when the Curreri formula was originally developed in the early 1970s.[55]

The equation in Table 7.12 developed by Allard and coworkers[53] has been shown to fairly accurately predict the energy requirements of burned patients, compared with energy expenditure measured by indirect calorimetry. Referred to as the "Toronto formula," it was derived by multiple-regression analysis of data collected from 23 patients with a mean burned body surface area of 39%.[56] Energy requirement is estimated by beginning with a negative value of 4343 kcal and adding or subtracting to this value various products. The equation requires information on the percent body surface area burned (estimated on admission and corrected where amputation was performed); the number of kilocalories the patient received in the previous 24 hours, including all dextrose infusions, and parenteral and enteral feedings; REE calculated from the Harris-Benedict equation; the average of the hourly rectal temperatures from the previous 24 hours expressed in degrees Celsius; and the number of postburn days as of the previous day. The Toronto formula has been shown to more closely predict the energy requirements of severely burned patients than the modified Curreri or the practice of doubling REE derived from the Harris-Benedict equation, both of which tend to overestimate energy requirements.[53] Energy expenditure predictions derived from the Toronto formula have also been shown to compare favorably with measured resting energy expenditure of clinically stable, mechanically ventilated burn patients.[60] The Toronto formula is unique in that it considers the thermic effect of food (which tends to be elevated in critically ill patients), the increased metabolic rate caused by elevations in body temperature, and the gradual fall in metabolic rate with time.

Energy Needs: Estimated or Measured?

Estimates of energy expenditure obtained from equations are just that—estimates. They are approximate and should be used only as rough guidelines.[49] However, for most hospital patients, estimates of energy expenditure are acceptable in providing the care their conditions demand. For these patients, the time and financial costs of measuring energy needs are not warranted. However, in some instances, it may be cost-effective to determine energy expenditure rather than to rely solely on estimates.[39,49] The use of total parenteral nutrition (TPN) is quite expensive; not only are the solutions themselves costly but their administration requires a considerable time investment by nurses, pharmacists, physicians,

and registered dietitians. Basing the administration of TPN solutions on measured energy expenditure may help prevent excessive use of TPN. Not only is undernutrition associated with increased morbidity and mortality, but overnutrition can have negative clinical outcomes as well. Measuring energy expenditure allows administration of TPN solutions to be based on physiologic need and promotes patient recovery. Thus, the cost of indirect calorimetry may be justified by both improved patient care and savings resulting from more judicious use of costly resources, such as TPN solutions and staff time and savings to the hospital because of shorter hospital stays.[49] In the case of burn patients, routine use of indirect calorimetry allows tailoring of nutritional support and is valuable in the early detection of significant undernutrition or overnutrition.[57] Considering the seriousness of thermal injury and the importance of nutritional support in its management, measuring the energy expenditure of severely burned patients should be standard practice.[57]

DETERMINING PROTEIN REQUIREMENTS

Protein serves as a functional component of body tissues and enzymes and as a fuel source. The protein needs of healthy, nonpregnant, nonlactating adults generally can be met with an intake of 0.8 g/kg body weight per day. In trauma or burn patients, protein catabolism increases markedly, as does protein loss, as indicated by urinary nitrogen excretion. Nitrogen makes up about 16% of protein and serves as a convenient way of measuring protein intake and losses.

Protein Losses in Disease and Injury

Figure 7.25 shows how urinary nitrogen losses vary over time among different conditions.[50] The normal range of

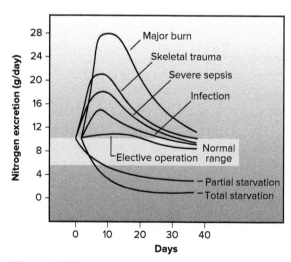

Figure 7.25   **Effect of various stresses on urinary nitrogen excretion in hospitalized patients.**

Source: Long CL, Schaffel N, et al. 1979. Metabolic response to injury and illness: Estimation of energy and protein needs from indirect calorimetry and nitrogen balance. *Journal of Parenteral and Enteral Nutrition* 3:452–456.

urinary nitrogen loss is represented by the figure's light horizontal bar. Partial or total starvation in the unstressed person often results in *reduced* nitrogen losses as the body attempts to spare protein. The opposite is true in trauma or burn patients, even though their energy and protein intakes often are reduced substantially. Trauma and burns are usually associated with increased protein catabolism and urinary nitrogen losses, although the patient's nutritional status before injury can affect the extent of loss. All other factors being equal, nitrogen losses after trauma and thermal injury are less in depleted persons and the elderly. Under these conditions, the protein reserves may be so depleted that the response is blunted or may not even be observed.

As with changes in REE seen in response to injury and illness (Figure 7.24), urinary nitrogen losses vary in degree and duration with the severity of the injury, may take several days after onset of the disease or trauma to reach their peak, and gradually return to the normal range.

Estimating Protein Needs

In practice, there is no single best method for conclusively determining the amount of protein that should be in the diet of patients suffering from trauma, burns, and other injuries. The protein requirements of these patients can only be estimated. Three approaches are commonly used—basing protein intake on body weight, caloric intake, or nitrogen balance.[50] Table 7.13 provides some suggested ranges of protein intake per kilogram of body weight for various injuries and situations. If the energy needs of a patient are reasonably well defined, these can be used to estimate protein requirements. Some authorities consider 1 g of nitrogen (or 6.25 g of protein) for every

TABLE 7.13	Suggested Ranges of Protein Intake per Kilogram of Body Weight During Peak Catabolic Response for Various Injuries and Conditions in Adults

Stress Level	Condition	Protein (g/kg/d)
Normal	Healthy	0.8
Mild	Minor surgery, mild infection	0.8–1.2
Moderate	Major surgery, moderate infection, moderate skeletal trauma	1.2–1.8
Severe	Severe infection, multiple injuries, severe trauma, major burns	1.6–2.2

Source: Ireton-Jones CS, Hasse JM. 1992. Comprehensive nutritional assessment: The dietitian's contribution to the team effort. *Nutrition* 8:75–81; Long CL. 1984. The energy and protein requirements of the critically ill patient. In Wright RA, Heymsfield SB, eds. *Nutritional assessment.* Boston: Blackwell Scientific Publications; Waymack JP, Herndon DN. 1992. Nutritional support of the burned patient. *World Journal of Surgery* 16:80–86; Mentegut WJ, Lowry SF. 1993. Nutrition in burn patients. *Seminars in Nephrology* 13:400–408.

150 nonprotein kilocalories to be an adequate daily protein intake for critically ill adults and adults with burns when the percent body surface area burned is ≤ 10.[50] When injuries are very severe or the burn involves more than 10% body surface area, 1 g of nitrogen is recommended for every 100 nonprotein kilocalories.

Nitrogen balance (discussed in Chapter 9) involves 24-hour measurement of protein intake and an estimate of nitrogen losses where N Bal = nitrogen balance; protein intake = protein intake in g/24 hours; and UUN = urine urea nitrogen in g/24 hours.

$$N\ Bal = \frac{Protein\ intake}{6.25} - UUN - 4$$

Protein intake is divided by 6.25 to arrive at an estimate of nitrogen intake. Because protein is 16% nitrogen, dividing grams of protein by 6.25 gives you grams of nitrogen. Nitrogen loss is *estimated* by measuring urine urea nitrogen (which accounts for 85% to 90% of total urinary nitrogen) and subtracting a constant (4 g in the equation, although this value can vary from 2 to 4 g) to account for dermal, fecal, and nonurea nitrogen losses, which cannot be easily measured.[61,62]

Measuring total urinary nitrogen (TUN) is more difficult, expensive, and time consuming than measuring urinary urea nitrogen (UUN). Consequently, estimating TUN from measurements of UUN is standard practice. However, some researchers question the appropriateness of this practice, suggesting that in trauma and burn patients UUN represents only about 65% of TUN, as opposed to 80% to 90% in healthy persons.[63,64] They suggest that TUN should be measured directly rather than estimated from UUN. Other researchers report that estimates of TUN based on UUN are significantly different from direct measures of TUN but that the differences are small and clinically insignificant to justify the added expense and trouble of directly measuring TUN.[65]

Despite the problems associated with measuring protein intake and nitrogen excretion, nitrogen balance is generally accepted as an appropriate and cost-effective way of monitoring the protein status of burn and other critically ill patients.[50,59,63,65] Although not an exact indicator of nutritional adequacy, nitrogen balance studies serve as an excellent guide to nutritional support when used in conjunction with changes in body weight and energy expenditure measured by indirect calorimetry.[65] However, even if more protein is provided a patient than is calculated from losses in the urine, nitrogen balance is difficult to achieve in the early stage of severe trauma and thermal injury. The catabolism associated with the stress of trauma and thermal injury, as well as the atrophy of muscle caused by immobilization and disuse, results in considerable urinary nitrogen losses. Given time and the provision of adequate energy and protein, the patient gradually will begin to retain more protein than is excreted and will replace lost body protein.[50,59]

SUMMARY

1. Malnutrition is common and associated with many adverse health, social, mental, and financial outcomes.

2. Health–care organizations should take specific actions to address prevention or treatment of acute or chronic disease-related malnutrition in hospitalized patients to improve the quality of patient care, improve clinical outcomes, and reduce costs.

3. The Academy of Nutrition and Dietetics (Academy) and the American Society for Parenteral and Enteral Nutrition (A.S.P.E.N.) recommend that a standardized set of diagnostic characteristics be used to identify and document adult malnutrition in routine clinical practice. The identification of two or more of the following six characteristics is recommended for diagnosing malnutrition: insufficient energy intake, weight loss, loss of muscle mass, loss of subcutaneous fat, localized or generalized fluid accumulation that may sometimes mask weight loss, and diminished functional status as measured by hand-grip strength.

4. Aging is accompanied by numerous physiologic changes that increase the odds for progressive undernutrition, which often goes undiagnosed. Early detection of malnutrition is important and is an important component of comprehensive geriatric assessment (CGA) (evaluation of physical health, mental health, social and economic status, and functional status).

5. Malnutrition assessment, depending on the patient and circumstances, can involve a variety of anthropometric measurements, including estimation of height from knee height, ulna length, half-arm span, and demispan; calf circumference to estimate BMI category; and various arm anthropometric measures to identify undernutrition, including the mid-upper arm circumference, mid-upper arm muscle circumference, and mid-upper arm muscle area. The hand-grip test is recommended to determine weakness and potential sarcopenia.

6. The quick, simple, and valid pediatric nutrition screening tool (PNST) consists of four simple questions: Has the child unintentionally lost weight lately? Has the child had poor weight gain over the last few months? Has the child been eating/feeding less in the last few weeks? Is the child obviously underweight/significantly overweight?

7. Energy needs are based on an individual's 24-hour energy expenditure, which is determined by resting energy expenditure, the thermic effect of food, energy expended in physical activity, and whether disease or injury is present. Resting energy expenditure is the largest component of 24-hour energy expenditure.

8. Twenty-four-hour energy expenditure can be determined through indirect calorimetry or roughly approximated from a variety of equations. Indirect calorimetry involves measurement of the body's oxygen consumption and carbon dioxide production and often uses a computerized metabolic monitor. The energy expenditure of patients usually is estimated. In critically ill persons or those receiving parenteral or enteral feedings, indirect calorimetry may be preferable to estimating energy expenditure.

9. Surgery, trauma, infection, burns, and various diseases can cause 24-hour energy expenditure and urinary excretion of nitrogen to increase markedly. Energy expenditure in patients can be obtained through indirect calorimetry or estimates using a variety of equations.

10. The degree and duration of increased protein catabolism following injury vary with the trauma's severity. Protein catabolism may take several days to peak before gradually returning to normal. Recommended protein intake can be based on nitrogen balance, body weight, or energy intake.

REFERENCES

1. Kubrak C, Jensen L. 2007. Malnutrition in acute care patients: A narrative review. *International Journal of Nursing Studies* 44:1036–1054.

2. Bally MR, Blaser Yildirim PZ, Bounoure L, Gloy VL, Mueller B, Briel M, Schuetz P. 2016. Nutritional support and outcomes in malnourished medical inpatients: A systematic review and meta-analysis. *JAMA Internal Medicine* 176:43–53.

3. Guenter P, Jensen G, Patel V, Miller S, Mogensen KM, Malone A,

Corkins M, Hamilton C, DiMaria-Ghalili RA. 2015. Addressing disease-related malnutrition in hospitalized patients: A call for a national goal. *The Joint Commission Journal on Quality and Patient Safety* 41:469–473.

4. White JV, Guenter P, Jensen G, Malone A, Schofield M; Academy Malnutrition Work Group; A.S.P.E.N. Malnutrition Task Force; A.S.P.E.N. Board of Directors. 2012. Consensus statement: Academy of Nutrition and Dietetics and American Society for Parenteral and Enteral Nutrition: Characteristics recommended for the identification and documentation of adult malnutrition (undernutrition). *JPEN Journal of Parenteral and Enteral Nutrition* 36:275–283.

5. Sauer AC, Alish CJ, Strausbaugh K, West K, Quatrara B. 2016. Nurses needed: Identifying malnutrition in hospitalized older adults. *NursingPlus Open* 2:21–25.

6. Moreira NC, Krausch-Hofmann S, Matthys C, Vereecken C, Vanhauwaert E, Declercq A, Bekkering GE, Duyck J. 2016. Risk factors for malnutrition in older adults: A systematic review of the literature based on longitudinal data. *Advanced Nutrition* 7:507–522.

7. Koren-Hakim T, Weiss A, Hershkovitz A, Otzrateni I, Anbar R, Gross Nevo RF, Schlesinger A, Frishman S, Salai M, Beloosesky Y. 2016. Comparing the adequacy of the MNA-SF, NRS-2002 and MUST nutritional tools in assessing malnutrition in hip fracture operated elderly patients. *Clinical Nutrition* 35:1053–1058.

8. Donini LM, Poggiogalle E, Molfino A, Rosano A, Lenzi A, Rossi Fanelli F, Muscaritoli M. 2016. Mini-Nutritional Assessment, Malnutrition Universal Screening Tool, and Nutrition Risk Screening Tool for the nutritional evaluation of older nursing home residents. *Journal of the American Medical Directors Association* 17:959.e11–8.

9. Christner S, Ritt M, Volkert D, Wirth R, Sieber CC, Gaßmann KG. 2016. Evaluation of the nutritional status of older hospitalized geriatric patients: A comparative analysis of a Mini Nutritional Assessment (MNA) version and the Nutritional Risk Screening (NRS 2002). *Journal of Human Nutrition and Dietetics* 29:704–713.

10. Vellas B, Villars H, Abellan G, Soto ME, Rolland Y, Guigoz Y, Morley JE, Chumlea W, Salva A, Rubenstein LZ, Garry P. Overview of the MNA—Its history and challenges. 2006. *The Journal of Nutrition, Health, and Aging* 10:456–463.

11. Rolland Y, Perrin A, Gardette V, Filhol N, Vellas B. 2012. Screening older people at risk of malnutrition or malnourished using the Simplified Nutritional Appetite Questionnaire (SNAQ): A comparison with the Mini-Nutritional Assessment (MNA) tool. *Journal of the American Medical Directors Association* 13:31–34.

12. Kaiser MJ, Bauer JM, Ramsch C, Uter W, Guigoz Y, Cederholm T, Thomas DR, Anthony P, Charlton KE, Maggio M, Tsai AC, Grathwohl D, Vellas B, Sieber CC, MNA-International Group. 2009. Validation of the Mini Nutritional Assessment short-form (MNA-SF): A practical tool for identification of nutritional status. *The Journal of Nutrition, Health & Aging* 13:782–788.

13. da Silva Fink J, Daniel de Mello P, Daniel de Mello E. 2015. Subjective global assessment of nutritional status—A systematic review of the literature. *Clinical Nutrition* 34:785–792.

14. Kondrup J, Allison SP, Elia M, Vellas B, Plauth M; Educational and Clinical Practice Committee, European Society of Parenteral and Enteral Nutrition (ESPEN). 2003. ESPEN guidelines for nutrition screening 2002. *Clinical Nutrition* 22:415–421.

15. van Bokhorst-de van der Schueren MA, Guaitoli PR, Jansma EP, de Vet HC. 2014. Nutrition screening tools: Does one size fit all? A systematic review of screening tools for the hospital setting. *Clinical Nutrition* 33:39–58.

16. Diekmann R, Winning K, Uter W, Kaiser MJ, Sieber CC, Volkert D, Bauer JM. 2013. Screening for malnutrition among nursing home residents—A comparative analysis of the Mini Nutritional Assessment, the nutritional risk screening, and the malnutrition universal screening tool. *The Journal of Nutrition, Health, & Aging* 17:326–331.

17. Webster-Grandy J, Madden A, Holdsworth M. 2012. *Oxford handbook of nutrition and dietetics,* 2nd ed. New York: Oxford University Press.

18. Chumlea WC. 1988. Methods of nutritional anthropometric assessment for special groups. In Lohman TG, Roche AF, Martorell R (eds.), *Anthropometric standardization reference manual.* Champaign, IL: Human Kinetics Books.

19. Kruizenga HM, Seidell JC, de Vet HC, Wierdsma NJ, van Bokhorst-de van der Schueren MA. 2005. Development and validation of a hospital screening tool for malnutrition: The short nutritional assessment questionnaire (SNAQ). *Clinical Nutrition* 24:75–82.

20. Wijnhoven HA, Schilp J, van Bokhorst-de van der Schueren MA, de Vet HC, Kruizenga HM, Deeg DJ, Ferrucci L, Visser M. 2012. Development and validation of criteria for determining undernutrition in community-dwelling older men and women: The Short Nutritional Assessment Questionnaire 65+. *Clinical Nutrition* 31:351–358.

21. Sheikh JI, Yesavage JA. 1986. Geriatric Depression Scale (GDS): Recent evidence and development of a shorter version. *Clinical Gerontology: A Guide to Assessment and Intervention.* New York: The Haworth Press, 165–173.

22. Bowling A, Hankins M, Windle G, Bilotta C, Grant R. 2013. A short measure of quality of life in older age: The performance of the brief Older People's Quality of Life questionnaire (OPQOL-brief). *Archives of Geriatrics and Gerontology,* 56:181–187.

23. Russell MK. Functional assessment of nutrition status. 2015. *Nutrition in Clinical Practice* 30:211–218.

24. Studenski SA, Peters KW, Alley DE, Cawthon PM, McLean RR, Harris TB, Ferrucci L, Guralnik JM, Fragala MS, Kenny AM, Kiel DP, Kritchevsky SB, Shardell MD, Dam TT, Vassileva MT. 2014. The FNIH sarcopenia project: Rationale, study description, conference recommendations, and final estimates. *The Journals of Gerontolgy. Series A, Biological Sciences and Medical Sciences* 69:547–558.

25. Alley DE, Shardell MD, Peters KW, McLean RR, Dam TT, Kenny AM, et al. 2014. Grip strength cutpoints for the identification of clinically relevant weakness. *The Journals of Gerontolgy. Series A, Biological Sciences and Medical Sciences* 69:559–566.

26. Looker AC, Wang CY. 2015. *Prevalence of reduced muscle strength in older U.S. adults: United States, 2011–2012.* NCHS data brief, no 179. Hyattsville, MD: National Center for Health Statistics.

27. National Health and Nutrition Examination Survey (NHANES). 2011. *Muscle strength procedures manual.* https://www.cdc.gov/nchs/data/nhanes/nhanes_11_12/muscle_strength_proc_manual.pdf.

28. Secker DJ, Jeejheebhoy KN. 2012. How to perform Subjective Global Nutritional assessment in children. *Journal of the Academy of Nutrition and Dietetics* 112:424–431.

29. White M, Lawson K, Ramsey R, Dennis N, Hutchinson Z, Soh XY, Matsuyama M, Doolan A, Todd A, Elliott A, Bell K, Littlewood R. 2016. Simple nutrition screening tool for pediatric inpatients. *JPEN Journal of Parenteral and Enteral Nutrition* 40:392–398.

30. Madden AM, Smith S. 2016. Body composition and morphological assessment of nutritional status in adults: A review of anthropometric variables. *Journal of Human Nutrition and Dietetics* 29:7–25.

31. Sungurtekin H, Sungurtekin U, Oner O, Okke D. 2008. Nutrition assessment in critically ill patients. *Nutrition in Clinical Practice* 23:635–641.

32. Landi F, Russo A, Liperoti R, Pahor M, Tosato M, Capoluongo E, Bernabei R, Onder G. 2010. Midarm muscle circumference, physical performance and mortality: Results from the aging and longevity study in the Sirente geographic area (ilSIRENTE study). *Clinical Nutrition* 29:441–447.

33. Heymsfield SB, McManus C, Smith J, Stevens V, Nixon DW. 1982. Anthropometric measurement of muscle mass: Revised equations for calculating bone-free arm muscle area. *American Journal of Clinical Nutrition* 36:680–690.

34. Frisancho AR. 2008. *Anthropometric standards: An interactive nutritional reference of body size and body composition for children and adults*, 2nd ed. Ann Arbor: University of Michigan Press.

35. Bishop CW. 1984. Reference values for arm muscle area, arm fat area, subscapular skinfold thickness, and sum of skinfold thicknesses for American adults. *Journal of Parenteral and Enteral Nutrition* 8:515–522.

36. Addo OY, Himes JH, Zemel BS. Reference ranges for midupper arm circumference, upper arm muscle area, and upper arm fat area in US children and adolescents aged 1–20 y. *American Journal of Clinical Nutrition* (in press).

37. Becker P, Carney LN, Corkins MR, Monczka J, Smith E, Smith SE, Spear BA, White JV; Academy of Nutrition and Dietetics; American Society for Parenteral and Enteral Nutrition. 2015. Consensus statement of the Academy of Nutrition and Dietetics/American Society for Parenteral and Enteral Nutrition: Indicators recommended for the identification and documentation of pediatric malnutrition (undernutrition). *Nutrition in Clinical Practice* 30:147–161.

38. Sims AH, Danforth E. 1987. Expenditure and storage of energy in man. *Journal of Clinical Investigation* 79:1019–1025.

39. Fullmer S, Benson-Davies S, Earthman CP, Frankenfield DC, Gradwell E, Lee PS, Piemonte T, Trabulsi J. Evidence analysis library review of best practices for performing indirect calorimetry in healthy and non-critically ill individuals. *Journal of the Academy of Nutrition and Dietetics* 115:1417–1446.

40. Villablanca PA, Alegria JR, Mookadam F, Holmes DR Jr., Wright RS, Levine JA. 2015. Nonexercise activity thermogenesis in obesity management. *Mayo Clinic Proceedings* 90:509–519.

41. Panel on Macronutrients, Panel on the Definition of Dietary Fiber, Subcommittee on Upper Reference Levels of Nutrients, Subcommittee on Interpretation and Uses of Dietary Reference Intakes, Standing Committee on the Scientific Evaluation of Dietary Reference Intakes. 2002. *Dietary reference intakes for energy, carbohydrate, fiber, fat, fatty acids, cholesterol, protein, and amino acids.* Washington, DC: National Academies Press.

42. World Health Organization. 1985. *Energy and protein requirements. Report of a joint FAO/WHO/UNU expert consultation.* Technical Report Series 724. Geneva, Switzerland: World Health Organization.

43. Roza AM, Shizgal HM. 1984. The Harris Benedict equation reevaluated: Resting energy requirements and the body cell mass. *American Journal of Clinical Nutrition* 40:168–182.

44. Ravussin E, Lillioja S, Anderson TE, Christin L, Bogardus C. 1986. Determinants of 24-hour energy expenditure in man. Methods and results using a respiratory chamber. *The Journal of Clinical Investigation* 78:1568–1578.

45. Committee on Metabolic Monitoring for Military Field Applications, Standing Committee on Military Nutrition Research, Food and Nutrition Board. 2004. *Monitoring metabolic status: Predicting decrements in*

physiological and cognitive performance. Washington, DC: National Academies Press.

46. Seale JL, Rumpler WV, Moe PW. 1991. Description of a direct indirect room-sized calorimeter. *American Journal of Physiology* 260:E306–E320.

47. Ainslie PN, Reilly T, Westerterp KR. 2003. Estimating human energy expenditure: A review of techniques with particular reference to doubly labelled water. *Sports Medicine* 33:683–698.

48. Hills AP, Mokhtar N, Byrne NM. 2014. Assessment of physical activity and energy expenditure: An overview of objective measures. *Frontiers in Nutrition* 1:5.

49. Schlein KM, Coulter SP. 2014. Best practices for determining resting energy expenditure in critically ill adults. *Nutrition in Clinical Practice* 29:44–55.

50. Long CL. 1984. The energy and protein requirements of the critically ill patient. In Wright RA, Heymsfield SB (eds.), *Nutritional assessment.* Boston: Blackwell Scientific Publications.

51. Damask MC, Schwarz Y, Weissman C. 1987. Energy measurements and requirements of critically ill patients. *Critical Care Clinics* 3:71–96.

52. Cunningham JJ, Lydon MK, Russell WE. 1990. Calorie and protein provision for recovery from severe burns in infants and young children. *American Journal of Clinical Nutrition* 51:533–537.

53. Allard JP, Pichard C, Hoshino E, Stechison S, Fareholm L, Peters WJ, Jeejeebhoy KN. 1990. Validation of a new formula for calculating the energy requirements of burn patients. *Journal of Parenteral and Enteral Nutrition* 14:115–118.

54. Hildreth MA, Herndon DN, Parks KH. 1987. Evaluation of a caloric requirement formula in burned children treated with early excision. *Journal of Trauma* 27:188–189.

55. Curreri PW, Richmond D, Marvin J, Baxter CR. 1974. Dietary requirements of patients with major burns. *Journal of the American Dietetic Association* 65:415–417.

56. Allard JP, Jeejeebhoy KN, Whitwell J, Pashutinski L, Peters WJ. 1988. Factors influencing energy expenditure in patients with burns. *Journal of Trauma* 28:199–202.

57. Lee JO, Benjamin D, Herndon DN. 2005. Nutrition support strategies for severely burned patients. *Nutrition in Clinical Practice* 20:325–330.

58. Curreri PW. 1990. Assessing nutritional needs for the burned patient. *Journal of Trauma* 30(12 suppl):S20–S23.

59. Waymack JP, Herndon DN. 1992. Nutritional support of the burned patient. *World Journal of Surgery* 16:80–86.

60. Royall D, Fairholm L, Peters WJ, Jeejeebhoy KJ, Allard JP. 1994. Continuous measurement of energy expenditure in ventilated burn patients: An analysis. *Critical Care Medicine* 22:399–406.

61. Benjamin DR. 1989. Laboratory tests and nutritional assessment: Protein-energy status. *Pediatric Clinics of North America* 36:139–161.

62. Alcock NW. Laboratory tests for assessing nutritional status. In Shils ME, Olson JA, Shike M, Ross AC (eds.), *Modern nutrition in health and disease,* 9th ed. Baltimore, MD: Williams & Wilkins.

63. Konstantinides FN, Radmer WJ, Becker WK, Herman VK, Warren WE, Solem LD, Williams JB, Cerra FB. 1992. Inaccuracy of nitrogen balance determinations in thermal injury with calculated total urinary nitrogen. *Journal of Burn Care and Rehabilitation* 13:254–260.

64. Loder PB, Kee AJ, Horsburgh R, Jones M, Smith RC. 1989. Validity of urinary urea nitrogen as a measure of total urinary nitrogen in adult patients requiring parenteral nutrition. *Critical Care Medicine* 17:309–312.

65. Milner EA, Cioffi WG, Mason AD, McManus WF, Pruitt BA. 1993. Accuracy of urinary urea nitrogen for predicting total urinary nitrogen in thermally injured patients. *Journal of Parenteral and Enteral Nutrition* 17:414–416.

ASSESSMENT ACTIVITY 7.1

Arm Anthropometry and Height Estimation

Carefully review the instructions given in this chapter for measuring MUAC, MAMC, and MAMA and for estimating height from ulnar length, half-arm span, and demispan. Take these measurements on a classmate under the guidance of your instructor, and enter the data below. You will need a nonstretchable tape measure, a skinfold caliper, and a stadiometer to measure actual height.

1. MUAC (cm) _____

2. Triceps skinfold (mm) _____

3. MAMC (cm)_____

4. MAMA (cm^2) _____

5. Ulna length (cm)_____

    Estimated height (cm) _____

6. Half-arm span (cm) _____

    Estimated height (cm) _____

7. Demispan (cm)_____

    Estimated height (cm) _____

8. Actual height (cm)_____

ASSESSMENT ACTIVITY 7.2

Malnutrition Assessment with the Mini Nutritional Assessment Short Form

As described in this chapter, malnutrition is most commonly assessed with the six-component Mini Nutritional Assessment Short Form (MNA-SF).®

First download the MNA-SF form at http://www.mna-elderly.com.

In this activity, you will use the MNA-SF to assess potential malnutrition in an elderly participant. You can make this assessment with an elderly individual whom you know, or make arrangements to meet with a patient at an assisted living facility or nursing home.

The six components of the MNA-SF include appetite, weight loss, mobility, psychological stress, neuropsychological problems, and BMI. Score each component from 0 to 2 or 3, and calculate the total score (range of 0–14) and classify the individual as well nourished, at risk of malnutrition, and malnourished (scores of 12–14, 8–11, and 0–7 points, respectively).

Turn in the completed MNA-SF to your instructor.

NUTRITIONAL ASSESSMENT IN PREVENTION AND TREATMENT OF CARDIOVASCULAR DISEASE

STUDENT LEARNING OUTCOMES

After studying this chapter, the student will be able to:

1. Identify the risk factors for cardiovascular disease.

2. Describe the 2013 ACC/AHA Guidelines on the Treatment of Blood Cholesterol to Reduce Atherosclerotic Cardiovascular Risk in Adults.

3. Explain the rationale for primordial and primary prevention of CVD in children and adolescents.

4. Describe the Cardiovascular Health Integrated Lifestyle Diet (CHILD 1) recommended by the NHLBI's Expert Panel on Integrated Guidelines for Cardiovascular Health and Risk Reduction in Children and Adolescents.

5. Describe the American Heart Association's specific definitions for ideal, intermediate, and poor cardiovascular health for each of the seven metrics in adults and children/adolescents.

6. Discuss the various preanalytical factors that influence a person's usual serum cholesterol level.

7. Describe the evidence-based guidelines for the management of high blood pressure in adults (JNC8).

8. Discuss the various modifiable risk factors for hypertension.

9. Identify the most recent diagnostic criteria for diabetes as established by the American Diabetes Association.

10. Define glycated hemoglobin A1C and discuss how it is used to assess and manage glycemic control.

INTRODUCTION

The prominent role of diet and nutritional status in several leading causes of death for North Americans gives nutritional assessment an important role to play in disease prevention. This chapter addresses nutritional assessment as it relates to cardiovascular disease, with an emphasis on dyslipidemia, hypertension, and diabetes.

Several risk factors of cardiovascular disease, the leading cause of death for North Americans, are related to diet. Among these are elevated serum total and low-density-lipoprotein cholesterol (LDL-C), low levels of high-density-lipoprotein cholesterol (HDL-C), obesity, hypertension, and diabetes. This chapter also discusses issues in measuring lipid and lipoprotein levels, which apply to practically all measurements in nutritional assessment.

The individual and societal burden imposed by cardiovascular disease can be mitigated through risk factor modification, early diagnosis, and research into more effective preventive measures. Nutritional assessment plays a prominent role in each of these.

CARDIOVASCULAR DISEASE

The heart and its blood vessels can become diseased, a common health problem called cardiovascular disease (CVD). The three major types of CVD are coronary heart disease (CHD), cerebrovascular disease (stroke), and peripheral artery disease (PAD).[1] Coronary heart disease accounts for nearly half of all CVD deaths and occurs when the coronary arteries supplying the heart with oxygen and nutrients become narrowed and inelastic because of atherosclerosis. There is substantial scientific evidence that atherosclerosis begins in childhood with the formation of fatty streaks as lipids (primarily cholesterol and its esters) become deposited in macrophages (large phagocytic cells located within connective tissue) and smooth muscle cells within the inner lining of large elastic and muscular arteries. These early lesions do not disturb blood flow in the affected artery. As more lipid collects within the artery wall during adolescence and early adulthood, a fibrous plaque develops that projects into the channel, or lumen, of the artery, resulting in ischemia, or impaired blood flow. Ischemia within the heart muscle or myocardium can result in angina pectoris, which is chest pain caused by insufficient blood flow to the heart. If the impaired blood flow is severe enough, the tissues fed by the obstructed artery may die. This is known as an **infarction.** When this process affects the coronary arteries, a heart attack, or **myocardial infarction,** occurs. When the cerebral arteries are affected (known as cerebrovascular disease), a **stroke** results. Atherosclerotic changes within the aorta and iliac and femoral arteries can result in **peripheral artery disease.**

Although death rates for CVD have decreased in the United States and many other developed countries around the world, CVD is still the leading global cause of death, accounting for more than 17.3 million deaths per year, or 31% of all deaths.[1] Over 800,000 people in the United States die from heart disease, stroke, and other CVD each year, accounting for one of every three deaths. About 86 million Americans are living with some form of CVD or the after-effects of stroke. Nearly 750,000 people in the United States have heart attacks each year, and of those, about 116,000 die. Strokes are also common, with a yearly incidence of 795,000 people and 129,000 deaths. Each year, 356,500 people experience out-of-hospital cardiac arrests, and survival rates could be improved by knowing heart attack warning signs (Box 8.1) and providing prompt medical care.

Death rates for cardiovascular disease have fallen dramatically since the 1950s (72% decrease for heart disease, 80% decrease for stroke) (Figure 8.1).[1-4] This is one of the greatest health success stories of the past half-century, and is due to improvements in American health habits and medical care. Cardiovascular disease, however, still remains the leading cause of death in the United States and costs $317 billion per year in direct and indirect health-care expenditures.[1] Certain sections of the country, such as the southern half of the Mississippi River, have CVD death

---

Box 8.1   Heart Attack Warning Signs

- **Chest discomfort or pain:** Most heart attacks involve discomfort or pain in the center of the chest that lasts more than a few minutes or that goes away and comes back. It can feel like uncomfortable pressure, tightness, squeezing, burning, heaviness, or pain.
- **Pain or discomfort in other regions of the upper body:** Symptoms can include pain or discomfort in one or both arms, the back, neck, jaw, or stomach.

- **Shortness of breath:** This feeling often comes along with chest discomfort. But it can occur before the chest discomfort.
- **Other signs:** Symptoms may include sweating, nausea, or dizziness. If you or someone you're with has chest discomfort, especially with one or more of the other signs, don't wait longer than a few minutes (no more than five) before calling for help or going to a hospital.

Source: American Heart Association, www.heart.org

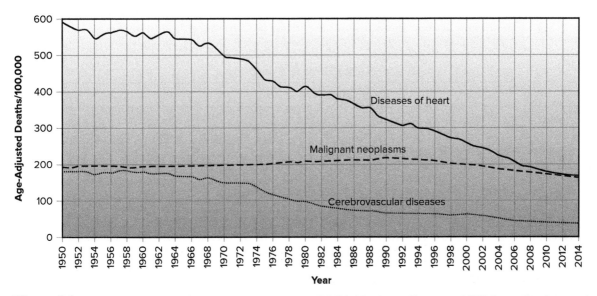

Figure 8.1   Death rates for cardiovascular disease have fallen 72% for heart disease and 80% for stroke since 1950.[1-4] This success is in sharp contrast to death rates for malignant neoplasms, which have fallen just 25% since peaking in 1990.

rates that are 10-fold higher than in central Colorado, for instance, and these differences exist because of contrasts in health behaviors and access to medical care.[5]

Cardiovascular Health Metrics

The American Heart Association's (AHA) 2020 goal is to reduce deaths from CVD and stroke by 20%.[1,6] As a part of this initiative, the AHA tracks seven key health factors and behaviors called "Life's Simple 7": not smoking, physical activity, healthy diet, body weight, and control of cholesterol, blood pressure and blood sugar.[1] Here are the ideal cardiovascular health metrics used by the AHA. They can be assessed for individuals at www.heart.org/mylifecheck/, and they require age, height, weight, gender, ethnicity, three measurements (blood pressure and two from a blood sample), and three lifestyle responses (smoking, physical activity, and dietary habits).

1. **Current smoking status:** Never or quit for more than one year
2. **Body mass index:** less than 25 kg/m² for adults or less than the 85th percentile for children and adolescents
3. **Physical activity:** at least 150 minutes per week of moderate or 75 minutes per week of vigorous for adults; 60 minutes per day of moderate to vigorous activity for children and adolescents
4. **Total cholesterol:** less than 200 mg/dL for adults; less than 170 mg/dL for children and adolescents
5. **Blood pressure:** less than 120/80 mm Hg for adults; less than the 90th percentile for children and adolescents
6. **Fasting plasma glucose:** less than 100 mg/dL for adults, children, and adolescents

7. **Health diet score:** meet four to five of these healthy diet goals (on the basis of a 2000-calorie/day diet):

   a. **Fruits and vegetables:** 4.5 cups per day or more
   b. **Fish:** two 3.5-ounce servings per week (preferably oily fish)
   c. **Fiber-rich whole grains:** three 1-ounce equivalents per day or more
   d. **Sodium:** less than 1500 mg per day
   e. **Sugar-sweetened beverages:** less than 450 calories (36 ounces) per week (one-fourth of a week's discretionary calories)

Tables 8.1 and 8.2 provide the specific definitions for ideal, intermediate, and poor cardiovascular health for each of the seven metrics in adults and children/adolescents. Body mass index (BMI) and blood pressure measurements for children/adolescents require using sex/height-specific percentile charts, and calculators are available:

- BMI-for-age percentile: https://nccd.cdc.gov/dnpabmi/calculator.aspx
- Blood pressure-for-age percentile: https://www.bcm.edu/bodycomplab/Flashapps/BPVAgeChartpage.html

Ideal cardiovascular health is defined by the AHA as the absence of clinically manifest CVD together with the simultaneous presence of optimal levels of all seven metrics.[1] Ideal cardiovascular health has become the new metric for population health since 2010, and many studies utilizing this standard have been published in all parts of the world.[1]

The top risk factor related to overall disease burden, according to data reviewed by the AHA, was suboptimal diet, followed by tobacco smoking, high BMI, raised

TABLE 8.1	Definitions of Poor, Intermediate, and Ideal Cardiovascular Health for Each Metric in the American Heart Association's 2020 Goals for Adults Aged ≥ 20 Years

	Level of Health for Each Metric		
	Poor	**Intermediate**	**Ideal**
Current smoking	Yes	Former ≤ 12 months	Never or quit > 12 months Never tried; never smoked whole cigarette
Body mass index (BMI)	≥ 30 kg/m²	25–29.9 kg/m²	18.5–25 kg/m²
Physical activity*	None	1–149 min/week moderate **or** 1–74 min/wk vigorous 1–149 min/wk moderate + 2x vigorous > 0 min < 60 min of moderate or vigorous every day	≥ 150 min/wk moderate **or** ≥ 75 min/wk vigorous ≥ 150 min/wk moderate + 2x vigorous ≥ 60 of moderate or vigorous every day
Healthy diet pattern, # components**	0–1	2–3	4–5
Total cholesterol	≥ 240 mg/dL	200–239 mg/dL or treated to goal	< 200 mg/dL
Blood pressure	SBP ≥ 140 mmHg or DBP ≥ 90 mmHg	SBP 120–139 mmHg **or** DBP 80–89 mmHg **or** treated to goal	< 120 mmHg/ < 80 mmHg
Fasting plasma glucose	≥ 126 mg/dL	100–125 mg/dL	< 100 mg/dL

DBP, diastolic blood pressure; SBP, systolic blood pressure

*Proposed questions to assess physical activity: (1) "On average, how many days per week do you engage in moderate to strenuous exercise (like a brisk walk)?" and (2) "On average, how many minutes do you engage in exercise at this level?"

**In the context of a healthy dietary pattern that is consistent with a Dietary Approaches to Stop Hypertension (DASH)–type eating pattern, to consume ≥ 4.5 cups/d of fruits and vegetables, ≥ 2 servings/wk of fish, and ≥ 3 servings/d of whole grains and no more than 36 oz/wk of sugar-sweetened beverages and 1500 mg/d of sodium.

TABLE 8.2	Poor, Intermediate, and Ideal Definitions: Health Metrics in Children and Adolescents

Metric	Poor	Intermediate	Ideal
Smoking status	Tried prior 30 days		Never tried; never smoked whole cigarette
Body mass index*	> 95th percentile	85–95th percentile	< 85th percentile
Physical activity level	None	> 0 and < 60 min/day moderate **or** vigorous activity every day	≥ 60 min/day moderate **or** vigorous activity every day
Healthy Diet Score	0–1 components	2–3 components	4–5 components
Total cholesterol	≥ 200 mg/dL	170–199 mg/dL	< 170 mg/dL
Blood pressure*	> 95th percentile	90–95th percentile	< 90th percentile
Fasting blood glucose	≥ 126 mg/dL	100–125 mg/dL	< 100 mg

*BMI and blood pressure require using sex/height-specific percentile charts. Calculators are available for determining the BMI-for-age percentile (https://nccd.cdc.gov/dnpabmi/calculator.aspx) and blood pressure-for-age percentile: https://www.bcm.edu/bodycomplab/Flashapps/BPVAgeChartpage.html.

blood pressure (i.e., hypertension), high fasting plasma glucose, and physical inactivity.[1] Risk of CVD mortality based on data from 45,000 individuals in the NHANES mortality study was 76% lower in individuals with six or seven ideal health metrics compared with zero ideal health metrics (Figure 8.2).[1,7] A meta-analysis showed that ideal cardiovascular health is associated with 80% lower risk of overall CVD, 69% lower risk of stroke, and 75% and 45% markedly lower risks for cardiovascular and all-cause mortality.[8]

Unfortunately, only a minority of Americans adhere to the ideal cardiovascular health metrics. NHANES data show that only 4.6% of adults have six or seven health metrics, and 18% have five or more, with children/adolescents at 11.2% and 45.5%, respectively.[1] Of the seven

health metrics, the lowest prevalence for ideal behavior is for the healthy dietary pattern, especially the standards for sodium, fruits and vegetables, and whole grains (Figure 8.3).

The AHA emphasizes that the development of childhood cardiovascular risk factors is accelerated in childhood, especially if accompanied by the onset of overweight/obesity.[1,9] The prevalence of overweight/obesity (now 32%) has risen dramatically over the past four decades for youth 2 to 19 years of age and has been linked to poor blood lipid profiles, elevated blood pressure and blood glucose, and early subclinical atherosclerosis.[9] Most children are born with ideal cardiovascular health but, over time, experience a decline in health factors and behaviors, resulting in a loss of ideal cardiovascular

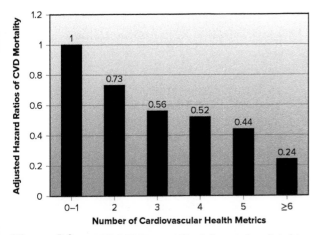

Figure 8.2   **Risk of CVD mortality is inversely related to the number of CVD health metrics in this study of 45,000 individuals in the NHANES mortality study.**

Source: Yang Q, Cogswell ME, Flanders WD, Hong Y, Zhang Z, Loustalot F, Gillespie C, Merritt R, Hu FB. 2012. Trends in cardiovascular health metrics and associations with all-cause and CVD mortality among US adults. *Journal of the American Medical Association* 307:1273–1283.

health as they reach adulthood. The AHA's 2020 goal of lowered CVD is directly linked to maintaining better levels of cardiovascular health for American youth, with the greatest challenge in the area of healthful eating, as depicted in Figure 8.3.[9]

The American Heart Association's Diet and Lifestyle Recommendations

The AHA urges that a healthy lifestyle and prudent dietary practices, at all stages of life, are central to CVD prevention and treatment.[1,10,11] Box 8.2 summarizes the current AHA diet and lifestyle recommendations (see www.heart.org).[10,11] These guidelines are based on heart-healthy nutrition-based practices, but they also focus on weight control, physical activity, and the avoidance of tobacco use.

The Dietary Guidelines for Americans (DGA) evolved from nutrient-based to food-based dietary patterns, improving the practical application to consumer-based tasks such as purchasing, preparing, and consuming foods.[12] The AHA recommends that adults who need to lower LDL-C and blood pressure should consume a dietary pattern that

- Emphasizes vegetables, fruits, and whole grains
- Includes low-fat dairy products, poultry, fish, legumes, nontropical vegetable oils, and nuts
- Limits intake of sweets, sugar-sweetened beverages, red meats, and processed foods

This dietary pattern should be adapted to meet appropriate calorie requirements and personal and cultural food

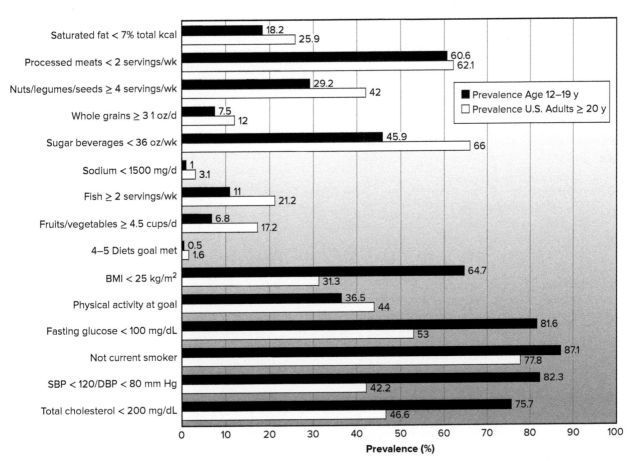

Figure 8.3   **Prevalence of ideal cardiovascular health components in U.S. adults and children/adolescents.[1]**

Box 8.2   **The American Heart Association's Diet and Lifestyle Recommendations**

1. USE UP AT LEAST AS MANY CALORIES AS YOU TAKE IN.

- Start by knowing how many calories you should be eating and drinking to maintain your weight. Nutrition and calorie information on food labels is typically based on a 2000-calorie diet. You may need fewer or more calories depending on several factors, including age, gender, and level of physical activity.
- If you are trying not to gain weight, don't eat more calories than you know you can burn up every day.
- Increase the amount and intensity of your physical activity to match the number of calories you take in.
- Aim for at least 150 minutes of moderate physical activity or 75 minutes of vigorous physical activity—or an equal combination of both—each week. Regular physical activity can help you maintain your weight, keep off weight that you lose, and help you reach physical and cardiovascular fitness. If it's hard to schedule regular exercise sessions, try aiming for sessions of at last 10 minutes spread throughout the week.
- If you would benefit from lowering your blood pressure or cholesterol, the American Heart Association recommends 40 minutes of aerobic exercise of moderate to vigorous intensity three to four times a week.

2. EAT A VARIETY OF NUTRITIOUS FOODS FROM ALL THE FOOD GROUPS.

You may be eating plenty of food, but your body may not be getting the nutrients it needs to be healthy. Nutrient-rich foods have minerals, protein, whole grains, and other nutrients but are lower in calories. They may help you control your weight, cholesterol, and blood pressure.

Eat an overall healthy dietary pattern that emphasizes

- A variety of fruits and vegetables
- Whole grains
- Low-fat dairy products
- Skinless poultry and fish
- Nuts and legumes
- Nontropical vegetable oils

Limit saturated fat, *trans* fat, sodium, red meat, sweets, and sugar-sweetened beverages. If you choose to eat red meat, compare labels and select the leanest cuts available.

One of the diets that fit this pattern is the DASH (Dietary Approaches to Stop Hypertension) eating plan. Most healthy eating patterns can be adapted based on calorie requirements and personal and cultural food preferences.

3. EAT LESS OF THE NUTRIENT-POOR FOODS.

The right number of calories to eat each day is based on your age and physical activity level and whether you're trying to gain, lose, or maintain your weight. You could use your daily allotment of calories on a few high-calorie foods and beverages, but you probably wouldn't get the nutrients your body needs to be healthy. Limit foods and beverages high in calories but low in nutrients. Also limit the amount of saturated fat, *trans* fat, and sodium you eat. Read Nutrition Facts labels carefully—the Nutrition Facts panel tells you the amount of healthy and unhealthy nutrients in a food or beverage.

4. AS YOU MAKE DAILY FOOD CHOICES, BASE YOUR EATING PATTERN ON THESE RECOMMENDATIONS:

- Eat a variety of fresh, frozen, and canned vegetables and fruits without high-calorie sauces or added salt and sugars. Replace high-calorie foods with fruits and vegetables.
- Choose fiber-rich whole grains for most grain servings.
- Choose poultry and fish without skin and prepare them in healthy ways without added saturated and *trans* fat. If you choose to eat meat, look for the leanest cuts available and prepare them in healthy and delicious ways.
- Eat a variety of fish at least twice a week, especially fish containing omega-3 fatty acids (for example, salmon, trout, and herring).
- Select fat-free (skim) and low-fat (1%) dairy products.
- Avoid foods containing partially hydrogenated vegetable oils to reduce *trans* fat in your diet.
- Limit saturated fat and *trans* fat and replace them with the better fats, monounsaturated and polyunsaturated. If you need to lower your blood cholesterol, reduce saturated fat to no more than 5% to 6% of total calories. For someone eating 2000 calories a day, that's about 13 grams of saturated fat.
- Cut back on beverages and foods with added sugars.
- Choose foods with less sodium and prepare foods with little or no salt. To lower blood pressure, aim to eat no more than 2400 milligrams of sodium per day. Reducing daily intake to 1500 mg is desirable because it can lower blood pressure even further. If you can't meet these goals right now, even reducing sodium intake by 1000 mg per day can benefit blood pressure.
- If you drink alcohol, drink in moderation. That means no more than one drink per day if you're a woman and no more than two drinks per day if you're a man.
- Follow the American Heart Association recommendations when you eat out, and keep an eye on your portion sizes.

5. ALSO, DON'T SMOKE TOBACCO—AND AVOID SECONDHAND SMOKE.

Sources: American College of Cardiology/American Heart Association Task Force on Practice Guidelines. 2014. 2013 AHA/ACC guideline on lifestyle management to reduce cardiovascular risk: A report of the American College of Cardiology/American Heart Association Task Force on Practice Guidelines. *Circulation* 129(25 Suppl 2): S76–S99. www.heart.org.

preferences. Additionally, this dietary pattern should incorporate relevant nutrition therapy to address multiple risk factors or medical conditions such as type 2 diabetes mellitus. This pattern can be achieved in a variety of ways, but both the DGA and AHA support the Dietary Approaches to Stop Hypertension (DASH) dietary pattern, the traditional Mediterranean-style diet, the healthy vegetarian eating pattern, and the healthy U.S.-style eating pattern.[10–12] The AHA dietary pattern incorporates all of the key principles advocated in the DGA. Although the AHA dietary pattern has been mistakenly referred to as a low-fat diet, it is more accurately described as an eating pattern low in saturated fatty acids (SFAs) and sodium, and moderate in unsaturated and total fat. The AHA dietary pattern can be readily adapted to individual tastes.

More specifically, the AHA recommends the following:[10,11]

- Reduction of SFA intake to less than 7% of total calorie intake (with a goal of less than 6% of total calorie intake for patients at cardiovascular risk)
- Avoidance of *trans* fats
- Reduction of sodium intake to less than 2300 mg per day, with further reduction to 1500 mg per day as needed for enhanced blood pressure lowering. Sodium reductions by at least 1000 mg per day are recommended even if the desired daily sodium intake is not yet achieved. The AHA urges that people limit intake of the "salty six" foods providing the most sodium in the U.S. diet, including bread and rolls, cured meats, pizza, poultry, soup, and sandwiches.

Currently, more than 80% of people in the United States consume greater than 2300 mg per day of sodium, and more than 60% of most people consume greater than 10% of energy from SFAs.[10,11] Excessive SFA intake should be replaced with polyunsaturated fatty acids and monounsaturated fatty acids without exceeding energy needs. Approximately 43% of total current energy intake in the United States comes from burgers, sandwiches, tacos, deserts and sweet snacks, sugar-sweetened beverages, rice- and pasta-mixed dishes, chips and crackers, and pizza.[1,11]

Table 8.3 summarizes the healthy U.S.-style eating pattern that has been adapted to meet AHA food-based and nutrient recommendations.[11] This dietary pattern achieves specified limits for three key dietary components of concern in the United States: added sugars (less than 10% of calories per day, with an AHA goal of less than 100 kcal/day for women and 150 kcal/day for men), saturated fats (less than 7% of calories per day), and sodium (less than 2300 mg per day).

Table 8.4 provides information on six tools for assessing and monitoring dietary pattern and physical activity behaviors.[11] Assessment of health behaviors improves awareness of lifestyle patterns that may need improvement. The AHA recommends that clients meet

TABLE 8.3	American Heart Association Eating Pattern Recommendations Based on the Healthy U.S.-Style Eating Pattern

Food Group (subgroups)	2000-Calorie Level	3000-Calorie Level
Fruits: fresh, frozen, canned unsweetened, cups	2	2.5
Vegetables: fresh, frozen, canned, cups/day	2.5	4
Dark green vegetables, cups/week	1.5	2.5
Red/orange vegetables, cups/week	5.5	7.5
Beans and peas, cups/week	1.5	3
Starchy vegetables, cups/week	5	8
Other vegetables, cups/week	4	7
Grains: emphasize whole grains high in dietary fiber, oz. eq./day	6	10
Whole grains	3	5
Other grains	3	5
Protein foods, oz. eq./day	5.5	7
Lean meat, poultry, eggs, oz. eq./week	26	33
Fish, preferably oily, oz. eq./week	8	10
Nuts, seeds, legumes, oz. eq./week (unsalted preferred)	5	6
Dairy: fat-free or low-fat, cups/day	3	3
Oils: unsaturated sources, g/day (Tbsp)	45 (3)	75 (5.5)
Fiber, g/day	31	48
Solid fats, g/day (% of total kcal)	13 (6)	20 (6)
Added sugars, g/day (kcal)	25 (100)	38 (150)
Sodium, mg/day	1787	2300

Source: Van Horn LV, et al. 2016. Recommended dietary pattern to achieve adherence to the American Heart Association/American College of Cardiology (AHA/ACC) guidelines: A scientific statement from the American Heart Association. *Circulation* 134:e505–e529.

with a registered dietitian or other qualified health-care professional to launch assessment activities in a timely and productive manner.[11] Self-monitoring can be challenging for people who have had no previous experience or who rarely purchase and prepare food. Mobile device applications can facilitate checking a food while in a social setting reviewing menus.

In general, achieving adherence to the AHA-recommended dietary pattern outlined in Table 8.3 is facilitated when individuals are counseled to choose foods that match guidelines and fit familiar cultural, economic, and social norms. Nutrient-dense food choices that meet but do not exceed calorie needs will facilitate weight-control goals, especially when combined with 30–60 minutes of physical activity on most days of the week. The goal is greater acceptance and sustained adherence to the AHA lifestyle and dietary patterns summarized in Table 8.3 and Box 8.2.

TABLE 8.4	Dietary Patterns: Tools for Assessing and Monitoring

One-Time Assessment Tools	Comments
Rate Your Plate	
http://www.dashdietoregon.org/Rate-Your-Plate	Simple evaluation of the DASH dietary pattern; provides tips
Your Med Diet Score	
http://oldwayspt.org/system/files/atoms/files/rateYourMedDietScore.pdf	Nine questions to calculate a Mediterranean diet score; provides feedback
Daily Food Plans	
https://www.choosemyplate.gov/myplate-daily-checklist-input/display	Menu planner based on the MyPlate food pattern based on personal characteristics and goals
Ongoing Tools For Dietary Self-Monitoring	
SuperTracker	
http://www.choosemyplate.gov/supertracker-tools/	Develop a personalized nutrition and physical activity plan, track foods and activity, and evaluate progress
MyFitnessPal	
https://www.myfitnesspal.com/	Record daily food intake and physical activity and follow progress to specified goals
Lose It	
https://www.loseit.com/how-it-works/	Self-monitoring tool to set a weight-loss goal and to record daily weight, food intake, and activity

Major Risk Factors That *Can* Be Modified, Treated, and Controlled	% U.S. Adults with Risk Prevalence
• Cigarette/tobacco smoke	15%
• High blood pressure	30% ($\geq$ 140/90 mm Hg or on meds)
• High blood cholesterol	28% ($\geq$ 240 mg/dL or on meds)
• Physical inactivity	32%
• Overweight and obesity	70% (BMI $\geq$ 25 kg/m^2)
• Diabetes	12%
Major Risk Factors That *Can't* Be Changed	
• Heredity	
• Male	
• Increasing age	15% (age 65 and over)
Other Factors That Contribute to Risk	
• Frequent mental distress	10%
• Excessive alcohol intake	6%
• Poor diet quality	41%

Figure 8.4   Risk factors for heart disease, according to the American Heart Association.

Sources: Risk factor list from the American Heart Association: https://www.heart.org. Prevalence data from National Center for Health Statistics. 2016. *Health, United States, 2015: With special feature on racial and ethnic health disparities.* Hyattsville, MD: National Center for Health Statistics. https://www.cdc.gov/nchs/data/hus/hus15.pdf.

Cardiovascular Disease Risk Factors

The AHA divides heart disease risk factors (Figure 8.4) into those that cannot be changed (heredity, male gender, age) and those that can be modified, treated, and controlled through lifestyle change (tobacco use, high blood pressure, high blood cholesterol, physical inactivity, obesity/overweight, diabetes, mental distress, excessive alcohol intake, and poor diet quality).[1–3] The three most prevalent of these AHA risk factors reflect the poor health behaviors of many U.S. adults: overweight/obesity, poor diet quality, and physical inactivity.

The AHA regards suboptimal diet quality as the leading risk factor for CVD death and mortality.[1] Major diet contributors to CVD risk are insufficient intakes of fruits, nuts/seeds, whole grains, vegetables, and seafood as well as excess intakes of sodium and saturated fat. Although tobacco use has declined substantially in the United States, almost one-third of CHD deaths are attributable to smoking and exposure to secondhand smoke, making this the second leading CVD risk factor.[1] Overweight/obesity and physical inactivity predispose individuals to most major risk factors, including high blood pressure, dyslipidemia, and diabetes mellitus.

AHA cardiovascular health metrics and risk factors are closely linked and represent a heightened disease prevention and health promotion focus for the AHA.[1] The AHA now places priority on both health behaviors (healthy diet pattern, appropriate energy balance, physical activity, and nonsmoking) and health factors that can be measured (optimal blood lipids, blood pressure, blood glucose levels) throughout the life span. To reach the 2020 AHA goal of lowered CVD death rates, strategies are based on shifting the majority of the public toward greater CVD health, with a focus on those individuals at greatest risk. The risk factors and CVD metrics with the greatest potential for improvement are health behaviors, including diet quality, physical activity, and body weight.[1]

The AHA supports three primary strategies to improve cardiovascular health:[1]

- Individual-focused approaches, which target lifestyle and treatments at the individual level
- Health-care systems approaches, which encourage, facilitate, and reward efforts by providers and patients to improve health behaviors and health factors
- Population approaches, which target lifestyle and treatments in schools or workplaces, local communities, and states, as well as throughout the nation

Risk Factors for Stroke

Stroke is currently the number five cause of death, but it is still a leading cause of serious, long-term disability. Each year, just under 800,000 people in the United States experience a new or recurrent stroke.[1] Most strokes occur because of atherosclerosis, the same underlying factor that causes CHD. Clots that form in the area of the narrowed brain blood vessels (thrombus) or ones that float in (embolus) can then totally block the blood flow, causing the ischemic stroke (87% of all strokes). When this happens, brain cells don't get the blood and oxygen that they need to survive, causing nerve cells to stop working and die within minutes along with control of specific, related body functions. The effects of stroke may be permanent depending on how many cells are lost, where they are in the brain, and other factors. Other strokes occur when a blood vessel ruptures and bleeds (hemorrhagic stroke), often in a brain artery that has been weakened from atherosclerosis or high blood pressure. Transient ischemic attack (TIA) is caused by a temporary clot and is sometimes called a "mini stroke," and it precedes about 15% of major strokes.

Stroke warning signs are very specific:

- Sudden numbness or weakness of the face, arm, or leg, especially on one side of the body
- Sudden confusion and trouble speaking or understanding
- Sudden trouble seeing in one or both eyes
- Sudden trouble walking, dizziness, and loss of balance or coordination
- Sudden severe headache with no known cause

Risk factors for stroke are similar to those for heart disease and include non-modifiable factors such as age, female sex, ethnicity, and personal or family history of stroke (Figure 8.5). The leading risk factor for stroke is high blood pressure, and much of the decrease in stroke death rates has been linked to improved detection and treatment of hypertension. Control of diabetes mellitus, high blood cholesterol, and cigarette smoking, particularly in combination with hypertension control and treatment, appear to have contributed to the decline in stroke mortality.[1] The "stroke belt" is located in the southeastern United States where obesity, hypertension, and CVD are highly prevalent. Other modifiable risk factors include cigarette smoking, physical inactivity and obesity, elevated blood cholesterol, diabetes mellitus, poor diet, alcohol and drug abuse, and various medical conditions such as CHD, PAD, carotid artery disease, atrial fibrillation, and sickle cell disease.

The Metabolic Syndrome

The metabolic syndrome is a multicomponent risk factor for CVD and type 2 diabetes mellitus, and it reflects the clustering of CVD and metabolic risk factors related to abdominal obesity and insulin resistance.[1,13] According to the AHA, the metabolic syndrome doubles the risk for CVD and should be considered largely a disease of an unhealthy lifestyle.[1] The AHA urges that identification of the metabolic syndrome represents a call to action for the health-care provider and patient to address the underlying lifestyle-related risk factors using a multidisciplinary team of health-care professionals to address all related issues.[1]

■ **Non-modifiable risk factors**
- Age (doubles for each decade after age 55), female sex (especially with birth control pills, pregnancy, history of preeclampsia/eclampsia or gestational diabetes, oral contraceptive use, smoking, and post-menopausal hormone therapy), ethnicity (African American), prior stroke, TIA, or heart attack, and personal or family history of stroke

■ **Well-documented modifiable risk factors**
- High blood pressure: the leading cause of stroke
- Cigarette smoking: nicotine and carbon monoxide damage the cardiovascular system in many ways
- Physical inactivity and obesity: increase risk of hypertension, high blood cholesterol, diabetes, CHD, and stroke
- Elevated blood cholesterol: people with high cholesterol have an elevated stroke risk
- Diabetes mellitus: typically combined with obesity, hypertension, and high blood cholesterol
- Carotid or other artery disease: carotid narrowing may become blocked by a clot
- Peripheral artery disease (PAD): people with PAD have a higher risk of carotid artery disease
- Atrial fibrillation: heart's upper chamber quiver *setting up clots*
- Other heart disease: people with CHD or heart failure have a higher stroke risk
- Sickle cell disease: genetic disorder leading to lower oxygen delivery and stickiness of cells to blood vessel walls
- Poor diet: *trans* fats, SFAs, sodium, and low fruit and vegetable intake increase risk

■ **Less well-documented modifiable risk factors**
- Geographic location (southeastern United States), socioeconomic factors (low income), alcohol abuse, drug abuse (cocaine, amphetamines, heroin)

Figure 8.5   Risk factors for stroke.
Source: www.strokeassociation.org.

Several different clinical definitions for the metabolic syndrome have been proposed, but the current harmonized definition backed by the AHA; the International Diabetes Federation; the National Heart, Lung, and Blood Institute (NHLBI); and others uses any three of five risk factors for diagnosis (see Figure 8.6):[1,13]

- Fasting plasma glucose ≥ 100 mg/dL or undergoing drug treatment for elevated glucose
- HDL-C < 40 mg/dL in men or < 50 mg/dL in women or undergoing drug treatment for reduced HDL-C
- Triglycerides ≥ 150 mg/dL or undergoing drug treatment for elevated triglycerides
- Waist circumference > 102 cm (> 40 inches) in men or > 88 cm (> 35 inches) in women for people of most ancestries living in the United States. Ethnicity and country-specific thresholds can be used for diagnosis in other groups, particularly Asians and

Metabolic Syndrome

Risk Factor	Defining Level
Abdominal obesity Men Women	Waist circumference > 40 inches > 35 inches
Plasma triglycerides	≥ 150 mg/dL
Plasma HDL cholesterol Men Women	< 40 mg/dL < 50 mg/dL
Blood pressure	≥ 130/≥ 85 mm Hg
Fasting plasma glucose	≥ 100 mg/dL

Figure 8.6   The metabolic syndrome is diagnosed when an individual has three or more of these five risk factors.

individuals of non-European ancestry who have predominantly resided outside the United States.
- BP ≥ 130 mm Hg systolic or ≥ 85 mm Hg diastolic or undergoing drug treatment for hypertension, or antihypertensive drug treatment in a patient with a history of hypertension

Using these criteria, the current prevalence of the metabolic syndrome in the United States is 34.7%, with a higher prevalence among women (36.6%) compared to men (32.8%).[14] The prevalence of metabolic syndrome rises sharply with age and approaches 50% among individuals 60 years of age and older.

The metabolic syndrome is related not only to CVD and type 2 diabetes mellitus but also to many other adverse health conditions, including nonalcoholic fatty liver disease, sexual/reproductive dysfunction (erectile dysfunction in men and polycystic ovarian syndrome in women), obstructive sleep apnea, certain forms of cancer, and possibly osteoarthritis, systemic inflammation, and the prothrombotic state.[1]

Individuals with a fasting glucose level ≥ 126 mg/dL or a casual glucose value ≥ 200 mg/dL or are taking hypoglycemic medication will normally be classified separately as having type 2 diabetes mellitus. Many of these will also have metabolic syndrome because of the clustering of two or more additional risk factors, listed in Figure 8.6.

Despite the high prevalence of the metabolic syndrome, the public's recognition of it is limited.[1] A diagnosis of metabolic syndrome may increase risk perception and motivation toward a healthier behavior. Although the metabolic syndrome has been linked with elevated CVD risk, the AHA does not recommend using the cluster of risk factors as a risk predictive assessment tool.[1]

HIGH BLOOD CHOLESTEROL

Despite an impressive drop from the 1960s, about 12% of Americans still have high-risk blood cholesterol levels (240 mg/dL and higher), with this proportion increasing to 28% when considering all individuals either with high blood cholesterol or on cholesterol-lowering medications.[3] The average American has a blood cholesterol level of 192 mg/dL, well below 1960s levels but substantially above the *Healthy People 2020* goal of 178 mg/dL (Figure 8.7). Most of the recent decline in cholesterol levels reflects greater intake of cholesterol-lowering medications.[1] The average cholesterol for children 6 to

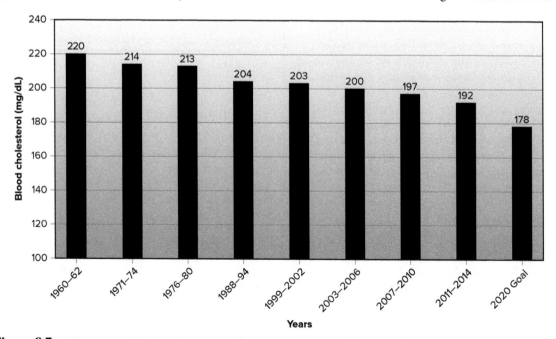

Figure 8.7   The average blood cholesterol level for U.S. adults has dropped from 220 mg/dL in the early 1960s to 192 mg/dL. The *Healthy People 2020* goal of 178 mg/dL will probably not be achieved.

Sources: National Center for Health Statistics. 2016. *Health, United States, 2015: With special feature on racial and ethnic health disparities.* Hyattsville, MD: National Center for Health Statistics. https://www.cdc.gov/nchs/data/hus/hus15.pdf. www.healthypeople.gov.

11 years of age is 160 mg/dL, and for adolescents 12 to 19 years the average is 158 mg/dL.[1]

High blood cholesterol is a major risk factor for CVD and stroke.[1] As reviewed previously in this chapter, the AHA has identified untreated total blood cholesterol levels below 170 mg/dL in children/adolescents and 200 mg/dL in adults as one of seven components of ideal cardiovascular health.[1-3] The AHA and National Center for Health Statistics (NCHS) report that 75.7% of children and 46.6% of adults have ideal cholesterol levels (untreated total cholesterol < 170 mg/dL for children and < 200 mg/dL for adults).[1,15] More than 100 million U.S. adults have total cholesterol levels ≥ 200 mg/dL, and almost 31 million have levels ≥ 240 mg/dL.

Use of cholesterol-lowering medication is widespread, with 28% of adults 40 years of age and older, and 48% of those 75 and over, reporting that they had used a cholesterol-lowering medication in the past 30 days.[1,16] Slightly more than 70% of adults with doctor-diagnosed CVD reported taking cholesterol-lowering medication in the past 30 days.[16] Among adults who used a prescription cholesterol-lowering medication, simvastatin was the most commonly used cholesterol-lowering medication, with 42% reporting its use. This was followed by atorvastatin (20.2%), pravastatin (11.2%), rosuvastatin (8.2%), and lovastatin (7.4%).[16]

According to the National Cholesterol Education Program (NCEP), every adult should know his or her cholesterol level and have it checked at least once every five years (or every year if heart disease risk is high).[17] CDC state survey data indicate that 76% of adults reported that they had been screened for high cholesterol in the previous five years.[1]

Cholesterol is transported through the blood by carriers called lipoproteins. Two specific types of cholesterol carriers are called low-density lipoproteins (LDL) and high-density lipoproteins (HDL). When cholesterol is carried in the LDL (called LDL-cholesterol or LDL-C), this is called "bad" cholesterol because it contributes to the buildup of atherosclerosis, increasing heart disease risk. In contrast, HDL-C is called the "good" cholesterol. The HDL carrier acts as a type of shuttle as it takes up cholesterol from the blood and body cells and transfers it to the liver, where it is used to form bile acids. Bile acids pass from the liver to the intestine to aid in fat digestion. Eventually, some of the bile acids pass out of the body in the stool, providing the body with a major route for excretion of cholesterol. HDLs have for this reason been called the "garbage trucks" of the body, collecting cholesterol and transporting it to the liver. Thus, if levels of HDL-C are high, the risk of heart disease is decreased. Blood fats or triglycerides predict increased risk of CHD when levels are elevated in combination with other CVD risk factors.

The total cholesterol is the sum of the cholesterol in the LDL, HDL, and very-low-density lipoproteins (VLDLs). VLDLs are about 60% triglycerides by weight

and contain 10% to 15% of the plasma's total cholesterol. LDLs transport cholesterol to the various cells of the body and contain approximately 70% of the plasma's total cholesterol. LDL is considered the most atherogenic (i.e., atherosclerosis-producing) lipoprotein, and low levels are predictive of reduced CVD risk. Isolation of LDL requires ultracentrifugation, a research technique not generally available in service laboratories. Most clinical laboratories estimate the LDL-C using the Friedewald equation from individuals who are overnight fasted:

$$LDL\text{-}C = TC - [HDL\text{-}C + (0.20 \times triglycerides)]$$

For example, if the total plasma cholesterol is 220 mg/dL, the plasma HDL-C is 50 mg/dL, and triglycerides are 100 mg/dL, then LDL-C = 220 − [50 + (0.20 × 100)] = 150 mg/dL. This equation is less reliable as triglyceride levels rise to very high levels.

Table 8.5 provides the National Cholesterol Education Program (NCEP) classification for total cholesterol, LDL-C, HDL-C, and triglycerides.[17] When total cholesterol and LDL-C are high, and HDL-C is low, the individual can be characterized as having a poor lipid profile, or

TABLE 8.5	**Classification of Total Blood Cholesterol, LDL-C, HDL-C, and Triglycerides**
Parameter (mg/dL)	**Classification**
Total Cholesterol	
< 200	Desirable
200–239	Borderline high
≥ 240	High
LDL Cholesterol	
< 100	Optimal
100–129	Near optimal/above optimal
130–159	Borderline high
160–189	High
≥ 190	Very high
HDL Cholesterol	
< 40	Low (undesirable)
≥ 60	High (desirable)
Triglycerides	
< 150	Normal
150–199	Borderline high
200–499	High
≥ 500	Very high

Note: Values given are in mg/dL. To convert to SI units, divide the results for total cholesterol (TC), low-density lipoprotein cholesterol (LDL-C), high-density lipoprotein cholesterol (HDL-C), and non-HDL-C by 38.6; for triglycerides (TG), divide by 88.6. **See Box 8.3 for a description of how to convert mg/dL to mmol/L.**

Source: National Cholesterol Education Program (NCEP) Expert Panel on Detection, Evaluation, and Treatment of High Blood Cholesterol in Adults (Adult Treatment Panel III). 2002. Third report of the National Cholesterol Education Program (NCEP) Expert Panel on Detection, Evaluation, and Treatment of High Blood Cholesterol in Adults (Adult Treatment Panel III) final report. *Circulation* 106:3143–3421.

Box 8.3   Using the SI Units

The International System of Units (abbreviated SI from the French *Le Systéme International d'Unités*) is the world's most widely used system of measurement, both for everyday commerce and for science. It was established in 1960 as an updated, modern form of the older metric system, and is periodically modified and updated through international agreement as the technology of measurement progresses, and as the precision of measurements improves. The SI units are nearly universally employed with the notable exception of the United States, which continues to use customary units in addition to SI.

Throughout Chapter 8, both conventional units and SI units are used to express the amounts of such laboratory components as serum lipids and lipoproteins, and plasma glucose. Below is a list of these components, the abbreviations of the conventional and SI units, and a factor for converting the values from the conventional unit to the SI unit. To convert values from conventional units to SI units, multiply the value in conventional units by the conversion factor. To convert values from SI units to conventional units, divide the SI value by the conversion factor.

Component	Conventional Unit	Conversion Factor	SI Unit
Cholesterol	mg/dL	0.0259	mmol/L
Glucose	mg/dL	0.0555	mmol/L
High-density-lipoprotein cholesterol	mg/dL	0.0259	mmol/L
Low-density-lipoprotein cholesterol	mg/dL	0.0259	mmol/L
Triglyceride	mg/dL	0.0113	mmol/L

Source: National Institute of Standards and Technology. 2008. *Guide for the use of the International System of Units (SI).* NIST Special Publication 811. Gaithersburg, MD: National Institute of Standards and Technology.

dyslipidemia. Table 8.6 summarizes the prevalence of dyslipidemia for each parameter. The average HDL-C for American adults 20 years of age and older is 53 mg/dL.[1] Approximately 19% of adults (28% of men and 10% of women) have HDL-C below 40 mg/dL.[15] The average LDL-C for American adults is 116 mg/dL, down from 126 mg/dL in 1999–2000.[1] About 32% of U.S. adults have high LDL-C (130 mg/dL and higher). The average triglyceride level for American adults is 109 mg/dL, with 25% of adults at 150 mg/dL and higher.[1]

Guidelines for the Treatment of High Blood Cholesterol

In 2013, the American College of Cardiology (ACC) and the American Heart Association (AHA) released updated guidelines for the treatment of high blood cholesterol.[18] These guidelines were designed to supersede the previous Adult Treatment Panel III (ATP III) report of the National Cholesterol Education Program (NCEP).[17] The NHLBI made a decision to discontinue the development of clinical guidelines and instead to provide its evidence review to the ACC and AHA. These two organizations transformed the NHLBI's evidence reviews into treatment guidelines.[16–18]

The 2013 ACC/AHA guidelines represent a major shift from prior cholesterol management guidelines, with a focus on atherosclerotic cardiovascular disease (ASCVD) risk reduction as opposed to targeting LDL-C levels, advocating for the use of evidence-based doses of statins as first line therapy and utilizing a new risk calculator and risk cut point to guide initiation of statin therapy. The 2013 ACC/AHA cholesterol guidelines focus on identifying groups of patients that are most likely to benefit from cholesterol treatment with HMG-CoA reductase inhibitors (statins), the therapy that has been consistently proven in randomized clinical trials to lower ASCVD risk.[18–20] Lovastatin became

TABLE 8.6	Prevalence of Dyslipidemia (High Total Cholesterol and LDL-C, Low HDL-C)				
	Total Cholesterol ≥ 200 mg/dL	Total Cholesterol ≥ 240 mg/dL	Total Cholesterol ≥ 240 mg/dL or on Medication	LDL-C ≥ 130 mg/dL	HDL-C < 40 mg/dL
All adults	42.8%	11.9%	27.8%	31.7%	18.7%
Males	40.4%	10.8%	28.4%	31.0%	27.9%
Females	44.9%	12.7%	27.3%	32.0%	10.0%

Sources: American Heart Association Statistics Committee, Stroke Statistics Subcommittee. 2016. Heart disease and stroke statistics—2016 update: A report from the American Heart Association. *Circulation* 133:e38–e360; National Center for Health Statistics. 2016. *Health, United States, 2015: With special feature on racial and ethnic health disparities.* Hyattsville, MD: National Center for Health Statistics. https://www.cdc.gov/nchs/data/hus/hus15.pdf. Carroll MD, Fryar CD, Kit BK. 2015. *Total and high-density lipoprotein cholesterol in adults: United States, 2011–2014.* NCHS Data Brief, no 226. Hyattsville, MD: National Center for Health Statistics.

the first commercially available statin medication in 1987, when it was given the United States Food and Drug Administration (FDA) approval.[20] Since then, the use of statins has proven to be advantageous for the primary prevention of CVD by reducing the risk and preventing the onset of the disease. In addition, statins are often used for secondary prevention, as they are effective in slowing disease progression and reducing cardiovascular-associated morbidities and mortalities. The 2013 ACC/AHA guidelines significantly expand the population of patients eligible for statin therapy. The scope of statin therapy is increasing in other directions, with the emergence of evidence that statins modulate immune and inflammation responses.[20] Statin therapy has potential applications to multiple sclerosis, inflammatory bowel diseases, rheumatoid arthritis, systemic lupus erythematosus, chronic obstructive pulmonary disease (COPD), cancer, strokes, Parkinson's and Alzheimer's diseases, bacterial infections, and HIV.[20]

Unlike ATP III, which recommended LDL-C goals based on a patient's risk category, the 2013 ACC/AHA guidelines recommended lipid measurement at baseline, at one to three months after statin initiation, and then annually to check for the expected percentage decrease of LDL-C levels (30% to 50% with a moderate-intensity statin and more than 50% with a high-intensity statin). The 2013 ACC/AHA guidelines identified four statin benefit groups (Figure 8.8):

1. Those with arteriosclerotic cardiovascular disease (ASCVD)
2. Those with LDL-cholesterol values of 190 mg/dL and higher
3. People with type 1 or 2 diabetes who are 40–75 years of age with LDL-C of 70–189 mg/dL
4. People without diabetes who are 40–75 years of age with LDL-C of 70–189 mg/dL and have an estimated ASCVD 10-year risk of 7.5% and higher

ASCVD 10-year risk can be assessed at http://tools.cardiosource.org/ASCVD-Risk-Estimator/. An Excel spreadsheet file can be downloaded that allows practitioners to estimate ASCVD on their personal computers. The estimator requires gender, total cholesterol, age, HDL cholesterol, race, systolic blood pressure, smoking status, diabetes history, and history of hypertension.

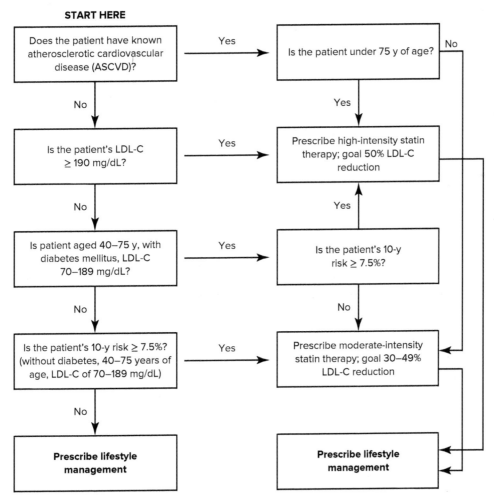

Figure 8.8   Simplified chart for the 2013 ACC/AHA guidelines on the treatment of blood cholesterol to reduce atherosclerotic cardiovascular risk in adults.[18]

High-intensity statin therapy (e.g., 40–80 mg atorvastatin, 20–40 mg rosuvastatin) is recommended for those with clinical ASCVD, as well as those with significant primary elevations in LDL-C, which are likely due to a genetic cholesterol disorder such as familial hypercholesterolemia. For diabetics, at least a moderate-intensity statin should be considered (e.g., 10–20 mg atorvastatin, 5–10 mg rosuvastatin, 20–40 mg simvastatin, 40–80 mg pravastatin), and high-intensity statin is recommended if the estimated 10-year risk using the Pooled Cohort Equations is 7.5% and higher. For other primary prevention patients with high 10-year risk, a moderate- or high-intensity statin is recommended, but only after an individualized clinician-patient discussion regarding risks and benefits of statin therapy. If the decision is still unclear, additional factors may be considered to aid in the risk assessment, including LDL-C of 160 mg/dL and higher, family history of premature ASCVD, high-sensitivity CRP 2.0 mg/L and higher, high lifetime risk of ASCVD, and other factors.[18-20]

Very importantly, lifestyle modification is encouraged for all risk groups, with diet, exercise, avoidance of tobacco products, and maintenance of a healthy weight serving as the platform upon which all other treatments are built.[10,18] The lifestyle recommendations are summarized in Box 8.2.[10] Lifestyle modification is a critical component of ASCVD risk reduction, both prior to and in concert with the use of cholesterol-lowering drug therapies. In individuals not receiving cholesterol-lowering drug therapy, the estimated 10-year ASCVD risk should be recalculated every 4–6 years in individuals aged 40–75 years without clinical ASCVD or diabetes and with LDL-C 70–189 mg/dL.[18]

Approximately 32% of the ASCVD-free, nonpregnant U.S. population between 40 and 79 years of age has a 10-year risk of a first hard CHD event of 10% and higher, or has diabetes mellitus.[1] As a result of the 2013 ACC/AHA guidelines, the number of people eligible for statin therapy has increased sharply, with most of the increase coming from adults 60 to 75 years old without CVD who have a 10-year ASCVD risk of 7.5% and higher.[1]

These major changes in guidelines for the treatment of high blood cholesterol and dyslipidemia have created controversy and confusion among the medical community, with some clinicians hesitant to embrace the shift.[19] The ASCVD risk calculator relies heavily on age, meaning that a high proportion of the elderly fall into the statin benefit group. While statins are generally well tolerated, adverse events include muscle pain and damage, increased blood glucose levels, liver damage, digestive problems, cognitive effects, and the development of rashes or flushing.[20] Simvastatin (Zocor) is the most widely used statin medication, and generic equivalents cost about $2.25 per day.[16,20] Nonetheless, the 2013 ACC/AHA cholesterol guidelines utilize a simple and accurate risk assessment method and should simultaneously help prevent undertreatment of higher-risk patients and overtreatment of lower-risk patients.

Screening for Dyslipidemia in Children and Adolescents

A series of studies have shown a clear relationship between dyslipidemia and the onset of atherosclerosis in children, adolescents, and young adults.[1,21] Obesity prevalence has increased sharply in American youth, increasing the proportion with dyslipidemia. Early identification and control of dyslipidemia throughout youth and into adulthood substantially reduces clinical CVD risk. In response to mounting evidence, an expert panel convened by the NHBLI in 2011 recommended universal dyslipidemia screening for all children between 9 and 11 years of age and again between 17 and 21 years of age, with more frequent testing for youth at high CVD risk.[21] The NHBLI Expert Panel did not recommend lipid screening in the first two years of life. This recommendation contrasted with earlier guidelines that reserved lipid profile testing only for children and adolescents at high CVD risk.

Table 8.7 summarizes the acceptable, borderline high, and high plasma lipid and lipoprotein levels for

TABLE 8.7	Acceptable, Borderline-High, and High Plasma Lipid and Lipoprotein Concentrations for Children and Adolescents (birth to age 19 years)
Parameter (mg/dL)	**Classification**
Total Cholesterol	
< 170	Acceptable
170–199	Borderline high
≥ 200	High
LDL Cholesterol	
< 110	Acceptable
110–129	Borderline high
≥ 130	High
Non-HDL Cholesterol	
< 120	Acceptable
120–144	Borderline high
≥ 145	High
HDL Cholesterol	
< 40	Low (undesirable)
40–45	Borderline
≥ 45	Acceptable
Triglycerides	
Ages 0–9 y *Ages 10–19 y*	
< 75 < 90	Acceptable
75–99 90–129	Borderline high
≥ 100 ≥ 130	High

Note: Values given are in mg/dL. To convert to SI units, divide the results for total cholesterol (TC), low-density lipoprotein cholesterol (LDL-C), high-density lipoprotein cholesterol (HDL-C), and non-HDL-C by 38.6; for triglycerides (TG), divide by 88.6.

Source: Expert Panel on Integrated Guidelines for Cardiovascular Health and Risk Reduction in Children and Adolescents. 2011. Expert Panel on Integrated Guidelines for Cardiovascular Health and Risk Reduction in Children and Adolescents: Summary report. *Pediatrics* 128(suppl 5):S213–S256.

children and adolescents.[21] Among children (ages 6 to 11 years) and adolescents (12 to 19 years), the average cholesterol is 160 mg/dL and 158 mg/dL, respectively.[1] The prevalence of dyslipidemia among adolescents is 20%, with this proportion increasing to 43% among obese youths. The average LDL-C among adolescents is 89 mg/dL, with HDL-C averaging 51 mg/dL and triglycerides 82 mg/dL.[1] Non-HDL-C has been identified as a significant predictor of the presence of atherosclerosis, as powerful as any other lipoprotein cholesterol measure in children and adolescents. For both children and adults, non-HDL-C (calculated by subtracting HDL-C from the total cholesterol) appears to be more predictive of persistent dyslipidemia and therefore atherosclerosis and future events than total cholesterol, LDL-C, or HDL-C alone.[21] A major advantage of non-HDL-C is that it can be accurately calculated in a non-fasting state and is therefore practical in clinical practice. The Expert Panel felt that non-HDL-C should be added as a screening tool for identification of a dyslipidemic state in childhood. The average non-HDL-C among adolescents is 112 mg/dL, which falls under the 120 mg/dL acceptable threshold (Table 8.7).[1,21]

The NHLBI Expert Panel developed comprehensive evidence-based guidelines addressing the known risk factors for CVD to assist all primary pediatric care providers in both the promotion of cardiovascular health and the identification and management of specific risk factors from infancy into young adult life. The recommendations addressed two goals: the prevention of risk factor development (sometimes called primordial prevention) and the prevention of future CVD by effective management of identified risk factors (or what is termed primary prevention). Specific recommendations are given for tobacco exposure, issues related to family CVD history, nutrition, obesity, lipids, blood pressure, physical activity, and diabetes. These guidelines are available at https://www.nhlbi.nih.gov/files/docs/peds_guidelines_sum.pdf.

Accompanying the Expert Panel's report is a set of evidence-based dietary recommendations for patients of pediatric care providers called the Cardiovascular Health Integrated Lifestyle Diet (CHILD 1), which is shown in Table 8.8. The Expert Panel stresses that good nutrition beginning at birth can have profound health

TABLE 8.8	Evidence-Based Dietary Recommendations for Patients of Pediatric Care Providers: Cardiovascular Health Integrated Lifestyle Diet (CHILD 1)

CHILD 1 is the recommended first step diet for all children and adolescents at elevated cardiovascular risk.

Birth–6 months	Infants should be exclusively breast-fed (no supplemental formula or other foods) until age 6 months. Infants who cannot be fed directly at the breast should be fed expressed milk. Infants for whom expressed milk is not available should be fed iron-fortified infant formula.
6–12 months	Continue breast-feeding until at least age 12 months while gradually adding solids. Transition to an iron-fortified formula until 12 months if reducing breast-feeding. Infants who cannot be fed directly at the breast should be fed expressed milk. Infants for whom expressed milk is not available should be fed iron-fortified infant formula.
	Fat intake in infants younger than 12 months of age should not be restricted without medical indication.
	Limit other drinks to 100% fruit juice ≤ 4 oz/d. No sweetened beverages. Encourage water.
12–24 months	Transition to reduced-fat (2% to fat-free) unflavored cow's milk. Toddlers 12–24 months of age with a family history of obesity, heart disease, or high cholesterol should discuss transition to reduced-fat milk with pediatric care provider after 12 months of age. Continued breast-feeding is still appropriate and nutritionally superior to cow's milk. Milk reduced in fat should be used only in the context of an overall diet that supplies 30% of calories from fat.
	Limit/avoid sugar-sweetened beverage intake. Encourage water.
	Transition to table food with: • Total fat 30% of daily kcal* • Saturated fat 8–10% of daily kcal* • Avoid *trans* fat as much as possible • Monounsaturated and polyunsaturated fat up to 20% of daily kcal* • Cholesterol < 300 mg/d
	Supportive actions: • The fat content of cow's milk to introduce at ages 12–24 months should be decided together by parents and health care providers based on the child's growth, appetite, intake of other nutrient-dense foods, intake of other sources of fat, and potential risk for obesity and CVD. • Limit 100% fruit juice (from a cup) to no more than 4 oz/d. • Limit sodium intake. • Consider DASH-type diet rich in fruits, vegetables, whole grains, low-fat/fat-free milk and milk products; lower in sugar.
2–10 years	Primary beverage: Fat-free unflavored milk.
	Limit/avoid sugar-sweetened beverages. Encourage water.

continued

TABLE 8.8	Evidence-Based Dietary Recommendations for Patients of Pediatric Care Providers: Cardiovascular Health Integrated Lifestyle Diet (CHILD 1)—*continued*

	Fat content: • Total fat 25–30% of daily kcal* • Saturated fat 8–10% of daily kcal* • Avoid *trans* fats as much as possible • Monounsaturated and polyunsaturated fat up to 20% of daily kcal* • Cholesterol < 300 mg/d Encourage high dietary fiber intake from foods. Naturally fiber-rich foods are recommended (fruits, vegetables, whole grains); fiber supplements are not advised. Limit refined carbohydrates (sugars, white rice, white bread). Supportive actions: • Teach portions based on EER for age/gender/activity. • Encourage moderately increased energy intake during periods of rapid growth and/or regular moderate-to-vigorous physical activity. • Encourage dietary fiber from foods: Age + 5 g/d. • Limit naturally sweetened juice (no added sugar) to 4 oz/d. • Limit sodium intake. • Support DASH-style eating plan.
11–21 years	Primary beverage: Fat-free unflavored milk. Limit/avoid sugar-sweetened beverages. Encourage water. Fat content: • Total fat 25–30% of daily kcal* • Saturated fat 8–10% of daily kcal* • Avoid *trans* fat as much as possible • Monounsaturated and polyunsaturated fat up to 20% of daily kcal* • Cholesterol < 300 mg/d Encourage high dietary fiber intake from foods. Naturally fiber-rich foods are recommended (fruits, vegetables, whole grains); fiber supplements are not advised. Limit refined carbohydrates (sugars, white rice, white bread). Supportive actions: • Teach portions based on EER for age/gender/activity. • Encourage moderately increased energy intake during periods of rapid growth and/or regular moderate-to-vigorous physical activity. • Advocate dietary fiber: Goal of 14 g/1000 kcal. • Limit naturally sweetened juice (no added sugar) to 4–6 oz/d. • Limit sodium intake. • Encourage healthy eating habits: Breakfast every day, eating meals as a family, limiting fast-food meals. • Support DASH-style eating plan.

*Kcal intake should be based on the Estimated Energy Requirement (EER) per day according to age and gender.

Source: Expert Panel on Integrated Guidelines for Cardiovascular Health and Risk Reduction in Children and Adolescents. 2011. *Expert Panel on Integrated Guidelines for Cardiovascular Health and Risk Reduction in Children and Adolescents: Full report.* National Heart, Lung, Blood Institute, National Institutes of Health, U.S. Department of Health and Human Services. www.nhlbi.nih.gov/guidelines/cvd_ped/index.htm.

benefits and potentially decrease future CVD risk, and it emphasizes the importance of exclusive breast-feeding for the first 6 months of life and continued breast-feeding for at least 12 months of age with the addition of appropriate complementary foods. Infants who cannot be fed directly from the breast should be fed expressed human milk from a bottle. Infants for whom expressed milk is not available should be fed an iron-fortified infant formula. Research has shown that individuals who were breast-fed during infancy have long-term cardiovascular health benefits such as lower risk of obesity, lower total cholesterol levels and carotid intima-media thickness in adulthood, and lower risk of type 2 diabetes mellitus.[21]

ISSUES IN MEASURING LIPID AND LIPOPROTEIN LEVELS

The public health impact of cardiovascular disease and the causal relationships between cardiovascular disease and serum lipid and lipoprotein levels make measurement of total cholesterol, low-density-lipoprotein cholesterol, and high-density-lipoprotein cholesterol among the most important in the clinical laboratory.[22] The presence of specific and detailed guidelines for detecting, evaluating, and treating elevated blood cholesterol levels in adults requires that serum lipid and lipoprotein measurement meet certain standards for *precision, accuracy,* and *total analytical error.* Although these three particularly important aspects apply to any measurement, whether a clinical laboratory test (such as serum total cholesterol) or measurement of weight or stature, they are discussed in this section as they relate to measurement of lipid and lipoprotein levels.

Precision (or reproducibility) relates to the difference in results when the same measurement is repeatedly performed. The difference, or variability, in results from repeated, or replicate, measurements should be within acceptable limits. *Accuracy* relates to the difference between the measured value as reported by a clinical laboratory and the "true," or "real," measurement value obtained by using the definitive analytical process known as the "reference method" of measurement. Accuracy is often expressed in terms of *bias,* which is defined as the average deviation of the measured value from the true, or real, value. *Total analytical error* is the National Cholesterol Education's primary criterion for evaluating the performance of an analytical test (e.g., measuring serum cholesterol), and it accounts for both accuracy and precision.[22,23]

Precision

Precision and its relationship to bias are illustrated in Figure 8.9. Precision is high when multiple analyses of the same sample result in values that are reasonably close. In Figure 8.9, high precision can be thought of as multiple shots at the target being in close proximity of each other, as seen in Figure 8.9a and 8.9b. Precision is low when multiple analyses performed on one sample result in values differing considerably, as illustrated in Figure 8.9c and 8.9d. Ideally, replicate analyses of a single sample would yield the same measurement result, but the reality is that these replicate measurements vary somewhat because of potential variation in sample preparation

(some analyses require precipitation and ultracentrifugation of the serum or plasma) and analytical variation inherent in the automatic analyzers used in clinical laboratories. Automatic analyzers are subject to slight variation in function over time. In addition, the reagents used in the analyzers can vary slightly from lot to lot. Obviously, the challenge to the clinical laboratory and the reagent manufacturer is to minimize such fluctuations.[23]

The importance of precision in diagnosing and monitoring persons with high cholesterol levels is illustrated in Figure 8.10. The figure shows the effect of differing degrees of imprecision (sometimes referred to as "random error" or "analytical noise") in cholesterol measurement. If a person's serum sample has a true cholesterol value of 240 mg/dL (6.21 mmol/L), values from replicate analyses of that sample could be scattered over a wide range, depending on the precision of the analytical method. Replicate analyses of a single specimen allow calculation of the measurement as represented by the coefficient of variation (CV). CV is a measure of imprecision and is calculated by dividing the standard deviation (SD) of replicate analyses by the mean of those replicate analyses and then multiplying them by 100 (CV = SD ÷ mean × 100).[22]

Figure 8.10 shows, for example, that, if the precision of an analytical method for serum total cholesterol were such that the CV were 10%, replicate cholesterol analyses of a single specimen having a true value of 240 mg/dL would yield values ranging from 192 to 288 mg/dL. Obviously, with this degree of imprecision, it would be very difficult to properly identify persons with elevated serum cholesterol. Surveys indicate that the analytical CV of clinical laboratories is in the range of 3% to 7%, with an average of 4%.[23] The National Cholesterol Education Program believes that a modern, well-controlled clinical laboratory should be able

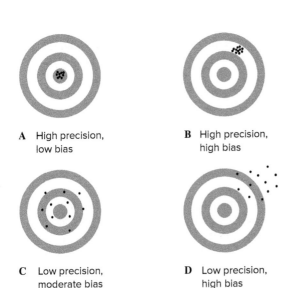

A High precision, low bias

B High precision, high bias

C Low precision, moderate bias

D Low precision, high bias

Figure 8.9
Multiple shots at a target can be used to illustrate precision and bias. Note that high precision is necessary for low bias to exist.

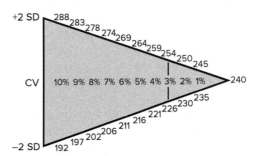

Figure 8.10 **Effect of differing degrees of imprecision in analysis of a blood specimen with a true cholesterol value of 240 mg/dL.**
An analytical method having a precision consistent with a coefficient of variation (CV) of 3% would yield, on repeat measurements of the same sample, values ranging from 226 to 254 mg/dL. SD = standard deviation.

Source: From National Cholesterol Education Program. 1988. *Current status of blood cholesterol measurement in clinical laboratories in the United States: A report from the Laboratory Standardization Panel of the National Cholesterol Education Program.* Bethesda, MD: U.S. Department of Health and Human Services, Public Health Service; National Institutes of Health; National Heart, Lung, and Blood Institute.

TABLE 8.9	Analytical Performance Goals for Lipid and Lipoprotein Measurements Established by the National Cholesterol Education Program

	Imprecision*	Bias†	Total Analytical Error‡
Total cholesterol	CV ≤ 3%	≤ ± 3%	≤ 8.9%
Triglyceride	CV ≤ 5%	≤ ± 5%	≤ 15.0%
HDL cholesterol	CV ≤ 6%	≤ ± 10%	≤ 22.0%
LDL cholesterol	CV ≤ 4%	≤ ± 4%	≤ 12.0%

Source: National Cholesterol Education Program. 1995. *Recommendations on lipoprotein measurement from the working group on lipoprotein measurement.* Bethesda, MD: U.S. Department of Health and Human Services, Public Health Service; National Institutes of Health; National Heart, Lung, and Blood Institute.

*CV = coefficient of variation.

†Percent difference between the measured value and the true value when analyzed using the reference method.

‡Total analytical error = percent bias + (1.96 × CV). Total analytical error is the National Cholesterol Education Program's primary criterion for analytical performance.

to maintain analytical CVs of less than 4%.[23] Analytical performance goals established by the National Cholesterol Education Program are shown in Table 8.9.

Accuracy

Accuracy and bias (also referred to as systematic error or overall inaccuracy) and their relationship to precision were illustrated in Figure 8.9. Bias is low when multiple shots at the target repeatedly hit the "bull's eye," as shown in Figure 8.9a. When bias is low, precision is simultaneously high. However, it is impossible for bias to be low when precision is low; thus, precision is a prerequisite for accuracy. Note, also, that high precision does not ensure accuracy, as illustrated in Figure 8.9b. Accuracy is necessary to correctly identify patients with elevated lipid and lipoprotein levels and to monitor their response to treatment. Clinical misdiagnosis can occur from inaccurate measurements, resulting in the reporting of false positive values (measurement results falsely classifying a person as having a condition) or false negative values (measurement results falsely classifying a person as not having a condition).

The true value of a measurement is determined using the reference method, which can be thought of as the "gold standard" measurement process. The U.S. Centers for Disease Control and Prevention (CDC) has established reference methods for measuring each of the lipids and lipoproteins. The CDC-sponsored Cholesterol Reference Method Laboratory Network has established a formal certification program for clinical laboratories, manufacturers of automated analyzers, and organizations providing laboratory standardization and proficiency testing. Laboratory standardization and proficiency testing programs provide clinical laboratories with an opportunity to determine the precision and accuracy of their instruments. The bias of a particular

analytical method or automated analyzer can be determined by comparing the mean value of replicate analyses performed on the particular analyzer with the mean value of replicate analyses of the same sample performed using the reference method. The percentage difference between the mean results of the clinical laboratory undergoing evaluation and that of the reference method is known as the relative bias.[22]

If a laboratory's particular analytical method of measuring serum total cholesterol has a *positive bias* of 10% and a subject's true cholesterol value is 200 mg/dL (5.17 mmol/L), the laboratory's reported value is 220 mg/dL (5.69 mmol/L), or 10% greater than the true value. If a person's true value is 240 mg/dL (6.21 mmol/L), a 10% negative bias results in a reported value of 216 mg/dL (5.59 mmol/L), or 10% less than the true value. If the true value is 240 mg/dL (6.21 mmol/L), a 10% positive bias yields a reported value of 264 mg/dL (6.83 mmol/L). Thus, at a given bias, the higher the true cholesterol value, the greater the magnitude of the error. The National Cholesterol Education Program's goals for bias were shown in Table 8.9.

Total Analytical Error

The National Cholesterol Education Program's primary criterion for analytical performance is expressed in terms of *total analytical error,* which takes into account both accuracy (represented as bias) and precision (represented as the coefficient of variation).[23] Total analytical error is calculated using the following equation: total analytical error = percent bias + (1.96 × coefficient of variation).[23] Because calculation of total analytical error includes both bias and the coefficient of variation, a greater inaccuracy (larger bias) can be tolerated if the measurements are very precise.[23] On the other hand, if the measurements are more accurate (bias is low), then a greater degree of imprecision (larger coefficient of variation) can be tolerated. The National Cholesterol Education Program's goals for total analytical error were shown in Table 8.9.

Sources of Error in Cholesterol Measurement

Approximately one-third of within-individual variability in cholesterol analyses is due to laboratory errors. These factors are beyond the scope of this text and will not be addressed.

The remaining two-thirds of within-individual variability is due to a variety of factors occurring before the sample is actually analyzed. These can be referred to as *preanalytical factors.*[22–24] Preanalytical factors operate before or during blood sampling or during sample storage or shipment to the laboratory. They can be divided into biological factors contributing to the patient's usual cholesterol level and those factors altering the patient's usual cholesterol level (Table 8.10).

TABLE 8.10	Preanalytical Factors Affecting Within-Individual Variability in Cholesterol Levels			
Biological	**Behavioral**	**Clinical (Disease-Induced)**	**Clinical (Drug-Induced)**	**Sample Collecting and Handling**
Age Individual biology Race	Usual diet Alcohol Caffeine	Acute and transient: burns, infections, recent myocardial infarction, recent stroke, trauma	Antihypertensives: beta-blockers, chlorothalidone, thiazides Immunosuppressives: cyclosporine, prednisolone, tacrolimus	Anticoagulants/preservatives Fasting status Diurnal variation/time of day
Sex	Exercise Smoking Stress	Endocrine: diabetes mellitus, hypothyroidism, hypopituitarism, pregnancy	Steroids: estrogen, progestin	Hemoconcentration Posture Specimen storage
		Hepatic: congenital biliary atresia		
		Renal: chronic renal failure, nephrotic syndrome		Venous vs. capillary blood Venous occlusion
		Storage diseases: Gaucher disease, glycogen storage disease, Tay-Sachs disease		
		Other: anorexia nervosa, systemic lupus erythematosus		

Source: Rifai N, Dufour R, Cooper GR. 1997. Preanalytical variation in lipid, lipoprotein, and apolipoprotein testing. In Rifai N, Warnick GR, Dominiczak MH (eds.), *Handbook of lipoprotein testing.* Washington, DC: American Association of Clinical Chemistry, 75–97; Warnick GR. 2000. Measurement of cholesterol and other lipoprotein constituents in the clinical laboratory. *Clinical Chemistry and Laboratory Medicine* 38:287–300.

As can be seen in Table 8.10, numerous factors have the potential for altering usual cholesterol level. Some of these can be controlled by those persons involved in the drawing, preparation, storage, and shipment of blood specimens. In addition, certain conditions call for postponing measurement of serum lipid and lipoprotein levels. Among those identified by the National Cholesterol Education Program are recent myocardial infarction, stroke, trauma, acute infections, and pregnancy.

Fasting

Total cholesterol and HDL-C levels can be measured in nonfasting persons. Recent food intake affects plasma total cholesterol levels by only about 1.5% or less.[25] The NCEP recommended that plasma triglyceride concentrations be measured only after a fast of at least 12 hours because absorption of fat after a meal elevates blood triglyceride levels. When a patient's LDL-C value is desired, a fast of at least 12 hours also is necessary because LDL-C typically is calculated from measurements of triglyceride, cholesterol, and HDL-C. If the triglyceride concentration is > 400 mg/dL (> 4.52 mmol/L), the LDL-C should be measured directly instead of being calculated.[25]

Posture

When a person sits or lies down after standing for several minutes, his or her plasma volume increases, and the concentration of cholesterol (and other nondiffusible

plasma components) decreases. Compared with values in blood drawn while a person is standing, cholesterol levels can be significantly lower in blood drawn from the same person after he or she has been lying down for 5 minutes and may be as much as 10% to 15% lower in blood drawn after the person has been lying down for 20 minutes. Cholesterol levels in blood drawn after a person has been sitting for 10 to 15 minutes have been shown to be 6% lower than those in blood drawn from the same person while standing. It is recommended that blood sampling conditions be standardized to the sitting position. The patient should sit quietly for about 5 minutes before the sample is drawn.[25]

Venous Occlusion

If a tourniquet is applied to a vein for a prolonged period, the concentration of cholesterol (and other nondiffusible plasma components) will increase. The cholesterol concentration of blood drawn from a vein following a 2-minute tourniquet application can be 2% to 5% higher than that of venous blood drawn after a 30- to 60-second tourniquet application. A 10% to 15% average increase can result from a 5-minute tourniquet application. Venipuncture should be completed as rapidly as possible, preferably within 1 minute.[25]

Anticoagulants

Plasma is derived from whole blood, which is treated with an anticoagulant. The anticoagulants heparin and ethylenediamine tetraacetic acid are preferred. Fluoride, citrate, and oxalate anticoagulants should not be used because they cause plasma components to be diluted (cholesterol concentration is lower when these are used).[25,26]

Recent Heart Attack and Stroke

When a person has suffered a heart attack or stroke, his or her total cholesterol and LDL-C should not be measured for eight weeks following the attack. These levels fall considerably in a heart attack or stroke victim and remain low for several weeks.

Trauma and Acute Infections

Cholesterol levels can fall by as much as 40% in a person who has suffered severe trauma and can fall temporarily in response to severe pain, surgery, and short-term physical strain. Cholesterol measurements should be performed no sooner than eight weeks after such conditions have occurred.

Pregnancy

Increases in LDL and VLDL during pregnancy can lead to increases in cholesterol levels by as much as 35%. It is recommended that lipid measurements not be made until three to four months after delivery.

HYPERTENSION

Hypertension (high blood pressure) is one of the most prevalent and serious risk factors for CVD (Figures 8.4, 8.5, 8.11). High blood pressure (HBP) usually doesn't give early warning signs and, for this reason, is known as the "silent killer." HBP increases the risk for CHD and other forms of heart disease, stroke, and kidney failure.[27–30] Figure 8.12 shows that as systolic blood pressure (SBP) or diastolic blood pressure (DBP) increases, there is an increased risk of CVD death.[31] Compared with other dietary, lifestyle, and metabolic risk factors, HBP is the leading cause of death in women and the second leading cause of death in men, behind smoking.[29] More than 360,000 American deaths in 2013 included HBP as a primary or contributing cause.[1] HBP increases the risk for dangerous health conditions, including[1]

- *First heart attack:* 7 of 10 people having their first heart attack have HBP.
- *First stroke:* 8 of 10 people having their first stroke have HBP.
- *Chronic (long-lasting) heart failure:* 7 of 10 people with chronic heart failure have HBP.
- *Kidney disease* is also a major risk factor for HBP.

About 80 million American adults (30.4%) have HBP, with the highest proportions found among the elderly and blacks/African Americans[1,3] (Figure 8.11a,b). NHANES data indicate that hypertension prevalence is currently higher than in 1988–1994[1,3] (Figure 8.11c). The year 2020 target for HBP prevalence is 27% (healthypeople.gov), but

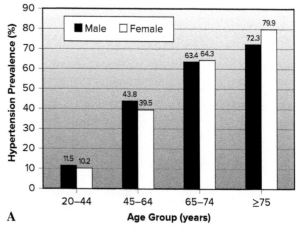

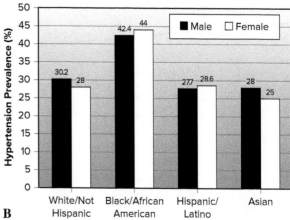

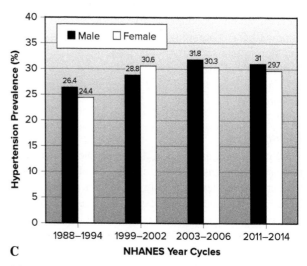

Figure 8.11   About 3 in 10 adults have high blood pressure, with proportions rising among (A) the elderly and (B) African-Americans. NHANES data show that hypertension prevalence is greater now than in 1988–1994.

Source: National Center for Health Statistics. 2016. *Health, United States, 2015: With special feature on racial and ethnic health disparities.* Hyattsville, MD: National Center for Health Statistics. https://www.cdc.gov/nchs/data/hus/hus15.pdf.

Note: Hypertension is defined as having measured high blood pressure and/or taking antihypertensive medication. High blood pressure is defined as having measured systolic pressure of at least 140 mm Hg or diastolic pressure of at least 90 mm Hg. Those with high blood pressure also may be taking prescribed medicine for high blood pressure. Those taking antihypertensive medication may not have measured high blood pressure but are still classified as having hypertension.

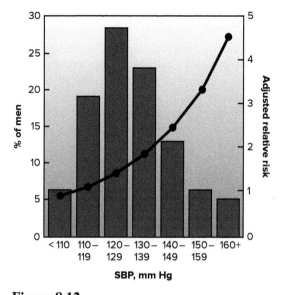 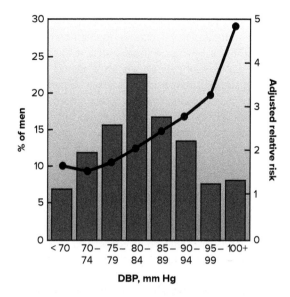

Figure 8.12

The bars in this figure represent the distribution of systolic blood pressure (chart on the left) and diastolic blood pressure (chart on the right) for males ages 35 to 57 years participating in the Multiple Risk Factor Intervention Trial ($N = 347,978$). The curved lines represent the 12-year rate of cardiovascular mortality for each level of systolic blood pressure (SBP) and diastolic blood pressure (DBP). As either SBP or DBP increases, risk of death from cardiovascular disease increases.

Source: National High Blood Pressure Education Program Working Group. 1993. National High Blood Pressure Education Program Working Group report on primary prevention of hypertension. *Archives of Internal Medicine* 153:186–208.

projections suggest that by 2030, 41.4% of U.S. adults will have hypertension.[1]

About 11% of children and adolescents aged 8 to 17 years have either HBP or borderline HBP.[1] High blood pressure costs the nation $50 billion each year, including health-care services, medications to treat high blood pressure, and missed days of work.[1]

Prehypertension is untreated SBP of 120 to 139 mm Hg or untreated DBP of 80 to 89 mm Hg and not having been told on two occasions by a physician or other health professional that one has hypertension. Among participants without a history of CVD or cancer in NHANES 1999–2006, the prevalence of prehypertension was 36.3%. Prevalence was higher in men than in women. Furthermore, prehypertension was correlated with an adverse cardiometabolic risk profile and the metabolic syndrome.[1]

Only about half (54%) of people with high blood pressure have their condition under control.[1] Data from NHANES 2009 to 2012 showed that of those with hypertension who were ≥ 20 years of age, 82.7% were aware of their condition, 76.5% were under current treatment, 54.1% had their hypertension under control, and 45.9% did not have it controlled.[1] As emphasized earlier in this chapter, the AHA has identified untreated and lower blood pressure (less than 90th percentile for youths, less than 120/80 mm Hg for adults) as one of the seven components of ideal cardiovascular health.[1] Approximately 82% of youths and 42% of adults meet this criteria.[1]

Arterial blood pressure is measured using a device called a sphygmomanometer ("blood pressure cuff") and is expressed in millimeters of mercury (mm Hg). Systolic blood pressure is the blood pressure following systole, the phase of cardiac contraction. Diastolic blood pressure is that following diastole, the phase of cardiac relaxation. Blood pressure is expressed as two numbers, as in 120/80. The first number (120 mm Hg) is systolic blood pressure, and the second is diastolic blood pressure (80 mm Hg). From the standpoint of cardiovascular disease, a normal blood pressure is one that is less than 120/80, although unusually low blood pressure readings should be evaluated for clinical significance.

There are three types of sphygmomanometers: mercury, aneroid, and electronic. Mercury sphygmomanometers are simple in design, accurate, reliable, and easy to calibrate; however, concerns about the potential of mercury spillage contaminating the environment have resulted in increased use of aneroid and electronic units, which do not contain mercury. Aneroid and electronic sphygmomanometers must be appropriately validated and regularly checked for accuracy.[28] The subject of a blood pressure measurement should be seated quietly in a chair (rather than on an examination table) for at least five minutes with both feet on the floor and the arms supported at heart level. To ensure accuracy, an appropriately sized cuff should be used; the bladder cuff should circle at least 80% of the arm. At least two measurements should be made and the average value recorded.[28] In ambulatory blood pressure monitoring (ABPM), the subject wears a device that periodically measures and records blood pressure over a period of 24 hours or longer. For some patients, ABPM is a better indicator of average blood pressure, particularly for patients who experience "white-coat hypertension," a temporary increase in blood pressure when it is measured in the medical care environment. Values obtained from ABPM are generally lower than those obtained when blood pressure is measured in a clinic setting. Self-monitoring of blood pressure is also a recommended approach, as long as the sphygmomanometer is reliable and properly calibrated and the subject is instructed in the correct operation of the unit.[28]

Table 8.11 shows the guidelines developed by the National High Blood Pressure Education Program for classifying blood pressure.[28] To be considered within the normal range, systolic blood pressure must be < 120 mm Hg and diastolic pressure must be < 80 mm Hg. The classification of *prehypertension* is defined as a systolic blood pressure ranging from 120 to 139 mm Hg and/or a diastolic blood pressure of 80 to 89 mm Hg. Introduction of the prehypertension category reflects the fact that the risk of cardiovascular and kidney disease is increased at levels of blood pressure previously thought to be normal. While prehypertension is not a disease category, it identifies high-risk persons who should modify their lifestyle practices to reduce their blood pressure, to decrease the risk that their blood pressure will progress to hypertensive levels with increasing age, or to prevent hypertension entirely.[28] Lifestyle modifications are generally sufficient to normalize the blood pressure in persons with prehypertension. However, persons with prehypertension who also have diabetes or kidney disease should be considered candidates for appropriate drug therapy if lifestyle modifications fail to normalize their blood pressure.[28]

Efforts to reduce morbidity and mortality related to hypertension can be grouped into two broad categories: the patient-based, or clinical, approach and the population-based, or public health, approach. Early efforts to reduce hypertension-related morbidity and mortality centered on the patient-based approach, which involves clinicians detecting and treating individual cases of hypertension. More recently, greater attention has been given to the population-based approach, which stresses increased public awareness of hypertension and encourages every adult to know his or her blood pressure and to avoid those behaviors identified as risk factors for hypertension.

Management of High Blood Pressure

For more than three decades, the NHLBI administered the National High Blood Pressure Education Program (NHBPEP) Coordinating Committee, a coalition of 39 major professional, public, and voluntary organizations and seven federal agencies.[27,28,31] One important function was to issue guidelines and advisories designed to increase awareness, prevention, treatment, and control of hypertension.

The prior Seventh Joint National Committee Guidelines on Prevention, Evaluation, Detection, and Treatment of High Blood Pressure (JNC7) established treatment goals for SBP and DBP of less than 130/80 mm Hg for individuals with diabetes mellitus or chronic kidney disease (CKD) and less than 140/90 mm Hg for individuals without these comorbidities.[28] In June 2013, NHLBI announced its decision to discontinue developing clinical guidelines, with a focus on partnering with selected organizations that would develop the guidelines. Toward this end, the 2014 Evidence-Based Guideline for the Management of High Blood Pressure in Adults from the Eight Joint National Committee Panel (JNC8) focused on blood pressure thresholds for pharmacological treatment.[27] After a critical review of the evidence, the JNC8 guidelines established less stringent thresholds for consideration of pharmacological intervention, setting a goal blood pressure of less than 150/90 mm Hg for aging individuals (60 years of age and older) without diabetes mellitus or CKD and less than 140/90 mm Hg for individuals with diabetes mellitus, CKD, or age of less than 60 years. Box 8.4 summarizes the nine major JNC8 recommendations. Concern has been raised that implementation of JNC8P guidelines will adversely affect the elderly population because of less aggressive treatment of hypertension, leading to an increase in CVD events. In response, defenders of the JNC8 panel reasoned that an evidence-based approach to the guidelines was used, and then adapted JNC7 guidelines accordingly.

TABLE 8.11	Classification of Blood Pressure for Persons Age 18 Years and Older*		
	Systolic BP (mm Hg)		Diastolic BP (mm Hg)
Normal[†]	< 120	and	< 80
Prehypertension	120–139	or	80–89
Stage 1 hypertension	140–159	or	90–99
Stage 2 hypertension	≥ 160	or	≥ 100

Source: National High Blood Pressure Education Program. 2004. *The seventh report of the Joint National Committee on Prevention, Detection, Evaluation, and Treatment of High Blood Pressure.* U.S. Department of Health and Human Services, National Institutes of Health, National Heart, Lung, and Blood Institute.

*Not taking antihypertensive drugs and not acutely ill.

[†]Based on the average of two or more properly measured, seated, blood pressure readings taken at each of two or more visits after an initial screening.

Lifestyle Guidelines to Manage Blood Pressure

Numerous risk factors and markers for development of hypertension have been identified, including age, race/

Box 8.4 | **2014 Evidence-Based Guideline for the Management of High Blood Pressure in Adults (JNC8)**

Recommendation 1: In the general population aged ≥ 60 years, initiate pharmacologic treatment to lower blood pressure (BP) at systolic blood pressure (SBP) ≥ 150 mm Hg or diastolic blood pressure (DBP) ≥ 90 mm Hg and treat to a goal SBP < 150 mm Hg and goal DBP < 90 mm Hg.

Recommendation 2: In the general population < 60 years, initiate pharmacologic treatment to lower BP at DBP ≥ 90 mm Hg and treat to a goal DBP < 90 mm Hg.

Recommendation 3: In the general population < 60 years, initiate pharmacologic treatment to lower BP at SBP ≥ 140 mm Hg and treat to a goal SBP < 140 mmHg.

Recommendation 4: In the population aged ≥ 18 years with chronic kidney disease (CKD), initiate pharmacologic treatment to lower BP at SBP ≥ 140 mm Hg or DBP ≥ 90 mm Hg and treat to goal SBP < 140 mm Hg and goal DBP < 90 mmHg.

Recommendation 5: In the population aged ≥ 18 years with diabetes, initiate pharmacologic treatment to lower BP at SBP ≥ 140 mm Hg or DBP ≥ 90 mm Hg and treat to a goal SBP < 140 mm Hg and goal DBP < 90 mm Hg.

Recommendation 6: In the general nonblack population, including those with diabetes, initial antihypertensive treatment should include a thiazide-type diuretic, calcium channel blocker (CCB), angiotensin-converting enzyme inhibitor (ACEI), or angiotensin receptor blocker (ARB).

Recommendation 7: In the general black population, including those with diabetes, initial antihypertensive treatment should include a thiazide-type diuretic or CCB.

Recommendation 8: In the population aged ≥ 18 years with CKD, initial (or add-on) antihypertensive treatment should include an ACEI or ARB to improve kidney outcomes. This applies to all CKD patients with hypertension regardless of race or diabetes status.

Recommendation 9: The main objective of hypertension treatment is to attain and maintain goal BP. If goal BP is not reached within a month of treatment, increase the dose of the initial drug or add a second drug from one of the classes in recommendation 6 (thiazide-type diuretic, CCB, ACEI, or ARB). The clinician should continue to assess BP and adjust the treatment regimen until goal BP is reached. If goal BP cannot be reached with two drugs, add and titrate a third drug from the list provided. Do not use an ACEI and an ARB together in the same patient. If goal BP cannot be reached using only the drugs in recommendation 6 because of a contraindication or the need to use more than three drugs to reach goal BP, antihypertensive drugs from other classes can be used. Referral to a hypertension specialist may be indicated for patients in whom goal BP cannot be attained using the above strategy or for the management of complicated patients for whom additional clinical consultation is needed.

Source: James PA, Oparil S, Carter BL, Cushman WC, Dennison-Himmelfarb C, Handler J, Lackland DT, LeFevre ML, MacKenzie TD, Ogedegbe O, Smith SC Jr., Svetkey LP, Taler SJ, Townsend RR, Wright JT Jr, Narva AS, Ortiz E. 2014. 2014 evidence-based guideline for the management of high blood pressure in adults: Report from the panel members appointed to the Eighth Joint National Committee (JNC 8). *Journal of the American Medical Association* 311:507–520.

ethnicity, family history of hypertension and genetic factors, lower education and socioeconomic status, greater weight, lower PA, tobacco use, psychosocial stressors, sleep apnea, and dietary factors (including dietary fats, higher sodium intake, lower potassium intake, and excessive alcohol intake).[1]

The 2014 JNC8 guidelines recommended lifestyle interventions for all persons with hypertension throughout the treatment and management process.[27] The JNC8 Expert Panel urged that the potential benefits of a healthy diet, weight control, and regular exercise could not be overemphasized and that lifestyle treatments have the potential to improve blood pressure control and even reduce medication needs. The JNC8 Expert Panel supported that the recommendations of the 2013 Lifestyle Work Group, and these are summarized in Box 8.2.[10]

In general, lifestyle treatments to improve blood pressure control are based on maintaining a healthy body weight, consuming a dietary pattern such as the DASH diet or the AHA diet (Table 8.3), lowering sodium intake, and engaging in regular physical activity. Specifically, the DASH and AHA dietary patterns emphasize vegetables, fruits, and whole grains, low-fat dairy products, poultry, fish, legumes, nontropical vegetable oils, and nuts while limiting sweets, sugar-sweetened beverages, and red meats. This diet is naturally low in sodium and high in potassium, and it is associated with lower blood pressure.

Energy intake should be adapted to appropriate calorie requirements, personal and cultural food preferences, and medical conditions (including diabetes). In general, adults should be advised to engage in three to four 40-minute sessions per week of moderate- to vigorous-intensity aerobic physical activity.[10] Energy balance and loss of excess weight are the most effective of all lifestyle strategies for management of blood pressure. Box 8.5 provides a summary of expected decreases in SBP with lifestyle modifications, including a 5–20 mm Hg reduction for every 10 kg weight loss.[28]

Box 8.5 | **Lifestyle Modifications to Prevent and Manage Hypertension**

MODIFICATION	RECOMMENDATION	APPROXIMATE SYSTOLIC BP REDUCTION (RANGE)*
Weight reduction	Maintain normal body weight (BMI 18.5–24.9 kg/m²)	5–20 mm Hg per 10 kg weight loss
Adopt DASH eating plan†	Consume a diet rich in fruits, vegetables, and low-fat dairy products with a reduced content of saturated and total fat.	8–14 mm Hg
Dietary sodium reduction	Reduce dietary sodium intake to no more than 100 mmol per day (2.4 g sodium or 6.0 g sodium chloride).	2–8 mm Hg
Physical activity	Engage in regular aerobic physical activity such as brisk walking (at least 30 min per day, most days of the week).	4–9 mm Hg
Moderation of alcohol consumption	Limit consumption to no more than two drinks per day in most men and to no more than one drink per day in women and lighter-weight persons	2–4 mm Hg

*The effects of implementing these modifications are dose and time dependent and could be greater for some individuals.
†DASH = Dietary Approaches to Stop Hypertension.
For overall cardiovascular risk reduction, stop smoking.

Source: National High Blood Pressure Education Program. 2004. *The seventh report of the Joint National Committee on Prevention, Detection, Evaluation, and Treatment of High Blood Pressure.* U.S. Department of Health and Human Services, National Institutes of Health, National Heart, Lung, and Blood Institute.

No more than 2400 mg of sodium should be consumed per day, with further reduction to 1500 mg per day for even greater reductions in blood pressure.[10] Most people consume a diet that contains well over 1 teaspoon of sodium per day, with about 75% of this from processed foods. This is far in excess of body needs and tends to elevate blood pressure as the salt habit is continued into old age.[28] Clinical trials have shown that lifestyle modifications involving these lifestyle factors can lower elevated blood pressure at little cost, with minimal risk, and to an extent equal to or greater than single-drug therapy.[27–31] Even when these modifications fail to control hypertension, they can reduce the number and dosage of antihypertensive medications needed to manage the condition—what is referred to as a "step-down" in therapy. Primary prevention is particularly helpful in lowering the elevated blood pressures of persons in groups at higher risk of hypertension, such as African Americans, older persons, and persons with hypertension or diabetes.[28]

Body Weight

The evidence linking body weight to blood pressure and overweight to hypertension is strong and consistent. A body mass index ≥ 30 kg/m² is closely correlated with increased blood pressure. Excess adipose tissue within the abdomen (abdominal fat) has been associated with increased risk of hypertension, dyslipidemia, type 2 diabetes, and coronary heart disease.[10,28] As discussed in Chapter 6, the best clinical approach to assessing abdominal adiposity is measuring waist circumference. A high-risk waist circumference in adult males and females as > 40 inches and > 35 inches, respectively. Several studies have shown that loss of excess body weight reduces both SBP and DBP and that the degree of blood pressure reduction is related to the extent of weight loss. A weight reduction of as little as 10 pounds is effective at reducing elevated blood pressure in overweight persons with hypertension, while enhancing the effectiveness of antihypertensive drugs and reducing cardiovascular disease risk by enhancing the management of type 2 diabetes and dyslipidemia.[10,28]

The largest randomized controlled trial to evaluate the impact of weight loss in persons with high-normal blood pressure, the Trials of Hypertension Prevention, showed that an average weight loss of 8.4 lb (3.8 kg) resulted in a 2.9 mm Hg and 2.3 mm Hg reduction in SBP and DBP, respectively.[32,33] Although this may seem like an insignificant decline in blood pressure, it has been estimated that a 2 mm Hg decline in the population mean SBP might reduce the annual mortality from stroke, CHD, and all causes by 6%, 4%, and 3%, respectively.[28] Not only is weight loss an effective means of lowering blood pressure, but it also tends to improve the lipid and lipoprotein profile and reduce the risk of developing noninsulin-dependent diabetes mellitus and possibly breast cancer.

Sodium

Research on the association between sodium intake and blood pressure has been hampered by several methodologic challenges. These include difficulty in measuring sodium intake, variable adherence to the prescribed reduction in sodium, the large day-to-day intraindividual (within-person) variation in sodium intake, the wide range of blood pressure values at any level of sodium intake, the small interindividual (between-person) variation in sodium intakes within a given population group, inadequate trial design, small numbers of subjects, and limitations in analysis and presentation of research findings. Despite these challenges, there is unequivocal evidence that a causal relationship exists between sodium intake and risk of hypertension, particularly from those studies that determine sodium intake by measuring 24-hour urinary sodium excretion, which is the definitive method for determining sodium intake.[10,28,34,35]

Sodium intake is far in excess of human physiologic need and is much greater than the typical intakes of people in less industrialized societies, who do not experience North America's age-related increase in blood pressure. The Adequate Intake (AI) (discussed in Chapter 2) for sodium for males and females ages 14 to 50 years is 1500 mg per day.[34] The AI for persons 51 to 70 years of age is 1300 mg per day, and for persons older than 70 years it is 1200 mg per day. The Tolerable Upper Intake Level (UL) (discussed in Chapter 2) for sodium for all age groups is 2300 mg per day.[34] The Dietary Guidelines for Americans recommend limiting sodium intake to less than 2300 mg per day. Adults with prehypertension and hypertension would benefit by further reducing sodium intake to 1500 mg per day (https://health.gov/dietaryguidelines/2015/). Research shows that for most people, a reduction in sodium intake to the current AI of 1500 mg per day is safe and is an effective way to reduce risk for hypertension.[10,28,30,34] Furthermore, the blood pressures of blacks, middle-aged and older persons, and those with hypertension are more responsive to changes in dietary sodium. A modest reduction in sodium intake to less than 2300 mg per day and adoption of some of the other lifestyle changes shown in Box 8.5 are sufficient to control mild hypertension in many patients. For those still needing antihypertensive medication, these steps will reduce their requirement for medication (result in a step-down in therapy).[10,28]

Data from the Dietary Approaches to Stop Hypertension (DASH) trial show that a further reduction in sodium intake to 1.5 g per day provides a safe and effective way to further reduce risk for hypertension. The DASH trial was a multicenter, randomized feeding trial testing the effects of certain dietary patterns on blood pressure. These and other data provide a scientific basis for a lower goal for dietary sodium than the level currently recommended.[35]

Maintaining a sodium intake of < 2300 mg per day is difficult, considering the high-salt food environment in the United States and the fact that approximately 77% of sodium in the U.S. diet comes from processed foods. Between the early 1970s and 2000, sodium intake in the United States rose 55%, primarily because of increased consumption of fast foods and convenience foods during that interval.[10,28] A sodium intake of < 2300 mg per day has been a "cornerstone" of the recommendations from the National Heart, Lung, and Blood Institute's National High Blood Pressure Education Program and other groups working to decrease the prevalence of hypertension in the United States. One of the *Healthy People 2020* objectives is for Americans 2 years of age and older to reduce their sodium intake to no more than 2300 mg per day.

Alcohol

Despite the difficulty of measuring the alcohol intake of study participants, there is consistent evidence of a strong positive relationship between alcohol consumption and blood pressure. It is estimated that as much as 5% to 7% of the overall prevalence of hypertension in the United States can be attributed to an alcohol intake of three drinks or more per day.[28] One drink of alcohol (0.5 fluid ounce of ethanol) is equivalent to 12 fluid ounces of beer, 4 fluid ounces of wine, or 1 ounce of 100-proof spirits. Furthermore, when alcohol intake is reduced, there is a subsequent reduction in blood pressure. A reduction in alcohol intake has been shown to be effective in lowering blood pressure in both hypertensive and normotensive individuals, and it may help prevent hypertension. Persons with hypertension should be advised to limit their alcohol intake to no more than two drinks per day.[28]

Physical Activity

Numerous studies have shown an inverse relationship between leisure-time and work-related physical activity and blood pressure. Other studies have shown that blood pressure tends to be lower in physically fit individuals. Although these studies have certain design limitations, they provide consistent evidence that increased physical activity results in an average reduction of approximately 6 to 7 mm Hg for both SBP and DBP. This reduction is not dependent on weight loss. A low to moderate exercise intensity (40% to 60% of maximum oxygen consumption) is as effective at lowering blood pressure in patients with mild to moderate hypertension as higher-intensity exercise. This can be achieved by brisk walking for 30 to 45 minutes most days of the week.[10,28]

Dietary Pattern

A number of studies have identified an inverse relationship between blood pressure and consumption of foods providing potassium, calcium, and magnesium. Persons consuming vegetarian diets, for example, tend to have a lower blood pressure than nonvegetarians. Aspects of the vegetarian diet believed to reduce blood pressure include minerals (potassium, calcium, and magnesium), reduced fat content, and possibly dietary fiber.[10,28,30] In studies investigating individual nutrients, often when provided in supplemental form, the reduction in blood pressure is typically small and inconsistent, probably because the blood pressure–lowering effect of a single nutrient is too small to detect in clinical trials. However, when these nutrients are consumed together, the cumulative effect is sufficient to bring about a statistically and clinically significant lowering of blood pressure. Food is incredibly complex and contains countless nutrients and components other than those few being examined in trials or measured in observational studies. When evaluating the blood pressure–lowering effects of foods, these nutrients and food components and the complex interactions among them must be considered.[30]

Consequently, increased attention is being given to the overall dietary pattern, rather than to a few individual nutrients. This is in large part due to results from the Dietary Approaches to Stop Hypertension (DASH) trial.[10,30,35] The DASH trial showed that a diet rich in fruits, vegetables, and fat-free or low-fat dairy products lowers elevated blood pressure, particularly when sodium intake is kept moderate.[30,35] The DASH diet, combined with a moderate sodium restriction and sustained efforts to modify the other factors associated with hypertension, which were listed in Box 8.5, is a safe, effective, and low-cost nonpharmacologic approach for promoting optimal to normal blood pressure.

Evaluating Blood Pressure in Children and Adolescents

As shown in Box 8.6, hypertension in children and adolescents age 1 to 17 years is defined as an average systolic blood pressure (SBP) and/or diastolic blood pressure (DBP) that is greater than or equal to the 95th percentile of blood pressure for a young person of a given sex, age, and height.[36] Prehypertension in children and adolescents age 1 to 17 years is defined as average SBP or DBP levels that are ≥ 90th percentile but < 95th percentile. This somewhat arbitrary definition of hypertension is based on the normative distribution of blood pressure in apparently

healthy children and adolescents in which those in the top 5% for a given sex, age, and height are categorized as hypertensive. In adults, blood pressure is categorized on the basis of clinical outcomes, with a normal blood pressure being one associated with a low-risk of disease and with hypertension associated with increasing risk of disease such as CHD, stroke, or kidney failure. Because these diseases are rarely *clinically evident* in young people, even those with hypertension, a different strategy must be used to establish categories of normal blood pressure, prehypertension, and hypertension.[36] It is important to identify and effectively treat children with hypertension because target-organ damage can occur at a young age in children and adolescents with hypertension.[1,36]

To evaluate the blood pressure of a child or adolescent, it is necessary to determine his or her percentile of height for sex and age. This is done using the sex- and age-appropriate CDC growth charts that provide the length-for-age percentiles (for children ≤ 3 years of age who are unable to stand on their own without assistance) or the stature-for-age percentiles (for those ≥ 2 years of age who are able to stand on their own without assistance). The CDC growth charts are discussed in Chapter 6 and shown in Appendix G. Once the subject's percentile of height is determined, Table 8.12 or 8.13 is used to determine the blood pressure percentile. Consider, for example, a 9-year-old male who is 53 inches tall and whose blood pressure, averaged from multiple measurements taken during three different visits to a physician's office, is shown to be 116/76 mm Hg. Using the appropriate CDC growth chart (2 to 20 years: boys, stature-for-age and weight-for-age percentiles) shown in Appendix G, it is determined that this youngster is at the 50th percentile of height (i.e., stature) for age. Table 8.12 is then used to categorize the systolic and diastolic blood pressure. For this youngster, an SBP of 116 mm Hg lies between the values of 114 and 118 mm Hg, which is between the 90th and 95th percentiles of SBP. The DBP of 76 mm Hg lies between the values of 75 and 79 mm Hg, which is between

Box 8.6	**Evaluating Blood Pressure in Children and Adolescents**

- Hypertension is defined as an average SBP and/or DBP that is greater than or equal to the 95th percentile for sex, age, and height on three or more occasions.
- Prehypertension in children is defined as average SBP or DBP levels that are greater than or equal to the 90th percentile but less than the 95th percentile.
- As with adults, adolescents with BP levels greater than or equal to 120/80 mm Hg but less

than the 95th percentile should be considered prehypertensive.
- A patient with BP levels above the 95th percentile in a physician's office or clinic but who is normotensive outside a clinical setting has white-coat hypertension. Ambulatory BP monitoring (ABPM) is usually required to make this diagnosis.

Source: National High Blood Pressure Education Program. 2005. *The fourth report on the diagnosis, evaluation, and treatment of high blood pressure in children and adolescents.* U.S. Department of Health and Human Services, National Institutes of Health, National Heart, Lung, and Blood Institute.

TABLE 8.12 | Blood Pressure Levels for Males by Age and Height Percentiles

Age, y	BP percentile	SBP, mm Hg							DBP, mm Hg						
		Percentile of height							Percentile of height						
		5th	10th	25th	50th	75th	90th	95th	5th	10th	25th	50th	75th	90th	95th
1	50th	80	81	83	85	87	88	89	34	35	36	37	38	39	39
	90th	94	95	97	99	100	102	103	49	50	51	52	53	53	54
	95th	98	99	101	103	104	106	106	54	54	55	56	57	58	58
	99th	105	106	108	110	112	113	114	61	62	63	64	65	66	66
2	50th	84	85	87	88	90	92	92	39	40	41	42	43	44	44
	90th	97	99	100	102	104	105	106	54	55	56	57	58	58	59
	95th	101	102	104	106	108	109	110	59	59	60	61	62	63	63
	99th	109	110	111	113	115	117	117	66	67	68	69	70	71	71
3	50th	86	87	89	91	93	94	95	44	44	45	46	47	48	48
	90th	100	101	103	105	107	108	109	59	59	60	61	62	63	63
	95th	104	105	107	109	110	112	113	63	63	64	65	66	67	67
	99th	111	112	114	116	118	119	120	71	71	72	73	74	75	75
4	50th	88	89	91	93	95	96	97	47	48	49	50	51	51	52
	90th	102	103	105	107	109	110	111	62	63	64	65	66	66	67
	95th	106	107	109	111	112	114	115	66	67	68	69	70	71	71
	99th	113	114	116	118	120	121	122	74	75	76	77	78	78	79
5	50th	90	91	93	95	96	98	98	50	51	52	53	54	55	55
	90th	104	105	106	108	110	111	112	65	66	67	68	69	69	70
	95th	108	109	110	112	114	115	116	69	70	71	72	73	74	74
	99th	115	116	118	120	121	123	123	77	78	79	80	81	81	82
6	50th	91	92	94	96	98	99	100	53	53	54	55	56	57	57
	90th	105	106	108	110	111	113	113	68	68	69	70	71	72	72
	95th	109	110	112	114	115	117	117	72	72	73	74	75	76	76
	99th	116	117	119	121	123	124	125	80	80	81	82	83	84	84
7	50th	92	94	95	97	99	100	101	55	55	56	57	58	59	59
	90th	106	107	109	111	113	114	115	70	70	71	72	73	74	74
	95th	110	111	113	115	117	118	119	74	74	75	76	77	78	78
	99th	117	118	120	122	124	125	126	82	82	83	84	85	86	86
8	50th	94	95	97	99	100	102	102	56	57	58	59	60	60	61
	90th	107	109	110	112	114	115	116	71	72	72	73	74	75	76
	95th	111	112	114	116	118	119	120	75	76	77	78	79	79	80
	99th	119	120	122	123	125	127	127	83	84	85	86	87	87	88
9	50th	95	96	98	100	102	103	104	57	58	59	60	61	61	62
	90th	109	110	112	114	115	117	118	72	73	74	75	76	76	77
	95th	113	114	116	118	119	121	121	76	77	78	79	80	81	81
	99th	120	121	123	125	127	128	129	84	85	86	87	88	88	89

TABLE 8.12 | Blood Pressure Levels for Males by Age and Height Percentiles—continued

Age, y	BP percentile	SBP, mm Hg — Percentile of height							DBP, mm Hg — Percentile of height						
		5th	10th	25th	50th	75th	90th	95th	5th	10th	25th	50th	75th	90th	95th
10	50th	97	98	100	102	103	105	106	58	59	60	61	61	62	63
	90th	111	112	114	115	117	119	119	73	73	74	75	76	77	78
	95th	115	116	117	119	121	122	123	77	78	79	80	81	81	82
	99th	122	123	125	127	128	130	130	85	86	86	88	88	89	90
11	50th	99	100	102	104	105	107	107	59	59	60	61	62	63	63
	90th	113	114	115	117	119	120	121	74	74	75	76	77	78	78
	95th	117	118	119	121	123	124	125	78	78	79	80	81	82	82
	99th	124	125	127	129	130	132	132	86	86	87	88	89	90	90
12	50th	101	102	104	106	108	109	110	59	60	61	62	63	63	64
	90th	115	116	118	120	121	123	123	74	75	75	76	77	78	79
	95th	119	120	122	123	125	127	127	78	79	80	81	82	82	83
	99th	126	127	129	131	133	134	135	86	87	88	89	90	90	91
13	50th	104	105	106	108	110	111	112	60	60	61	62	63	64	64
	90th	117	118	120	122	124	125	126	75	75	76	77	78	79	79
	95th	121	122	124	126	128	129	130	79	79	80	81	82	83	83
	99th	128	130	131	133	135	136	137	87	87	88	89	90	91	91
14	50th	106	107	109	111	113	114	115	60	61	62	63	64	65	65
	90th	120	121	123	125	126	128	128	75	76	77	78	79	79	80
	95th	124	125	127	128	130	132	132	80	80	81	82	83	84	84
	99th	131	132	134	136	138	139	140	87	88	89	90	91	92	92
15	50th	109	110	112	113	115	117	117	61	62	63	64	65	66	66
	90th	122	124	125	127	129	130	131	76	77	78	79	80	80	81
	95th	126	127	129	131	133	134	135	81	81	82	83	84	85	85
	99th	134	135	136	138	140	142	142	88	89	90	91	92	93	93
16	50th	111	112	114	116	118	119	120	63	63	64	65	66	67	67
	90th	125	126	128	130	131	133	134	78	78	79	80	81	82	82
	95th	129	130	132	134	135	137	137	82	83	83	84	85	86	87
	99th	136	137	139	141	143	144	145	90	90	91	92	93	94	94
17	50th	114	115	116	118	120	121	122	65	66	66	67	68	69	70
	90th	127	128	130	132	134	135	136	80	80	81	82	83	84	84
	95th	131	132	134	136	138	139	140	84	85	86	87	87	88	89
	99th	139	140	141	143	145	146	147	92	93	93	94	95	96	97

SBP = systolic blood pressure; DBP = diastolic blood pressure; age is in years.

National High Blood Pressure Education Program. 2005. *The fourth report on the diagnosis, evaluation, and treatment of high blood pressure in children and adolescents.* Bethesda, MD: U.S. Department of Health and Human Services, National Institutes of Health, National Heart, Lung, and Blood Institute.

TABLE 8.13 | **Blood Pressure Levels for Females by Age and Height Percentiles**

Age, y	BP percentile	SBP, mm Hg							DBP, mm Hg						
		Percentile of height							Percentile of height						
		5th	10th	25th	50th	75th	90th	95th	5th	10th	25th	50th	75th	90th	95th
1	50th	83	84	85	86	88	89	90	38	39	39	40	41	41	42
	90th	97	97	98	100	101	102	103	52	53	53	54	55	55	56
	95th	100	101	102	104	105	106	107	56	57	57	58	59	59	60
	99th	108	108	109	111	112	113	114	64	64	65	65	66	67	67
2	50th	85	85	87	88	89	91	91	43	44	44	45	46	46	47
	90th	98	99	100	101	103	104	105	57	58	58	59	60	61	61
	95th	102	103	104	105	107	108	109	61	61	62	63	64	65	65
	99th	109	110	111	112	114	115	116	69	69	70	70	71	72	72
3	50th	86	87	88	89	91	92	93	47	48	48	49	50	50	51
	90th	100	100	102	103	104	106	106	61	62	62	63	64	64	65
	95th	104	104	105	107	108	109	110	65	66	66	67	68	68	69
	99th	111	111	113	114	115	116	117	73	73	74	74	75	76	76
4	50th	88	88	90	91	92	94	94	50	50	51	52	52	53	54
	90th	101	102	103	104	106	107	108	64	64	65	66	67	67	68
	95th	105	106	107	108	110	111	112	68	68	69	70	71	71	72
	99th	112	113	114	115	117	118	119	76	76	76	77	78	79	79
5	50th	89	90	91	93	94	95	96	52	53	53	54	55	55	56
	90th	103	103	105	106	107	109	109	66	67	67	68	69	69	70
	95th	107	107	108	110	111	112	113	70	71	71	72	73	73	74
	99th	114	114	116	117	118	120	120	78	78	79	79	80	81	81
6	50th	91	92	93	94	96	97	98	54	54	55	56	56	57	58
	90th	104	105	106	108	109	110	111	68	68	69	70	70	71	72
	95th	108	109	110	111	113	114	115	72	72	73	74	74	75	76
	99th	115	116	117	119	120	121	122	80	80	80	81	82	83	83
7	50th	93	93	95	96	97	99	99	55	56	56	57	58	58	59
	90th	106	107	108	109	111	112	113	69	70	70	71	72	72	73
	95th	110	111	112	113	115	116	116	73	74	74	75	76	76	77
	99th	117	118	119	120	122	123	124	81	81	82	82	83	84	84
8	50th	95	95	96	98	99	100	101	57	57	57	58	59	60	60
	90th	108	109	110	111	113	114	114	71	71	71	72	73	74	74
	95th	112	112	114	115	116	118	118	75	75	75	76	77	78	78
	99th	119	120	121	122	123	125	125	82	82	83	83	84	85	86
9	50th	96	97	98	100	101	102	103	58	58	58	59	60	61	61
	90th	110	110	112	113	114	116	116	72	72	72	73	74	75	75
	95th	114	114	115	117	118	119	120	76	76	76	77	78	79	79
	99th	121	121	123	124	125	127	127	83	83	84	84	85	86	87

TABLE 8.13 | **Blood Pressure Levels for Females by Age and Height Percentiles—continued**

Age, y	BP percentile	SBP, mm Hg							DBP, mm Hg						
		Percentile of height							Percentile of height						
		5th	10th	25th	50th	75th	90th	95th	5th	10th	25th	50th	75th	90th	95th
10	50th	98	99	100	102	103	104	105	59	59	59	60	61	62	62
	90th	112	112	114	115	116	118	118	73	73	73	74	75	76	76
	95th	116	116	117	119	120	121	122	77	77	77	78	79	80	80
	99th	123	123	125	126	127	129	129	84	84	85	86	86	87	88
11	50th	100	101	102	103	105	106	107	60	60	60	61	62	63	63
	90th	114	114	116	117	118	119	120	74	74	74	75	76	77	77
	95th	118	118	119	121	122	123	124	78	78	78	79	80	81	81
	99th	125	125	126	128	129	130	131	85	85	86	87	87	88	89
12	50th	102	103	104	105	107	108	109	61	61	61	62	63	64	64
	90th	116	116	117	119	120	121	122	75	75	75	76	77	78	78
	95th	119	120	121	123	124	125	126	79	79	79	80	81	82	82
	99th	127	127	128	130	131	132	133	86	86	87	88	88	89	90
13	50th	104	105	106	107	109	110	110	62	62	62	63	64	65	65
	90th	117	118	119	121	122	123	124	76	76	76	77	78	79	79
	95th	121	122	123	124	126	127	128	80	80	80	81	82	83	83
	99th	128	129	130	132	133	134	135	87	87	88	89	89	90	91
14	50th	106	106	107	109	110	111	112	63	63	63	64	65	66	66
	90th	119	120	121	122	124	125	125	77	77	77	78	79	80	80
	95th	123	123	125	126	127	129	129	81	81	81	82	83	84	84
	99th	130	131	132	133	135	136	136	88	88	89	90	90	91	92
15	50th	107	108	109	110	111	113	113	64	64	64	65	66	67	67
	90th	120	121	122	123	125	126	127	78	78	78	79	80	81	81
	95th	124	125	126	127	129	130	131	82	82	82	83	84	85	85
	99th	131	132	133	134	136	137	138	89	89	90	91	91	92	93
16	50th	108	108	110	111	112	114	114	64	64	65	66	66	67	68
	90th	121	122	123	124	126	127	128	78	78	79	80	81	81	82
	95th	125	126	127	128	130	131	132	82	82	83	84	85	85	86
	99th	132	133	134	135	137	138	139	90	90	90	91	92	93	93
17	50th	108	109	110	111	113	114	115	64	65	65	66	67	67	68
	90th	122	122	123	125	126	127	128	78	79	79	80	81	81	82
	95th	125	126	127	129	130	131	132	82	82	83	84	85	85	86
	99th	133	133	134	136	137	138	139	90	90	91	91	92	93	93

SBP = systolic blood pressure; DBP = diastolic blood pressure; age is in years.

National High Blood Pressure Education Program. 2005. *The fourth report on the diagnosis, evaluation, and treatment of high blood pressure in children and adolescents.* Bethesda, MD: U.S. Department of Health and Human Services, National Institutes of Health, National Heart, Lung, and Blood Institute.

the 90th and 95th percentiles of DBP. Based on the information given in Box 8.6, this youngster's blood pressure would be categorized as prehypertension.[36]

The National High Blood Pressure Education Program recommends that after 3 years of age, all children and adolescents have their blood pressure measured every time they are seen in a health-care setting.[36] Measuring blood pressure in children less than 3 years of age is not recommended unless special circumstances exist, such as a previous neonatal complication that required intensive care, congenital heart disease, recurrent urinary tract problems, treatment with drugs known to raise blood pressure, or the presence of some other disease associated with hypertension.[36] Blood pressure should be measured after the subject has been quietly and comfortably seated for five minutes with both feet on the floor and the back supported. Subjects should avoid consuming stimulant drugs or foods prior to the visit with the health-care provider. Using the appropriate size cuff is important, and specific recommendations on cuff size have been published.[13] If the cuff size is too small, the blood pressure measurement will be erroneously high. A cuff that is too large will cause blood pressure to be underestimated, but not to the extent that an inappropriately small cuff will cause blood pressure to be overestimated.[13] An instance of elevated systolic and/or diastolic blood pressure must be confirmed by repeat measurement on at least two additional occasions in order to confirm a diagnosis of prehypertension or hypertension. Blood pressure should be measured two or more times per health-care visit, and values obtained over the course of at least three different visits should be averaged.

DIABETES MELLITUS

Diabetes mellitus is a group of diseases characterized by a defect in insulin secretion and/or increased cellular resistance to insulin, resulting in elevated plasma (or serum) glucose levels, abnormalities of carbohydrate and lipid metabolism, characteristic pathologic changes in the nerves and small blood vessels, and aggravation of atherosclerosis.[37–39] Since 1932, diabetes mellitus has been among the top 10 leading causes of death in America. It is a major cause of blindness, renal failure, congenital malformation, and lower extremity amputation. The prevalence of coronary artery disease and peripheral vascular disease is twice as common among persons with diabetes, compared with those without diabetes. Over 29 million Americans, or 11.9% of the population, have diabetes. As shown in Figure 8.13, diabetes prevalence is highest in the elderly and various ethnic groups (blacks/African Americans, Hispanics/Latinos, and Asian Americans). Another 35% of adults (81 million) have prediabetes, with this proportion rising to 51% among the elderly. Approximately 186,000 children and adolescents have diabetes mellitus, with over 18,000 and 5000 new cases of type 1 and type 2 diabetes, respectively, diagnosed yearly.[37]

Types of Diabetes

Diabetes can be classified into the following general categories:[37,38]

1. Type 1 diabetes (due to autoimmune β-cell destruction, usually leading to absolute insulin deficiency)
2. Type 2 diabetes (due to a progressive loss of β-cell insulin secretion frequently on the background of insulin resistance)
3. Gestational diabetes mellitus (GDM) (diabetes diagnosed in the second or third trimester of pregnancy that was not clearly overt diabetes prior to gestation)
4. Specific types of diabetes due to other causes—for instance, monogenic diabetes syndromes (such as neonatal diabetes and maturity-onset diabetes of the young [MODY]), diseases of the exocrine pancreas (such as cystic fibrosis), and drug- or chemical-induced diabetes (such as with glucocorticoid use, in the treatment of HIV/AIDS, or after organ transplantation)

Type 1 diabetes and type 2 diabetes are heterogeneous diseases that vary in progression and clinical expression and occur in both children and adults.[37,38] Children with type 1 diabetes typically present with the hallmark symptoms of polyuria (excessive urination) and polydipsia (excessive thirst and fluid intake), and approximately one-third present with diabetic ketoacidosis (DKA) (severe insulin deficiency leading to overproduction of ketones and resulting acidosis). Occasionally, patients with type 2 diabetes may have DKA, and this occurs more frequently in ethnic minorities. For adults, the onset of type 1 diabetes may be more variable and without the classic symptoms seen in children. Diagnosing the type of diabetes can be difficult in all age groups but becomes more obvious over time. Box 8.7 summarizes the common symptoms of diabetes, within the context that some people with type 2 diabetes have symptoms so mild that they go unnoticed (www.diabetes.org).

In both type 1 and type 2 diabetes, genetic and environmental factors contribute to the progressive loss of β-cell mass and/or function that results in high blood glucose (i.e., hyperglycemia). Once hyperglycemia occurs, patients with all forms of diabetes are at risk for developing the same complications, but often at different rates of progression. Autoantibodies, plasma glucose, and glycated hemoglobin (A1C) levels rise well before the clinical onset of type 1 diabetes, making diagnosis feasible well before the onset of DKA.[37,38]

The paths to β-cell dysfunction are less well defined in type 2 diabetes but often include deficient insulin secretion from pancreatic β-cells, insulin resistance (i.e., resistance of body cells to the normal actions of insulin due to changes in surface receptors), inflammation, metabolic stress, and genetic factors.[37,38] Type 2 is the most

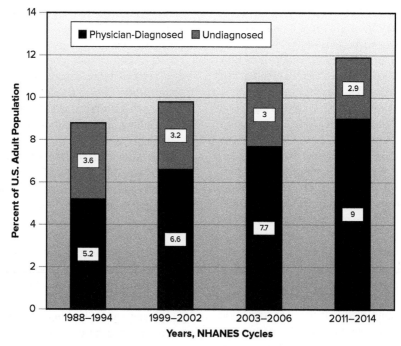

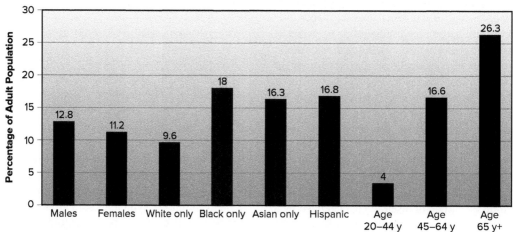

Figure 8.13 a,b

Diabetes prevalence (physician diagnosed and undiagnosed) has risen to 11.9% of the adult U.S. population, with proportions highest among the elderly and various ethnic groups (Blacks/African Americans, Hispanics/Latinos, Asian Americans).

Source: National Center for Health Statistics. 2016. *Health, United States, 2015.* Hyattsville, MD.

Box 8.7   Common Symptoms of Diabetes

1. The following symptoms of diabetes are typical. However, some people with type 2 diabetes have symptoms so mild that they go unnoticed.

   a. Urinating often (polyuria)
   b. Feeling very thirsty (polydipsia)
   c. Feeling very hungry—even though you are eating (polyphagia)

   d. Extreme fatigue
   e. Blurry vision
   f. Cuts/bruises that are slow to heal
   g. Weight loss—even though you are eating more (type 1)
   h. Tingling, pain, or numbness in the hands/feet (type 2)

Source: American Diabetes Association. www. Diabetes.org.

common form of diabetes, seen in 90% to 95% of persons with diabetes. Most patients with type 2 diabetes are obese and have other related risk factors.

Risk Factors and Screening Criteria for Diabetes Mellitus

Risk factors and screening criteria for type 2 diabetes are summarized in Box 8.8. Type 2 diabetes risk factors include non-modifiable criteria (older age, family history, race/ethnicity) and many modifiable factors (BMI, physical activity levels, unhealthy eating, cigarette smoking, hypertension, HDL-C and triglycerides, and blood glucose levels).

Approximately one-quarter of people with diabetes in the United States and nearly half of Asian and Hispanic Americans with diabetes are undiagnosed.[37] The American Diabetes Association recommends screening for prediabetes and risk for future diabetes with an informal assessment of risk factors or validated tools in asymptomatic adults (see http://www.diabetes.org/are-you-at-risk/diabetes-risk-test/) and should be considered in adults of any age who are overweight or obese (BMI $\geq$ 25 kg/m^2) and have one or more additional risk factors for diabetes.[37] For all people, testing should begin at age 45 years, regardless of risk factor status, and if tests are normal, repeat testing should be carried out at a minimum of three-year intervals. To test for

---

Box 8.8 | **Risk Factors and Screening Criteria for Diabetes Mellitus and Gestational Diabetes Mellitus (GDM)**

DIABETES RISK FACTORS*

1. Older age
2. Body mass index (BMI)* of 25 kg/m^2 and higher
3. Physical inactivity
4. First-degree relative with diabetes
5. High-risk race/ethnicity (African American, Latino, Native American, Asian American, Pacific Islander)
6. Women who were diagnosed with gestational diabetes mellitus (GDM)
7. Women with polycystic ovary syndrome
8. Hypertension ($\geq$ 140/90 mm Hg or on therapy for hypertension)
9. HDL-C < 35 mg/dL and/or a triglyceride level > 250 mg/dL
10. A1C $\geq$ 5.7%, prediabetes, impaired glucose tolerance (IGT), or impaired fasting glucose (IFG) on previous testing
11. Other clinical conditions associated with insulin resistance, such as severe obesity, acanthosis nigricans
12. History of cardiovascular disease (CVD)
13. Cigarette smoking
14. Unhealthy eating

SCREENING CRITERIA FOR PREDIABETES OR DIABETES MELLITUS IN ASYMPTOMATIC ADULTS

1. Testing at age 45 years for ALL ADULTS
2. Consider testing (screening) all adults with a BMI* $\geq$ 25 kg/m^2 and additional risk factors
   - If no risk factors, consider screening no later than age 45 years
3. If normal results, repeat testing (screening) at $\geq$ 3-year intervals
   - More frequently depending on initial test results and risk factors
   - Test yearly if tested with prediabetes

CHILD ($\leq$ 18 Y) SCREENING CRITERIA FOR DIABETES MELLITUS

1. Consider screening for all children who are overweight (BMI > 85th percentile) and have two of any of the following risk factors:
   - Family history of type 2 diabetes in first- or second-degree relatives
   - High-risk race/ethnicity (African American, Latino, Native American, Asian American, Pacific Islander)
   - Signs of insulin resistance or conditions associated with insulin resistance
   - Maternal history of diabetes or gestational diabetes mellitus (GDM) during child's gestation
2. Begin screening at age 10 years or at the onset of puberty
3. Screen every three years
4. The A1C test is recommended for diagnosis in children

TESTING RECOMMENDATIONS FOR GDM

1. Test for undiagnosed diabetes at the first prenatal visit in those with risk factors, using standard diagnostic criteria
2. Test for gestational diabetes mellitus at 24–28 weeks of gestation in pregnant women not previously known to have diabetes
3. Test women with gestational diabetes mellitus for persistent diabetes at 4–12 weeks postpartum, using the oral glucose tolerance test and clinically appropriate nonpregnancy diagnostic criteria
4. Women with a history of gestational diabetes mellitus should have lifelong screening for the development of diabetes or prediabetes at least every three years
5. Women with a history of gestational diabetes mellitus found to have prediabetes should receive intensive lifestyle interventions or metformin to prevent diabetes

Note: See http://www.diabetes.org/are-you-at-risk/diabetes-risk-test/ for the type 2 diabetes risk test.

*At-risk BMI may be lower in some ethnic groups (use $\geq$ 23 kg/m^2 in Asian Americans).

Source: www.diabetes.org; Adapted from American Diabetes Association. 2017. *Diabetes Care* 40:S1–S143.

prediabetes, fasting plasma glucose, two-hour plasma glucose after the 75-g oral glucose tolerance test, and A1C are equally appropriate.[37] In patients with prediabetes, the American Diabetes Association recommends that other CVD risk factors be identified and treated. The American Diabetes Association recommends that testing be conducted within a health-care setting because of the need for follow-up and treatment.[37] Community screening outside a health-care setting is not recommended by the American Diabetes Association because people with positive tests may not seek, or have access to, appropriate follow-up testing and care. Community testing may also fail to reach the groups most at risk.

The incidence and prevalence of type 2 diabetes in adolescents have increased dramatically, especially in racial and ethnic minority populations. Testing for prediabetes should be considered in children and adolescents who are overweight or obese and who have two or more additional risk factors for diabetes.[37] The American Diabetes Association recommends that testing start at age 10 or at onset of puberty and be repeated every three years. Although some studies question the validity of A1C in the pediatric population, the American Diabetes Association continues to recommend A1C for diagnosis of type 2 diabetes in children and adolescents.[37]

The ongoing epidemic of obesity has led to more diagnosed and undiagnosed cases of type 2 diabetes in women of childbearing age. Because of the number of pregnant women with undiagnosed type 2 diabetes, the American Diabetes Association recommends testing women with risk factors for type 2 diabetes at their initial prenatal visit, using standard diagnostic criteria.[37] Women diagnosed with diabetes in the first trimester should be classified as having preexisting pregestational diabetes (type 2 diabetes or, very rarely, type 1 diabetes). GDM is diabetes that is first diagnosed in the second or third trimester of pregnancy that is not clearly either preexisting type 1 or type 2 diabetes. The true prevalence of GDM is unknown but may be as high as 9.2%.

Shortly after pregnancy, 5% to 10% of women with GDM continue to have high blood glucose levels and are diagnosed as having diabetes, usually type 2. The risk factors for GDM are similar to those for type 2 diabetes, and GDM is a risk factor itself for developing recurrent GDM and subsequent development of type 2 diabetes. Also, the children of women who had GDM during pregnancies may be at risk of developing obesity and diabetes. Women with GDM are at high risk for pregnancy and delivery complications, including infant macrosomia (i.e., a large baby), neonatal hypoglycemia, and cesarean delivery.

Diagnosis of Diabetes and Prediabetes

Criteria for the diagnosis of diabetes mellitus is summarized in Box 8.9.[37,38] Diabetes may be diagnosed based on plasma glucose criteria, either the fasting plasma glucose (FPG) or the two-hour plasma glucose (2-h PG) value after a 75-g oral glucose tolerance test (OGTT) or A1C criteria. All of these are equally appropriate for diagnostic testing for diabetes, according to the American Diabetes Association.[37] In the absence of unequivocal hyperglycemia, criteria 1–3 in Box 8.9 should be confirmed by repeat testing. Beginning in 2010, the American Diabetes Association added to this set of diagnostic criteria a hemoglobin A1C value ≥ 6.5%.

A normal fasting plasma glucose level is considered < 100 mg/dL. Prediabetes is diagnosed when the fasting plasma glucose is 100–125 mg/dL (also called impaired fasting glucose, or IFG), or the two-hour plasma glucose during the oral glucose tolerance test is 140–199 mg/dL (also called impaired glucose tolerance, or IGT), or the

---

 Box 8.9   Diagnostic Criteria for Diabetes

1. **Glycated hemoglobin A1C ≥ 6.5%.** The test should be performed by a laboratory using a method that is certified by the National Glycohemoglobin Standardization Program (NGSP) and standardized or traceable to the Diabetes Control and Complication Trial reference assay.*

2. **Fasting plasma glucose (FPG) ≥ 126 mg/dL (7.0 mmol/L).** Fasting is defined as no caloric intake for at least eight hours.*

3. **An oral glucose tolerance test (OGTT) with a two-hour plasma glucose ≥ 200 mg/dL (11.1 mmol/L).** The test should adhere to World Health Organization protocol with a glucose load containing the equivalent of 75 g of anhydrous glucose dissolved in water.*

4. **Presence of the classic symptoms of hyperglycemia or hyperglycemic crisis plus a random (nonfasting) plasma glucose ≥ 200 mg/dL (11.1 mmol/L).** Classic symptoms of diabetes include polyuria (excessive urination), polydipsia (excessive thirst), polyphagia (excessive consumption of food), unexplained weight loss, blurred vision, and recurrent infections.

In the absence of unequivocal hyperglycemia, criteria 1–3 should be confirmed by repeat testing.

Source: American Diabetes Association. 2014. Diagnosis and classification of diabetes mellitus. *Diabetes Care* 37(suppl 1):S81–S90.

Fasting Plasma Glucose		**2-hour Plasma Glucose On OGTT**		**Hemoglobin A1C (glycated)**	
Diabetes Mellitus	126 mg/dL	Diabetes Mellitus	200 mg/dL	Diabetes Mellitus	6.5%
Prediabetes Impaired Fasting Glucose	100 mg/dL	Prediabetes Impaired Glucose Tolerance	140 mg/dL	Prediabetes	5.7%
Normal		Normal		Normal	

Diagnosis of diabetes can also be made based on unequivocal symptoms and a random glucose > 200 mg/dL; any abnormality must be repeated and confirmed on a separate day

Figure 8.14

Classification of diabetes mellitus using test results from the fasting plasma glucose, 2-hour plasma glucose from the oral glucose toterance test (OGTT), and the hemoglobin A1C.

Source: American Diabetes Association. 2014. Diagnosis and classification of diabetes mellitus. *Diabetes Care* 37(Suppl 1): S81–S90.

hemoglobin A1C is 5.7% to 6.4%.[37,38] Figure 8.14 summarizes this information. For the purpose of some glucose measurements, fasting can be defined as no consumption of food or beverage other than water for at least 8 hours before testing.[37,38]

Oral Glucose Tolerance Test

The oral glucose tolerance test (OGTT) involves having the patient who is fasting drink a beverage containing a known amount of glucose, usually 75 grams for adults or 1.75 g/kg for children.[37,38] A fasting venous blood sample is drawn immediately before the glucose beverage is consumed and then at set intervals following consumption to monitor changes in blood sugar level. In preparing for the

OGTT, it is best for the patient to consume more than 150 g of carbohydrate per day, abstain from alcohol, and have unrestricted activity for three days before the test.[37,38] On the morning of the test, the fasting subject consumes the glucose beverage within a 5- to 10-minute period. Plasma glucose is measured while fasting and usually at one-hour intervals for two or three hours.

A plasma glucose level ≥ 200 mg/dL (≥ 11.1 mmol/L) at two hours is diagnostic of diabetes. Figure 8.15 shows examples of how plasma glucose might respond to an OGTT in a person with diabetes, a person with impaired glucose tolerance, and a person without diabetes. In the curve representing the person with diabetes, the plasma glucose exceeds 200 mg/dL at two hours after consuming the glucose load. Impaired glucose tolerance is diagnosed when plasma glucose level is 140 mg/dL but is < 200 mg/dL.

In the one-step strategy for screening and diagnosis of GDM, perform a 75-g OGTT, with plasma glucose measurement when the patient is fasting, at 1 and 2 h, and at 24 to 28 weeks of gestation in women not previously diagnosed with overt diabetes.[37,38] The OGTT should be performed in the morning after an overnight fast of at least 8 h. The diagnosis of GDM is made when any of the following plasma glucose values are met or exceeded:

- Fasting: 92 mg/dL
- 1 h: 180 mg/dL
- 2 h: 153 mg/dL

In the two-step strategy for screening and diagnosis of GDM, first perform a 50-g glucose load test (GLT) (nonfasting), with plasma glucose measurement at 1 h, at 24 to 28 weeks of gestation in women not previously diagnosed with overt diabetes.[37,38] If the plasma glucose level measured 1 h after the load is ≥ 130 mg/dL, 135 mg/dL, or 140 mg/dL, proceed to a 100-g OGTT. In step 2, the 100-g OGTT should be performed when the

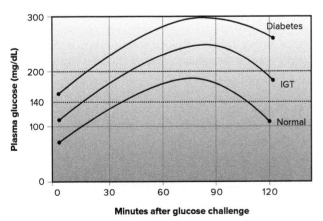

Figure 8.15   Diagnosis of diabetes using the oral glucose tolerance test (OGTT).

Normally, plasma glucose should be < 140 mg/dL two hours after ingesting 75 g of glucose (the so-called glucose challenge). A diagnostic criterion for impaired glucose tolerance (IGT) is a two-hour plasma glucose ≥ 140 mg/dL and < 200 mg/dL. A two-hour plasma glucose ≥ 200 mg/dL is a diagnostic criterion for diabetes.

patient is fasting. The diagnosis of GDM is made if at least two of the following four plasma glucose levels (measured fasting and 1 h, 2 h, 3 h after the OGTT) are met or exceede

- Fasting: 95–105 mg/dL
- 1 h: 180–190 mg/dL
- 2 h: 155–165 mg/dL
- 3 h: 140–145 mg/dL

Self-Monitoring of Blood Glucose

In self-monitoring of blood glucose (SMBG), persons with diabetes periodically measure the amount of glucose in a small sample of their blood. It allows patients to evaluate their response to therapy and to assess whether their treatment goals are being met. It is valuable in preventing hypoglycemia and adjusting medical nutrition therapy, physical activity, and medications, especially insulin doses given immediately before meals.[37] Self-monitoring of blood glucose can be accurately and precisely done using a commercially available blood glucose meter. A test strip is inserted into the meter, the side of a fingertip is pricked using a lancet to draw a drop of blood for testing, and the tip of the test strip is touched to the drop of blood. Capillary action draws the blood into the strip for analysis by the meter, which provides a digital readout of the blood glucose level. Before testing, patients should be instructed to wash their hands using soap and warm water. Gently massaging the tip of the finger that will be lanced improves blood flow to that area and makes the lancing more successful.

The frequency of SMBG depends primarily on the type of diabetes and a person's overall therapy. It is especially important for preventing hypoglycemia and hyperglycemia in patients treated with insulin. For most patients with type 1 diabetes and pregnant women taking insulin, monitoring as often as three or more times a day is appropriate. More frequent testing may be required in order to reach targets for A1C without experiencing hypoglycemia. In patients attempting tight glycemic control, testing might be recommended before performing critical tasks such as driving. In a large study of children and adolescents with type 1 diabetes, each additional test per day up to a maximum of five tests per day was associated with a reduction in A1C of 0.2%. Testing should be more frequent when there are changes in a person's schedule, exercise habits, medications, diet, and body weight and during illness. There is uncertainty about the optimal frequency of SMBG in patients with type 2 diabetes who are not treated with insulin. Some research suggests that in patients not treated with insulin, SMBG may not be cost-effective. Because many of the studies investigating the benefits of SMBG on improved glycemic control also included patient education on diet and physical activity, separating the effect of SMBG from these other efforts is difficult.

The accuracy and precision of blood glucose measurements using a commercially available meter are dependent on the instrument and the user. Patients need to be instructed on the correct use of the instrument and monitored initially and periodically to ensure that they are using proper technique. Patients also need to be instructed on how to use the SMBG data to adjust their diet and physical activity and any medications they are taking.[37]

Glycated Hemoglobin

During the average life span of a red blood cell (approximately 120 days), glucose in the blood binds to the major form of hemoglobin (Hb) in the red blood cell, hemoglobin A (HbA). When this occurs, the hemoglobin is said to be glycated. There are several forms of HbA in the red blood cell. The form of glycated HbA that most closely correlates with mean blood glucose levels is referred to as hemoglobin $A1_C$ (A1C).[37,38] The binding of glucose to HbA is almost irreversible during the life span of the red blood cell. Consequently, HbA_{1C} reflects average blood glucose levels during the past 8 to 12 weeks or 2 to 3 months. The proportion of A1C does not decline with a temporary fall in blood glucose. It decreases only when glycemic control has been consistent over a period of several weeks, and older red blood cells with a high proportion of A1C are replaced by new red blood cells with a lower proportion of A1C. Consequently, the test is a good way to assess a patient's adherence to his or her program of blood glucose control. It can also serve as a check on the accuracy of the patient's glucose meter and how accurately the patient is reported results from SMBG. The A1C has several advantages compared with the fasting plasma glucose and OGTT, including greater convenience (fasting not required), greater preanalytical stability, and less day-to-day perturbations during stress and illness.[37]

The American Diabetes Association recommends that A1C testing be done routinely in all patients with diabetes during their initial assessment and then periodically, depending on the patient's clinical situation, the treatment regimen used, and the judgment of the clinician.[37] Testing approximately every three months is useful in determining whether a patient's glycemic targets have been reached and are maintained. For patients meeting treatment goals and maintaining stable glycemic control, testing twice a year is considered sufficient. For patients whose therapy has changed or who are not meeting glycemic goals, quarterly testing may be warranted.[37,38] There are limitations to A1C testing. It does not serve as a measure of glycemic variability or hypoglycemia. In conditions that accelerate red blood cell turnover such as anemia from hemolysis, blood loss, and iron deficiency, plasma glucose levels must be used in diagnosing and monitoring patients. Some A1C tests may give inaccurately high or low readings in patients with hemoglobin variants such as sickle cell trait, in which case a testing method that yields accurate results should be specifically selected.[36,37] NHANES data indicate that an A1C cut point of $\geq 6.5\%$ identifies one-third fewer cases of undiagnosed diabetes than a fasting glucose cut point of ≥ 126 mg/dL.[37]

Lifestyle Management

Lifestyle management is a fundamental aspect of diabetes care and includes[37]

- Diabetes self-management education (DSME)
- Diabetes self-management support (DSMS)
- Nutrition therapy
- Physical activity
- Smoking cessation counseling
- Psychosocial care

Lifestyle management begins at the time of the initial comprehensive medical evaluation, should be patient centered and individualized, and is integral to all subsequent evaluations and follow-up.[37]

One of the most challenging parts of the lifestyle treatment plan is the development of an individualized eating plan.[37,39] The American Diabetes Association recommends that each person with diabetes should be actively engaged with a registered dietitian in all aspects of medical nutrition therapy (MNT). Emphasis should be on healthful eating patterns containing nutrient-dense, high-quality foods with less focus on specific nutrients. The Mediterranean, Dietary Approaches to Stop Hypertension (DASH), and plant-based diets are all examples of healthful eating patterns. See Box 8.10 for specific nutrition recommendations.[39]

There are four goals of MNT for adults with diabetes:[37,39]

1. To promote and support healthful eating patterns, emphasizing a variety of nutrient-dense foods in appropriate portion sizes, in order to improve overall health and specifically to

   - Achieve and maintain body weight goals
   - Attain individualized glycemic, blood pressure, and lipid goals
   - Delay or prevent the complications of diabetes

2. To address individual nutrition needs based on personal and cultural preferences, health literacy and numeracy, access to healthful foods, willingness and ability to make behavioral changes, and barriers to change
3. To maintain the pleasure of eating by providing nonjudgmental messages about food choices
4. To provide an individual with diabetes the practical tools for developing healthy eating patterns rather than focusing on individual macronutrients, micronutrients, or single foods

Body weight management is the primary focus for overweight and obese people with type 1 and type 2 diabetes. There is strong and consistent evidence that modest persistent weight loss of 5% to 7% can delay the progression from prediabetes to type 2 diabetes and is beneficial to the management of type 2 diabetes.[37,39] Lifestyle weight management intervention programs should be intensive (16 sessions or more during a six-month period) and have

 Box 8.10   **American Diabetes Association Medical Nutrition Therapy (MNT) Recommendations**

The American Diabetes Association recommends several key nutrition guidelines for persons with diabetes:

- **Energy balance:**
  - Aim for at least 5% to 7% weight loss with an intensive lifestyle intervention program.
  - To lose weight, reduce caloric intake 500–750 kcal/day.
  - Aim for at least 150 minutes per week of moderate to vigorous physical activity (with two to three sessions per week of resistance exercise).

- **Eating patterns, macronutrient distribution:**
  - Individualize macronutrient distribution of carbohydrates, fats, and proteins.
  - Emphasize healthy eating patterns such as the Mediterranean, DASH, and plant-food based diets. Emphasize nutrient-dense foods/dietary patterns (whole grains, vegetables, fruits, legumes, low-fat dairy, lean meats, nuts, seeds).

- Avoid sugar-sweetened beverages, and minimize added sugars.
- Don't use carbohydrate sources high in protein to treat or prevent hypoglycemia.
- Limit intake of refined carbohydrates, added sugars, and sodium.
- Dietary fat: The Mediterranean eating pattern is rich in monounsaturated fats and may improve glucose metabolism and lower CVD risk. Eating fatty fish, nuts, and seeds with omega-3 fats can lower CVD risk (no benefit of omega-3 dietary supplements).

- **Alcohol, sodium, nonnutritive sweeteners:**
  - Guidelines are the same as for the general population.

- **Supplements:**
  - Vitamin and mineral supplements, herbal products, or spices to manage diabetes are not recommended due to lack of evidence.

Source: Evert AB, Boucher JL, Cypress M, et al. 2014. Nutrition therapy recommendations for the management of adults with diabetes. *Diabetes Care* 37(suppl 1): S120–S143.

frequent follow-up to achieve significant reductions in excess body weight and improve clinical indicators.

Patients with diabetes should be advised not to smoke or use tobacco products. Counseling on smoking prevention and cessation should be a part of routine clinical care. The level of nicotine dependence should be assessed, with pharmacologic therapy offered as appropriate.[37]

Psychological and social problems can impair the individual's ability to carry out the lifestyle management plan. The clinician should integrate psychosocial care into the clinical support plan and consider assessing for symptoms of diabetes distress, depression, anxiety, disordered eating, cognitive capacities. Diabetes distress can occur when treatment targets are not met and/or at the onset of complications.[37]

SUMMARY

1. Cardiovascular disease (CVD) remains the leading cause of death in the United States and is causally associated with risk factors that are modifiable and nonmodifiable.

2. Because cholesterol, triglycerides, and other lipids are fat soluble, they are transported in the blood by lipoproteins. CHD risk is directly related to serum levels of total cholesterol and low-density-lipoprotein cholesterol (LDL-C) and inversely related to levels of high-density-lipoprotein cholesterol (HDL-C). The National Cholesterol Education Program (NCEP) has set desirable levels of total cholesterol in adults at < 200 mg/dL.

3. Although clinically manifest CVD is rare in children and adolescents, risk factors during childhood initiate and accelerate the development of CVD, which is then manifest in adulthood. According to the Expert Panel on Integrated Guidelines for Cardiovascular Health and Risk Reduction in Children and Adolescents, preventing CVD must begin in childhood and address two fundamental goals: preventing development of CVD risk factors (*primordial prevention*) and preventing future CVD by managing any identified risk factors (*primary prevention*).

4. The Expert Panel developed dietary recommendations for children and adolescents called the Cardiovascular Health Integrated Lifestyle Diet (CHILD 1). These are consistent with the Dietary Guidelines for Americans and provide additional guidance specifically targeting children and adolescents at increased risk of CVD. The Expert Panel also recommends universal lipid screening in all children at 9 to 11 years of age and then again for all adolescents at 17 to 21 years of age.

5. Two ways of addressing the problem of high serum cholesterol levels are the population-based and the patient-based approaches. The former emphasizes dietary and lifestyle changes for all people to lower average cholesterol levels in the entire population. The latter promotes identification and treatment of

individuals with elevated cholesterol levels by physicians.

6. The American Heart Association's (AHA) 2020 goal is to reduce deaths from CVD and stroke by 20%. As a part of this initiative, the AHA tracks seven key health factors and behaviors: not smoking, physical activity, healthy diet, body weight, and control of cholesterol, blood pressure, and blood sugar.

7. The AHA urges that a healthy lifestyle and prudent dietary practices, at all stages of life, are central to CVD prevention and treatment. AHA guidelines are based on heart-healthy nutrition-based practices, but also focus on weight control, physical activity, and the avoidance of tobacco use.

8. Precision, or reproducibility, relates to the difference in results when the same blood sample is measured repeatedly. The coefficient of variation (CV) is a measure of precision and is calculated by dividing the standard deviation (SD) by the mean and multiplying by 100 ($CV = SD \div mean \times 100$). The NCEP recommends that laboratories achieve a $CV \leq 3\%$.

9. The 2013 ACC/AHA guidelines represent a major shift from prior cholesterol management guidelines, with a focus on atherosclerotic cardiovascular disease (ASCVD) risk reduction as opposed to targeting LDL-C levels, advocating for the use of evidence-based doses of statins as first line therapy, and utilizing a new risk calculator and risk cut point to guide initiation of statin therapy. The 2013 ACC/AHA cholesterol guidelines focus on identifying groups of patients that are most likely to benefit from cholesterol treatment with HMG-CoA reductase inhibitors (statins), the therapy that has been consistently proven in randomized clinical trials to lower ASCVD risk.

10. Hypertension is one of the most common risk factors for cardiovascular and renal diseases. One of every three Americans has hypertension or is taking antihypertensive medication. As systolic blood pressure increases above 120 mm Hg and

diastolic blood pressure increases above 80 mm Hg, risk for death from cardiovascular disease increases.

11. The 2014 Evidence-Based Guideline for the Management of High Blood Pressure in Adults from the Eight Joint National Committee Panel (JNC8) focused on blood pressure thresholds for pharmacological treatment. The 2014 JNC8 guidelines recommended lifestyle interventions for all persons with hypertension throughout the treatment and management process. The JNC8 Expert Panel urged that the potential benefits of a healthy diet, weight control, and regular exercise could not be overemphasized, and that lifestyle treatments have the potential to improve blood pressure control and even reduce medication needs.

12. In both type 1 and type 2 diabetes, genetic and environmental factors contribute to the progressive loss of β-cell mass and/or function that results in high blood glucose (i.e., hyperglycemia). Once hyperglycemia occurs, patients with all forms of diabetes are at risk for developing the same complications, but often at different rates of progression.

13. Despite its public health significance, diabetes is undiagnosed in about 30% of people who have the disease. Diagnostic criteria for diabetes include the presence of symptoms of diabetes and fasting glucose measurements of ≥ 126 mg/dL (≥ 7.0 mmol/L) on two occasions. The oral glucose tolerance test also can be used to diagnose diabetes, especially gestational diabetes.

14. Glycated hemoglobin, or simply called an A1C test, is useful for assessing a person's mean glucose levels during the past 8 to 12 weeks. Self-monitoring blood glucose is helpful in evaluating how changes in diet, exercise, and medications affect glycemic control. Glycemic control has been shown to be effective in reducing the risk of microvascular complications in persons with type 1 diabetes.

15. Lifestyle management is a fundamental aspect of diabetes care and includes diabetes self-management education (DSME), diabetes self-management support (DSMS), nutrition therapy, physical activity, smoking cessation counseling, and psychosocial care.

16. There are four goals of medical nutrition therapy (MNT) for adults with diabetes. In general, an individualized eating plan should be developed with an RD and an emphasis on healthful eating patterns containing nutrient-dense, high-quality foods and less focus on specific nutrients.

REFERENCES

1. Writing Group Members, Mozaffarian D, Benjamin EJ, Go AS, Arnett DK, Blaha MJ, Cushman M, Das SR, de Ferranti S, Després JP, Fullerton HJ, Howard VJ, Huffman MD, Isasi CR, Jiménez MC, Judd SE, Kissela BM, Lichtman JH, Lisabeth LD, Liu S, Mackey RH, Magid DJ, McGuire DK, Mohler ER 3rd, Moy CS, Muntner P, Mussolino ME, Nasir K, Neumar RW, Nichol G, Palaniappan L, Pandey DK, Reeves MJ, Rodriguez CJ, Rosamond W, Sorlie PD, Stein J, Towfighi A, Turan TN, Virani SS, Woo D, Yeh RW, Turner MB; American Heart Association Statistics Committee; Stroke Statistics Subcommittee. 2016. Heart disease and stroke statistics—2016 update: A report from the American Heart Association. *Circulation* 133:e38–e360.

2. Mozaffarian D, Benjamin EJ, Go AS, Arnett DK, Blaha MJ, Cushman M, de Ferranti S, Després JP, Fullerton HJ, Howard VJ, Huffman MD, Judd SE, Kissela BM, Lackland DT, Lichtman JH, Lisabeth LD, Liu S, Mackey RH, Matchar DB, McGuire DK, Mohler ER 3rd, Moy CS, Muntner P, Mussolino ME, Nasir K, Neumar RW, Nichol G, Palaniappan L, Pandey DK, Reeves MJ, Rodriguez CJ, Sorlie PD, Stein J, Towfighi A, Turan TN, Virani SS, Willey JZ, Woo D, Yeh RW, Turner MB; American Heart Association Statistics Committee and Stroke Statistics Subcommittee. 2015. Heart disease and stroke statistics—2015 update: A report from the American Heart Association. *Circulation* 131:e29–e322.

3. National Center for Health Statistics. 2016. *Health, United States, 2015: With special feature on racial and ethnic health disparities.* Hyattsville, MD: National Center for Health Statistics. https://www.cdc.gov/nchs/data/hus/hus15.pdf.

4. Kochanek KD, Murphy SL, Xu JQ, Tejada-Vera B. 2016. Deaths: Final data for 2014. *National Vital Statistics Reports* 65 (no 4). Hyattsville, MD: National Center for Health Statistics.

5. Dwyer-Lindgren L, Bertozzi-Villa A, Stubbs RW, Morozoff C, Kutz MJ, Huynh C, Barber RM, Shackelford KA, Mackenbach JP, van Lenthe FJ, Flaxman AD, Naghavi M, Mokdad AH, Murray CJ. 2016. US county-level trends in mortality rates for major causes of death, 1980–2014. *Journal of the American Medical Association* 316:2385–2401.

6. Lloyd-Jones DM, Hong Y, Labarthe D, Mozaffarian D, Appel LJ,

Van Horn L, Greenlund K, Daniels S, Nichol G, Tomaselli GF, Arnett DK, Fonarow GC, Ho PM, Lauer MS, Masoudi FA, Robertson RM, Roger V, Schwamm LH, Sorlie P, Yancy CW, Rosamond WD; American Heart Association Strategic Planning Task Force and Statistics Committee. 2010. Defining and setting national goals for cardiovascular health promotion and disease reduction: The American Heart Association's strategic impact goal through 2020 and beyond. *Circulation* 121:586–613.

7. Yang Q, Cogswell ME, Flanders WD, Hong Y, Zhang Z, Loustalot F, Gillespie C, Merritt R, Hu FB. 2012. Trends in cardiovascular health metrics and associations with all-cause and CVD mortality among US adults. *Journal of the American Medical Association* 307:1273–1283.

8. Fang N, Jiang M, Fan Y. 2016. Ideal cardiovascular health metrics and risk of cardiovascular disease or mortality: A meta-analysis. *International Journal of Cardiology* 214:279–283.

9. Steinberger J, Daniels SR, Hagberg N, Isasi CR, Kelly AS, Lloyd-Jones D, Pate RR, Pratt C, Shay CM, Towbin JA, Urbina E, Van Horn LV, Zachariah JP; American Heart Association Atherosclerosis, Hypertension, and Obesity in the Young Committee of the Council on Cardiovascular Disease in the Young; Council on Cardiovascular and Stroke Nursing; Council on Epidemiology and Prevention; Council on Functional Genomics and Translational Biology; and Stroke Council. 2016. Cardiovascular health promotion in children: Challenges and opportunities for 2020 and beyond: A scientific statement from the American Heart Association. *Circulation* 134:e236–e255.

10. Eckel RH, Jakicic JM, Ard JD, de Jesus JM, Houston Miller N, Hubbard VS, Lee IM, Lichtenstein AH, Loria CM, Millen BE, Nonas CA, Sacks FM, Smith SC Jr, Svetkey LP, Wadden TA, Yanovski SZ, Kendall KA, Morgan LC, Trisolini MG,

Velasco G, Wnek J, Anderson JL, Halperin JL, Albert NM, Bozkurt B, Brindis RG, Curtis LH, DeMets D, Hochman JS, Kovacs RJ, Ohman EM, Pressler SJ, Sellke FW, Shen WK, Smith SC Jr., Tomaselli GF; American College of Cardiology/American Heart Association Task Force on Practice Guidelines. 2014. 2013 AHA/ACC guideline on lifestyle management to reduce cardiovascular risk: A report of the American College of Cardiology/American Heart Association Task Force on Practice Guidelines. *Circulation* 129(25 suppl 2):S76–S99.

11. Van Horn L, Carson JA, Appel LJ, Burke LE, Economos C, Karmally W, Lancaster K, Lichtenstein AH, Johnson RK, Thomas RJ, Vos M, Wylie-Rosett J, Kris-Etherton P; American Heart Association Nutrition Committee of the Council on Lifestyle and Cardiometabolic Health; Council on Cardiovascular Disease in the Young; Council on Cardiovascular and Stroke Nursing; Council on Clinical Cardiology; and Stroke Council. 2016. Recommended dietary pattern to achieve adherence to the American Heart Association/American College of Cardiology (AHA/ACC) guidelines: A scientific statement from the American Heart Association. *Circulation* 134:e505–e529.

12. U.S. Department of Health and Human Services and U.S. Department of Agriculture. 2015. *2015–2020 dietary guidelines for Americans.* 8th ed. http://health.gov/dietaryguidelines/2015/guidelines.

13. Alberti KG, Eckel RH, Grundy SM, Zimmet PZ, Cleeman JI, Donato KA, Fruchart JC, James WP, Loria CM, Smith SC Jr.; International Diabetes Federation Task Force on Epidemiology and Prevention; National Heart, Lung, and Blood Institute; American Heart Association; World Heart Federation; International Atherosclerosis Society; International Association for the Study of Obesity. 2009. Harmonizing the metabolic syndrome: A joint interim statement of the International

Diabetes Federation Task Force on Epidemiology and Prevention; National Heart, Lung, and Blood Institute; American Heart Association; World Heart Federation; International Atherosclerosis Society; and International Association for the Study of Obesity. *Circulation* 120:1640–1645.

14. Aguilar M, Bhuket T, Torres S. 2015. Prevalence of the metabolic syndrome in the United States, 2003–2012. *Journal of the American Medical Association* 313:1973–1974.

15. Carroll MD, Fryar CD, Kit BK. 2015. Total and high-density lipoprotein cholesterol in adults: United States, 2011–2014. *NCHS Data Brief*, no 226. Hyattsville, MD: National Center for Health Statistics.

16. Gu Q, Paulose-Ram R, Burt VL, Kit BK. 2014. Prescription cholesterol-lowering medication use in adults aged 40 and over: United States, 2003–2012. *NCHS Data Brief*, no 177. Hyattsville, MD: National Center for Health Statistics.

17. National Cholesterol Education Program (NCEP) Expert Panel on Detection, Evaluation, and Treatment of High Blood Cholesterol in Adults (Adult Treatment Panel III). 2002. Third report of the National Cholesterol Education Program (NCEP) Expert Panel on Detection, Evaluation, and Treatment of High Blood Cholesterol in Adults (Adult Treatment Panel III) final report. *Circulation* 106:3143–3421.

18. Stone NJ, Robinson JG, Lichtenstein AH, Bairey Merz CN, Blum CB, Eckel RH, Goldberg AC, Gordon D, Levy D, Lloyd-Jones DM, McBride P, Schwartz JS, Shero ST, Smith SC Jr, Watson K, Wilson PW, Eddleman KM, Jarrett NM, LaBresh K, Nevo L, Wnek J, Anderson JL, Halperin JL, Albert NM, Bozkurt B, Brindis RG, Curtis LH, DeMets D, Hochman JS, Kovacs RJ, Ohman EM, Pressler SJ, Sellke FW, Shen WK, Smith SC Jr., Tomaselli GF; American College of Cardiology/American Heart Association Task Force on Practice Guidelines. 2014. 2013 ACC/AHA

guideline on the treatment of blood cholesterol to reduce atherosclerotic cardiovascular risk in adults: A report of the American College of Cardiology/American Heart Association Task Force on Practice Guidelines. *Circulation* 129(25 suppl 2):S1–45.

19. Finkel JB, Duffy D. 2015. 2013 ACC/AHA cholesterol treatment guideline: Paradigm shifts in managing atherosclerotic cardiovascular disease risk. *Trends in Cardiovascular Medicine* 25:340–347.

20. Davies JT, Delfino SF, Feinberg CE, Johnson MF, Nappi VL, Olinger JT, Schwab AP, Swanson HI. 2016. Current and emerging uses of statins in clinical therapeutics: A review. *Lipid Insights* 9:13–29.

21. Expert Panel on Integrated Guidelines for Cardiovascular Health and Risk Reduction in Children and Adolescents. 2011. Expert Panel on Integrated Guidelines for Cardiovascular Health and Risk Reduction in Children and Adolescents: Summary report. *Pediatrics* 128(suppl 5):S213–S256.

22. Warnick GR. 2000. Measurement of cholesterol and other lipoprotein constituents in the clinical laboratory. *Clinical Chemistry and Laboratory Medicine* 38:287–300.

23. National Cholesterol Education Program. 1995. *Recommendations on lipoprotein measurement from the Working Group on Lipoprotein Measurement.* Bethesda, MD: U.S. Department of Health and Human Services, Public Health Service; National Institutes of Health; National Heart, Lung, and Blood Institute.

24. Rifai N, Dufour R, Cooper GR. 1997. Preanalytical variation in lipid, lipoprotein, and apolipoprotein testing. In Rifai N, Warnick GR, Dominiczak MH (eds.), *Handbook of lipoprotein testing.* Washington, DC: American Association of Clinical Chemistry, 75–97.

25. National Cholesterol Education Program. 1990. *Recommendations for improving cholesterol measurement: A report from the Laboratory Standardization Panel of the National Cholesterol Education Program.* Bethesda,

MD: U.S. Department of Health and Human Services, Public Health Service; National Institutes of Health; National Heart, Lung, and Blood Institute.

26. Cooper GR, Myers GL, Smith SJ, Schlant RC. 1992. Blood lipid measurements: Variations and practical utility. *Journal of the American Medical Association* 267:1652–1660.

27. James PA, Oparil S, Carter BL, Cushman WC, Dennison-Himmelfarb C, Handler J, Lackland DT, LeFevre ML, MacKenzie TD, Ogedegbe O, Smith SC Jr., Svetkey LP, Taler SJ, Townsend RR, Wright JT Jr., Narva AS, Ortiz E. 2014. 2014 evidence-based guideline for the management of high blood pressure in adults: Report from the panel members appointed to the Eighth Joint National Committee (JNC 8). *Journal of the American Medical Association* 311:507–520.

28. Chobanian AV, Bakris GL, Black HR, Cushman WC, Green LA, Izzo JL Jr., Jones DW, Materson BJ, Oparil S, Wright JT Jr., Roccella EJ; Joint National Committee on Prevention, Detection, Evaluation, and Treatment of High Blood Pressure; National Heart, Lung, and Blood Institute; National High Blood Pressure Education Program Coordinating Committee. 2003. Seventh report of the Joint National Committee on Prevention, Detection, Evaluation, and Treatment of High Blood Pressure. *Hypertension* 42:1206–1252.

29. Danaei G, Ding EL, Mozaffarian D, Taylor B, Rehm J, Murray CJ, Ezzati M. 2009. The preventable causes of death in the United States: Comparative risk assessment of dietary, lifestyle, and metabolic risk factors. *PLoS Medicine* 6(4):e1000058.

30. Ndanuko RN, Tapsell LC, Charlton KE, Neale EP, Batterham MJ. 2016. Dietary patterns and blood pressure in adults: A systematic review and meta-analysis of randomized controlled trials. *Advances in Nutrition* 7:76–89.

31. National High Blood Pressure Education Program Working Group. 1993. National High Blood Pressure Education Program

Working Group report on primary prevention of hypertension. *Archives of Internal Medicine* 153:186–208.

32. Stevens VJ, Obarzanek E, Cook NR, Lee IM, Appel LJ, et al. 2001. Long-term weight loss and changes in blood pressure: Results of the Trials of Hypertension Prevention, phase II. *Annals of Internal Medicine* 134:1–11.

33. The Trials of Hypertension Prevention Collaborative Research Group. 1992. The effects of nonpharmacologic interventions on blood pressure of persons with high normal levels: Results of the Trials of Hypertension Prevention. Phase I. *Journal of the American Medical Association* 267:1213–1220.

34. Panel on Dietary Reference Intakes for Electrolytes and Water, Standing Committee on the Scientific Evaluation of Dietary Reference Intakes, Food and Nutrition Board. 2004. *Dietary Reference Intakes for water, potassium, sodium, chloride, and sulfate.* Washington, DC: National Academies Press.

35. Greenland P. 2001. Beating high blood pressure with low-sodium DASH. *New England Journal of Medicine* 344:53–55.

36. National High Blood Pressure Education Program. 2005. *The fourth report on the diagnosis, evaluation, and treatment of high blood pressure in children and adolescents.* U.S. Department of Health and Human Services, National Institutes of Health; National Heart, Lung, and Blood Institute.

37. American Diabetes Association. 2017. Standards of medical care in diabetes—2017. *Diabetes Care* 40(suppl 1):S1–S135.

38. American Diabetes Association. 2014. Diagnosis and classification of diabetes mellitus. *Diabetes Care* 37(suppl 1):S81–S90.

39. Evert AB, Boucher JL, Cypress M, et al. 2014. Nutrition therapy recommendations for the management of adults with diabetes. *Diabetes Care* 37 (suppl 1):S120–S143.

ASSESSMENT ACTIVITY 8.1

Lipid and Lipoprotein Levels and Coronary Heart Disease Risk

The National Cholesterol Education Program recommends that all adults 20 years of age or older know their serum total cholesterol. Values < 200 mg/dL (5.17 mmol/L) can be repeated at least every five years. Values of 200 mg/dL (5.17 mmol/L) or greater should be verified by a repeat measurement within one to eight weeks. If the second value is within 30 mg/dL (0.8 mmol/L) of the first, the average of the two can be used as a guide for subsequent decisions. Otherwise, a third test should be obtained in another one to eight weeks and the average of the three values used.

You are encouraged to have your blood lipid and lipoprotein levels measured and to know these values. There are several ways you can do this. Your professor may be able to arrange with student health services or a local hospital or clinical laboratory to have cholesterol and lipoprotein measurements performed on all interested students in your class. If measurements are done on several members of your class, they may be done at a reduced price. Some hospitals offer low-priced testing as a community service.

When you receive your results, answer the following questions:

1. How do your values compare with the classifications summarized in Table 8.5?

2. How do these compare with the population norms given in Appendix M?

3. Review the AHA lifestyle recommendations in Box 8.2, and discuss changes that may influence your results.

ASSESSMENT ACTIVITY 8.2

Calculating ASCVD Risk

The 2013 ACC/AHA guidelines represent a major shift from prior cholesterol management guidelines, with a focus on atherosclerotic cardiovascular disease (ASCVD) risk reduction as opposed to targeting LDL-C levels, advocating for the use of evidence-based doses of statins as first line therapy, and utilizing a new risk calculator and risk cut point to guide initiation of statin therapy. The 2013 ACC/AHA cholesterol guidelines focus on identifying groups of patients that are most likely to benefit from cholesterol treatment with HMG-CoA reductase inhibitors (statins), the therapy that has been consistently proven in randomized clinical trials to lower ASCVD risk.

ASCVD 10-year risk can be assessed at http://tools.cardiosource.org/ASCVD-Risk-Estimator/. An Excel spreadsheet file can be downloaded that allows practitioners to estimate ASCVD on their personal computers. The estimator requires gender, total cholesterol, age, HDL cholesterol, race, systolic blood pressure, smoking status, diabetes history, and history of hypertension. Go to this website, enter the requested information (either for yourself or a case study provided by your instructor), and obtain the 10-year ASCVD calculated risk percentile (e.g., 4.7%) and the lifetime ASCVD calculated risk (e.g., 5.0%). Also print and save recommendations provided at the website based on the data entered, especially whether or not statin therapy is recommended. Bring to your class and discuss with the instructor and classmates.

Here is a recommended case study for a male patient that has no clinical ASCVD and an LDL-C of 70–189 mg/dL. These data can be entered:

- Gender: Male
- Age: 59
- Race: White/Other
- Total cholesterol: 205
- HDL cholesterol: 39
- Systolic blood pressure: 146
- Hypertension treatment: No
- Diabetes: No
- Smoker: No

ASSESSMENT ACTIVITY 8.3

Categorizing Blood Pressure in Children and Adolescents

As discussed in this chapter, an entirely different approach is used to categorize blood pressure (BP) in children and adolescents than that used to categorize blood pressure in adults. As shown in Box 8.6, in children and adolescents 1 to 17 years of age, hypertension is defined as an average systolic blood pressure (SBP) and/or diastolic blood pressure (DBP) that is ≥ 95th percentile of BP for a young person of a given sex, age, and stature or height. Prehypertension is defined as average SBP or DBP levels that are ≥ 90th percentile but < 95th percentile. To categorize the BP of a person in this age group, it is necessary to determine his or her percentile of stature for sex and age using the sex- and age-appropriate CDC growth chart that provides the length-for-age percentiles or stature-for-age percentiles. The CDC growth charts are discussed in Chapter 6 and shown in Appendix G. Once the subject's percentile of length or stature is determined, Table 8.12 or 8.13 is used to determine the BP percentile that is then used to categorize BP.

Keep in mind that following proper technique is critical to measuring BP in any age group. Categorization of BP in children and adolescents is based on the average of multiple BP measurements. At each visit with a health-care provider, BP should be measured two or three times following the protocol discussed in this chapter. Furthermore, categorization of BP is done on an average of multiple BP measurements taken during at least three different visits with the health-care provider. A diagnosis of hypertension cannot be made on the basis of a single BP measurement or on values taken during a single visit with a health-care provider.

Working through the following three cases will help you understand how to categorize blood pressure in children and adolescents.

1. A 7-year-old female is 4 feet tall. Using multiple measurements of BP taken during three different visits with a health-care provider, it was determined that this child's average BP is 110/72 mm Hg. What is this child's percentile of stature for sex and age?

_____

This child's BP would be categorized as

A. normal
B. prehypertension
C. hypertension

2. A 14-year-old female is 156 cm tall and has an average BP of 127/83 mm Hg. What is this adolescent's percentile of stature for sex and age?

_____

This adolescent's BP would be categorized as

A. normal
B. prehypertension
C. hypertension

3. What would be the 50th to 90th percentile range of BP for 10-year-old males who are at the 50th percentile of stature-for-age?

_____ to _____ / _____ to _____

ASSESSMENT ACTIVITY 8.4

Cardiovascular Health Metrics

As discussed in this chapter, the American Heart Association's (AHA) 2020 goal is to reduce deaths from CVD and stroke by 20%. As a part of this initiative, the AHA tracks seven key health factors and behaviors called "Life's Simple 7": not smoking, physical activity, healthy diet, body weight, and control of cholesterol, blood pressure, and blood sugar. The ideal cardiovascular health metrics can be assessed for individuals at www.heart.org/mylifecheck/. Go to this website and input all of the required information: age, height, weight, gender, ethnicity, three measurements (blood pressure, fasting plasma glucose, total blood cholesterol), and three lifestyle responses (smoking, physical activity, and dietary habits). Discover your heart score, a number from 0 to 10, which is an indication of your overall cardiovascular health based on the information you've given. Print or save your results (My Life Check Report), and discuss the process and results with your instructor and classmates.

9 BIOCHEMICAL ASSESSMENT OF NUTRITIONAL STATUS

STUDENT LEARNING OUTCOMES

After studying this chapter, the student will be able to:

1. Discuss the biochemical tests for assessing visceral and somatic protein status.

2. Recall the formula for determining nitrogen balance and calculate nitrogen balance given a patient's protein intake and urine urea nitrogen value.

3. Discuss the advantages and disadvantages of using serum proteins for assessing nutritional status.

4. Discuss the strengths and weaknesses of the models used for assessing iron status.

5. Describe the state of iron nutriture in the United States using data from NHANES.

6. Describe the state of iodine nutriture in the United States using data from NHANES.

7. Explain how vitamin D status is assessed.

8. Describe how indicators of folate status have changed since the FDA required the addition of folate to refined cereal products.

INTRODUCTION

Compared with the other methods of nutritional assessment (anthropometric, clinical methods, and dietary), biochemical tests can potentially provide more objective and quantitative data on nutritional status. Biochemical tests, also known as biomarkers, often can detect nutrient deficits long before anthropometric measures are altered and clinical signs and symptoms appear. Some of these tests are useful indicators of recent nutrient intake and can be used in conjunction with dietary methods to assess food and nutrient consumption.

This chapter discusses the topic of biochemical methods in nutritional assessment, reviews the more commonly encountered tests for those nutrients of public health importance, and provides examples of various biochemical techniques in nutritional assessment.

Nutritional science is a relatively young discipline, and use of biochemical methods as indicators of nutritional status is still in development. This, along with all that yet remains unknown about the human body, makes the use of these measures in nutritional assessment a rapidly developing field and one with many research opportunities.

USE OF BIOCHEMICAL MEASURES

Biochemical tests available for assessing nutritional status can be grouped into two general and somewhat arbitrary categories: *static tests* and *functional tests*. These are sometimes referred to as *direct* and *indirect tests,* respectively. Static tests are also referred to as qualitative and quantitative biochemical indicators. Functional tests are also referred to as biological, functional, and histologic indicators.[1]

Static tests are based on measurement of a nutrient or its metabolite in the blood, urine, or body tissue—for example, serum measurements of folate, retinol, vitamin B_{12}, vitamin D. These are among the most readily available tests, but they have certain limitations. Although they may indicate nutrient levels in the particular tissue or fluid sampled, they often fail to reflect the overall nutrient status of an individual or whether the body as a whole is in a state of nutrient excess or depletion.[2] For example, the amount of calcium in serum can be easily determined, but that single static measurement is a poor indicator of the body's overall calcium status or of bone mineral content.

Functional tests of nutritional status are based on the ultimate outcome of a nutrient deficiency, which is the failure of the physiologic processes that rely on that nutrient for optimal performance. Included among these functional tests are measurement of dark adaptation (assesses vitamin A status) and urinary excretion of xanthurenic acid in response to consumption of tryptophan (assesses vitamin B_6 status). Although many functional tests remain in the experimental stage, this is an area of active research and one that is likely to be fruitful. One drawback of some functional tests, however, is a tendency to be nonspecific; they may indicate general nutritional status but not allow identification of specific nutrient deficiencies.

Biochemical tests can also be used to examine the validity of various methods of measuring dietary intake or to determine if respondents are underreporting or overreporting what they eat. The ability of a food frequency questionnaire to accurately measure protein intake, for example, can be assessed by comparing reported protein intake with 24-hour urine nitrogen excretion. When properly used, this method is sufficiently accurate to use as a validation method in dietary surveys. As with any test requiring a 24-hour urine sample, however, each collection must be complete (i.e., respondents must collect all

urine during an exact 24-hour period). Urinary nitrogen is best estimated using multiple 24-hour urine samples, and any extrarenal nitrogen losses must be accounted for.[3] The doubly labeled water technique, as mentioned in Chapters 3 and 7, is another biochemical test useful for determining validity and accuracy of reporting. It can be an accurate way of measuring energy expenditure without interfering with a respondent's everyday life.[4] If reported energy and protein consumption fail to match estimates of energy and protein intake derived from these properly performed biochemical tests, then the dietary assessment method may be faulty or the respondent did not accurately report food intake.

Biochemical tests are a valuable adjunct in assessing and managing nutritional status; however, their use is not without problems. Most notable among these is the influence that nonnutritional factors can have on test results. A variety of pathologic conditions, use of certain medications, and technical problems in a sample collection or assay can affect test results in ways that make them unusable. Another problem with some biochemical tests is their nonspecificity. A certain test may indicate that a patient's general nutritional status is impaired yet lack the specificity to indicate which nutrient is deficient. Additionally, no single test, index, or group of tests by itself is sufficient for monitoring nutritional status. Biochemical tests must be used in conjunction with measures of dietary intake, anthropometric measures, and clinical methods.

PROTEIN STATUS

Assessing protein status can be approached by use of anthropometric (Chapters 6 and 7), biochemical, clinical (Chapter 10), and dietary data (Chapters 3 and 4).

Biochemical assessment of protein status has typically been approached from the perspective of the two-compartment model: evaluation of somatic protein and visceral protein status. The body's somatic protein is found within skeletal muscle. Visceral protein can be regarded as consisting of protein within the organs or viscera of the body (liver, kidneys, pancreas, heart, and so on), the erythrocytes (red blood cells), and the granulocytes and lymphocytes (white blood cells), as well as the serum proteins.[5,6] The somatic and visceral pools contain the metabolically available protein (known as body cell mass), which can be drawn on, when necessary, to meet various bodily needs. The somatic and visceral protein pools comprise about 75% and 25% of the body cell mass, respectively. Together, they comprise about 30% to 50% of total body protein.[5] The remaining body protein is found primarily in the skin and connective tissue (bone matrix, cartilage, tendons, and ligaments) and is not readily exchangeable with the somatic and visceral protein pools. Division of the body's protein into these two compartments is somewhat arbitrary and artificial. Although the somatic compartment is homogeneous, the visceral protein pool is composed of hundreds of different proteins serving many structural and functional roles.

Although protein is not considered a public health issue among the general population of developed nations, protein-energy malnutrition (PEM), also known as protein-calorie malnutrition, can be a result of certain diseases and is clearly a pressing concern in many developing nations. Protein-energy malnutrition can be seen in persons with cancer and acquired immune deficiency syndrome (AIDS), children who fail to thrive, those with anorexia nervosa, and homeless persons.

Because of its high prevalence and relationship to infant mortality and impaired physical growth, PEM is considered the most important nutritional disease in developing countries.[7] It is also of concern in developed nations. According to some reports, PEM has been observed in nearly half of the patients hospitalized in medical and surgical wards in the United States. In more recent studies, the prevalence of PEM ranged from 30% to 40% among patients with hip fractures, patients undergoing thoracic surgery for lung cancer, patients receiving ambulatory peritoneal dialysis, and children and adolescents with juvenile rheumatoid arthritis.[2,7–9]

Assessment of protein status is central to the prevention, diagnosis, and treatment of PEM. The causes of PEM can be either primary (inadequate food intake) or secondary (other diseases leading to insufficient food intake, inadequate nutrient absorption or utilization, increased nutritional requirement, and increased nutrient losses).[7–9] The protein and energy needs of hospitalized patients can be two or more times those of healthy persons as a result of hypermetabolism accompanying trauma, infection, burns, and surgical recovery. PEM can result in kwashiorkor (principally a protein deficiency), marasmus (predominantly an energy deficiency), or marasmic kwashiorkor (a combination of chronic energy deficit and chronic or acute protein deficiency).[7] Clinical findings pertinent to kwashiorkor and marasmus are discussed in Chapter 10.

Body weight is a readily obtained indicator of energy and protein reserves. However, it must be carefully interpreted because it fails to distinguish between fat mass and fat-free mass, and losses of skeletal muscle and adipose tissue can be masked by water retention resulting from edema and ascites. The creatinine-height index is also well suited to the clinical setting but has limited precision and accuracy. Use of midarm muscle circumference and midarm muscle area are two other approaches to assessing somatic protein status.[7] These are discussed in Chapter 7.

Rather than relying on any single indicator, a combination of measures can produce a more complete picture of protein status. The choice of approaches depends on methods available to the particular facility. Biochemical data on nutritional status constitute only part of the necessary information to evaluate the severity of nutritional depletion and PEM. Data relating to dietary intake, pertinent anthropometric measures, and clinical findings are necessary as well.

Creatinine Excretion and Creatinine-Height Index

A biochemical test sometimes used for estimating body muscle mass is 24-hour urinary creatinine excretion. Creatinine, a product of skeletal muscle, is excreted in a relatively constant proportion to the mass of muscle in the body. It is readily measured by any clinical laboratory. Lean body mass can be estimated by comparing 24-hour urine creatinine excretion with a standard based on stature (Table 9.1) or from reference values of 23 and 18 mg/kg of recommended body weight for males and females, respectively. Another approach is using the creatinine-height index (CHI), a ratio of a patient's measured 24-hour urinary creatinine excretion and the expected excretion of a reference adult of the same sex and stature. The CHI is expressed by the following formula:

$$CHI = \frac{24\text{-hr urine creatinine(mg)} \times 100}{\text{Expected 24-hr urine creatinine (mg)}}$$

Expected 24-hour urine creatinine values are shown in Table 9.1. These should be matched to the subject's sex and height.

The CHI is expressed as a percent of expected value. A CHI of 60% to 80% is considered indicative of mild protein depletion; 40% to 60% reflects moderate protein depletion; and a value under 40% represents severe depletion.[5–7]

TABLE 9.1	**Expected 24-Hour Urinary Creatinine Values for Height for Adult Males and Females**

Adult Males*		Adult Females†	
Height (cm)	Creatinine (mg)	Height (cm)	Creatinine (mg)
157.5	1288	147.3	830
160.0	1325	149.9	851
162.6	1359	152.4	875
165.1	1386	154.9	900
167.6	1426	157.5	925
170.2	1467	160.0	949
172.7	1513	162.6	977
175.3	1555	165.1	1006
177.8	1596	167.6	1044
180.3	1642	170.2	1076
182.9	1691	172.7	1109
185.4	1739	175.3	1141
188.0	1785	177.8	1174
190.5	1831	180.3	1206
193.0	1891	182.9	1240

Source: Blackburn GL, Bistrian BR, Maini BS, Schlamm HT, Smith MR. 1977. Nutritional and metabolic assessment of the hospitalized patient. *Journal of Parenteral and Enteral Nutrition* 1:11–12.

*Creatinine coefficient for males = 23 mg/kg of "ideal" body weight.

†Creatinine coefficient for females = 18 mg/kg of "ideal" body weight.

As mentioned in the section "Use of Biochemical Measures," a major concern when using any test requiring a 24-hour urine sample is obtaining a complete urine sample collected during an exact 24-hour period. The value of protein status measurements based on urinary creatinine measurements can also be compromised by the effect of diet on urine creatinine levels, variability in creatinine excretion, and the use of height-weight tables for determining expected creatinine excretion based on sex and stature.[5] These limitations are discussed in Chapter 6.

Nitrogen Balance

A person is said to be in nitrogen balance when the amount of nitrogen (consumed as protein) equals the amount excreted by the body. It is the difference between nitrogen intake and the amount excreted from the body in urine and feces or lost in miscellaneous ways such as the sloughing of skin cells and blood loss.[10] Nitrogen balance is the expected state of the healthy adult. It occurs when the rate of protein synthesis, or anabolism, equals the rate of protein degradation, or catabolism. Positive nitrogen balance occurs when nitrogen intake exceeds nitrogen loss and is seen in periods of anabolism, such as childhood or recovery from trauma, surgery, or illness. Negative nitrogen balance occurs when nitrogen losses exceed nitrogen intake and can result from insufficient protein intake, catabolic states (for example, sepsis, trauma, surgery, and cancer), or periods of excessive protein loss (as a result of burns or certain gastrointestinal and renal diseases characterized by unusual protein loss). Nutritional support can help return a patient to positive nitrogen balance or at least prevent severe losses of energy stores and body protein.[5–7]

Nitrogen balance studies involve 24-hour measurement of protein intake and an estimate of nitrogen losses from the body. The following formula is used:

$$N_2 \text{ Balance} = \frac{PRO}{6.25} - UUN - 4$$

where N_2 Balance = nitrogen balance; PRO = protein intake (g/24 h); and UUN = urine urea nitrogen (g/24 h).

Protein intake, measured by dietary assessment methods, is divided by 6.25 to arrive at an estimate of nitrogen intake. Nitrogen loss is generally estimated by measuring urine urea nitrogen (which accounts for 85% to 90% of nitrogen in the urine) and adding a constant (for example, 4 g) to account for nitrogen losses from the skin, stool, wound drainage, nonurea nitrogen, and so on, which cannot be easily measured.[5–7,10]

Problems associated with measuring protein intake and nitrogen excretion limit the usefulness of this approach. For example, it is difficult to account for the unusually high nonurine nitrogen losses seen in some patients with burns, diarrhea, vomiting, or fistula drainage. In such cases, this approach to calculating nitrogen balance may not yield accurate results.

Serum Proteins

Serum protein concentrations can be useful in assessing protein status, in determining whether a patient is at risk of experiencing medical complications, and for evaluating a patient's response to nutritional support. The serum proteins of primary interest in nutritional assessment are shown in Table 9.2.[2] In most instances, their measurement is simple and accurate. Use of serum protein measurements is based on the assumption that decreases in serum concentrations are due to decreased liver production (the primary site of synthesis). This is considered a consequence of a limited supply of amino acids from which the serum proteins are synthesized or a decrease in the liver's capacity to synthesize serum proteins. The extent to which nutritional status or liver function affects serum protein concentrations cannot always be determined. A number of factors other than inadequate protein intake affect serum protein concentrations. These are noted in Table 9.2.

Albumin

The most familiar and abundant of the serum proteins, as well as the most readily available clinically, is albumin. Serum albumin level has been shown to be an indicator of depleted protein status and decreased dietary protein intake. Measured over the course of several weeks, it has been shown to correlate with other measures of protein status and to respond to protein repletion. Low concentrations of serum albumin are associated with increased morbidity and mortality in hospitalized patients.[2,5–7,11] Despite these correlations, the value of albumin as a protein status indicator is severely limited by several factors. Its relatively long half-life (14 to 20 days) and large body pool (4 to 5 g/kg of body weight) cause serum levels to respond very slowly to nutritional change.[2,5–7,11] Because it is neither sensitive to, nor specific for, acute PEM or a patient's response to nutritional support, it is not a useful indicator of protein depletion or repletion.[2,11]

Serum albumin level is determined by several factors: the rate of synthesis, its distribution in the body, the rate at which it is catabolized, abnormal losses from the body, and altered fluid status.[2,11] About 60% of the body's albumin is found outside the bloodstream. When serum concentrations begin falling during early PEM, this extravascular albumin moves into the bloodstream, helping maintain normal serum concentrations despite protein and energy deficit. During the acute catabolic phase of an injury, an infection, or surgery, there is increased synthesis of substances known as acute-phase reactants. Included among these are C-reactive protein, fibrinogen, haptoglobin, and alpha-1-acid glycoprotein. Acute-phase reactants decrease synthesis of albumin, prealbumin, and transferrin. Consequently, levels of these serum proteins may remain low during this catabolic phase despite the provision of adequate nutritional

TABLE 9.2	Serum Proteins Used in Nutritional Assessment

Serum Protein		Half-Life	Function	Comments*
Albumin		18–20 days	Maintains plasma oncotic pressure; carrier for small molecules	In addition to protein status, other factors affect serum concentrations.
Normal:	3.5–5.0 g/L			
Mild depletion:	3.0–3.4 g/L			
Moderate depletion:	2.4–2.9 g/L			
Severe depletion:	< 2.4 g/L			
Transferrin		8–9 days	Binds iron in plasma and transports to bone marrow	Iron deficiency increases hepatic synthesis and plasma levels; increases during pregnancy, during estrogen therapy, and in acute hepatitis; reduced in protein-losing enteropathy and nephropathy, chronic infections, uremia, and acute catabolic states; often measured indirectly by total iron-binding capacity; equations for indirect prediction should be developed locally.
Normal:	200–400 mg/dL			
Mild depletion:	150–200 mg/dL			
Moderate depletion:	100–149 mg/dL			
Severe depletion:	< 100 mg/dL			
Prealbumin (transthyretin)		2–3 days	Binds T_3 and, to a lesser extent, T_4; carrier for retinol-binding protein	Level is increased in patients with chronic renal failure on dialysis due to decreased renal catabolism; reduced in acute catabolic states, after surgery, in hyperthyroidism, in protein-losing enteropathy; increased in some cases of nephrotic syndrome; serum level determined by overall energy balance as well as nitrogen balance.
Normal:	16–40 mg/dL			
Mild depletion:	10–15 mg/dL			
Moderate depletion:	5–9 mg/dL			
Severe depletion:	< 5 mg/dL			
Retinol-binding protein (RBP)		12 hours	Transports vitamin A in plasma; binds noncovalently to prealbumin	It is catabolized in renal proximal tubular cell; with renal disease, RBP increases and half-life is prolonged; low in vitamin A deficiency, acute catabolic states, after surgery, and in hyperthyroidism.
Normal:	2.1–6.4 mg/dL			

Source: Heimburger DC. 2012. Malnutrition and nutritional assessment. In Longo DL, Fauci AS, Kasper DL, Hauser SL, Jameson JL, Loscalzo J (eds.), *Harrison's principles of internal medicine,* 18th ed. New York: McGraw-Hill, 605–612; and Charney P, Malone AM. 2009. *ADA pocket guide to nutrition assessment,* 2nd ed. Chicago: American Dietetic Association.

*All the listed proteins are influenced by hydration and the presence of hepatocellular dysfunction.

support.[14] The practice of administering albumin to severely ill patients also can interfere with its use as an indicator of protein status.

Transferrin

Serum transferrin is a β-globulin synthesized in the liver that binds and transports iron in the plasma. Because of its smaller body pool and shorter half-life, it has been considered a better index of changes in protein status compared with albumin.[2,11] Although serum transferrin has been shown to be associated with clinical outcome in children with kwashiorkor and marasmus, its use to predict morbidity and mortality outcomes in hospitalized patients has produced conflicting results.[5]

Serum transferrin can be measured directly (by radial immunodiffusion and nephelometry), but it is frequently estimated indirectly from total iron-binding capacity (TIBC) using a prediction formula suited to the particular facility's method for measuring TIBC.[5]

The use of transferrin as an index of nutritional status and repletion is limited by several factors other than protein status that affect its serum concentration. As outlined in Table 9.2, transferrin levels decrease in chronic infections, protein-losing enteropathy, chronically draining wounds, nephropathy, acute catabolic states (e.g., surgery and

trauma), and uremia. Serum levels can be increased during pregnancy, estrogen therapy, and acute hepatitis.[14,18]

Prealbumin

Prealbumin, also known as transthyretin and thyroxine-binding prealbumin, is synthesized in the liver and serves as a transport protein for thyroxine (T_4) and as a carrier protein for retinol-binding protein. Because of its short half-life (two to three days) and small body pool (0.01 g/kg body weight), it is considered a more sensitive indicator of protein nutriture and one that responds more rapidly to changes in protein status than albumin or transferrin.

Prealbumin decreases rapidly in response to deficits of either protein or energy and is sensitive to the early stages of malnutrition. Because serum concentration quickly returns to expected levels once adequate nutritional therapy begins, it is not recommended as an endpoint for terminating nutritional support. It may prove to be better suited as an indicator of recent dietary intake than as a means of assessing nutritional status.[2] Serum concentration also will return to expected levels in response to adequate energy in the absence of sufficient protein intake. Its use as an indicator of protein status appears to be preferable to the use of albumin or transferrin. However, like the other serum proteins outlined in

Table 9.2, several factors other than protein status affect its concentration in serum. Levels are reduced in liver disease, sepsis, protein-losing enteropathies, hyperthyroidism, and acute catabolic states (e.g., following surgery or trauma). Serum prealbumin can be increased in patients with chronic renal failure who are on dialysis due to decreased renal catabolism.[2,11]

Retinol-Binding Protein

Retinol-binding protein, a liver protein, acts as a carrier for retinol (vitamin A alcohol) when complexed with prealbumin. It circulates in the blood as a 1:1:1 trimolecular complex with retinol and prealbumin.[13] Retinol-binding protein shares several features with prealbumin. It responds quickly to protein-energy deprivation and adequate nutritional therapy, as well as to ample energy in the absence of sufficient protein. Like prealbumin, it may be a better indicator of recent dietary intake than of overall nutritional status. It has a much shorter half-life (about 12 hours) than prealbumin. Its smaller body pool (0.002 g/kg body weight), however, complicates its precise measurement. There is no convincing evidence that its use in nutritional assessment is preferred over prealbumin. Because it is catabolized in the renal proximal tubule cell, serum levels are increased in renal disease and its half-life is prolonged. Serum levels can be decreased in vitamin A deficiency, acute catabolic states, and hyperthyroidism.[2,13]

IRON STATUS

Iron deficiency is the most common single nutrient deficiency in the United States and the most common cause of anemia. Preschool children and women of childbearing age are at highest risk of iron deficiency.[14] Globally, 43% of preschool children and 33% of nonpregnant women are anemic, with the highest burden in Africa and South Asia.[15]

Iron deficiency results when ingestion or absorption of dietary iron is inadequate to meet iron losses or iron requirements imposed by growth or pregnancy. Considerable iron can be lost from heavy menstruation, frequent blood donations, early feeding of cow's milk to infants, frequent aspirin use, or disorders characterized by gastrointestinal bleeding. Risk of iron deficiency increases during periods of rapid growth—notably, in infancy (especially in premature infants), adolescence, and pregnancy. The consequences of iron deficiency include reduced work capacity, impaired body temperature regulation, impairments in behavior and intellectual performance, increased susceptibility to lead poisoning, and decreased resistance to infections. During pregnancy, iron deficiency increases risk of maternal death, prematurity, low birth weight, and neonatal mortality. During early childhood it can have adverse effects on cognitive, motor, and emotional development that may be only partially reversible.[15,16] The public health significance of iron deficiency is underscored by the fact that two of the objectives for *Healthy People 2020* relate to reducing iron deficiency among young children and females of childbearing age and among pregnant females.[14]

Clinicians typically request the complete blood count (CBC) as a first-step approach to assessing iron status (see Box 9.1). Anemia is a hemoglobin level below the normal reference range for individuals of the same sex and age. Descriptive terms such as *microcytic, macrocytic,* and *hypochromic* are sometimes used to describe anemias. *Microcytic* refers to abnormally small red blood cells defined by a mean corpuscular volume (MCV) < 80 femtoliters (fL), whereas *macrocytic* describes unusually large red blood cells defined as an MCV > 100 fL. Hypochromic cells are those with abnormally low levels of hemoglobin as defined by a mean corpuscular hemoglobin concentration < 320 g of hemoglobin/L or by a mean corpuscular hemoglobin < 27 picograms (pg, 10^{-12} grams).

Although the most common cause of anemia is iron deficiency, other common causes include inflammation, infection, tissue injury, and cancer, which are collectively referred to as anemia of inflammation.[15] Anemia can also result from deficiencies of folate and vitamin B_{12}. Of particular concern to physicians working with individual patients and nutritional epidemiologists attempting to estimate the prevalence of iron deficiency in populations is differentiating iron-deficiency anemia from anemia caused by inflammatory disease, infection, chronic diseases, and thalassemia traits.[17,18]

Stages of Iron Depletion

The risk of iron deficiency increases as the body's iron stores are depleted. Iron depletion can be divided into three stages. These stages and the biochemical tests used in identifying them are shown in Table 9.3. Figure 9.1 illustrates how values for these tests change throughout the stages of iron deficiency.

The first stage of iron depletion, depleted iron stores, is not associated with any adverse physiologic effects, but it does represent a state of vulnerability.[16,18] Low stores occur in healthy persons and appear to be the usual physiologic condition for growing children and menstruating women.[18,19] As shown in Figure 9.1, during this first stage, low iron stores are reflected by decreased serum ferritin levels, but values for the other biochemical tests remain within normal limits.

The second stage of iron depletion, early functional iron deficiency without anemia, can be considered representative of early or mild iron deficiency because, at this point, adverse physiologic consequences can begin to occur. This stage is characterized by changes indicating insufficient iron for normal production of hemoglobin and other essential iron compounds (for example, myoglobin and iron-containing enzymes).[16,18,19] As shown in Figure 9.1, this stage is characterized by decreased

Box 9.1   The Complete Blood Count (CBC)

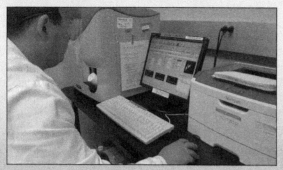

©David C. Nieman

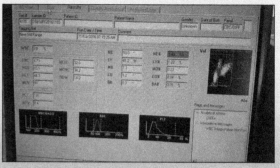

©David C. Nieman

A complete blood count (CBC) is a blood test used to evaluate overall health and detect a wide range of disorders, including anemia, infection, inflammation, bleeding disorder, and leukemia. Abnormal increases or decreases in cell counts as revealed in a complete blood count may indicate an underlying medical condition that calls for further evaluation.

A phlebotomist collects the sample through venipuncture, drawing the blood into a test tube containing an anticoagulant (EDTA, sometimes citrate) to stop it from clotting. The sample is then transported to a laboratory, where automated hematology analyzers perform the cell counts, measurements, and calculations. The three main physical technologies used in hematology analyzers are electrical impedance, flow cytometry, and fluorescent flow cytometry. These are used in combination with chemical reagents that lyse or alter blood cells to perform the measurable parameters.

The CBC is a panel of tests that evaluates the three types of cells (red blood cells, white blood cells, and platelets) that circulate in the blood compartment.

1. **Red blood cells and iron status: red blood cells (RBC), which carry oxygen; hemoglobin, the oxygen-carrying protein in red blood cells; and hematocrit, the proportion of red blood cells to the fluid component, or plasma, in blood.** If measures in these three areas are lower than normal, anemia is typically diagnosed (with follow-up tests to confirm). High RBC counts (erythrocytosis) or high hemoglobin or hematocrit levels could indicate an underlying medical condition, such as polycythemia vera or heart disease. (See Tables 9.4 and 9.5 and www. labtestsonline.org for normal ranges.)

   RBC indices, often included in the CBC, are calculations that provide information on the physical characteristics of the RBCs. (See Tables 9.4 and 9.5 for

normal ranges.) Mean corpuscular volume (MCV) is a measurement of the average size of a single red blood cell. Mean corpuscular hemoglobin (MCH) is a calculation of the average amount of hemoglobin inside a single red blood cell. Mean corpuscular hemoglobin concentration (MCHC) is a calculation of the average concentration of hemoglobin inside a single red blood cell. Red cell distribution width (RDW) is a calculation of the variation in the size of RBCs. The CBC may also include reticulocyte count, which is a measurement of the absolute count or percentage of young red blood cells in blood.

2. **White blood cells:** A low white blood cell (WBC) count (leukopenia) may be caused by a medical condition such as an autoimmune disorder that destroys WBCs, bone marrow disease, or cancer. Certain medications can cause WBCs to drop. High WBC counts (leukocytosis) may indicate an infection or inflammation, an immune system disorder, bone marrow disease, or a reaction to medication. The normal WBC range is 3.5–10.5 billion cells/L.

   The WBC differential, which may or may not be included in the CBC test, identifies and counts the number of five different types of WBCs: neutrophils, lymphocytes, monocytes, eosinophils, and basophils.

3. **Platelets:** Platelets are cell fragments that are vital for normal blood clotting. A platelet count that is lower than normal (thrombocytopenia) or higher than normal (thrombocytosis) may indicate an underlying disease condition or a side effect from medication. Further testing is needed to diagnose the cause. The normal platelet count is 150–450 billion/L.

Mean platelet volume (MPV) and platelet distribution width (PDW) may be reported with a CBC (calculations of the average size of platelets and how uniform platelets are in size, respectively).

transferrin saturation and increased erythrocyte protoporphyrin levels. A precursor of hemoglobin, erythrocyte protoporphyrin increases when too little iron is available for optimal hemoglobin synthesis. Although hemoglobin

may be decreased at this stage, it may not fall below the lowest levels seen in normal subjects. Consequently, hemoglobin is not a useful indicator of either stage 1 or stage 2 iron depletion.[16]

TABLE 9.3	The Three Stages of Iron Deficiency and the Indicators Used to Identify Them	

Stage of Iron Deficiency	Indicator	Diagnostic Range
1. Depleted stores	Serum ferritin concentration	< 12 µg/L
	Total iron-binding capacity	> 400 µg/dL
2. Early functional iron deficiency (without anemia)	Transferrin saturation	< 16%
	Free erythrocyte protoporphyrin	> 70 µg/dL erythrocyte
	Serum transferrin receptor	> 8.5 mg/L
3. Iron-deficiency anemia	Hemoglobin concentration	< 130 g/L in males
		< 120 g/L in females
	Mean corpuscular volume	< 80 fL

Source: Panel on Micronutrients, Subcommittee on Upper Reference Levels of Nutrients and of Interpretation and Uses of Dietary Reference Intakes, Standing Committee on the Scientific Evaluation of Dietary Reference Intakes. 2001. *Dietary Reference Intakes for vitamin A, vitamin K, arsenic, boron, chromium, copper, iodine, iron, manganese, molybdenum, nickel, silicon, vanadium, and zinc.* Washington, DC: National Academies Press.

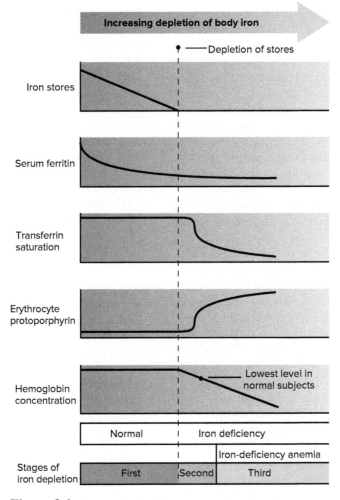

Figure 9.1 Changes in body iron compartments and laboratory assessments of iron status during the stages of iron depletion.

The third stage of iron depletion, iron-deficiency anemia, is characterized by decreased serum ferritin, transferrin saturation, hemoglobin, and MCV and increased erythrocyte protoporphyrin.[18,19]

No single biochemical test is diagnostic of impaired iron status. Several different static tests used together provide a much better measure of iron status.[16,18,19]

Serum Ferritin

When the protein apoferritin combines with iron, ferritin is formed. Ferritin, the primary storage form for iron in the body, is found primarily in the liver, spleen, and bone marrow. In healthy persons, approximately 30% of all iron in the body is in the storage form, most of this as ferritin but some as hemosiderin. As iron stores become depleted, tissue ferritin levels decrease. This is accompanied by a fall in serum ferritin concentration.[18–20] Although low serum ferritin concentration is a sensitive indicator of early iron deficiency, it does not necessarily reflect the severity of the depletion as it progresses. Because ferritin is an acute-phase protein, serum concentration is increased in acute and chronic diseases, potentially masking iron deficiency.[20]

Soluble Transferrin Receptor

Cells acquire iron when the iron transport protein transferrin forms a complex with a highly specific transferrin receptor (TfR) located on the plasma membrane surfaces of cells. Intracellular iron is regulated by the number of transferrin receptors on the plasma membrane, and the number of transferrin receptors on the plasma membrane is proportional to the cell's requirement for iron. When cellular iron content is low, more transferrin receptors appear on cell surfaces as a mechanism for cells to sequester the iron they need.[16,17,20–22] Soluble transferrin receptor (sTfR) is a shortened form of the membrane-bound TfR that is cleaved from TfR and released into the serum. The concentration of sTfR is proportional to the concentration of TfR on the plasma membranes of cells, especially the erythrocyte-producing cells of bone marrow. The sTfR concentration begins to increase in early iron deficiency with the onset of iron-deficient erythropoiesis (red blood cell production) before anemia develops and continues to increase as iron-deficient erythropoiesis worsens. Serum sTfR concentration is not affected by concurrent inflammation or infection. Measurement of serum sTfR concentration is now regarded as a valuable tool in diagnosing iron deficiency and monitoring erythropoiesis. During the first stage of iron depletion, when there are residual iron stores in the body, serum ferritin is the most sensitive index of iron status. However, sTfR concentration is a more sensitive index of iron status when iron stores are depleted and before anemia develops.[20–22] NHANES began measuring serum sTfR concentration in 2003, and it is one of the key variables in the model now used by NHANES to assess iron status in children 1 to 5 years of age and in women of childbearing age.[14,20]

Transferrin, Serum Iron, and Total Iron-Binding Capacity

Iron is transported in the blood bound to transferrin, a β-globulin protein molecule synthesized in the liver. Transferrin accepts iron from sites of hemoglobin destruction (the primary source for iron bound to transferrin), from storage sites, and from iron absorbed through the intestinal tract. It then delivers the iron to sites where it is used—primarily the bone marrow for hemoglobin synthesis, as well as to storage sites, to the placenta for fetal needs, and to all cells for incorporation into iron-containing enzymes. Each molecule of transferrin has the capacity to transport two atoms of iron, but under most circumstances only about 30% of the available iron-binding sites are occupied or saturated.[34]

Because iron is carried in the blood by transferrin, serum iron level is a measure of the amount of iron bound to transferrin. Levels fall sometime between depletion of tissue iron stores and development of anemia, although they may actually be normal in persons with iron deficiency.[18,19]

Total iron-binding capacity measures the amount of iron capable of being bound to serum proteins and provides an estimate of serum transferrin. It is usually measured by adding an excess of iron to serum (thus saturating iron-binding proteins in serum), removing all iron not bound to protein in the serum, and then measuring serum iron. Because it is assumed that most serum iron is bound to transferrin, TIBC is an indirect measure of serum transferrin. Because other serum proteins can bind iron, TIBC is not an exact measure of transferrin, especially in cases of iron overload and certain other conditions. In about 30% to 40% of persons with iron-deficiency anemia, TIBC is not elevated.[18,19]

Transferrin saturation is the ratio of serum iron to TIBC and is calculated using the following formula:

$$TS = \frac{Serum\ iron\ (\mu mol/L)}{TIBC\ (\mu mol/L)} \times 100$$

where TS = percent transferrin saturation and TIBC = total iron-binding capacity.

Transferrin saturation is the percent of transferrin that is saturated with iron. In uncomplicated iron-deficiency anemia, serum iron levels decrease and TIBC increases, resulting in a decreased transferrin saturation.

Measures of serum iron, TIBC, transferrin saturation, and serum ferritin concentration are useful in distinguishing iron deficiency from other disorders capable of causing microcytic anemias (anemias in which the erythrocytes are smaller than normal).[18,19] Transferrin saturation, however, is considered to be a more sensitive indicator of iron deficiency than either serum iron or TIBC.[35]

Erythrocyte Protoporphyrin

Protoporphyrin is a precursor of heme and accumulates in red blood cells (erythrocytes) when the amount of heme that can be produced is limited by iron deficiency. Protoporphyrin concentration is generally reported in the range of 0.622 ± 0.27 μmol/L of red blood cells, although the value can vary depending on the analytic method. Iron deficiency can lead to a more than twofold increase over normal values. Erythrocyte protoporphyrin increases as iron depletion worsens, as can be seen in Figure 9.1. Lead poisoning also can result in increased erythrocyte protoporphyrin levels.

Hemoglobin

Hemoglobin is an iron-containing molecule found in red blood cells that is capable of carrying oxygen and carbon dioxide. It also acts as an important acid-base buffer system. It is used as an index of the blood's oxygen-carrying capacity. The amount of hemoglobin in blood depends primarily on the number of red blood cells and to a lesser extent on the amount of hemoglobin in each red blood cell.[12,18,19] Despite its use as a screening test for iron-deficiency anemia, isolated measurements of hemoglobin concentration or hematocrit level are not suitable as the sole indicator of iron status.[17] They tend not to become abnormal until the late stages of iron deficiency and are not good indicators of early iron deficiency. In addition, hemoglobin fails to distinguish between iron-deficiency anemia and anemia of inflammation.[17] Normal ranges for hemoglobin and hematocrit are shown in Table 9.4.

The use of cutoff points (as in Table 9.4) to evaluate laboratory values inevitably results in some degree of misclassification. For example, no matter where the cutoff value is placed in Figure 9.2, there will be some individuals with adequate iron status whose hemoglobin levels fall below the cutoff value. These are the false positives. There will be some, on the other hand, with an inadequate iron status whose hemoglobin levels fall above the cutoff value. These are the false negatives.

Hematocrit

Hematocrit (also known as *packed cell volume*) is defined as the percentage of red blood cells making up the entire

TABLE 9.4	Normal Ranges for Hemoglobin and Hematocrit	
Age Group	**Hemoglobin (g/dL)**	**Hematocrit (%)**
Newborn	14–24	44–64
2–8 weeks	12–20	39–59
2–6 months	10–17	35–50
6–12 months	9.5–14	29–43
1–6 years	9.5–14	30–40
6–18 years	10–15.5	32–44
Adult male	14–18	42–52
Adult female	12–16	37–47
Pregnant female	> 11	> 33

Source: Pagana KD, Pagana TJ. 2010. *Mosby's manual of diagnostic and laboratory tests*, 4th ed. St. Louis: Mosby Elsevier.

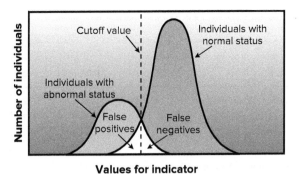

Figure 9.2 **Effect of applying a cutoff value for an indicator of nutritional status to the distributions of values for individuals with adequate status and individuals with inadequate status.**

volume of whole blood. It can be measured manually by comparing the height of whole blood in a capillary tube with the height of the RBC column after the tube is centrifuged. In automated counters, it is calculated from the RBC count (number of RBCs per liter of blood) and the mean corpuscular volume. Hematocrit depends largely on the number of red blood cells and to a lesser extent on their average size. Normal ranges for hematocrit are shown in Table 9.4. As is the case with hemoglobin, isolated measurement of hematocrit is not suitable as a sole indicator of iron status.[17]

Mean Corpuscular Hemoglobin

The mean corpuscular hemoglobin (MCH) is the amount of hemoglobin in red blood cells. It is calculated by dividing hemoglobin level by the red blood cell count. Reference values are approximately 26 to 34 pg. MCH is influenced by the size of the red blood cell and the amount of hemoglobin in relation to the size of the cell.[18,19]

A similar measure, mean corpuscular hemoglobin concentration (MCHC) is the average concentration of hemoglobin in the average red blood cell. It is calculated by dividing the hemoglobin value by the value for hematocrit. Normal values lie in the range of 320 to 360 g/L (32 to 36 g/dL).[18,19]

Mean Corpuscular Volume

Mean corpuscular volume (MCV) is the average volume of red blood cells. It is calculated by dividing the hematocrit value by the RBC count. Values for MCV are normally in the range of 80 to 100 fL for both males and females.

Factors increasing MCV (resulting in macrocytosis) include deficiencies of folate or vitamin B_{12}, chronic liver disease, alcoholism, and cytotoxic chemotherapy. Among factors decreasing MCV (resulting in microcytosis) are chronic iron deficiency, thalassemia, anemia of chronic diseases, and lead poisoning.[18,19] Reference blood cell values for adults are shown in Table 9.5.

TABLE 9.5	Reference Blood Cell Values for Adults

	Males	Females
Hemoglobin (g/dL of blood)	14–18	12–16
Hematocrit (%)	40–54	37–47
Red cell count ($\times 10^{12}$/L blood)	4.7–6.1	4.2–5.4
Mean corpuscular hemoglobin (pg)	27–33	27–33
Mean corpuscular hemoglobin concentration (g/dL of blood)	31–35	31–35
Mean corpuscular volume (fL)	82–98	82–98

Source: Ravel R. 1994. *Clinical laboratory medicine: Clinical application of laboratory data,* 6th ed. St. Louis: Mosby.

Assessing Iron Status

One of the challenges of addressing iron deficiency has been uncertainty about the best approach for assessing iron status.[17] Because no single biochemical test exists for reliably assessing iron status, models using two or more different indicators of iron status have been developed. Three of these models are shown in Table 9.6. The two most commonly used are the ferritin model and the body iron model. The ferritin model (also known as the three-indicator model) uses three indicators: serum ferritin, transferrin saturation, and erythrocyte protoporphyrin.[14,16,23,24] The body iron model uses two indicators: serum ferritin and soluble transferrin receptor (sTfR).[14,15,17,20–23] Another model, the mean corpuscular volume (MCV) model, uses MCV, transferrin saturation, and erythrocyte protoporphyrin as indicators.[25] Both the ferritin model and the MCV model require that at least two of the three indicators be abnormal.[23–25] The ferritin model tends to overestimate the presence of iron deficiency because it includes ferritin, which reflects stores in the first stage of iron depletion. The MCV model, on the other hand, includes three biochemical tests, all of which reflect altered red blood cell formation.[26] Both models are capable of identifying persons in the second and third stages of iron depletion, but they may fail to distinguish iron-deficiency anemia from the other common causes of anemia, such as inflammation, acute and chronic disease, and lead poisoning, because they include erythrocyte protoporphyrin as a variable.[24–26]

The MCV model was employed to assess iron status using data from NHANES II (1976–1980).[25] The ferritin model was used in NHANES III as well as the first few years of the continuous NHANES survey that began in 1999.[20] Beginning in 2003, NHANES limited its interest in assessing iron status to children 1–5 years of age and to women of childbearing age (12–49 years of age) and introduced the measurement of sTfR. Since 2003, NHANES has used the body iron model to assess body iron in the two groups of interest (children 1–5 years and women 12–49 years).[20] Of the three models, the body iron model is considered superior because it is less affected by inflammation than are the ferritin and MCV models. In addition, only two measures are used in the body model, whereas three measures are used in the other models. The greater simplicity of the body iron model makes it more suitable for use in areas where resources are limited and where anemia due to inflammation, chronic disease, and nutrient deficiencies other than iron are relatively common.[14,15,20–22] Using the body iron model, body iron can be estimated from the ratio of sTfR to serum ferritin. Body iron is in positive balance (≥ 0 mg of iron per kg of body weight or ≥ 0 mg/kg) when there is residual storage iron or in a negative balance (< 0 mg of iron per kg of body weight or < 0 mg/kg) during functional iron deficiency when there is a lack of iron required to maintain a normal hemoglobin concentration.[20] Both sTfR and serum ferritin can be measured using a small capillary blood specimen. Body iron is expressed in mg of iron per kg of body weight, controlling for the effect of body weight when estimating body iron and increasing the utility of this model for assessing the iron status of younger persons. Figure 9.3 shows the age-adjusted prevalence estimates of low body iron stores (< 0 mg/kg) in U.S. children and women by race/ethnicity using data from NHANES 2003–2006. The highest prevalence of low body iron assessed using the body iron model was seen in Mexican American children 1–5 years of age and in non-Hispanic black women 12–49 years of age.[20]

TABLE 9.6	Models for Assessing Iron Status

Model	Measurements Used
Body iron model*	Soluble transferrin receptor (sTfR) Serum ferritin
Ferritin model[†]	Serum ferritin Transferrin saturation Erythrocyte protoporphyrin
Mean corpuscular volume (MCV) model[†]	MCV Transferrin saturation Erythrocyte protoporphyrin

*Measurements used to calculate the sTfR to serum ferritin ratio.

[†]Two of three values must be abnormal.

Iron Overload

A second disorder of iron metabolism is iron overload, which is the accumulation of excess iron in body tissues. Iron overload is most often the result of hemochromatosis, a group of genetic diseases characterized by excessive intestinal iron absorption and deposition of excessive amounts of iron in parenchymal cells with eventual tissue

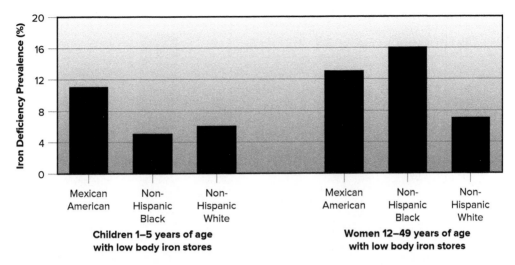

Figure 9.3 **Age-adjusted prevalence estimates of low body iron stores (< 0 mg/kg) in U.S. children and women by race/ethnicity, NHANES 2003–2006.**
The highest prevalence of low body iron assessed using the body iron model was seen in Mexican American children 1–5 years of age and in non-Hispanic Black women 12–49 years of age.

Source: U.S. Centers for Disease Control and Prevention. 2012. *Second national report on biochemical indicators of diet and nutrition in the U.S. population.* Atlanta: National Center for Environmental Health. www.cdc.gov/nutritionreport.

damage. Organs particularly affected by hemochromatosis are the liver, heart, and pancreas, leading to the failure of these organs and possibly death. Iron overload can also result from multiple blood transfusions and the excessive intake of iron from fortified foods and supplements.[16,17,20,27] Among North Americans of European extraction, it is estimated that more than 10% have a mild form of hemochromatosis resulting in a slight to moderate increase in serum ferritin concentration and transferrin saturation, and that 0.3–0.5% have the more severe form causing organ damage and possibly death.[17,27]

The degree of increase in total body iron is an elevated serum ferritin concentration. Figure 9.4 shows age-adjusted prevalence estimates of low (< 15 ng/mL) and high serum ferritin (> 200 ng/mL for men and > 150 ng/mL for women) in U.S. men and women 12–49 years of age, based on data collected by NHANES between 1999 and 2006. As shown in Figure 9.4, women are at risk of iron deficiency, while men are at risk of iron excess, and there are marked differences in the prevalence of low and high serum ferritin concentrations between the two sexes.[20,27]

CALCIUM STATUS

Calcium is essential for bone and tooth formation, muscle contraction, blood clotting, and cell membrane integrity.[28,29] Of the 1200 g of calcium in the adult body, approximately 99% is contained in the bones. The remaining 1% is found in extracellular fluids, intracellular structures, and cell membranes.[28,29]

Interest in osteoporosis prevention and treatment, coupled with data showing low calcium intakes in certain groups, especially women, has made calcium a current

public health issue. This has sparked interest in assessing the body's calcium status.

At the current time, there are no appropriate biochemical indicators for assessing calcium status. This is due in large part to the biological mechanisms that tightly control serum calcium levels despite wide variations in dietary intake and the fact that the skeleton serves as a calcium reserve so large that calcium deficiency at the cellular or tissue level is essentially never encountered, at least for nutritional reasons.[28,31] Potential approaches to assessing calcium status can be categorized in three areas: bone mineral content measurement, biochemical markers, and measures of calcium metabolism.[28] Of these three approaches, measurement of bone mineral content by such methods as quantitative computed tomography, single- and dual-photon absorptiometry, and dual-energy X-ray absorptiometry is currently the most feasible approach to assessing calcium status. DXA testing for body composition and bone mineral content is described in Chapter 6. However, fewer biochemical markers and measures of calcium metabolism are available. Attempts to identify a calcium status indicator in blood have been unsuccessful.

Serum Calcium Fractions

Serum calcium exists in three fractions: protein-bound, ionized, and complexed.[28] These and other values for calcium in body fluids are shown in Table 9.7. The protein-bound calcium is considered physiologically inactive, whereas the ionized fraction is considered physiologically active and functions as an intracellular regulator.[30–32] Complexed calcium is complexed with small negative ions, such as citrate, phosphate, and lactate. Its biological role is uncertain. Because the ionized and complexed

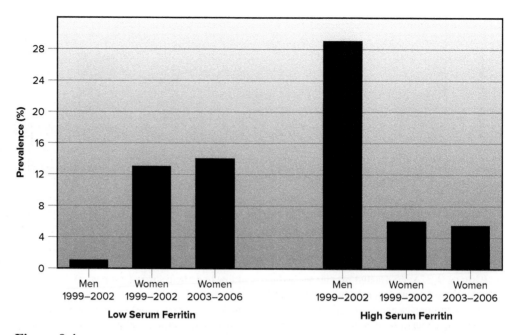

Figure 9.4 **Age-adjusted prevalence estimates of low (< 15 ng/mL) and high serum ferritin (> 200 ng/mL for men and > 150 ng/mL for women) in U.S. men and women 12–49 years of age, NHANES 1999–2006.**

Women are at risk of iron deficiency, while men are at risk of iron excess, as shown by the marked differences in the prevalence of low and high serum ferritin concentrations between the two sexes.

Source: U.S. Centers for Disease Control and Prevention. 2012. *Second national report on biochemical indicators of diet and nutrition in the U.S. population.* Atlanta: National Center for Environmental Health. www.cdc.gov/nutritionreport.

TABLE 9.7	Normal Values for Calcium in Body Fluids	
	Mean	Normal Range
Plasma		
Total calcium (mmol/L)	2.5	2.3–2.75
Ionized (mmol/L)	1.18	1.1–1.28
Complexed (mmol/L)		0.15–0.30
Protein-bound (mmol/L)		0.93–1.08
Urine		
24-hour calcium (mmol/L)		
Women	4.55	1.25–10
Men	6.22	1.25–12.5
Fasting calcium: creatinine ratio (molar)		
Postmenopausal women	0.341 ± 0.183*	
Men	0.169 ± 0.099*	

Source: Weaver CM. 1990. Assessing calcium status and metabolism. *Journal of Nutrition* 120:1470–1473.
*Mean ± SD.

calcium are diffusible across semipermeable membranes, these two fractions can be collectively referred to as *ultrafilterable calcium.* Serum levels of calcium are so tightly controlled by the body that there is little, if any, association between dietary calcium intake and serum levels.[32] Altered serum calcium levels are rare and indicate serious metabolic problems rather than low or high dietary intakes. Low serum calcium, or hypocalcemia (serum calcium concentration < 2.3 mmol/L), can result from a variety of conditions, including hypoparathyroidism (deficient or absent levels of parathyroid hormone), renal disease, and acute pancreatitis. High serum calcium concentrations, or hypercalcemia (serum calcium > 2.75 mmol/L), can be due to increased intestinal absorption, bone resorption, or renal tubular reabsorption resulting from such conditions as hyperparathyroidism, hyperthyroidism, and hypervitaminosis D (excessive intake of vitamin D).[30,31]

Urinary Calcium

Urinary calcium levels are more responsive to changes in dietary calcium intake than are serum levels.[31] However, urinary calcium is affected by a number of other factors, including those factors leading to hypercalcemia. When serum levels are high, more calcium is available to be excreted through the urine. There is a diurnal variation in urinary calcium, with concentrations higher during the day and lower in the evening.[30] Calcium output tends to be increased when the diet is rich in dietary protein and is low in phosphate and tends to be decreased by high-protein diets rich in phosphate.[30] Urinary calcium losses are increased when the volume of urine output is higher and when the kidneys' ability to reabsorb calcium is impaired.[31,32] Hypocalciuria can result from those factors leading to hypocalcemia as well as from renal failure.[36,37]

Use of the ratio of calcium to creatinine calculated from two-hour fasting urine samples has been suggested as a possible indicator of calcium status but requires further research. The calcium level in an overnight urine sample shows potential as an indicator of compliance with calcium supplementation.[31]

ZINC STATUS

Zinc's most important physiologic function is as a component of numerous enzymes.[16,33–35] Consequently, zinc is involved in many metabolic processes, including protein synthesis, wound healing, immune function, and tissue growth and maintenance. Severe zinc deficiency characterized by hypogonadism and dwarfism has been observed in the Middle East. Evidence of milder forms of zinc deficiency (detected by biochemical and clinical measurements) has been found in several population groups in the United States. In humans and laboratory animals, a reduction or cessation of growth is an early response to zinc deficiency, and supplementation in growth-retarded infants and children who are mildly zinc deficient can result in a growth response.[33,34]

Because there is concern about the adequacy of zinc intake among certain groups, especially females, zinc is considered a potential public health issue for which further study is needed. Nutrient intake data and other specific findings suggest that several U.S. population groups may have marginal zinc intakes. According to NHANES data, the average intake of zinc among females ages 20 to 49 years (approximately 9.6 mg/d) is roughly 80% of the RDA. Biochemical and clinical data derived from U.S. government nutritional monitoring activities, however, show no impairment of zinc status.

Plasma Zinc Concentrations

There is currently no specific sensitive biochemical or functional indicator of zinc status.[33] Static measurements of plasma zinc are available, but their use is complicated by the body's homeostatic control of zinc levels and by factors influencing serum zinc levels that are unrelated to nutritional status.[33,34]

There is little, if any, functional reserve of zinc in the body, as there is of some other nutrients (for example, iron, calcium, and vitamin A). The body's zinc levels are maintained by both conservation and redistribution of tissue zinc. In mild zinc deficiency, conservation is manifested by reduction or cessation of growth in growing organisms and by decreased excretion in nongrowing organisms. In most instances of mild deficiency, this appears to be the extent of clinical and biochemical changes. If the deficiency is severe, however, additional clinical signs soon appear.[16,33]

Mature animals and humans have a remarkable capacity to conserve zinc when intakes are low. As a result, inducing zinc deficiency in full-grown animals can be difficult.[33] Several mechanisms are responsible for this. Fecal zinc excretion, for example, can be cut by as much as 60% when dietary intake is low. Not only is the efficiency of intestinal absorption of zinc increased, but losses via the gastrointestinal tract, urine, and sweat are diminished.[33–38]

In laboratory animals, deficiency can lead to selective redistribution of zinc from certain tissues to support other, higher-priority tissues. In mild zinc deficiency, plasma zinc levels apparently can be maintained at the expense of zinc from other tissues.[33,34] Some evidence suggests that redistribution of total body zinc also occurs in humans.

The result of the body's conservation of and ability to redistribute zinc is that measurements of plasma zinc are not a reliable indicator of dietary zinc intake or changes in whole-body zinc status.[38] This is especially the case in mild zinc deficiency. For example, plasma zinc concentrations in growth-retarded children whose growth responded to zinc supplementation were not significantly different from concentrations in normally developed children either before or after supplementation.[38] Despite these limitations, measurement of plasma zinc concentration may be a useful, albeit late, indicator of the size of the body's exchangeable zinc pool. Less than expected values may signal a loss of zinc from bone and liver and increased risk for clinical and metabolic signs of zinc deficiency.[37,38]

Several factors unrelated to nutritional status can influence plasma zinc levels. Decreased levels can result from stress, infection or inflammation, and use of estrogens, oral contraceptives, and corticosteroids.[16,33,34] Plasma zinc can fall by 15% to 20% following a meal.[35] Increased plasma zinc concentrations can result from fasting and red blood cell hemolysis.

Metallothionen and Zinc Status

Metallothionen is a protein found in most tissues but primarily in the liver, pancreas, kidney, and intestinal mucosa. Metallothionen holds promise as a potential indicator of zinc status, particularly when used in conjunction with plasma zinc levels.[35,38] Measurable amounts are found in serum and in red blood cells. Metallothionen has the capacity of binding zinc and copper, and tissue metallothionen concentrations often are proportional to zinc status. In animals, levels are almost undetectable in zinc deficiency and are responsive to zinc supplementation. Whereas plasma zinc levels fall in response to acute stimuli (for example, stress, infection, and inflammation), hepatic and serum metallothionen levels are increased in response to these stimuli. Thus, when plasma levels of zinc fall and of metallothionen rise, it is likely that tissue zinc has been redistributed in response to acute stimuli and that a zinc deficiency is not present because metallothionen is not responsive to acute stimuli in zinc-deficient animals. If plasma zinc and metallothionen are both below expected levels, it is likely that zinc deficiency is present. Erythrocyte metallothionen (which is not affected by stress) also can be used as an indicator of zinc status.[35]

Hair Zinc

Several researchers have investigated the use of zinc in hair as an indicator of body zinc status.[36,38] Decreased concentration of zinc in hair has been reported in zinc-deficient dwarfs, in marginally deficient children and adolescents, and in conditions related to zinc deficiency, such as celiac disease, acrodermatitis enteropathica, and sickle cell disease. Because hair grows slowly (about 1 cm per month), levels of zinc and other trace elements in hair reflect nutritional status over many months and thus are not affected by diurnal variations or short-term fluctuations in nutritional status. Because of this, hair zinc levels may not be correlated with measurements of zinc in serum or erythrocytes, which reflect shorter-term zinc status.[36,38] Obtaining a sample is noninvasive, and analyzing hair for zinc and other trace elements is relatively easy.

It is important to note that trace elements in hair can come from endogenous sources (those that are ingested or inhaled by the subject and then enter the hair through the hair follicle) and exogenous sources (contamination from trace elements in dust, water, cosmetics, and so on).[39] A major drawback in using hair as an indicator of trace element status is its susceptibility to contamination from these exogenous sources. Some exogenous contaminants can be removed by carefully washing the hair sample before analysis, and several standardized washing procedures have been suggested.[39] However, some contaminants may be difficult or impossible to remove. Selenium, an ingredient in some antidandruff shampoos, is known to increase the selenium content of hair and cannot be removed by the recommended washing procedures.[39]

A variety of other nonnutritional factors may affect the trace element content of hair. Included among these are certain diseases, rate of hair growth, hair color, sex, pregnancy, and age.[39] It has been reported, for example, that higher concentrations of zinc, iron, nickel, and copper can be found in red hair, compared with brown hair, and that iron and manganese are found in higher concentrations in brown hair than in blonde hair.[36,38,39] These factors limit the usefulness of hair as an index of zinc and other trace element status.

Urinary Zinc

Lower than expected concentrations of zinc have been reported in the urine of zinc-depleted persons.[35,36] However, factors other than nutritional status can influence urinary zinc levels, such as liver cirrhosis, viral hepatitis, sickle cell anemia, surgery, and total parenteral nutrition. Problems associated with obtaining 24-hour urine collections can also complicate use of this indicator. Consequently, urine measurements of zinc are not the preferred approach to assessing zinc status.

IODINE STATUS

Iodine is a trace element essential for the synthesis of thyroid hormones that regulate metabolic processes related to normal growth and development in humans and animals.[24,40] Inadequate intake of iodine leads to insufficient production of thyroid hormones, resulting in a variety of adverse effects collectively referred to as iodine-deficiency disorders. In humans these include mental retardation, hypothyroidism, cretinism, goiter, and varying degrees of other growth and developmental abnormalities (see Box 9.2). Thyroid hormones are particularly important for central nervous system development during uterine development and the first two years of life, making this the most critical period for adequate

 Box 9.2   **Manifestations of Iodine Deficiency Disorder Throughout the Life Span**

Fetal Period
Spontaneous abortion
Stillbirth
Congenital anomalies in offspring
Increased perinatal mortality

Neonatal Period
Increased infant mortality
Cretinism

Childhood and Adolescence
Impaired mental function
Cretinism
Delayed physical development

Adulthood
Impaired mental function
Decreased ability to learn
Apathy
Reduced work productivity

All Ages
Goiter
Hypothyroidism
Increased susceptibility of the thyroid gland to nuclear radiation

Source: Zimmermann MB, Jooste PL, Pandav CS. 2008. Iodine-deficiency disorders. *Lancet* 372:1251–1262; and Zimmermann MB. 2009. Iodine deficiency. *Endocrine Reviews* 30:376–408.

iodine intake. Deficiency during pregnancy can lead to spontaneous abortion, stillbirth, congenital anomalies in offspring, and increased perinatal and infant mortality. Severe iodine deficiency in utero can result in a condition known as cretinism, which is characterized by gross mental retardation, short stature, deaf-mutism, and spasticity.[41,42] According to the World Health Organization, iodine deficiency is the leading cause of mental retardation in the world. Studies of moderately to severely iodine-deficient populations indicate that chronic iodine deficiency can reduce the intelligence quotient (IQ) by 12.5 to 13.5 points.[24,41] The provision of an iodine supplement to moderately iodine-deficient children has been shown to improve cognitive functioning, suggesting that in some instances cognitive impairment can be at least partly reversed by iodine repletion.[41]

The classic sign of iodine deficiency is thyroid gland enlargement, or goiter, which can occur at any age, including infancy. Goiter is the earliest and most obvious manifestation of iodine deficiency but certainly not its most devastating consequence.[40,41] When iodine intake is insufficient, the anterior pituitary gland increases its secretion of thyroid-stimulating hormone (TSH) in an effort to maximize the thyroid gland's uptake of available iodine, which stimulates thyroid hypertrophy and hyperplasia. Initially goiters are a small, diffuse, and uniform enlargement of the thyroid gland, increasing in size as the iodine deficiency continues. Over time they can develop nodules or lumps and become massive enough to compress neighboring structures, such as the trachea, esophagus, and nerves, as shown in Figure 9.5. In some instances, surgical removal is required.[40–42] In younger patients and

those with relatively small, diffuse, and soft goiters, iodine repletion can result in a variable degree of shrinkage of the goiter. However, in older patients and those with nodular or fibrotic goiters, fewer than one-third experience any significant shrinkage of the goiter.[43] Paradoxically, excessive iodine intake can cause goiter, as well as hyperthyroidism and hypothyroidism, and increases the risk of thyroid cancer.[20]

Assessing Iodine Status

Because more than 90% of dietary iodine is eventually excreted in the urine, urinary iodine (UI) is the most widely used indicator of recent iodine intake and nutrition status.[24,41,42,44] For individuals, a 24-hour urine collection is necessary to estimate iodine intake using UI concentration. Because 24-hour urine collections are impractical in field studies involving large numbers of subjects, spot urine collections from a representative sample of the target population can be used to calculate median UI in nanograms of iodine per milliliter of urine (ng/mL). Variations in UI concentrations due to differences in hydration among the subjects and the day-to-day variation in iodine intake by individuals will be evened out when a sufficiently large number of spot urine samples are collected from each group or subgroup. The categories for median UI concentrations developed by the World Health Organization (WHO) for assessing iodine status in school-age children and adults (excluding pregnant and lactating women) are shown in Table 9.8. The WHO's categories for median UI concentrations for assessing iodine status in pregnant and lactating women and children less than 2 years of age are shown in Table 9.9. Because of hydration status and day-to-day variation in iodine intake, UI concentrations of spot urine samples are not a reliable indicator of an individual's iodine status. Therefore, it would be a mistake to assume that an individual is iodine deficient based on a UI concentration < 100 ng/mL in a single spot urine sample collected from that individual.[24,45]

In addition to UI concentration, other methods for assessing iodine status include serum thyroglobulin, the goiter rate, and serum concentration of thyroid-stimulating hormone (TSH). While UI concentration is a sensitive indicator of recent iodine intake (days), serum thyroglobulin reflects iodine status over an intermediate period of time spanning weeks to months, and the goiter rate reflects long-term iodine status spanning months to years. TSH is a sensitive indicator of iodine status during the neonatal period. Thyroid hormone concentrations are considered unreliable indicators of iodine status.[41]

Iodine Status in the United States

In the early part of the 20th century, prior to the iodization of table salt, iodine-deficiency diseases, particularly goiter, were common and a significant problem. Goiter

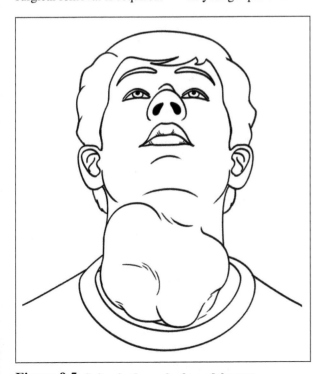

Figure 9.5 Goiter in the neck of an adolescent.

TABLE 9.8	World Health Organization Criteria for Assessing Iodine Nutrition Based on Median Urinary Iodine Concentrations of School-age Children (≥ 6 Years of Age) and Adults*

Median Urinary Iodine (ng/mL)	Category of Iodine Intake	Iodine Status
< 20	Insufficient	Severe iodine deficiency
20–49	Insufficient	Moderate iodine deficiency
50–99	Insufficient	Mild iodine deficiency
100–199	Adequate	Adequate iodine nutrition
200–299	Above requirements	Likely to provide adequate intake for pregnant/lactating women but may pose a slight risk of more than adequate intake in the overall population
≥ 300	Excessive	Risk of adverse health consequences (e.g., iodine-induced hyperthyroidism, autoimmune thyroid disease)

Source: Adapted from U.S. Department of Health and Human Services. 2012. *Second national report on biochemical indicators of diet and nutrition in the U.S. population.* National Center for Environmental Health, Centers for Disease Control and Prevention. www.cdc.gov/nutritionreport.

*These criteria do not apply to pregnant or lactating women or to children less than 2 years of age.

TABLE 9.9	World Health Organization Categories for Median UI Concentrations for Assessing Iodine Status in Pregnant and Lactating Women and Children Less Than 2 Years of Age

Population Group	Median Urinary Iodine (ng/mL)	Category of Iodine Intake
Pregnant women	< 150	Insufficient
	150–249	Adequate
	250–499	More than adequate
	≥ 500	Excessive
Lactating women	< 100	Insufficient
	≥ 100	Adequate
Children < 2 years of age	< 100	Insufficient
	≥ 100	Adequate

Source: Andersson M, de Benoist B, Rogers L. 2010. Epidemiology of iodine deficiency: Salt iodisation and iodine status. *Best Practices & Research Clinical Endocrinology & Metabolism* 24:1–11.

was endemic in the United States and Canada, particularly the Great Lakes region, the interior, the U.S. Pacific Northwest, and British Columbia. Voluntary iodization of table salt was introduced in the United States in the 1920s, but it is not mandatory. In Canada, the iodization of table salt is mandatory. The level of iodization is 100 parts per million (PPM), with 1 g of table salt providing 100 μg of iodine. The RDA for adults of 150 μg/d can be met by less than 2 grams of iodized table salt. The RDA for women who are pregnant or lactating, 220 μg/d and 290 μg/d, respectively, can be met by less than 3 g of iodized table salt per day. By the mid-1900s, the iodine status of people in North America had dramatically improved, goiter was rare, and iodine deficiency

disorders were no long considered a public health problem.[24,46] However, in 1970 the U.S. population was thought to have an excessive iodine intake, with iodine-induced hypothyroidism, autoimmune thyroiditis, and hyperthyroidism becoming more of a problem than iodine-deficiency disorders.[46–48] Data from NHANES I, conducted in 1971–1974, found a median UI concentration of 320 ng/mL, representing excessive iodine intake, according to WHO criteria shown in Table 9.8. Since then, UI concentrations in Americans have declined and stabilized. Recent data from NHANES, shown in Figure 9.6, indicate that iodine intake for the overall U.S. population is adequate, with median UI concentrations within the 100 to 200 ng/mL range, indicating adequate iodine intake and with no group with a median UI concentration representing excessive intake.[20]

In addition to iodized table salt, other adventitious food sources of iodine, such as dairy products and breads, contributed to the excessive iodine intake shown by the NHANES I data. During this period of excessive iodine intake, much of the iodine in milk was from iodine added as a supplement to animal feed and residues of iodine-containing sanitizing agents (disinfectant iodophors) used by the dairy industry to sanitize the teats of cows before milking and for cleaning milk-processing equipment.[24,46,48] Concerns about excessive iodine intake led the dairy industry to switch from iodine-based sanitizing agents to chlorine-based agents, thus reducing the amount of iodine in milk in recent decades. Much of the iodine in bread and other baked goods came from the use of iodine-containing dough conditioners. The baking industry has reduced its use of iodine-containing dough conditioners in recent years, further contributing to the decline in iodine intake to more adequate levels.

While median UI concentrations indicate that iodine intake is adequate for the overall U.S. population, including

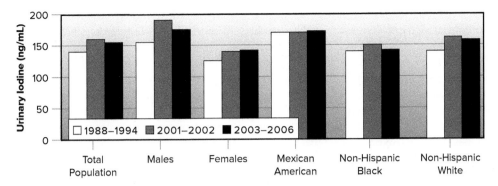

Figure 9.6 **Age-adjusted mean concentrations of urinary iodine in the U.S. population aged 6 years and older by sex or race/ethnicity, National Health and Nutrition Examination Survey, 1988–2006.**

Between 1988 and 2006, urinary iodine concentrations remained relatively stable and within the range of adequacy, which is 100 to 200 nanograms of iodine per milliliter of urine (ng/mL).

Source: U.S. Department of Health and Human Services. 2012. *Second national report on biochemical indicators of diet and nutrition in the U.S. population.* National Center for Environmental Health, Centers for Disease Control and Prevention. www.cdc.gov/nutritionreport.

children, women 20 to 39 years of age have the lowest UI concentrations, just slightly above the range representing insufficient.[24,47,49] Because requirements increase during pregnancy and lactation, the American Thyroid Association recommends that pregnant women in the United States and Canada take a prenatal supplement containing 150 µg of iodine daily and that all prenatal supplements contain 150 µg of iodine. Approximately half (49%) of commercially available prenatal supplements marketed in the United States contain iodine, and < 20% of women of childbearing age are consuming supplements containing iodine.[24,50] Mandatory iodization of all table salt sold in the United States would also help ensure adequate iodine intakes in women of childbearing age. Iodization of table salt in the United States is voluntary, and iodized salt is chosen by only 50% to 60% of the U.S. population. In addition, approximately 75% of all sodium consumed by Americans is that added in the processing and manufacturing of food, little of which is iodized. Consequently, efforts to reduce the amount of sodium in processed foods will have little, if any, adverse impact on iodine intakes in the United States. In fact, if the amount of sodium added during the manufacturing and processing of foods were reduced as some groups recommend, Americans would increase their use of iodized table salt during cooking and at the table, thus ensuring that more Americans have adequate iodine intakes. Efforts to prevent iodine deficiency and efforts to reduce salt consumption to prevent chronic disease do not conflict. As long as all salt consumed is iodized, adequate iodine intake is certain, even at levels of salt intake currently recommended by the Dietary Guidelines for Americans for persons 51 years of age and older and those of any age who are African American or have hypertension, diabetes, or chronic kidney disease.[48,51,52]

VITAMIN A STATUS

Vitamin A status can be grouped into five categories: deficient, marginal, adequate, excessive, and toxic. In the deficient and toxic states, clinical signs are evident, while biochemical or static tests of vitamin A status must be relied on in the marginal, adequate, and excessive states.[53] Biochemical assessment of vitamin A status generally involves measurements of plasma concentrations of retinol or the vitamin A carrier protein, retinol-binding protein (RBP), retinol isotope dilution, and dose-response tests. Used less frequently are examination of epithelial cells of the conjunctiva, assessment of dark adaptation, and liver biopsy.[1,16,53,54] These approaches are best used when assessing the vitamin A status of populations. The approaches for diagnosing vitamin A deficiency in an individual are limited to retinol isotope dilution, assessment of dark adaptation, and liver biopsy.[54] Vitamin A levels in breast milk can also be used as an index of vitamin A status in lactating women and in detecting response to maternal supplementation.[55]

Plasma Levels

Measurement of plasma concentration of retinol is the most common biochemical measure of vitamin A in a population group.[1,16,53,54] Under normal conditions, about 95% of plasma vitamin A is in the form of retinol and bound to retinol-binding protein, and about 5% is unbound and in the form of retinyl esters.[53,54] Serum measurements are predictive of vitamin A status only when the body's reserves are either critically depleted or overfilled. Because plasma concentration of retinol may be within the expected range despite low vitamin A concentrations within the liver, test results should be interpreted with caution.[54] However, data from plasma measurements can be of some value in drawing conclusions about the relationship of plasma measurements to clinical signs of deficiency, dietary intake data, and various socioeconomic factors. Plasma concentrations < 10 μg/dL (0.35 μmol/L) are considered severely deficient, and values < 20 μg/dL (0.70 μmol/L) are considered deficient.[20] Serum values > 20 μg/dL (> 0.70 μmol/L) are indicative of adequate status, while serum levels > 300 μg/dL are diagnostic of chronic hypervitaminosis A.[20] Using these criteria, data from NHANES indicate that the likelihood of being vitamin A deficient was very low throughout the U.S. population and that the likelihood of vitamin A excess was also very low, but it increased with increasing age. For the past two decades, more than 95% of the U.S. population have had adequate serum concentrations of vitamin A.[20] The plasma concentration of retinol-binding protein (RBP) can be used as a surrogate measure of plasma retinol, but it is affected by conditions other than vitamin A status. It is likely to be low during conditions of malnutrition and inflammation.[53]

Relative Dose Response

The relative dose-response test (RDR) and modified relative dose-response test (MRDR) are based on the principle that, when stores of retinol are high, plasma retinol concentration is little affected by oral administration of vitamin A. But when reserves are low, the plasma retinol concentration increases markedly, reaching a peak five hours after an oral dose. As hepatic vitamin A stores become depleted, retinol-binding protein (RBP) accumulates in the liver in an unbound state known as *apo-RBP*. When vitamin A is given to a subject whose stores are depleted, the vitamin A is absorbed from the intestinal tract; is taken up by the liver, where it binds to the apo-RBP; and then is released from the liver in the form of *holo-RBP* (the complex of RBP and vitamin A). In the RDR, a fasting blood sample is taken, followed by oral administration of vitamin A as retinyl palmitate. Another blood sample is drawn five hours later. Comparison of the fasting and postdosing holo-RBP measurements represents the extent of apo-RBP accumulation, which is directly related to the shortage of vitamin A.[1,16,53,54]

The RDR is calculated using the following formula:[1]

$$RDR = \frac{Vit\ A_5 - vit\ A_0}{Vit\ A_5} \times 100$$

where vit A_5 = serum vitamin A level five hours after receiving the dose of vitamin A and vit A_0 = fasting serum vitamin A level.

An RDR > 50% is considered indicative of acute deficiency, values between 20% and 50% indicate marginal status, and values < 20% suggest adequate intake.[1] Limitations of the RDR include the five-hour waiting period and the need to draw two blood samples.[1]

The MRDR is based on the same principle but uses only one blood sample five hours after administration of

the test dose of dehydroretinol, a naturally occurring form of vitamin A but one rarely present in most diets.[1] The measured response is the molar ratio of dehydroretinol to retinol in the serum sample. A ratio > 0.06 indicates marginal or poorer vitamin A status. A ratio < 0.03 indicates adequate vitamin A status.[1]

The assay is limited by the fact that there currently is no commercial source of dehydroretinol, and the assay requires the use of high-pressure liquid chromatography to distinguish between the two forms of vitamin A. The assay is still under development but does have the advantage of requiring only one blood sample.[1]

Conjunctival Impression Cytology

Vitamin A deficiency can result in morphologic changes in epithelial cells covering the body and lining its cavities. It can result in a decline in the number of mucus-producing goblet cells in the epithelium of the conjunctiva of the eye. The epithelial cells also may take on a more squamous appearance—flatter cells, smaller nuclei, and the cytoplasm making up a greater proportion of the total cell. The conjunctival impression cytology test involves the microscopic examination of the conjunctival epithelial cells to determine morphologic changes indicative of vitamin A deficiency.[1,16]

A minute sample of epithelial cells can be obtained by touching a strip of cellulose ester filter paper to the outer portion of the conjunctiva for three to five seconds and then gently removing it. The filter paper with the adherent epithelial cells is placed in a fixative solution, where it can be stored until being stained and examined by ordinary light microscopy.[1]

The test is limited by several factors and is not widely used.[1] It is difficult to get tissue samples from children under 3 years of age, and the cytologists must follow standardized criteria in evaluating samples. The sensitivity of the test is limited by conjunctival and systemic infections and possibly by severe malnutrition.[1,16]

Dark Adaptation

The best-defined function of vitamin A is its role in the visual process. The visual pigment rhodopsin is generated when the protein opsin in the rods of the retina combines with a *cis*-isomer of retinol. When light strikes the eye, rhodopsin is split into opsin and a *trans*-isomer of retinol, generating the visual-response signal. The *trans*-isomer is then converted back to the *cis*-isomer, which then combines with opsin to reform rhodopsin. During this process, some of the retinol isomer is lost and must be replaced by vitamin A present in the retina. Under normal conditions, sufficient retinol is present, and rhodopsin is readily formed. When vitamin A is in short supply, less rhodopsin is formed, and the eye fails to adapt as readily to low light levels after exposure to bright light levels.[1,16]

Tests are available to directly measure the level of rhodopsin and its rate of regeneration. Field tests measuring visual acuity in dim light after exposure to bright light also can be used.[1] However, the relative dose response, when available, is a more specific and objective test of vitamin A status and is preferred over functional tests of dark adaptation.

Direct Measurement of Liver Stores

Direct measurement of hepatic vitamin A stores in liver tissue is considered the "gold standard" of vitamin A status, but its invasive nature limits its usefulness.[53] In many countries, the median vitamin A concentration in liver tissue of well-nourished persons is approximately 100 μg of retinol/g of liver tissue. A concentration > 20 μg of retinol/g of liver tissue is considered adequate for both children and adults of all ages.[53] Concentrations < 5 μg of retinol/g of liver tissue are associated with vitamin A deficiency.

The assay can be done on a very small amount of liver tissue obtained by inserting a biopsy needle through the abdominal wall. Because of the invasiveness of the biopsy procedure, assaying liver tissue for vitamin A is limited to situations when a liver biopsy is necessary for diagnostic purposes or when liver tissue can be obtained from postmortem examinations.[16,53]

Retinol Isotope Dilution

The best way to represent vitamin A status is in terms of total body stores of vitamin A. Approximately 90% of the body's vitamin A stores are in the liver, but direct measurement of vitamin A concentration in the liver is not practical in most instances because a liver biopsy is a highly invasive surgical procedure. A noninvasive, indirect approach to measuring total body stores of vitamin A is retinol isotope dilution, which is considered the best approach currently available for assessing vitamin A status with the least risk to subjects.[1,16,56] The procedure involves administering to a subject a known amount of vitamin A that is labeled with a nonradioactive isotope. This is ingested with an adequate amount of fat to ensure suitable absorption. After a period of approximately two to three weeks, the isotopically labeled vitamin A mixes with the body's existing total pool of unlabeled vitamin A. A sample of blood is then removed from the subject and the plasma concentrations of the labeled and unlabeled vitamin A are measured. Using a mathematical formula, the ratio of the labeled vitamin A to the unlabeled vitamin A is calculated. This ratio is used to estimate the size of the subject's total vitamin A pool.[56,57] Limitations of this method include the high cost of the isotopically labeled vitamin A and the sophisticated laboratory techniques needed to measure the plasma concentrations of the labeled and unlabeled vitamin A. However, it is the only noninvasive method currently available for assessing the full range of vitamin A status, from deficient to toxic (hypervitaminosis A).[1,56,57]

VITAMIN D STATUS

The major physiological function of vitamin D in vertebrates, including humans, is to maintain serum calcium and phosphorus concentrations in a range that supports bone mineralization, neuromuscular function, and various cellular processes. Vitamin D increases serum concentrations of calcium and phosphorus by promoting their absorption by the small intestine, promoting their reabsorption by the kidney, and stimulating bone resorption with the release of calcium and phosphorus from bone.[58] The role of vitamin D in maintaining skeletal health is well established.[30] Deficiency of vitamin D causes growth retardation and rickets in children. In adults vitamin D deficiency causes osteomalacia, and precipitates and exacerbates bone demineralization, leading to osteopenia, osteoporosis, and increased fracture risk.[58] What is less certain and a matter of debate is whether vitamin D exposure at levels sufficient to prevent clinically evident bone disease is optimal in terms of reducing risk of a variety of other conditions not traditionally linked to vitamin D. Research suggests that increasing vitamin D exposure decreases risk of certain types of cancer, type 1 and type 2 diabetes, respiratory tract infections, and influenza and asthma in children.[59–61]

In general, the available data support that adequate vitamin D supplementation and sensible sunlight exposure to achieve optimal vitamin D status are important in the prevention of cardiovascular disease and other chronic diseases.[58]

Vitamin D (calciferol) is a fat-soluble sterol found in a limited number of foods, including fish-liver oils, fatty fishes, mushrooms, egg yolks, and liver.[20] The two major forms of vitamin D are cholecalciferol (D_3) and ergocalciferol (D_2). Vitamin D_3 is synthesized in the skin of vertebrates by the action of ultraviolet B (UVB) radiation on 7-dehydrocholesterol present in the skin. Vitamin D_2 is produced by UV irradiation of ergosterol, as sterol occurring in molds, yeast, mushrooms, and higher-order plants. Vitamin D in humans comes from two sources: from that present in the foods we eat and from that synthesized in the body by sun exposure. If sun exposure is sufficient, dietary intake is not necessary. However, cutaneous synthesis of vitamin D_3 is decreased by such factors as living at a higher latitude, older age, darker skin pigmentation, less skin exposed to sunlight, and sunscreen use. Major dietary sources of vitamin D in the United States are foods fortified with vitamin D, including milk products, some citrus juices, and ready-to-eat breakfast cereals.[20] Practically all fortified foods and supplements in the United States use vitamin D_3 instead of vitamin D_2.[62]

Assessing Vitamin D Status

Vitamin D status is best assessed by measuring the serum concentration of 25-hydroxyvitamin D [25(OH)D], the major circulating form of the vitamin, which reflects total

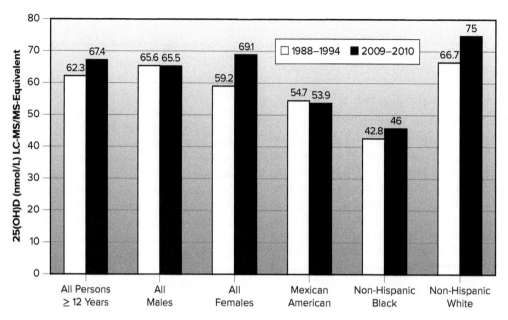

Figure 9.7 **LC-MS/MS-equivalent serum 25(OH)D concentrations for persons aged 12 years and older stratified by NHANES cycle and grouped by demographic variables.**

The vitamin D status of the U.S. population showed modest increases in from 1988–1994 to 2009–2010 and corresponded in time with an increase in the use of supplements containing higher amounts of vitamin D.

Source: Graph developed using data from Schleicher RL, Sternberg MR, Lacher DA, Sempos CT, Looker AC, Durazo-Arvizu RA, Yetley EA, Chaudhary-Webb M, Maw KL, Pfeiffer CM, Johnson CL. 2016. The vitamin D status of the US population from 1988 to 2010 using standardized serum concentrations of 25-hydroxyvitamin D shows recent modest increases. *American Journal of Clinical Nutrition* 104:454–461.

vitamin D exposure from food, supplements, and synthesis.[20,30] Although serum concentration of 25(OH)D is not considered a validated health outcome indicator, it is the measure preferred by clinicians to assess total vitamin D exposure and allows comparisons to be made between exposure and health outcomes. What serum concentrations of 25(OH)D represent an optimal vitamin D exposure is a matter of some disagreement. There has been no systematic, evidence-based development process to establish 25(OH)D cutpoints for defining what is indicative of vitamin D deficiency or adequacy.[20,30,62] Based on its review of the available data, the Institute of Medicine's Committee to Review Dietary Reference Intakes for Vitamin D and Calcium concluded that persons are at risk of deficiency relative to bone health when the serum concentration of 25(OH)D is < 30 nmol/L (nanomoles per liter). The Committee concluded that some, but not all, persons are potentially at risk of inadequate vitamin D exposure when their serum 25(OH)D is between 30 and 50 nmol/L. Practically all persons have a sufficient exposure with serum 25(OH)D between 50 and 75 nmol/L. The Committee concluded that serum concentrations between 75 and 125 nmol/L were not consistently associated with increased benefits and that there may be reason for concern at concentrations > 125 nmol/L.[30] The Committee concluded that a serum 25(OH)D of 40 nmol/L represented a vitamin D exposure that met the average requirement and was consistent with the Estimated Average Requirement (EAR). A serum 25(OH)D

concentration of approximately 50 nmol/L represented a vitamin D exposure that was associated with benefit for nearly all the population and was consistent with the Recommended Dietary Allowance (RDA).[30]

Beginning with NHANES III in 1988, the vitamin D status of the U.S. population has been monitored. NHANES collects survey information and biological samples during the summer from people living at higher latitudes and in the winter from those living in lower latitudes. Serum 25(OH)D concentration data from NHANES are shown in Figure 9.7. When 25(OH)D was expressed in LC-MS/MS equivalents (the most accurate method of measurement), the vitamin D status of the U.S. population 12 years of age and older showed modest increases in 2009–2010. The increase in 25(OH)D corresponded in time with an increase in the use of supplements containing higher amounts of vitamin D. Marked race-ethnic differences in 25(OH)D concentrations, however, are apparent, with the lowest levels found in non-Hispanic Blacks.[62] NHANES data indicate that 46% of non-Hispanic Blacks have serum 25(OH)D concentrations below 40 nmol/L in comparison to 6.6% of non-Hispanic Whites (Figure 9.8).[62]

VITAMIN C STATUS

Vitamin C is a generic term for compounds exhibiting the biological activity of *ascorbic acid,* the reduced form of

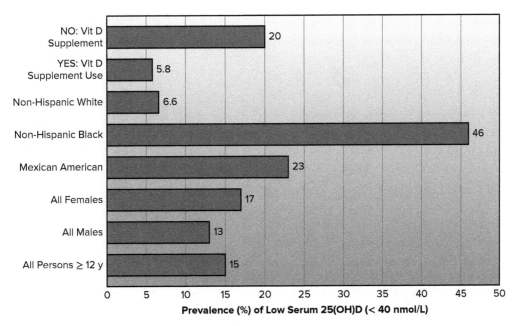

Figure 9.8 Prevalence of LC-MS/MS–equivalent serum 25(OH)D concentrations below 40 nmol/L for persons aged 12 years and older, grouped by demographic variables or vitamin D supplement use: NHANES 2009–2010.

Forty nmol/L is the concentration consistent with an intake equivalent to the Estimated Average Requirement, which is useful for evaluating the possible adequacy of nutrient intakes of population groups. Vitamin D supplement use was defined as the use of any vitamin D–containing supplements in the month preceding the household interview.

Source: Graph developed using data from Schleicher RL, Sternberg MR, Lacher DA, Sempos CT, Looker AC, Durazo-Arvizu RA, Yetley EA, Chaudhary-Webb M, Maw KL, Pfeiffer CM, Johnson CL. 2016. The vitamin D status of the US population from 1988 to 2010 using standardized serum concentrations of 25-hydroxyvitamin D shows recent modest increases. *American Journal of Clinical Nutrition* 104:454–461.

vitamin C. The oxidized form of vitamin C is known as *dehydroascorbic acid.* The sum of ascorbic acid and dehydroascorbic acid constitutes all the naturally occurring biologically active vitamin C.[63,64] When used in this chapter, the term *vitamin C* refers to total vitamin C—the sum of ascorbic acid and dehydroascorbic acid.

Vitamin C is necessary for the formation of collagen; the maintenance of capillaries, bone, and teeth; the promotion of iron absorption; and the protection of vitamins and minerals from oxidation. Evidence from several large cohort studies suggests a protective effect against certain cancers and CHD, but these observations are not supported by most randomized clinical trials.[65] Deficiency of vitamin C results in scurvy, a condition characterized by weakness, hemorrhages in the skin and gums, and defects in bone development in children.

Vitamin C status is assessed by measuring total ascorbic acid in serum (or plasma) and in leukocytes (white blood cells). The serum concentration of ascorbic acid is considered an index of the circulating vitamin available to the tissues. The leukocyte concentration is considered an index of tissue stores.[20] Vitamin C deficiency is generally defined as a serum (or plasma) concentration < 11.4 micromoles per liter (μmol/L) or the level at which signs and symptoms of scurvy begin to

appear. A low serum (or plasma) concentration is 11.4 to 23.0 μmol/L.[20]

Data collected by NHANES in 2003–2006 show that the prevalence of low serum concentrations among all individuals in the United States 6 years of age and older is 6%. As shown in Figure 9.9, the prevalence of vitamin C deficiency (serum concentration < 11.4 μmol/L) and low serum vitamin C (serum concentrations 11.4–23.0 μmol/L) is lowest in children and adolescents. As shown in Figure 9.10, U.S. females are at lower risk of vitamin C deficiency than U.S. males, and non-Hispanic Whites have a greater prevalence of low vitamin C than non-Hispanic Blacks and Mexican Americans.[20]

Serum and Leukocyte Vitamin C

Measurement of serum (or plasma) vitamin C is the most commonly used biochemical procedure for assessing vitamin C status.[20,64,66,67] However, in recent years, there has been increasing interest in using the level of vitamin C in polymorphonuclear leukocytes (the granular leukocytes: neutrophils, eosinophils, and basophils) and the mononuclear leukocytes (the agranular leukocytes: lymphocytes and monocytes) as indicators of vitamin C status.[63,64] Serum levels of ascorbic acid have been shown to correlate

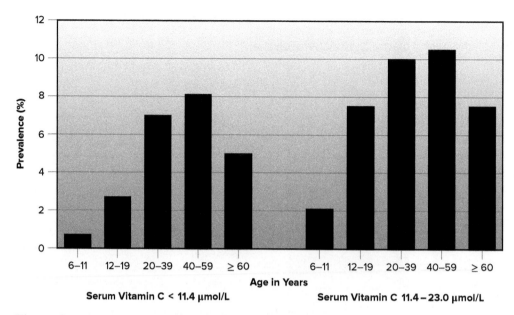

Figure 9.9 Prevalence estimates of vitamin C deficiency (serum concentrations < 11.4 μmol/L) and of low vitamin C concentrations (11.4–23.0 μmol/L) in the U.S. population aged 6 years and older by age groups, NHANES 2003–2006.

Source: U.S. Department of Health and Human Services. 2012. *Second national report on biochemical indicators of diet and nutrition in the U.S. population.* National Center for Environmental Health, Centers for Disease Control and Prevention. www.cdc.gov/nutritionreport.

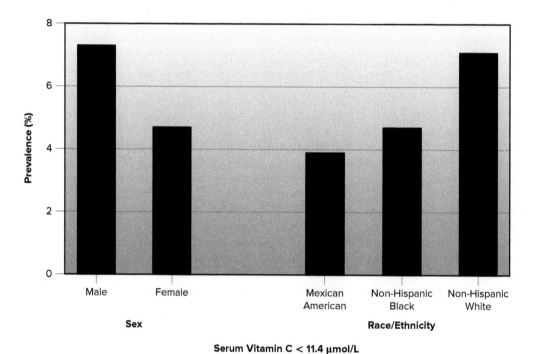

Figure 9.10 Age-adjusted prevalence estimates of vitamin C deficiency (serum concentrations < 11.4 μmol/L) in the U.S. population aged 6 years and older by sex and race/ethnicity, NHANES 2003–2006.

Source: U.S. Department of Health and Human Services. 2012. *Second national report on biochemical indicators of diet and nutrition in the U.S. population.* National Center for Environmental Health, Centers for Disease Control and Prevention. www.cdc.gov/nutritionreport.

with dietary vitamin C intake and with vitamin C levels in leukocytes (white blood cells).[20] However, research suggests that vitamin C concentration in serum is a better indicator of recent dietary intake of vitamin C than leukocyte

levels and that leukocyte vitamin C levels better represent cellular stores and the total body pool of the vitamin.

Factors affecting vitamin C levels in tissues and fluids include cigarette smoking and sex.[66,67] Compared with nonsmokers, cigarette smokers tend to have lower vitamin C levels in serum and leukocytes even after correcting for vitamin C intake.[67] The metabolic turnover of vitamin C in smokers has been estimated to be 35 mg/d greater than that of nonsmokers. However, evidence suggests that smokers may need to ingest > 200 mg of vitamin C daily to achieve serum ascorbic acid levels typically seen in nonsmokers meeting the RDA currently set at 90 mg/d for adult males and 75 mg/d for adult females.[67]

After correcting for vitamin C intakes, females consistently show higher vitamin C levels in tissues and fluids than males.[64,71,75] Age does not appear to influence vitamin C levels in adults.[64,69]

VITAMIN B_6 STATUS

The vitamin B_6 group is composed of three naturally occurring compounds related chemically, metabolically, and functionally: pyridoxine (PN), pyridoxal (PL), and pyridoxamine (PM). Within the liver, erythrocytes, and other tissues of the body, these forms are phosphorylated into pyridoxal 5'-phosphate (PLP) and pyridoxamine phosphate (PMP). PLP and PMP primarily serve as coenzymes in a large variety of reactions.[68,69] Especially important among these are the transamination reactions in protein metabolism. PLP also is involved in other metabolic transformations of amino acids and in the metabolism of carbohydrates, lipids, and nucleic acids.[68,69] Because of its role in protein metabolism, the requirement for vitamin B_6 is directly proportional to protein intake.[70]

Although frank vitamin B_6 deficiency resulting in clinical manifestations is not considered widespread in the general U.S. population, there is evidence of impaired status among certain groups—most notably, the elderly and alcoholic individuals. There is also concern about excessive vitamin B_6 intake and the possibility of resulting peripheral nervous system damage.[70]

Vitamin B_6 status can be assessed by several methods. Static measurements can be made of vitamin B_6 concentrations in blood or urine, and functional tests can measure the activity of several enzymes dependent on vitamin B_6.[68,71,72]

Plasma and Erythrocyte Pyridoxal 5'-Phosphate

The most frequently used biochemical indicator of vitamin B_6 status is plasma PLP.[68,71,72] PLP accounts for approximately 70% to 90% of the total vitamin B_6 present in plasma.[68,72] PL is the next most abundant form in plasma, followed by lower levels of PN and PM.[71]

Fasting measurements of plasma PLP are considered the single most informative indicator of vitamin B_6 status for healthy persons. Use of this single measure is limited by the fact that abnormally low concentrations of plasma PLP may result from asthma, coronary heart disease, and

TABLE 9.10	Factors Affecting Plasma PLP* Concentrations
Factors	**Effect**
Increased vitamin B_6 intake	Increases
Increased protein intake	Decreases
Increased glucose	Decreases (a)†
Increased plasma volume	Decreases
Increased physical activity	Increases (a)
Decreased uptake into nonhepatic tissues	Increases
Increased age	Decreases

Source: Leklem JE. 1990. Vitamin B_6: A status report. *Journal of Nutrition* 120:1503–1507.

*PLP = pyridoxal 5'-phosphate.

†(a) indicates that the effect is an acute effect.

pregnancy and may not reflect a true vitamin B_6 deficiency.[71] Dietary intake of vitamin B_6 and protein can affect plasma PLP concentrations as well. As shown in Table 9.10, increases in dietary vitamin B_6 intake raise plasma PLP, and plasma levels fall in response to increased protein consumption.[70,72] Thus, although plasma PLP is a valuable measure, the assessment of vitamin B_6 status is best accomplished by using several indicators in conjunction with each other—for example, measures of other vitamin B_6 forms and/or functional tests.[70–72] Table 9.11 lists expected biochemical values for adults with adequate vitamin B_6 status for various measures of the vitamin.

Measurement of PLP in erythrocytes has been suggested as another approach to assessing vitamin B_6 status. Certain characteristics of the erythrocyte may make it unrepresentative of other body tissues. The ability of hemoglobin to bind tightly to PLP and PL, along with the relatively long life of red blood cells (about 120 days), may make red blood cells a significant reservoir for vitamin B_6 and may complicate the use of erythrocyte PLP levels as a useful indicator of vitamin B_6 status.[70–72]

Plasma Pyridoxal

Measurement of plasma PL has been suggested as an additional indicator of B_6 status to use with plasma PLP. PL is the major dietary form of the vitamin, crosses all membranes on absorption from the gastrointestinal tract, and comprises about 8% to 30% of the total plasma vitamin B_6. There are questions about how well plasma PL represents vitamin B_6 status, and further research is needed on this indicator. Despite these questions, plasma PL is recommended in the assessment of B_6 status.[72]

Urinary 4-pyridoxic Acid

4-pyridoxic acid (4-PA) is the major urinary metabolite of vitamin B_6. Urinary excretion of 4-PA has been shown

TABLE 9.11	Indices for Evaluating Vitamin B$_6$ Status and Suggested Values for Adequate Status in Adults

Indices	Suggested Values for Adequate Status*
Direct	
Blood	
Plasma pyridoxal 5′-phosphate (PLP)	> 30 nmol/L
Plasma pyridoxal	NV†
Plasma total vitamin B$_6$	> 40 nmol/L
Erythrocyte PLP	NV
Urine	
4-pyridoxic acid	> 3.0 µmol/day
Indirect	
Urine	
3-g methionine load; cystathionine	< 350 µmol/day
Oxalate excretion	NV
Diet Intake	
Vitamin B$_6$ intake, weekly average	> 1.2–1.5 mg/day
Vitamin B$_6$: protein ratio	> 0.020
Other	
Electroencephalogram pattern	NV

Source: Leklem JE. 1990. Vitamin B$_6$: A status report. *Journal of Nutrition* 120:1503–1507.

*These values are dependent on sex, age, and, for most, protein intake.

†NV = no value established; limited data are available.

‡The index value for each transaminase represents the ratio of the enzyme activity with added PLP to the activity without PLP added.

to change rapidly in response to alterations in vitamin B$_6$ intake and to be indicative of immediate dietary intake. Thus, it is considered useful as a short-term index of vitamin B$_6$ status. In studies of subjects whose usual dietary intake of vitamin B$_6$ was known, males had a 4-PA excretion of 3.5 µmol/day, and females had a 4-PA excretion of > 3.2 µmol/day. Urinary excretions of 4-PA of ≥ 3.0 µmol/day appear to be indicative of acceptable vitamin B$_6$ status.[1] 4-PA is likely to be absent from urine of persons with a marked vitamin B$_6$ deficiency. The value of this method is limited by the need for a complete 24-hour urine collection.[20,68,72]

Methionine Load Test

The principle of the methionine load test is similar to that of the tryptophan load test. PLP is required in the metabolism of the amino acid methionine. Compared with persons with adequate vitamin B$_6$ status, those with impaired vitamin B$_6$ status have higher urine levels of the metabolites cystathionine and cysteine sulfonic acid following consumption of 3 g of methionine.[72]

Use of this test is limited by the required 24-hour urine sample and factors other than vitamin B$_6$ status that can affect test results (for example, protein intake). Because this test has been used in a limited number of studies, no definitive values for urinary cystathionine are available. The value of < 350 µmol/day given in Table 9.11 is based on three studies.[72]

FOLATE STATUS

Folate, or folacin, is a group of water-soluble compounds with properties and chemical structures similar to those of folic acid, or pteroylglutamic acid. Folate functions as a coenzyme transporting single carbon groups from one compound to another in amino acid metabolism and nucleic acid synthesis. One of the most significant of folate's functions appears to be purine and pyrimidine synthesis. Folate deficiency can lead to inhibition of DNA synthesis, impaired cell division, and alterations in protein synthesis. It is especially important during periods of rapid cell division and growth, such as occurs during pregnancy and infancy.[20,70,73,74] Clinical trials have shown that a marginal folate intake during pregnancy increases the risk of an infant being born with a neural tube defect (i.e., spina bifida, encephalocele, and anencephaly) and that folate supplementation reduces the number of pregnancies affected by neural tube defects (NTDs). This led the U.S. Food and Drug Administration to require the addition of folic acid to enriched cereal products beginning in 1998.[20] Since then, the rate of NTDs has declined by 36%.[75] The Dietary Guidelines for Americans recommend that women who are capable of becoming pregnant or who are pregnant pay special attention to folic acid. The RDAs for folate are based on the prevention of folate deficiency, not on the prevention of neural tube defects. The RDA for adult women is 400 micrograms (mcg) Dietary Folate Equivalents (DFE) and, for women during pregnancy, 600 mcg DFE daily from all sources. To prevent birth defects, all women capable of becoming pregnant are advised to consume 400 mcg of synthetic folic acid daily, from fortified foods and/or supplements. This recommendation is for an intake of synthetic folic acid in addition to the amounts of food folate contained in a healthy eating pattern. All enriched grains are fortified with synthetic folic acid. Sources of food folate include beans and peas, oranges and orange juice, and dark-green leafy vegetables, such as spinach and mustard greens.[51]

The recommended measurements for assessing folate status are serum folate concentration and red blood cell (RBC) folate concentration.[20,73] Serum folate is largely the product of absorbed dietary folate and fluctuates daily. It provides information about recent folate intake and does not necessarily represent tissue stores. Nonnutritional factors that can increase serum folate concentrations include acute renal failure, active liver

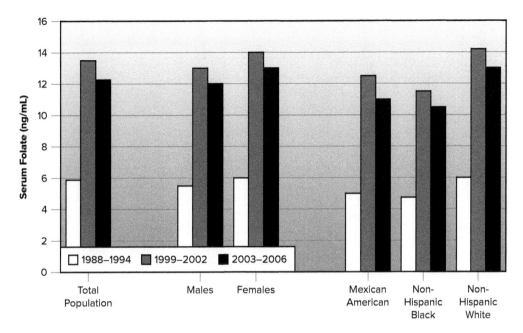

Figure 9.11 Age-adjusted mean concentrations of serum folate in the U.S. population aged 4 years and older by sex or race/ethnicity, NHANES 1988–2006.
Serum folate concentrations more than doubled after the FDA required the addition of folic acid to enriched cereal products beginning in 1998.

Source: U.S. Department of Health and Human Services. 2012. *Second national report on biochemical indicators of diet and nutrition in the U.S. population.* National Center for Environmental Health, Centers for Disease Control and Prevention. www.cdc.gov/nutritionreport.

disease, and hemolysis of red blood cells. Alcohol consumption, cigarette smoking, and oral contraceptive use may lower serum folate levels.[70,73] RBC folate concentration is considered the best clinical index of folate stores in the tissues of the body. RBC folate concentration reflects folate status at the time the erythrocyte was synthesized, because only young cells in the bone marrow take up folate.[70] Unlike serum folate, RBC folate is less subject to transient fluctuations in dietary intake. It decreases after tissue stores are depleted because erythrocytes have a 120-day average life span and reflect folate status at the time of their synthesis. It has been shown to correlate with liver folate stores and to reflect total body stores.[70,73]

The monitoring of serum folate concentration in the U.S. population began with NHANES I (1974–1975). The measurement of RBC folate concentration began with NHANES II (1978–1980). NHANES has continued measuring these biomarkers since then.[74] Figure 9.11 shows the age-adjusted mean concentrations of serum folate in the U.S. population aged 4 years and older by sex or race/ethnicity from 1988 to 2006.[20] Based on the assay method consistently used throughout this time period, a low serum folate concentration is considered < 2 ng/mL. As can be seen in Figure 9.11, serum folate concentrations more than doubled after the FDA required the addition of folic acid to enriched cereal products beginning in 1998.

Figure 9.12 shows the age-adjusted mean concentrations of RBC folate in the U.S. population aged 4 years and older by sex or race/ethnicity from 1988 to 2006.[20] Based on the assay method consistently used throughout this time

period, a low RBC folate concentration is considered < 95 ng/mL. The cutoff values for defining low values will vary depending on the assay used to measure folate concentrations.[20,73,74] The plasma concentration of homocysteine, an amino acid naturally found in the blood, can be elevated by folate deficiency, but plasma homocysteine is not specific for folate deficiency because it is also elevated during deficiency of vitamin B_6 and vitamin B_{12}.[20]

VITAMIN B_{12} STATUS

Vitamin B_{12}, or cobalamins, includes a group of cobalt-containing molecules that can be converted to methylcobalamin or 5′-deoxyadenosylcobalamin, the two coenzyme forms of vitamin B_{12} that are active in human metabolism.[70,76] Vitamin B_{12} is synthesized by bacteria, fungi, and algae, but not by yeast, plants, and animals. Vitamin B_{12} synthesized by bacteria accumulates in the tissues of animals that are then consumed by humans. Thus, animal products serve as the primary dietary source of vitamin B_{12}. Although plants are essentially devoid of vitamin B_{12} (unless they are contaminated by microorganisms or soil containing vitamin B_{12}), foods such as breakfast cereals, soy beverages, and plant-based meat substitutes are often fortified with vitamin B_{12}.

The diets of most Americans supply more than adequate amounts of vitamin B_{12}. The average vitamin B_{12} intake is well above the RDA for all sex-age groups, including pregnant and lactating females; however, after age 40 the risk of low vitamin B_{12} status increases due to

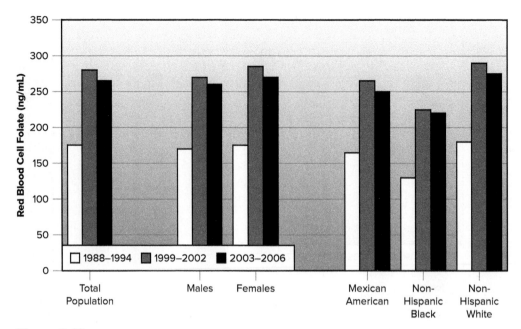

Figure 9.12 **Age-adjusted mean concentrations of red blood cell folate in the U.S. population aged 4 years and older by sex or race/ethnicity, NHANES 1988–2006.**
Red blood cell folate concentrations increased by approximately 50% after the FDA required the addition of folic acid to enriched cereal products beginning in 1998.

Source: U.S. Department of Health and Human Services. 2012. *Second national report on biochemical indicators of diet and nutrition in the U.S. population.* National Center for Environmental Health, Centers for Disease Control and Prevention. www.cdc.gov/nutritionreport.

diminished vitamin B_{12} absorption in older persons.[20,70,77,78] Vegans, or strict vegetarians (persons eating no animal products), could become vitamin B_{12} deficient, although this is unlikely because many commercially available foods such as soy beverages, ready-to-eat breakfast cereals, and plant-based meat substitutes are fortified with vitamin B_{12}. Despite these facts, vitamin B_{12} deficiency does occur, although rarely because of a dietary deficiency. Approximately 95% of the cases of vitamin B_{12} deficiency seen in the United States are due to inadequate absorption of the vitamin, generally because of pernicious anemia caused by inadequate production of intrinsic factor. Approximately 2% of elderly people in the United States have clinical vitamin B_{12} deficiency and 10–20% have subclinical deficiency.[78] Because most vitamin B_{12} absorption occurs in the distal ileum, B_{12} malabsorption could also result from surgical resection of the distal ileum, bacterial overgrowth in the small intestine ("blind loop" syndrome), or damage to the ileum from such causes as tropical sprue or regional enteritis.[70,77]

Intrinsic factor is a glycoprotein produced by the parietal cells of the gastric glands, located in the body of the stomach. Intrinsic factor (IF) combines with vitamin B_{12} in the upper small intestine. The B_{12}-IF complex is carried to the ileum (the distal part of the small intestine), where it attaches to B_{12}-IF receptors on the brush border of ileal mucosal cells. The B_{12}-IF complex is then taken up by the ileal mucosal cells and makes its way into the blood for distribution to the rest of the body.[70,77] Under normal circumstances, most vitamin B_{12} is absorbed by this mechanism;

however, approximately 1% of ingested vitamin B_{12} can be absorbed through passive diffusion along the entire length of the small intestine.[77] Approximately 56% of a 1-mcg oral dose of vitamin B_{12} is absorbed, but absorption decreases sharply when the capacity of intrinsic factor is exceeded (at 1–2 mcg of vitamin B_{12}). The usual cause of inadequate IF production is atrophy of the gastric mucosa, a condition most often seen in older persons. Thus, pernicious anemia is a disease of the elderly, with an average age at diagnosis of 60 years. The Institute of Medicine recommends that adults older than 50 years obtain most of their vitamin B_{12} from vitamin supplements or fortified foods. In dietary supplements, vitamin B_{12} is usually present as cyanocobalamin, a form that the body readily converts to the active forms of methylcobalamin and 5-deoxyadenosylcobalamin. Vitamin B_{12} can also be administered by intramuscular injection or in a gel formulation as a prescription medication. Other causes of inadequate IF production include total gastrectomy and extensive damage to the gastric mucosa caused by ingestion of corrosive agents.[70,77]

Clinical features of vitamin B_{12} deficiency involve the blood, the gastrointestinal tract, and the nervous system. An early feature of vitamin B_{12} deficiency is megaloblastic anemia, which is characterized by the presence of abnormally large cells (megaloblasts) in the peripheral blood and a low hemoglobin level. A mean corpuscular volume (MCV) > 100 fL is suggestive of megaloblastic anemia. The tongue may become sore, smooth, and beefy red. Anorexia with moderate weight loss and diarrhea may also be present. The most troublesome consequences of B_{12} deficiency occur in the nervous system. Neurologic manifestations include demyelination and axonal degeneration of the peripheral nerves, spinal cord, and cerebrum. Eventually, irreversible neuronal death can occur in these areas. The earliest symptoms of these changes are numbness and paresthesias (abnormal sensations, such as burning, prickling, or the feeling that ants are crawling on the skin) in the extremities. This can progress to weakness, muscular incoordination (ataxia), irritability, forgetfulness, severe dementia, and even psychosis.[77]

Biochemical Indicators of B_{12} Status

Currently recommended biomarkers for assessing vitamin B_{12} status are those that directly measure vitamin B_{12} in the blood and functional biomarkers measuring metabolites that accumulate when vitamin B_{12} status is inadequate.[78,79] Direct measures of circulating vitamin B_{12} are serum or plasma total cobalamin and serum holo-transcobalamin II (holo-TC II), the transport protein of absorbed vitamin B_{12}. These measures reflect the broad range of vitamin B_{12} status from severe deficiency to adequacy.[20,78] Vitamin B_{12} status is typically assessed via serum or plasma vitamin B_{12} levels, with values below 170–250 pg/mL indicating a vitamin B_{12} deficiency. Serum vitamin B_{12} concentrations, however, might not accurately reflect intracellular concentrations. A functional biomarker specific to vitamin B_{12} status is urinary or serum methylmalonic acid (MMA), which is increased when vitamin B_{12} status is inadequate. Another functional biomarker is the plasma concentration of total homocysteine (tHcy), which increases when vitamin B_{12} status is inadequate but is also increased during folate and vitamin B_6 deficiency.[20,70,78,79] Both MMA and tHcy reflect early changes in vitamin B_{12} status and are useful for identifying subclinical B_{12} deficiency. But the fact that tHcy is increased by folate deficiency limits its usefulness as a biomarker for vitamin B_{12}.[79] Elevated MMA (values > 0.4 micromol/L) might be a more reliable indicator of vitamin B_{12} status because of the linkage to a metabolic change that is highly specific to vitamin B_{12} deficiency.

Factors unrelated to vitamin B_{12} status can affect all four of the biomarkers. MMA and tHcy are increased by impaired renal function, even when it is mild as evidenced by minor changes in creatinine and indices of glomerular filtration, which is common in older persons.[20] Elevation of cobalamin and holo-TC II are generally only seen in advanced renal failure. Genetics can influence serum concentrations, transport, and metabolism. Serum cobalamin concentration is decreased in pregnancy and folate deficiency. There are also concerns about suboptimal laboratory monitoring and proficiency testing.[79] Because there is no single biomarker that is considered a "gold standard" for vitamin B_{12} status assessment, information from two or more tests should be used to assess vitamin B_{12} status.[79]

Data on the age-adjusted mean concentrations of serum vitamin B_{12} in the U.S. population aged 4 years and older collected by NHANES in 1991–2006 are shown in Figure 9.13. In these data, a low serum vitamin B_{12} concentration is defined as < 200 pg/mL, indicating that for all groups, mean serum vitamin B_{12} concentrations were adequate. Figure 9.14 shows prevalence estimates of low serum vitamin B_{12}, high plasma methylmalonic acid (MMA), and high plasma total homocysteine (tHcy) concentrations in persons in the United States 60 years of age and older based on data collected by NHANES in 2003–2006.[20] Assessing the extent of inadequate vitamin B_{12} status is complicated by the fact that serum tHcy is not specific to vitamin B_{12} deficiency (it is also increased by folate deficiency) and tHcy and MMA are both elevated when renal function is impaired, a common condition in elderly people.[20]

BLOOD CHEMISTRY TESTS

Blood chemistry tests include a variety of assays performed on plasma or serum that are useful in the diagnosis and management of disease. They include electrolytes, enzymes, metabolites, and other miscellaneous substances, which are discussed in this section. When run at one time, blood chemistry tests often are known by such names as the *chemistry profile, chemistry panel, chem profile,* and *chem panel.* To perform these tests, clinical laboratories use automated analyzers capable of performing several thousand blood tests per hour. The patient's plasma or serum sample is placed into the analyzer, which performs the desired tests and provides a printout of the patient's results, including reference ranges and flagged abnormal results. A related series of tests, often known as the *coronary risk profile,* measures levels of triglyceride, total cholesterol, and HDL-C (cholesterol carried by high-density lipoproteins) and calculates LDL-C (cholesterol carried by low-density lipoproteins) and, in some instances, the total cholesterol/HDL-C ratio. These are discussed in Chapter 8.

Following is a brief overview of the major blood chemistry tests. Normal adult serum levels (known as reference ranges) are given. These reference ranges vary, depending on the individual biochemical and analytic method used. It is generally best, however, to use reference ranges suggested by the laboratory performing the analyses.

Alanine Aminotransferase

Alanine aminotransferase (ALT), also known as serum glutamic pyruvic transaminase (SGPT), is an enzyme found in large concentrations in the liver and to a lesser extent in the kidneys, skeletal muscles, and myocardium (heart muscle). Injury to the liver caused by such conditions as hepatitis (viral, alcoholic, and so on), cirrhosis, and bile duct obstruction or by drugs toxic to the liver is the usual cause of elevated serum ALT levels.

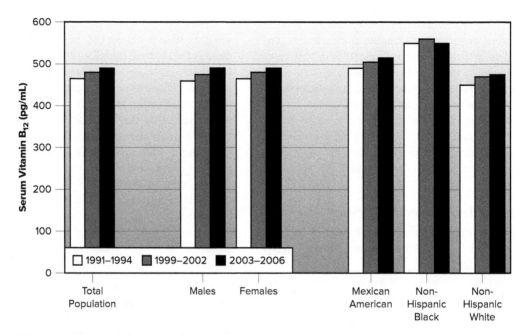

Figure 9.13 **Age-adjusted mean concentrations of serum vitamin B_{12} in the U.S. population aged 4 years and older by sex or race/ethnicity, NHANES 1991–2006.**

A low serum vitamin B_{12} concentration is defined as < 200 pg/mL, indicating that for all groups, serum vitamin B_{12} concentrations were adequate.

Source: U.S. Department of Health and Human Services. 2012. *Second national report on biochemical indicators of diet and nutrition in the U.S. population.* National Center for Environmental Health, Centers for Disease Control and Prevention. www.cdc.gov/nutritionreport.

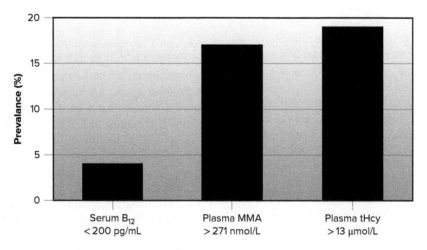

Figure 9.14 **Prevalence estimates of low serum vitamin B_{12}, high plasma methylmalonic acid (MMA), and high plasma total homocysteine (tHcy) concentrations in persons in the United States who were 60 years of age and older, NHANES 2003–2006.**

Source: U.S. Department of Health and Human Services. 2012. *Second national report on biochemical indicators of diet and nutrition in the U.S. population.* National Center for Environmental Health, Centers for Disease Control and Prevention. www.cdc.gov/nutritionreport.

Levels may be elevated to a lesser extent in myocardial infarction, musculoskeletal diseases, and acute pancreatitis. Decreased levels may result from chronic renal dialysis.[12,80] The adult reference range is 4 to 36 IU/L or 4 to 36 U/L.[12]

Albumin and Total Protein

Albumin is a serum protein produced in the liver. Total protein is the sum of all serum proteins, but the vast majority of total protein is composed of albumin and globulin. Once total protein and albumin are known, an estimate of globulin can be calculated. Levels of albumin and total protein reflect nutritional status, and alterations suggest the need for further diagnostic testing. The adult reference range for albumin is 3.5 to 5.0 g/dL or 35 to 50 g/L; for globulin, 2.3 to 3.5 g/dL or 23 to 35 g/L; and for total protein, 6.4 to 8.3 g/dL or 64 to 83 g/L.[12]

Alkaline Phosphatase

Alkaline phosphatase (ALP) is an enzyme found in the liver, bone, placenta, and intestine and is useful in detecting diseases in these organs. Expected values are higher in children, during skeletal growth in adolescents, and during pregnancy.[12] Elevated levels can be seen in conditions involving increased deposition of calcium in bone (hyperparathyroidism, healing fractures, certain bone tumors) and certain liver diseases. Low levels of ALP usually are not clinically significant. The adult reference range is 30 to 120 U/L or 0.5 to 2.0 µkat/L.[12]

Aspartate Aminotransferase

Aspartate aminotransferase (AST), also known as serum glutamic oxaloacetic transaminase (SGOT), is an enzyme found in large concentrations in the myocardium, liver, skeletal muscles, kidneys, and pancreas. Within 8 to 12 hours following injury to these organs, AST is released into the blood. Serum levels peak in 24 to 36 hours and then return to normal in about 4 to 6 days following injury.[12,80] Elevated levels are seen in such conditions as myocardial infarction (blood levels reflect the size of the infarct), liver diseases (for example, acute viral hepatitis), pancreatitis, musculoskeletal injuries, and exposure to drugs toxic to the liver. The adult reference range is 0 to 35 U/L or 0 to 0.58 µkat/L.[12]

Bilirubin

Bilirubin, the major pigment of bile, is produced by the spleen, liver, and bone marrow from the breakdown of the heme portion of hemoglobin and is released into the blood. Most of the bilirubin combines with albumin to form what is called free, or unconjugated, bilirubin. Free bilirubin then is absorbed by the liver, where it is conjugated (joined) to other molecules to form what is called conjugated bilirubin and is then excreted into the bile. Serum bilirubin levels can be reported as direct bilirubin, indirect bilirubin, or total bilirubin. Direct bilirubin is a measure of conjugated bilirubin in serum. Indirect bilirubin is a measure of free, or unconjugated, bilirubin in serum. Total bilirubin is a measure of both direct and indirect bilirubin.[12]

Serum bilirubin rises when the liver is unable to either conjugate or excrete bilirubin. Elevated conjugated (direct) bilirubin suggests obstruction of bile passages within or near the liver. Elevated free, or unconjugated (indirect), bilirubin is indicative of excessive hemolysis (destruction) of red blood cells. Elevated indirect bilirubin also is seen in neonates whose immature livers are unable to adequately conjugate bilirubin. A serum bilirubin concentration greater than about 2 mg/dL results in jaundice. The adult reference ranges for adults are 0.3 to 1.0 mg/dL or 5.1 to 17.0 µmol/L for total bilirubin, 0.1 to 0.3 mg/dL or 1.7 to 5.1 µmol/L for direct (conjugated), and 0.2 to 0.8 mg/dL or 3.4 to 12.0 µmol/L for indirect (unconjugated) bilirubin.[12]

Blood Urea Nitrogen

Urea, the end product of protein metabolism and the primary method of nitrogen excretion, is formed in the liver and excreted by the kidneys in urine. An increased blood urea level usually indicates renal failure, although it may also result from dehydration, gastrointestinal bleeding, congestive heart failure, high protein intake, insufficient renal blood supply, or blockage of the urinary tract.[12,80] Blood urea nitrogen (BUN) is more easily measured than urea and is used as an index of blood urea levels. Elevated BUN is referred to as azotemia. Decreased BUN can result from liver disease, overhydration, malnutrition, or anabolic steroid use. In the absence of other signs, elevated BUN is probably insignificant. The adult reference range is 10 to 20 mg/dL or 3.6 to 7.1 mmol/L.[12]

Calcium

Serum levels of calcium, an important cation (positively charged ion), are helpful in detecting disorders of the bones and parathyroid glands, kidney failure, and certain cancers. Calcium is discussed at length in the earlier section "Calcium Status." The adult reference range for total calcium is 9.0 to 10.5 mg/dL or 2.25 to 2.75 mmol/L, and for ionized calcium it is 4.5 to 5.6 mg/dL or 1.05 to 1.30 mmol/L.[12]

Carbon Dioxide

Measurement of carbon dioxide (CO_2) in serum helps assess the body's acid-base balance. Elevated CO_2 is seen in metabolic alkalosis, and decreased levels reflect metabolic acidosis. The adult reference range in serum or plasma is 23 to 30 mEq/L or 23 to 30 mmol/L.[12]

Chloride

Chloride, an electrolyte, is the primary anion (negatively charged ion) within the extracellular fluid. It works in conjunction with sodium to help regulate acid-base balance, osmotic pressure, and fluid distribution within the body. It often is measured along with sodium, potassium, and carbon dioxide. Low serum chloride levels (hypochloremia) are associated with alkalosis and low serum potassium levels (hypokalemia). Hypokalemia may not accompany hypochloremia if the patient receives a potassium supplement that does not contain chloride or takes a potassium-sparing diuretic. Hyperchloremia (elevated serum chloride) may be seen in kidney disease, overactive thyroid, anemia, or heart disease. The adult reference range is 100 to 106 mEq/L or 100 to 106 mmol/L.[12]

Cholesterol

According to the National Cholesterol Education Program, a desirable serum total cholesterol level is < 200 mg/dL (5.17 mmol/L). Chapter 8 discusses recommended levels of serum cholesterol and its relationship to coronary heart disease. Population reference values for serum total cholesterol are shown in Appendix M.

Creatinine

Measurement of serum creatinine, like measurement of blood urea nitrogen, is used for evaluating renal function. Elevated serum levels are seen when 50% or more of the kidney's nephrons are destroyed. The reference range for adult males is 0.6 to 1.2 mg/dL or 53 to 106 μmol/L, and for adult females it is 0.6 to 1.2 mg/dL or 53 to 106 μmol/L.[12]

Glucose

Measurement of serum glucose is of interest in the diagnosis and management of diabetes mellitus. This is discussed in detail in Chapter 8. Use of serum glucose to diagnose diabetes is discussed at length in Chapter 8. Serum glucose can also be used to diagnose hypoglycemia, or low blood sugar. Glycosylated hemoglobin (A1C), an index of long-term blood sugar control, and the oral glucose tolerance test (OGTT) are also discussed in Chapter 8.

Lactic Dehydrogenase

Lactic dehydrogenase (LDH), an enzyme found in the cells of many organs (skeletal muscles, myocardium, liver, pancreas, spleen, and brain), is released into the blood when cellular damage to these organs occurs. Serum levels of LDH rise 12 to 24 hours following a myocardial infarction and are often measured to determine whether an infarction has occurred. Increased LDH may result from a number of other conditions, including hepatitis, cancer, kidney disease, burns, and trauma. Measurement of five forms of LDH, known as isoenzymes, allows a more definitive diagnosis to be made. Low serum LDH is of no clinical significance. The adult reference range for serum LDH is 100 to 190 U/L.[12]

Phosphorus

The serum level of phosphorus (also known as inorganic phosphorus) is closely correlated with serum calcium level. Elevated serum phosphorus (hyperphosphatemia) is seen in renal failure, hypoparathyroidism, hyperthyroidism, and increased phosphate intake (use of phosphate-containing laxatives and enemas). Low serum phosphorus (hypophosphatemia) can be seen in hyperparathyroidism, rickets, osteomalacia, and chronic use of antacids containing aluminum hydroxide or calcium carbonate, which binds phosphorus in the gastrointestinal tract and prevents its absorption. The adult reference range is 3.0 to 4.5 mg/dL or 0.97 to 1.45 mmol/L.[12]

Potassium

Potassium, the major intracellular cation, is involved in the maintenance of acid-base balance, the body's fluid balance, and nerve impulse transmission. Elevated serum potassium (hyperkalemia) is most often due to renal failure but also may result from inadequate adrenal gland function (Addison's disease), severe burns, or crushing injuries. Low serum potassium (hypokalemia) can result from a number of causes, including use of diuretics or intravenous fluid administration without adequate potassium supplementation, vomiting, diarrhea, and eating disorders.[12] The reference range for adults is 3.5 to 5.0 mEq/L or 3.5 to 5.0 mmol/L.[12]

Sodium

Sodium, the major extracellular cation, is primarily involved in the maintenance of fluid balance and acid-base balance. Elevated serum levels (hypernatremia) are most frequently seen in dehydration resulting from insufficient water intake, excessive water output (for example, severe diarrhea or vomiting, profuse sweating, burns), or loss of antidiuretic hormone control. Hypernatremia suggests the need for water. Hyponatremia may be due to conditions resulting in excessive sodium loss from the body (vomiting, diarrhea, gastric suctioning, diuretic use), conditions resulting in fluid retention (congestive heart failure or renal disease), or water intoxication. The adult reference range is 135 to 145 mEq/L or 135 to 145 mmol/L.[12]

Triglyceride

Triglyceride (TG) is a useful indicator of lipid tolerance in patients receiving total parenteral nutrition. Fasting serum TG provides a good estimate of very-low-density lipoprotein levels. Factors contributing to increased fasting serum TG include genetic factors, obesity, physical inactivity, cigarette smoking, excess alcohol intake, very-high-carbohydrate diets, type 2 diabetes, chronic renal failure, nephrotic syndrome, and use of such drugs as corticosteroids, protease inhibitors, beta-adrenergic blocking agents, and estrogen. Elevated serum TG is considered a risk factor for coronary heart disease and an indicator of persons needing coronary heart disease risk-reduction intervention. According to the National Cholesterol Education Program, a normal serum TG is < 150 mg/dL (< 1.69 mmol/L). Borderline-high and high TG are 150 to 199 mg/dL (1.69 to 2.25 mmol/L) and 200 to 499 mg/dL (2.26 to 5.63 mmol/L), respectively. Very-high serum TG is considered ≥ 500 mg/dL (5.64 mmol/L). Population reference values for serum TG are shown in Appendix M.

SUMMARY

1. Biochemical tests to assess nutritional status can be grouped into two general categories: static and functional tests. Static tests are based on measurement of a nutrient or specific metabolite in the blood, urine, or body tissue. Functional tests involve the physiologic processes that rely on the presence of adequate quantities of a nutrient.

2. The value of biochemical tests is limited by nonnutritional factors affecting test results and the occasional inability of tests to identify the nutrient deficiency. Monitoring nutritional status requires the use of several biochemical tests used in conjunction with each other and with data derived from dietary, anthropometric, and clinical methods. Compared with other assessment methods, biochemical tests have the advantage of being somewhat more objective and quantitative.

3. Protein-energy malnutrition can be either primary (insufficient intake of protein and calories) or secondary (resulting from other diseases). When severe, it results in kwashiorkor (principally a protein deficiency), marasmus (predominantly an energy deficiency), or marasmic kwashiorkor (a combination of chronic energy deficit and chronic or acute protein deficiency).

4. Creatinine is a muscle metabolite excreted in urine used to quantitate muscle mass. Creatinine is excreted in a relatively constant proportion to the body's muscle mass. Muscle mass can be estimated by comparing 24-hour urine creatinine excretion with certain standards. The creatinine-height index is a ratio of a patient's measured 24-hour urinary creatinine excretion and the expected excretion by a reference adult of the same sex and stature expressed as a percent of expected value.

5. Included among the serum proteins used to assess protein nutriture are albumin, transferrin, prealbumin, and retinol-binding protein. Considerations in their use include their body pool amount, half-life, and responsiveness to protein and energy depletion and repletion. Other considerations include how serum proteins are affected by nutritional and nonnutritional factors and how they correlate with morbidity and mortality.

6. Iron deficiency is the most common single nutrient deficiency in the United States and the most common cause of anemia. Serum ferritin is the most useful index of the body's iron stores. Hemoglobin is the most widely used screening test for iron-deficiency anemia but is not an early indicator of iron depletion. Hematocrit is defined as the percentage of red blood cells making up the entire volume of whole blood.

7. Models that combine several indicators of iron status are better at predicting the presence of iron deficiency. Among these are the body iron model, the ferritin model, and the MCV model. These models allow better discrimination between iron-deficiency anemias and those caused by infection, inflammation, and chronic disease than do single measurements.

8. Biochemical tests for assessing calcium status are hampered by the body's tight control of serum calcium levels. Measurement of urinary calcium, which is more responsive to dietary calcium change than serum calcium, is limited by the need for 24-hour urine samples and several nonnutritional factors that affect results.

9. Despite changes in dietary intake, the body maintains tight metabolic control of zinc status through conservation and redistribution of tissue zinc. Consequently, there are no sensitive biochemical or functional indicators of zinc status. Serum zinc level is not reflective of dietary changes and is only a late indicator of the body's exchangeable zinc pool size.

10. Iodine is a trace element essential for the synthesis of thyroid hormones, which regulate metabolic processes related to normal growth and development. Although iodine status is adequate in North American populations, it is a significant public health problem in much of the world, resulting in goiter, cretinism, and impaired mental and physical development.

11. Assessing vitamin A status involves measurement of plasma concentrations of retinol or the vitamin A carrier protein, retinol-binding protein (RBP), retinol isotope dilution, and dose-response tests.

12. The major function of vitamin D is to maintain serum calcium and phosphorus concentrations in a range that supports bone mineralization, neuromuscular function, and various cellular processes. Vitamin D status is best assessed by measuring the serum concentration of 25-hydroxyvitamin D [25(OH)D], the major circulating form of the vitamin, which reflects total vitamin D exposure from food, supplements, and synthesis.

13. Measurements of vitamin C in serum and leukocytes can be used for assessing vitamin C

status. Serum vitamin C is a good indicator of recent vitamin C intake, whereas leukocyte vitamin C better represents cellular stores and the total body pool.

14. Assays for assessing vitamin B_6 status include measurement of plasma pyridoxal 5'-phosphate (PLP), plasma pyridoxal, and urine 4-pyridoxic acid. A functional measure is the methionine load test.

15. Plasma PLP appears to be the single most informative indicator of vitamin B_6 status for healthy persons, but results must sometimes be interpreted with caution because values can be affected by several diseases. 4-pyridoxic acid is the major urinary metabolite of vitamin B_6. It is considered a useful indicator of immediate dietary intake and of short-term vitamin B_6 status.

16. Measures for assessing folate status include measurement of serum folate and erythrocyte folate. Serum folate provides information about recent folate intake and does not necessarily represent tissue stores. Erythrocyte folate is considered to be the best clinical index of depleted tissue stores.

17. The primary cause of vitamin B_{12} deficiency is inadequate absorption, usually because of inadequate gastric production of intrinsic factor, although ileal resection or ileal dysfunction can also cause B_{12} malabsorption. Vitamin B_{12} is assessed by directly measuring serum concentrations of vitamin B_{12} or its transport protein, or by measuring metabolites in the blood that are increased when B_{12} status is compromised.

18. Blood chemistry tests are assays performed on the substances in plasma or serum that are useful in diagnosing and managing disease. They include electrolytes, enzymes, metabolites, and other substances present in serum or plasma. These tests usually are performed using an automated chemistry analyzer capable of performing several thousand blood tests per hour.

References

1. Tanumihardjo SA. 2011. Vitamin A: Biomarkers of nutrition for development. *American Journal of Clinical Nutrition* 94:658S–665S.

2. Heimburger DC. 2012. Malnutrition and nutritional assessment. In Longo DL, Fauci AS, Kasper DL, Hauser SL, Jameson JL, Loscalzo J (eds.), *Harrison's principles of internal medicine,* 18th ed. New York: McGraw-Hill, 605–612.

3. Bingham SA. 1994. The use of 24-h urine samples and energy expenditure to validate dietary assessments. *American Journal of Clinical Nutrition* 59:S227–S231.

4. Tran KM, Johnson RK, Soultanakis RP, Matthews DE. 2000. In-person vs telephone administered multiple-pass 24-hour recalls in women: Validation with doubly labeled water. *Journal of the American Dietetic Association* 100:777–780, 783.

5. Gibson RS. 2005. *Nutritional assessment,* 2nd ed. New York: Oxford University Press.

6. Mosby TT, Barr RD, Pencharz PB. 2009. Nutritional assessment of children with cancer. *Journal of Pediatric Oncology Nursing* 26:186–197.

7. Torun B. 2006. Protein-energy malnutrition. In Shils ME, Shike M, Ross AC, Cabellero B, Cousins RJ (eds.), *Modern nutrition in health and disease,* 10th ed. Philadelphia: Lippincott Williams & Wilkins, 881–908.

8. Hoffer LJ. 2001. Clinical nutrition: 1. Protein-energy malnutrition in the inpatient. *Canadian Medical Association Journal* 165: 1345–1349.

9. McKnight K, Farmer A, Zuberbuhler L, Mger D. 2010. Identification and treatment of protein-energy malnutrition in renal disease. *Canadian Journal of Dietetic Practice and Research* 71:27–32.

10. Panel on Macronutrients, Panel on the Definition of Dietary Fiber, Subcommittee on Upper Reference Levels of Nutrients, Subcommittee on Interpretation and Uses of Dietary Reference Intakes, Standing Committee on the Scientific Evaluation of Dietary Reference Intakes. 2002. *Dietary Reference Intakes for energy, carbohydrate, fiber, fat, fatty acids, cholesterol, protein, and amino acids.* Washington, DC: National Academies Press.

11. Charney P, Malone AM. 2009. *ADA pocket guide to nutrition assessment,* 2nd ed. Chicago: American Dietetic Association.

12. Pagana KD, Pagana TJ. 2010. *Mosby's manual of diagnostic and laboratory tests,* 4th ed. St. Louis: Mosby Elsevier.

13. Ross CA. 2006. Vitamin A and carotenoids. In Shils ME, Shike M, Ross AC, Cabellero B, Cousins RJ (eds.), *Modern nutrition in health and disease,* 10th ed. Philadelphia: Lippincott Williams & Wilkins, 351–375.

14. Mei Z, Cogswell ME, Looker AC, Pfeiffer CM, Cusick SE, Lacher DA, Grummer-Strawn LM. 2011.

Assessment of iron status in US pregnant women from the National Health and Nutrition Examination Survey (NHANES), 1999–2006. *American Journal of Clinical Nutrition* 93:1312–1320.

15. Suchdev PS, Namaste SML, Aaron GJ, Raiten DJ, Brown KH, Flores-Ayala R. 2016. Overview of the Biomarkers Reflecting Inflammation and Nutritional Determinants of Anemia (BRINDA) Project. *Advances in Nutrition* 7:349–356.

16. Panel on Micronutrients, Subcommittee on Upper Reference Levels of Nutrients and of Interpretation and Uses of Dietary Reference Intakes, Standing Committee on the Scientific Evaluation of Dietary Reference Intakes. 2001. *Dietary Reference Intakes for vitamin A, vitamin K, arsenic, boron, chromium, copper, iodine, iron, manganese, molybdenum, nickel, silicon, vanadium, and zinc.* Washington, DC: National Academies Press.

17. Cook JD, Flowers CH, Skikne BS. 2003. The quantitative assessment of body iron. *Blood* 101:3359–3364.

18. Adamson JW. 2012. Iron deficiency and other hypoproliferative anemias. In Longo DL, Fauci AS, Kasper DL, Hauser SL, Jameson JL, Loscalzo J (eds.), *Harrison's principles of internal medicine,* 18th ed. New York: McGraw-Hill, 844–851.

19. Wood RJ, Ronnenbeg AG. 2006. Iron. In Shils ME, Shike M, Ross AC, Cabellero B, Cousins RJ (eds.), *Modern nutrition in health and disease,* 10th ed. Philadelphia: Lippincott Williams & Wilkins, 248–270.

20. U.S. Centers for Disease Control and Prevention. 2012. *Second national report on biochemical indicators of diet and nutrition in the U.S. population.* Atlanta: National Center for Environmental Health. www.cdc.gov/nutritionreport.

21. Skikne BS, Flowers CH, Cook JD. 1990. Serum transferrin receptor: A quantitative measure of tissue iron deficiency. *Blood* 75:1870–1878.

22. Skikne BS. 2008. Serum transferrin receptor. *American Journal of Hematology* 83:872–875.

23. Cogswell ME, Looker AC, Pfeiffer CM, Cook JD, Lacher DA, Beard JL, Lynch SR, Grummer-Strawn LM. 2009. Assessment of iron deficiency in US preschool children and nonpregnant females of childbearing age: National Health and Nutrition Examination Survey 2003–2006. *American Journal of Clinical Nutrition* 89:1334–1342.

24. U.S. Centers for Disease Control and Prevention. 2008. *National report on biochemical indicators of diet and nutrition in the U.S. population 1999–2002.* Atlanta: National Center for Environmental Health.

25. Expert Scientific Working Group. 1985. Summary of a report on assessment of the iron nutritional status of the United States population. *American Journal of Clinical Nutrition* 42:1318–1330.

26. Life Sciences Research Office, Federation of American Societies for Experimental Biology. 1989. *Nutrition monitoring in the United States: An update report on nutrition monitoring.* Washington, DC: U.S. Department of Health and Human Services, Public Health Service.

27. Powell LW. 2012. Hemochromatosis. In Longo DL, Fauci AS, Kasper DL, Hauser SL, Jameson JL, Loscalzo J (eds.), *Harrison's principles of internal medicine,* 18th ed. New York: McGraw-Hill, 3162–3167.

28. Weaver CM, Heaney RP. 2006. Calcium. In Shils ME, Shike M, Ross AC, Cabellero B, Cousins RJ (eds.), *Modern nutrition in health and disease,* 10th ed. Philadelphia: Lippincott Williams & Wilkins, 194–210.

29. Weaver CM. 2006. Calcium. In Bowman BA, Russell RM (eds.), *Present knowledge in nutrition,* 9th ed. Washington, DC: International Life Sciences Institute, 373–382.

30. Committee to Review Dietary Reference Intakes for Vitamin D and Calcium, Food and Nutrition Board. Ross AC, Taylor CL, Yaktine AL, Del Valle HB, eds.

2011. *Dietary Reference Intakes for calcium and vitamin D.* Washington, DC: National Academies Press.

31. Weaver CM. 1990. Assessing calcium status and metabolism. *Journal of Nutrition* 120:1470–1473.

32. Nordin BEC, Need AG, Hartley TF, Philcox JC, Wilcox M, Thomas DW. 1989. Improved method for calculating calcium fractions in plasma: Reference values and effects of menopause. *Clinical Chemistry* 35:14–17.

33. King JC, Cousins RJ. 2006. Zinc. In Shils ME, Shike M, Ross AC, Cabellero B, Cousins RJ (eds.), *Modern nutrition in health and disease,* 10th ed. Philadelphia: Lippincott Williams & Wilkins, 271–285.

34. Cousins RJ. 2006. Zinc. In Bowman BA, Russell RM (eds.), *Present knowledge in nutrition,* 9th ed. Washington, DC: International Life Sciences Institute, 445–457.

35. King JC. 2011. Zinc: An essential but elusive nutrient. *American Journal of Clinical Nutrition* 94:679S–684S.

36. Lowe NM, Fekete K, Decsi T. 2009. Methods of assessment of zinc status in humans: A systematic review. *American Journal of Clinical Nutrition* 89:2040S–2051S.

37. Hotz C, Lowe NM, Araya M, Brown KH. 2003. Assessment of the trace element status of individuals and populations: The example of zinc and copper. *Journal of Nutrition* 133:1563S–1568S.

38. Hambidge M. 2003. Biomarkers of trace mineral intake and status. *Journal of Nutrition* 133:948S–955S.

39. Taylor A. 1986. Usefulness of measurements of trace elements in hair. *Annals of Clinical Biochemistry* 23:364–378.

40. Dunn JT. 2006. Iodine. In Shils ME, Shike M, Ross AC, Cabellero B, Cousins RJ (eds.), *Modern nutrition in health and disease,* 10th ed. Philadelphia: Lippincott Williams & Wilkins, 300–310.

41. Zimmermann MB, Jooste PL, Pandav CS. 2008. Iodine-deficiency disorders. *Lancet* 372:1251–1262.

42. Zimmermann MB. 2009. Iodine deficiency. *Endocrine Reviews* 30:376–408.

43. Jameson JL, Weetman AP. 2012. Disorders of the thyroid gland. In Longo DL, Fauci AS, Kasper DL, Hauser SL, Jameson JL, Loscalzo J (eds.), *Harrison's principles of internal medicine*, 18th ed. New York: McGraw-Hill, 2911–2939.

44. Ristic-Medic D, Piskackova Z, Hooper L, Ruprish J, Casgrain A, Ashton K, Pavlovic M, Glibetic M. 2009. Methods of assessment of iodine status in humans: A systematic review. *American Journal of Clinical Nutrition* 89:2052S–2069S.

45. Zimmermann MB. 2006. Iodine and the iodine deficiency disorders. In Bowman BA, Russell RM (eds.), *Present knowledge in nutrition*, 9th ed. Washington, DC: International Life Science Institute, 471–479.

46. Lee K, Bradley R, Dwyer J, Lee SL. 1999. Too much versus too little: The implication of current iodine intake in the United States. *Nutrition Reviews* 57:177–181.

47. Hollowell JG, Haddow JE. 2007. The prevalence of iodine deficiency in women of reproductive age in the United States of America. *Public Health Nutrition* 10:1532–1539.

48. Zimmermann MB. 2011. Iodine deficiency in industrialized countries. *Clinical Endocrinology* 75:287–288.

49. Zimmermann MB. 2007. The impact of iodised salt or iodine supplements on iodine status during pregnancy, lactation and infancy. *Public Health Nutrition* 10:1584–1595.

50. Perrine CG, Kerrick K, Serdula MK, Sullivan KM. 2010. Some subgroups of reproductive age women in the United States may be at risk for iodine deficiency. *Journal of Nutrition* 140:1489–1494.

51. U.S. Department of Health and Human Services and U.S. Department of Agriculture. 2015. *2015–2020 dietary guidelines for Americans*, 8th ed. http://health.gov/dietaryguidelines/2015/guidelines/.

52. Appel LJ, Frohlich ED, Hgall JE, Pearson TA, Sacco RL, et al. 2011. The importance of population-wide sodium reduction as a means to prevent cardiovascular disease and stroke: A call to action from the American Heart Association. *Circulation* 123:1138–1143.

53. Ross AC. 2006. Vitamin A and carotenoids. In Shils ME, Shike M, Ross AC, Cabellero B, Cousins RJ (eds.), *Modern nutrition in health and disease*, 10th ed. Philadelphia: Lippincott Williams & Wilkins, 351–375.

54. Solomons NW. 2006. Vitamin A. In Bowman BA, Russell RM (eds.), *Present knowledge in nutrition*, 9th ed. Washington, DC: International Life Sciences Institute, 157–183.

55. Rice AL, Stoltzfus RJ, de Francisco A, Kjolhede CL. 2000. Evaluation of serum retinol, the modified-relative-dose-response ratio, and breast-milk vitamin A as indicators of response postpartum maternal vitamin A supplementation. *American Journal of Clinical Nutrition* 71:799–806.

56. Furr HC, Green MH, Haskell M, Mokhtar N, Nestel P, Newton S, Ribaya-Mercado JD, Tang G, Tanumihardjo S, Wasantwisut E. 2005. Stable isotope dilution techniques for assessing vitamin A status and bioavailability of provitamin A carotenoids in humans. *Public Health Nutrition* 8:596–607.

57. Olson JA. Isotope-dilution techniques: A wave of the future in human nutrition. *American Journal of Clinical Nutrition* 66:186–187.

58. Wimalawansa SJ. Vitamin D and cardiovascular diseases: Causality. *Journal of Steroid Biochemistry and Molecular Biology* (in press).

59. Holick MF. 2011. Health benefits of vitamin D and sunlight: A D-bate. *Nature Reviews Endocrinology* 7:73–75.

60. Heaney RP, Holick MF. 2011. Why the IOM recommendations for vitamin D are deficient. *Journal of Bone and Mineral Research* 26:455–457.

61. Holick MF, Chen TC. 2008. Vitamin D deficiency: A worldwide problem with health consequences. *American Journal of Clinical Nutrition* 87:1080S–1086S.

62. Schleicher RL, Sternberg MR, Lacher DA, Sempos CT, Looker AC, Durazo-Arvizu RA, Yetley EA, Chaudhary-Webb M, Maw KL, Pfeiffer CM, Johnson CL. 2016. The vitamin D status of the US population from 1988 to 2010 using standardized serum concentrations of 25-hydroxyvitamin D shows recent modest increases. *America Journal of Clinical Nutrition* 104:454–461.

63. Levine M, Katz A, Padayatty SJ. 2006. Vitamin C. In Shils ME, Shike M, Ross AC, Cabellero B, Cousins RJ (eds.), *Modern nutrition in health and disease*, 10th ed. Philadelphia: Lippincott Williams & Wilkins, 507–524.

64. Jacob RA. 1990. Assessment of human vitamin C status. *Journal of Nutrition* 120:1480–1485.

65. Lykkesfeldt J, Poulsen HE. 2010. Is vitamin C supplementation beneficial? Lessons learned from randomised controlled trials. *British Journal of Nutrition* 103:1251–1259.

66. Johnston CS. 2006. Vitamin C. In Bowman BA, Russell RM (eds.), *Present knowledge in nutrition*, 9th ed. Washington, DC: International Life Sciences Institute, 233–241.

67. Standing Committee on the Scientific Evaluation of Dietary Reference Intakes, Food and Nutrition Board, Institute of Medicine. 2000. *Dietary Reference Intakes for vitamin C, vitamin E, selenium, and carotenoids*. Washington, DC: National Academies Press.

68. Mackey AD, Davis SR, Gregory JF. 2006. Vitamin B_6. In Shils ME, Shike M, Ross AC, Cabellero B, Cousins RJ (eds.), *Modern nutrition in health and disease*, 10th ed. Philadelphia: Lippincott Williams & Wilkins, 452–461.

69. McCormick DB. 2006. Vitamin B_6. In Bowman BA, Russell RM (eds.), *Present knowledge in nutrition,* 9th ed. Washington, DC: International Life Sciences Institute, 269–277.

70. Standing Committee on the Scientific Evaluation of Dietary Reference Intakes, Food and Nutrition Board, Institute of Medicine. 1998. *Dietary Reference Intakes for thiamin, riboflavin, niacin, vitamin B6, folate, vitamin B12, pantothenic acid, biotin, and choline.* Washington, DC: National Academies Press.

71. Leklem JE. 1988. Vitamin B_6 metabolism and function in humans. In Leklem JE, Reynolds RD (eds.), *Clinical and physiological applications of vitamin B_6.* New York: Alan R. Liss.

72. Leklem JE. 1990. Vitamin B_6: A status report. *Journal of Nutrition* 120:1503–1507.

73. Carmel R. 2006. Folic acid. In Shils ME, Shike M, Ross AC, Cabellero B, Cousins RJ (eds.), *Modern nutrition in health and disease,* 10th ed. Philadelphia: Lippincott Williams & Wilkins, 470–481.

74. Yetley EA, Pfeiffer CM, Phinney KW, et al. 2011. Biomarkers of folate status in NHANES: A roundtable summary. *American Journal of Clinical Nutrition* 94:303S–312S.

75. U.S. Centers for Disease Control and Prevention. 2010. CDC grand rounds: Additional opportunities to prevent neural tube defects with folic acid fortification. *Morbidity and Mortality Weekly Report* 59:980–984.

76. Carmel R. 2006. Cobalamin (vitamin B_{12}). In Shils ME, Shike M, Ross AC, Cabellero B, Cousins RJ (eds.), *Modern nutrition in health and disease,* 10th ed. Philadelphia: Lippincott Williams & Wilkins, 482–497.

77. Hofafbrand AV. 2012. Megaloblastic anemias. In Longo DL, Fauci AS, Kasper DL, Hauser SL, Jameson JL, Loscalzo J (eds.), *Harrison's principles of internal medicine,* 18th ed. New York: McGraw-Hill, 862–872.

78. Yetley EA, Pfeiffer CM, Phinney KW, et al. 2011. Biomarkers of vitamin B-12 status in NHANES: A roundtable summary. *American Journal of Clinical Nutrition* 94:313S–321S.

79. Carmel R. 2011. Biomarkers of cobalamin (vitamin B-12) status in the epidemiologic setting: A critical overview of context, applications, and performance characteristics of cobalamin, methylmalonic acid, and holotranscobalamin II. *American Journal of Clinical Nutrition* 94:348S–358S.

80. Malarkey LM, McMorrow ME. 2012. *Saunders nursing guide to laboratory and diagnostic tests,* 2nd ed. St. Louis: Elsevier/Saunders.

ASSESSMENT ACTIVITY 9.1

Visiting a Clinical Laboratory

Every hospital or clinic has a clinical laboratory where at least some of the facility's biochemical tests are performed. Specimens are sometimes sent to an outside clinical laboratory because it has specialized instruments and expertise or because its automated analyzers allow certain tests to be performed more economically. However, all hospitals have facilities for performing certain basic tests, especially those required in emergency situations. Among these are tests for electrolytes, blood gases, enzymes diagnostic of cardiac or liver disease, and glucose.

Your class can arrange to visit a clinical laboratory to see how some of these tests are performed. You may be surprised by the capability of various automated instruments used to perform the chemistry profile and complete blood count on a single specimen of serum or whole blood.

ASSESSMENT ACTIVITY 9.2

Chemistry Profile, Complete Blood Count, and Coronary Risk Profile

The chemistry profile, complete blood count (CBC), and coronary risk profile are among the most basic series of tests performed by clinical laboratories. Generally included in the chemistry profile are those tests listed in the section entitled "Blood Chemistry Tests." Included in the CBC are the red blood cell count, white blood cell count, and measurements of hemoglobin, hematocrit, mean corpuscular volume, mean corpuscular hemoglobin, and mean corpuscular hemoglobin concentration (see Box 9.1). The coronary risk profile measures levels of triglyceride, total cholesterol, and HDL-C (cholesterol carried by high-density lipoproteins) and calculates LDL-C (cholesterol carried by low-density lipoproteins) and the total cholesterol/HDL-C ratio. These tests are discussed in Chapter 8. These measurements are routinely performed using automated instruments capable of performing several thousand tests per hour.

Members of your class may want to have their blood drawn by a qualified venipuncturist and have the samples sent to a clinical laboratory for analysis. Tests that might be performed include the CBC, chemistry profile, and coronary risk profile.

Another example of a simple test that can be done in the classroom is the hematocrit. The necessary equipment includes a centrifuge, capillary tubes, lancets, alcohol wipes, gloves, and some way of comparing the volume of whole blood in the capillary tube with the volume of packed cells after the tube is spun down. Whatever approach your class takes, compare your test results with the reference values given in this chapter and Chapter 8. Obtain an average value for the class and compare this with the reference values.

Remember, in handling blood specimens or any bodily fluid, precautions must be taken to protect patients and laboratory staff from infectious agents, especially those causing hepatitis as well as the human immunodeficiency virus (HIV). All bodily fluids must be regarded as being infectious and handled with the utmost care. All syringes, lancets, needles, tubes, and other materials that have come in contact with blood or other bodily fluids must be handled safely and disposed of properly. Gloves should be worn whenever drawing blood or handling other bodily fluids.

CLINICAL ASSESSMENT OF NUTRITIONAL STATUS

STUDENT LEARNING OUTCOMES

After studying this chapter, the student will be able to:

1. Name the components of a patient's medical history that are relevant to nutritional assessment.

2. Explain the advantages and limitations of Subjective Global Assessment.

3. Use Subjective Global Assessment to assess a patient's nutritional status.

4. Differentiate between kwashiorkor and marasmus.

5. Calculate and interpret percent weight for height.

6. Calculate and interpret percent height for age.

7. Describe the body composition changes that result from lipodystrophy in HIV patients.

8. Discuss the diagnostic criteria for anorexia nervosa and bulimia.

INTRODUCTION

Clinical assessment of nutritional status involves a detailed history, a thorough physical examination, and the interpretation of the signs and symptoms associated with malnutrition. It can be an efficient and effective way for an experienced and astute clinician to evaluate a patient's nutritional status without having to depend entirely on laboratory and diagnostic tests that may delay initiation of nutritional support and increase the time and cost of hospitalization. **Signs** are defined as observations, made by a qualified examiner, of which the patient is usually unaware. **Symptoms** are clinical manifestations reported by the patient. This chapter discusses clinical assessment of nutritional status and gives examples of clinical indicators of impaired nutritional status. As a dietitian or nutritionist, you will likely see some of the conditions discussed and illustrated in this chapter. For example, protein-energy malnutrition and severe wasting are common features of certain cancers, acquired immunodeficiency syndrome (AIDS), and advanced disease of the gastrointestinal tract. However, some of the other conditions discussed in this chapter, such as clinical signs of advanced nutrient deficiency, are not often seen in developed countries but occur more frequently in less industrialized nations. But given the global nature of the work of health-care professionals, understanding how to evaluate advanced malnutrition and starvation will be of interest to students and practitioners of nutrition. Because many of the clinical findings are not specific for a particular nutrient deficiency, they often must be integrated with anthropometric, biochemical, and dietary data before arriving at a definitive diagnosis. The information in this chapter complements information provided in Chapter 1 on the Nutrition Care Process and in Chapter 7 on assessment of the hospitalized patient. The focus in this chapter will be on protein-energy malnutrition (PEM), human immunodeficiency virus (HIV) infection, and eating disorders.

MEDICAL HISTORY

Obtaining a patient's history is the first step in the clinical assessment of nutritional status.[1] A good way to begin is by reviewing the patient's medical record, giving careful attention to the patient's medical history.[2,3] Components from the medical history to consider in nutritional assessment are shown in Box 10.1.

Essential components of a patient's history include pertinent facts about past and current health and use of medications, as well as personal and household information.[1,2] A variety of diseases can affect nutritional status. Among these are diabetes, kidney disease, various cancers, coronary heart disease, stroke, liver disease (e.g., hepatitis and cirrhosis), gallbladder disease, AIDS, ulcers, and colitis, as well as recent or past surgical procedures. Other conditions affecting nutritional status also should be explored: the ability to chew and swallow; appetite; and the presence of vomiting, diarrhea, constipation, flatulence, belching, or indigestion. An inquiry should be made about the patient's usual weight and any recent changes (gains or losses) in weight. A systematic approach to the detection of deficiency syndromes based on findings from the history is shown in Table 10.1.

Information on the use of medications will provide clues about the patient's actual or perceived medical condition. This will include prescription and over-the-counter medications, vitamin and mineral supplements, and nontraditional medications, such as herbal and folk remedies. This information can also be helpful in identifying drug-nutrient interactions potentially having an adverse effect on the patient's nutritional status.[3]

Psychosocial factors include the patient's age; occupation; educational level; marital status; income; living arrangements; number of dependents; use of alcohol, tobacco, and illicit drugs; degree of social and emotional support; and access to and ability to pay for health care. These factors are summarized in Box 10.2.

Box 10.1   Components of the Medical History to Consider in Nutritional Assessment

- Past and current diagnoses of nutritional consequence
- Diagnostic procedures
- Surgeries
- Chemotherapy and radiation therapy
- History of nutrition-related problems
- Existing nutrient deficiencies

- Medications and their nutrient interactions
- Psychosocial history—alcohol, smoking, finances, social support
- Signs or symptoms suggestive of vitamin deficiency
- Signs or symptoms suggestive of mineral deficiency

Source: Phinney SD. 1981. The assessment of protein nutrition in the hospitalized patient. *Clinics in Laboratory Medicine* 1:767–774; McLaren DS. 1992. *A colour atlas and text of diet-related disorders,* 2nd ed. London: Mosby Europe; Jeejeebhoy KN. 1994. Clinical and functional assessments. In Shils ME, Olson JA, Shike M (eds.), *Modern nutrition in health and disease,* 8th ed. Philadelphia: Lea & Febiger.

Box 10.2   Factors to Consider in Taking a Patient's Dietary History

- Weight changes
- Usual meal pattern
- Appetite
- Satiety
- Discomfort after eating
- Chewing/swallowing ability
- Likes/dislikes
- Taste changes/aversions
- Allergies
- Nausea/vomiting

- Bowel habits—diarrhea, constipation, steatorrhea
- Living conditions
- Snack consumption
- Vitamin/mineral supplement use
- Alcohol/drug use
- Previous diet restrictions
- Surgery/chronic diseases
- Ability to purchase and prepare food
- Access to and ability to pay for health care

TABLE 10.1	Nutritional History Screens—a Systematic Approach to the Detection of Deficiency Syndromes	

Mechanism of Deficiency	If History Of	Suspect Deficiency Of
Inadequate intake	Alcoholism	Energy, protein, thiamin, niacin, folate, pyridoxine, riboflavin
	Avoidance of fruit, vegetables, grains	Vitamin C, thiamin, niacin, folate
	Avoidance of meat, dairy products, eggs	Protein, vitamin B_{12}
	Constipation, hemorrhoids, diverticulosis	Dietary fiber
	Isolation, poverty, dental disease, food idiosyncrasies	Various nutrients
	Weight loss	Energy, other nutrients
Inadequate absorption	Drugs (especially antacids, anticonvulsants, cholestyramine, laxatives, neomycin, alcohol)	Various nutrients, depending on drug/nutrient interaction
	Malabsorption (diarrhea, weight loss, steatorrhea)	Vitamins A, D, K; energy; protein; calcium; magnesium; zinc
	Parasites	Iron, vitamin B_{12} (fish tapeworm)
	Pernicious anemia	Vitamin B_{12}
	Surgery	
	Gastrectomy	Vitamin B_{12}, iron
	Small bowel resection	Vitamin B_{12} (if distal ileum), others as in malabsorption
Decreased utilization	Drugs (especially anticonvulsants, antimetabolites, oral contraceptives, isoniazid, alcohol)	Various nutrients, depending on drug/nutrient interaction
	Inborn errors of metabolism (by family history)	Various nutrients
Increased losses	Alcohol abuse	Magnesium, zinc
	Blood loss	Iron
	Centesis (ascitic, pleural taps)	Protein
	Diabetes, uncontrolled	Energy
	Diarrhea	Protein, zinc, electrolytes
	Draining abscesses, wounds	Protein, zinc
	Nephrotic syndrome	Protein, zinc
	Peritoneal dialysis or hemodialysis	Protein, water-soluble vitamins, zinc
Increased requirements	Fever	Energy
	Hyperthyroidism	Energy
	Physiologic demands (infancy, adolescence, pregnancy, lactation)	Various nutrients
	Surgery, trauma, burns, infection	Energy, protein, vitamin C, zinc
	Tissue hypoxia	Energy (inefficient utilization)
	Cigarette smoking	Vitamin C, folic acid

The necessary detail of the history will vary depending on circumstances and will be influenced by the patient's ability to respond to questioning. In some instances, the necessary information might need to be obtained from a surrogate (a parent, a companion, a sibling, or another person knowledgeable about the patient's life habits). Much of this information can be obtained from the history and physical examination performed by the admitting physician, from the notes of nurses or social workers, and from previous medical records. Remember that this and all information about the patient should be dealt with in a confidential and strictly professional manner.

DIETARY HISTORY

Included with the dietary history is information about the patient's eating practices. This includes a wide range of information about usual eating patterns (timing and location of meals and snacks), food preferences and aversions, intolerances and allergies, amount of money available for purchasing food, ability to obtain and prepare food, eligibility for and access to food assistance programs, and use of vitamin, mineral, and other supplements. These and other factors are included in Box 10.2.

For example, when inquiring about appetite, satiety, or discomfort, it is important to ask if the patient has experienced any changes in desire for food, if he or she experiences satiety earlier or later than usual, and if there is any pain or discomfort associated with eating. Questions about the ability to chew and swallow food are important. Are there dental or oral problems making it difficult to chew certain foods or to consume adequate energy to support normal body weight? If the patient wears dentures, are they well fitting? If swallowing is painful or difficult, for what foods?

Questioning the patient about bowel habits can often provide information pertinent to the diagnosis of gastrointestinal disease. The patient should be asked about changes in bowel habits, such as constipation, diarrhea, or unusual amounts of flatus (gas), and about stool consistency and color. Obviously, the presence of bright red blood in the stool is an important finding. Stools containing digested blood (e.g., from a bleeding peptic ulcer) may appear black or tarry. The finding of frothy, watery, and foul-smelling stools suggests the possibility of fat malabsorption. Table 10.2 gives a listing of clinical findings and links their presence with either an excess or a deficiency of various nutrients.

SUBJECTIVE GLOBAL ASSESSMENT

Subjective Global Assessment (SGA) is a clinical technique for assessing the nutritional status of a patient based on features of the patient's history and physical examination.[4] Unlike traditional methods that rely heavily on objective anthropometric and biochemical data, SGA is based on four elements of the patient's history (recent loss of body weight, changes in usual diet, presence of significant gastrointestinal symptoms, and the patient's functional capacity) and three elements of the physical examination (loss of subcutaneous fat, muscle wasting, and presence of edema or ascites).[4] Information obtained from the history and physical examination can be entered into a form, such as the one shown in Figure 10.1, to arrive at an SGA rating of nutritional status. The Academy of Nutrition and Dietetics recommends that dietitians participate in the SGA process with nurses, physicians, and other clinicians. The website http://pt-global.org/ provides more information on SGA and an online application to facilitate the process.

Elements of the History

The first of the four elements of the SGA history is the percent and pattern of weight loss within six months prior to examination. A weight loss < 5% is considered small. A 5% to 10% weight loss is considered potentially significant. A weight loss > 10% is considered definitely significant. The pattern of weight loss is also important. A patient who has lost 12% of his or her weight in the past six months but has recently gained 6% of it back is considered better nourished than a patient who has lost 6% of his or her weight in the past six months and continues to lose weight. Information about the patient's maximum weight and what it was six months ago can be compared with the patient's current weight. Questions about changes in the way clothing fits may confirm reports of weight change. Information about changes in body weight in the past two weeks (increase, no change, decrease) should be elicited as well. These data can be entered or noted in the appropriate places in Figure 10.1.

Dietary intake, the second element of the history, is classified as either normal (i.e., what the patient usually eats) or abnormal (i.e., a change from the patient's usual diet). If intake is abnormal, the duration in weeks is entered, and the appropriate box is checked to indicate the type of dietary intake abnormality (i.e., increased intake, suboptimal solid, full-liquid, IV or hypocaloric liquids, or starvation). The patient can be asked if the amount of food consumed has changed and, if so, by how much and why. If the patient is eating less, it would be valuable to know what happens when he or she tries to eat more. Ask for a description of a typical breakfast, lunch, and dinner and how that compares with what the patient typically ate 6 or 12 months ago.

Information about any gastrointestinal symptoms persisting more than two weeks (the third history element) should be elicited and noted on the form. Diarrhea or occasional vomiting lasting only a few days is not considered significant. The presence or absence of any dysfunction in the patient's ability to attend to activities of daily living (the last history element) should also be noted on the form. If a dysfunction is present, its duration and type should be noted.

Elements of the Physical Examination

The first of the three elements of the physical examination is loss of subcutaneous fat. The four anatomic areas listed in Figure 10.1 (shoulders, triceps, chest, and hands) should be checked for loss of fullness or loose-fitting skin, although the latter may appear in older persons who are not malnourished. Illustrations of subcutaneous fat loss in the arm, chest wall, and hands are shown in Figure 10.2 and Figure 10.3. Loss of subcutaneous fat should be noted as normal (0), mild loss (1+), moderate loss (2+), or severe loss (3+).

According to Detsky, the presence of muscle wasting (the second element of the physical examination) is best assessed by examining the deltoid muscles (located at the sides of the shoulders) and the quadriceps femoris muscles (the muscles of the anterior thigh).[4] Loss of subcutaneous fat in the shoulders and deltoid muscle wasting gives the shoulders a squared-off appearance, similar to that shown in Figure 10.4. These areas can be assessed as being normal or mildly, moderately, or severely wasted.

The presence of edema at the ankle or sacrum can also be assessed as absent, mild, moderate, or severe. The presence of "pitting" edema can be checked by momentarily pressing the area with a finger and then looking for a persistent depression (more than five seconds) where the finger was. Ankle edema and ascites can be assessed as absent, mild, moderate, or severe. When considerable edema or ascites are present, weight loss is a less important variable.

The final step in SGA is arriving at a rating of nutritional assessment. Instead of an explicit numerical

TABLE 10.2	Clinical Nutrition Examination

Clinical Findings	Consider Deficiency Of	Consider Excess Of	Frequency
Hair, Nails			
Flag sign (traverse depigmentation of hair)	Protein		Rare
Easily pluckable hair	Protein		Common
Sparse hair	Protein, biotin, zinc	Vitamin A	Occasional
Corkscrew hairs and unemerged coiled hairs	Vitamin C		Common
Traverse ridging of nails	Protein		Occasional
Skin			
Scaling	Vitamin A, zinc, essential fatty acids	Vitamin A	Occasional
Cellophane appearance	Protein		Occasional
Cracking (flaky paint or crazy pavement dermatosis)	Protein		Rare
Follicular hyperkeratosis	Vitamins A, C		Occasional
Petechiae (especially perifollicular)	Vitamin C		Occasional
Purpura	Vitamins C, K		Common
Pigmentation, desquamation of sun-exposed areas	Niacin		Rare
Yellow pigmentation-sparing sclerae (benign)		Carotene	Common
Eyes			
Papilledema		Vitamin A	Rare
Night blindness	Vitamin A		Rare
Perioral			
Angular stomatitis	Riboflavin, pyridoxine, niacin		Occasional
Cheilosis (dry, cracking, ulcerated lips)	Riboflavin, pyridoxine, niacin		Rare
Oral			
Atrophic lingual papillae (slick tongue)	Riboflavin, niacin, folate, vitamin B_{12}, protein, iron		Common
Glossitis (scarlet, raw tongue)	Riboflavin, niacin, pyridoxine, folate, vitamin B_{12}		Occasional
Hypogeusesthesia, hyposmia	Zinc		Occasional
Swollen, retracted, bleeding gums (if teeth are present)	Vitamin C		Occasional
Bones, Joints			
Beading of ribs, epiphyseal swelling, bowlegs	Vitamin D		Rare
Tenderness (subperiosteal hemorrhage in child)	Vitamin C		Rare
Neurologic			
Headache		Vitamin A	Rare
Drowsiness, lethargy, vomiting		Vitamins A, D	Rare
Dementia	Niacin, vitamin B_{12}		Rare
Confabulation, disorientation	Thiamin (Korsakoff's psychosis)		Occasional
Ophthalmoplegia	Thiamin, phosphorus		Occasional
Peripheral neuropathy (e.g., weakness; paresthesia; ataxia; decreased tendon reflexes; fine tactile sense, vibratory sense, and position sense)	Thiamin, pyridoxine, vitamin B_{12}	Pyridoxine	Occasional
Tetany	Calcium, magnesium		Occasional
Other			
Parotid enlargement	Protein (also consider bulimia)		Occasional
Heart failure	Thiamin (wet beriberi), phosphorus		Occasional
Sudden heart failure, death	Vitamin C		Rare
Hepatomegaly	Protein	Vitamin A	Rare
Edema	Protein, thiamin		Common
Poor wound healing, pressure ulcers	Protein, vitamin C, zinc		Common

HISTORY

1. Weight Change

Maximum body weight _____

Weight 6 months ago _____

Current weight _____

Overall weight loss in past 6 months _____

Percent weight loss in past 6 months _____

Change in 2 past weeks: _____ increase _____ no change _____ decrease

$$\% \text{ Wt change} = \frac{\text{wt 6 months ago} - \text{current wt}}{\text{wt 6 mos ago}} \times 100$$

2. Dietary Intake (relative to normal)

_____ No change

_____ Change   Duration: _____ Weeks

Type: _____ Increased intake

_____ Suboptimal solid diet

_____ Full liquid diet

_____ IV or hypocaloric liquids

_____ Starvation

3. Gastrointestinal Symptoms (lasting > 2 weeks)

_____ None

_____ Nausea   _____ Vomiting   _____ Diarrhea   _____ Anorexia

4. Functional Capacity

_____ No dysfunction

_____ Dysfunction   Duration: _____ Weeks

Type: _____ Works suboptimally

_____ Ambulatory

_____ Bedridden

PHYSICAL EXAMINATION

(For each trait specify: 0 = normal; 1+ = mild; 2+ = moderate; 3+ = severe)

_____ Loss of subcutaneous fat (shoulders, triceps, chest, hands)

_____ Muscle wasting (quadriceps, deltoids)

_____ Ankle edema

_____ Ascites

Subjective Global Assessment Rating (select one)

_____ A = well nourished

_____ B = moderately (or suspected of being) malnourished

_____ C = severely malnourished

Figure 10.1 Form for rating nutritional status based on Subjective Global Assessment.

Source: Adapted from Detsky AS, McLaughlin JR, Baker JP, Johnston N, Whittaker S, Mendelson RA, Jeejeebhoy KN. 1987. What is Subjective Global Assessment of nutritional status? *Journal of Parenteral and Enteral Nutrition* 11:8–13; Detsky AS, Smalley PS, Change J. 1994. Is this patient malnourished? *Journal of the American Medical Association* 271:54–58.

weighting scheme, SGA depends on the clinician's subjectively combining the various elements to arrive at an overall, or global, assessment. Patients with weight loss > 10% that is continuing, poor dietary intake, and severe loss of subcutaneous fat and muscle wasting fall within the severely malnourished category (class C rank). Patients with at least a 5% weight loss, reduced dietary intake, and mild to moderate loss of subcutaneous fat and muscle wasting fall within the moderately malnourished category (class B rank). Patients are generally ranked as well nourished when they have had a recent improvement in appetite or the other historical features of SGA. A class A rank would be given to patients having a recent increase in weight (that is not fluid retention), even if their net loss for the past six months was between 5% and 10%. Using this approach, very few well-nourished patients are classified as malnourished, but some patients with mild malnutrition may be missed.[4]

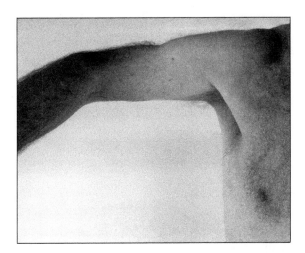

Figure 10.2 **Subcutaneous tissue loss from the arm and chest wall.**
©McGraw-Hill Education/Mark Dierker, photographer

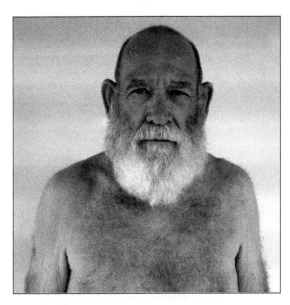

Figure 10.4
The squared-off appearance of the shoulders indicates the loss of subcutaneous tissue and wasting of the deltoid muscle. Loss of subcutaneous fat and muscle wasting are also apparent in the upper arms.
©McGraw-Hill Education/Mark Dierker, photographer

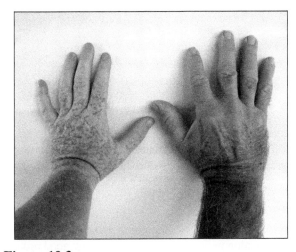

Figure 10.3
Loss of subcutaneous tissue can be clearly seen in the hand on the left, compared with the hand of a healthy person on the right.
©McGraw-Hill Education/Mark Dierker, photographer

Despite this subjective nature, clinicians (nurses and residents) trained to use SGA were shown to have arrived at very similar rankings when comparing their evaluations of a series of 109 patients.[4] The method has also been shown to be a powerful predictor of postoperative complications.[4,5] SGA has been shown to be a simple, safe, effective, and inexpensive tool for clinicians to identify patients who are malnourished or at risk of malnutrition. It is regarded by many as the most reliable and efficient method to assess nutritional status at the bedside and is considered the gold standard for bedside assessment tools.[6,7]

PROTEIN-ENERGY MALNUTRITION

Clinical Signs

In its most severe states, protein-energy malnutrition (PEM) takes the form of kwashiorkor or marasmus. Kwashiorkor is predominantly a protein deficiency, whereas marasmus is mainly an energy deficiency.[8] Kwashiorkor (Figure 10.5) is characterized by a relatively normal weight, generally intact skeletal musculature, and decreased concentrations of serum proteins.[8-10] A common feature is soft, pitting, painless edema in the feet and legs, extending into the perineum, upper extremities, and face in severe cases. The hair can become dry, brittle, dull, and easily pulled out without pain. The marasmic patient typically presents with significant loss of body weight, skeletal muscle, and adipose tissue mass but with serum protein concentrations relatively intact. Patients are often seen at 60% or less of their expected weight for height, and marasmic children have a marked reduction in their longitudinal growth. Patients are described as having a "skin and bones" appearance. General characteristics of kwashiorkor and marasmus are outlined in Table 10.3.

Although such obvious cases of kwashiorkor and marasmus as illustrated in Figure 10.5 will not often be seen in developed countries, severe cases of protein-energy malnutrition and wasting still occur, especially as a result of AIDS, certain cancers, some gastrointestinal diseases, and alcoholism and other instances of substance abuse. The emaciated condition of the body and general ill health resulting from these and other diseases are also

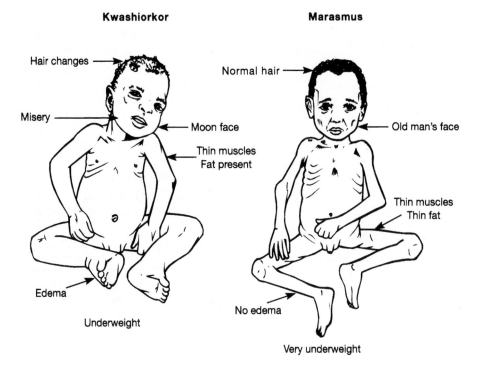

Figure 10.5 **Differences in clinical signs between kwashiorkor and marasmus.**

Source: Adapted from Jellife DB. 1968. *Clinical nutrition in developing countries.* Washington, DC: U.S. Department of Health and Human Services.

called **cachexia.** Many patients presenting with protein-energy malnutrition and wasting will have diagnostic features in common with either marasmus or kwashiorkor. Diagnostic features of marasmus include considerable loss of skeletal muscle, adipose tissue, and body weight, without edema. The wasting is particularly apparent in the neck, shoulders, and upper arms. With three months of nutritional support, increases in skeletal muscle, adipose tissue, and body weight can be measured, with a fuller face and less wasting in the neck, shoulders, and upper arms.

With kwashiorkor, edema can be clearly seen, especially in the legs and feet. Some wasting is also experienced in

the neck, shoulders, and upper arms. After three months of nutritional support and medical treatment, patients will experience a fuller appearance to the face, neck, shoulders, and upper arms and no apparent edema.

Other clinical signs of PEM include the "flag sign" and growth failure. In the flag sign, there are alternating bands of depigmented and normal-colored hair produced by alternating periods of poor and relatively good protein intake. Hair grown during periods of poor protein intake can become depigmented and turn a dull brown, red, or even yellowish white. Hair grown during periods of more adequate protein intake returns to its normal color. The flag sign is especially noticeable in persons with long, dark-colored hair. An example of the flag sign is shown in Figure 10.6.

Growth failure (or failure to thrive) is the most common sign of malnutrition in children. It is a failure to gain weight and height at the expected rate. Growth failure can result from one or any combination of factors, such as inadequate nutrient intake, nutrient malabsorption, failure to utilize nutrients, increased nutrient losses, and increased nutrient requirements. Major contributing factors to growth failure include poverty, inadequate emotional and social nurturing, and infections, especially parasitic gut infestations. Children with growth failure can have a markedly reduced height for age and weight for age, but with a normal weight-to-height ratio and no other signs of clinical malnutrition.

TABLE 10.3	Characteristics of Kwashiorkor and Marasmus	
Variable	**Kwashiorkor**	**Marasmus**
Skeletal muscle	No major losses	Significant losses
Serum proteins	Significantly decreased	Relatively normal
Adipose tissue	Preserved	Significant loss
Body weight	Relatively normal	Significant loss
Edema	Pitting edema common	Absent
Predisposing factors	Ample energy with little or no protein	Starvation, lack of both protein and total energy

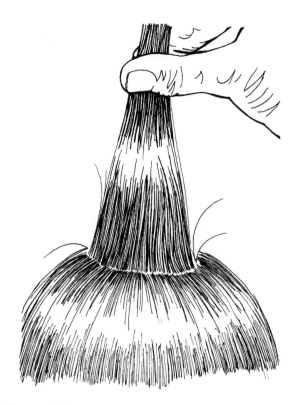

Figure 10.6
The flag sign is characterized by bands of depigmented hair that grew during periods of inadequate protein intake. The normally colored hair grew during periods of relatively adequate protein intake.

Classifying Protein-Energy Malnutrition

The severity of PEM in children and adolescents can be classified using records of age and measurements of weight and height or length.[8] From these, weight for height (or length) and height for age can be calculated.

Weight for height is a convenient index of current nutritional status, while height for age better represents past nutritional status. In this context of classifying the severity of PEM, **wasting** has been suggested as a term for a deficit in weight for height, and the term **stunting** has been suggested for a deficit in height for age. Patients with PEM can be placed in one of four categories: normal; wasted but not stunted (indicating acute PEM); wasted and stunted (indicating acute and chronic PEM); or stunted but not wasted (indicating past PEM with adequate nutrition at present).[6] The severity of wasting can be determined by calculating weight as a percentage of the reference median weight for height using the following equation:

$$\% \text{ weight for height} = \frac{\text{Actual body weight}}{\text{Reference weight for height}} \times 100$$

where reference weight for height = the median (or 50th percentile) weight for height for the subject's age and sex. To determine the severity of stunting, calculate the height as a percentage of the reference height for age using the following equation:

$$\% \text{ height for age} = \frac{\text{Actual height or length}}{\text{Reference height for age}} \times 100$$

where reference height for age = the median (or 50th percentile) height for the subject's age and sex. The values derived from these equations can then be compared with the reference values shown in Table 10.4 to classify the severity of wasting or stunting.

A simple approach to assessing the severity of PEM in an adult is to compare his or her body mass index (kg/m^2) (see Chapter 6) with the reference values shown in Table 10.5. The table also gives values for determining the presence of PEM in adolescents but does not allow the

TABLE 10.4	Reference Values for Classifying Deficits in Weight for Height and Height for Age*	
Classification	**Weight for Height[†]** **(Deficit = Wasting)**	**Height for Age[†]** **(Deficit = Stunting)**
Normal	90% to 110%	95% to 105%
Mild deficit	80% to 89%	90% to 94%
Moderate deficit	75% to 79%	85% to 89%
Severe deficit	< 75% or with edema	< 85%

Source: Torun B. 2006. Protein-energy malnutrition. In Shils ME, Shike M, Ross AC, Cabellero B, Cousins RJ (eds.), *Modern nutrition in health and disease,* 10th ed. Philadelphia: Lippincott Williams & Wilkins, 881–908.

*Reference values for classifying the severity of deficits in weight for height (wasting) are derived using the percentage of reference median weight for height, and deficits in height for age (stunting) are derived using the percentage of reference median height for age. Median weight for height and median height for age are derived from the CDC growth charts (see Chapter 6).

[†]Percentage calculated from equations discussed in the text.

TABLE 10.5	Reference Values for Classifying the Severity of Protein-Energy Malnutrition (PEM) in Adult Males and Females and the Presence of PEM in Adolescent Males and Females	
Subject Age	**Body Mass Index**	**PEM**
18 years and older	< 16.0	Severe
	16.0–16.9	Moderate
	17.0–18.4	Mild
	≥ 18.5	Not present
14–17 years old	14.5– < 16.5	Present
	< 14.5	Severe
11–13 years old	13.5– < 15.0	Present
	< 13.5	Severe

Source: Torun B. 2006. Protein-energy malnutrition. In Shils ME, Shike M, Ross AC, Cabellero B, Cousins RJ (eds.), *Modern nutrition in health and disease,* 10th ed. Philadelphia: Lippincott Williams & Wilkins, 881–908.

severity of PEM in this age group to be assessed.[8] These values can be used for either males or females.

HIV INFECTION

Nutritional alterations are common in persons infected with the human immunodeficiency virus (HIV), the cause of acquired immunodeficiency syndrome, or AIDS. Since the height of the epidemic in the mid-1980s, the annual number of new HIV infections in the United States has been reduced by more than two-thirds. At the same time, treatment advances since the late 1990s have dramatically increased the number of people living with HIV (www.aids.gov). Of the 1.2 million Americans living with HIV, an estimated 87% have been diagnosed, but less than half have their virus under control.

Before the development of HIV antiretroviral drugs for treating HIV infection, a common feature of patients with AIDS was PEM characterized by marked weight loss and depletion of body cell mass, a condition known as HIV wasting syndrome.[11-13] During this era, more than 60% of HIV-positive patients presented with PEM, and, in roughly 80% of deaths attributed to AIDS, protein-energy malnutrition was considered a concurrent cause of death.[13] Since AIDS was first recognized in 1981, remarkable progress has been made in developing antiretroviral agents for treating HIV infection and AIDS. Nearly half of the 37 million people worldwide living with HIV/AIDS are accessing antiretroviral therapy (www.aids.gov). These drugs have improved the quality and duration of life of HIV-infected persons in the industrialized world and have led to decreased incidence of the severe malnutrition characteristic of HIV wasting syndrome, although altered body fat distribution, loss of lean body mass or fat-free mass, and metabolic alterations are still common in these HIV patients. In some older HIV-infected patients, overweight and obesity with loss of fat-free mass occurs.[11-15]

HIV wasting syndrome is typically characterized by the disproportionate loss of lean body mass and muscle wasting with relative preservation of fat mass.[15,16] The U.S. Centers for Disease Control and Prevention's definition of HIV wasting syndrome is shown in Box 10.3 within the context of the 2007 World Health Organization's clinical staging of HIV/AIDS for adults and adolescents. Wasting is of considerable concern because it is associated with increased morbidity in people with AIDS.[12] It results in physical impairment, psychologic stress, decreased tolerance of therapeutic agents, increased susceptibility to infection, and overall diminished quality of life. The known adverse effects of malnutrition on immune function also suggest that wasting may independently affect the progression of AIDS. Prevention of HIV wasting and preservation of body weight (both adipose tissue and lean tissue mass) may enhance survival, enhance physical and social functioning, and enrich the quality of life of people with AIDS.[11,12,14] Although HIV wasting is a multifactorial condition, the causes can be categorized under three general headings: decreased food intake, increased nutrient requirements, and nutrient malabsorption. These are outlined in Table 10.6.

Wasting syndrome can be treated by a proper diet, medications to stimulate appetite and control diarrhea, and hormonal therapy to build muscle (www.aids.gov). Good nutrition is especially important to those living with and being treated for HIV because of the potential for related conditions (wasting syndrome, diarrhea, nausea, vomiting, lipodystrophy, lipid abnormalities, insulin resistance, and immune suppression) and the need to maintain strength, energy, and a healthy immune system. Food safety and proper hygiene are a concern to prevent infections.

With the introduction of protease inhibitors in 1996 and even newer antiretroviral therapies in more recent years, the number of patients dying from AIDS in developed countries has decreased, the prognosis of HIV-infected patients in these countries has dramatically improved, and HIV wasting syndrome is no longer the AIDS terminal phase.[13] Despite these dramatic improvements, some people with AIDS experience marked changes in body fat distribution (referred to as lipodystrophy) and certain metabolic alterations, such as hyperlipidemia, insulin resistance, and diabetes mellitus.[13,15,16] These changes in body fat distribution include fat accumulation (lipohypertrophy) in the abdominal region (truncal and visceral obesity), in the axillary pads (bilateral symmetric lipomatosis), and in the dorsocervical pads at the posterior base of the neck (referred to by some as "buffalo hump" or "bull neck") and loss of fat (lipoatrophy) in the arms, legs, and nasolabial and cheek pads (peripheral lipodystrophy).[13] It appears that these alterations in body fat distribution are due, at least in part, to certain metabolic changes brought about by the multiple drugs used to treat HIV infection.[13-18] The so-called buffalo hump is also a clinical feature of Cushing's syndrome, a combination of symptoms and signs resulting from a persistent elevation of serum glucocorticosteroids. Unlike the loss of facial fat seen in patients presenting with peripheral lipodystrophy, a characteristic feature of Cushing's syndrome is a fullness or roundness of the face, which is referred to as "moon face."

Because changes in the distribution of body fat and increased adiposity can occur at the same time as decreased fat-free mass in patients with HIV/AIDS, changes in weight and BMI alone may not be suitable indicators of nutritional status. Approaches to assessing body fat distribution, somatic muscle status, and body composition will be required in some instances to evaluate a patient's nutritional status and response to HIV/AIDS therapy and

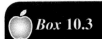

| Box 10.3 | 2007 WHO Clinical Staging of HIV/AIDS for Adults and Adolescents |

The clinical staging and case definition of HIV for resource-constrained settings were developed by the WHO in 1990 and revised in 2007. Staging is based on clinical findings that guide the diagnosis, evaluation, and management of HIV/AIDS, and it does not require a CD4 cell count (the basis of the CDC system). This staging system is used in many countries to determine eligibility for antiretroviral therapy, particularly in settings in which CD4 testing is not available. Clinical stages are categorized as 1 through 4, progressing from primary HIV infection to advanced HIV/AIDS. These stages are defined by specific clinical conditions or symptoms. For the purpose of the WHO staging system, adolescents and adults are defined as individuals aged ≥ 15 years.

PRIMARY HIV INFECTION

- Asymptomatic
- Acute retroviral syndrome

CLINICAL STAGE 1

- Asymptomatic
- Persistent generalized lymphadenopathy
- Moderate unexplained weight loss (< 10% of presumed or measured body weight)
- Recurrent respiratory infections (sinusitis, tonsillitis, otitis media, and pharyngitis)
- Herpes zoster

CLINICAL STAGE 2

- *Constellation of symptoms and medical problems, including* angular cheilitis, recurrent oral ulceration, papular pruritic eruptions, seborrheic dermatitis, fungal nail infections, unexplained severe weight loss (> 10% of presumed or measured body weight), unexplained chronic diarrhea for more than one month, unexplained persistent fever for more than one month (> 37.6°C, intermittent or constant), persistent oral candidiasis (thrush), oral hairy leukoplakia

CLINICAL STAGE 3

- *Constellation of symptoms and medical problems, including* pulmonary tuberculosis (current), severe presumed bacterial infections (e.g., pneumonia, empyema, pyomyositis, bone or joint infection, meningitis, bacteremia), acute necrotizing ulcerative stomatitis, gingivitis, or periodontitis, unexplained anemia (hemoglobin < 8 g/dL), neutropenia (neutrophils < 500 cells/μL), chronic thrombocytopenia (platelets < 50,000 cells/μL), **HIV wasting syndrome,** * pneumocystis pneumonia, recurrent severe bacterial pneumonia, chronic herpes simplex infection (orolabial, genital, or anorectal site for more than one month or visceral herpes at any site), esophageal candidiasis (or candidiasis of trachea, bronchi, or lungs), extrapulmonary tuberculosis, Kaposi sarcoma, cytomegalovirus infection (retinitis or infection of other organs), central nervous system toxoplasmosis, HIV encephalopathy, cryptococcosis, extrapulmonary (including meningitis)

CLINICAL STAGE 4

- *Constellation of symptoms and medical problems, including* disseminated nontuberculosis mycobacteria infection; progressive multifocal leukoencephalopathy; candida of the trachea, bronchi, or lungs; chronic cryptosporidiosis (with diarrhea); chronic isosporiasis; disseminated mycosis (e.g., histoplasmosis, coccidioidomycosis, penicilliosis); recurrent nontyphoidal *Salmonella* bacteremia; lymphoma (cerebral or B-cell non-Hodgkin); invasive cervical carcinoma; atypical disseminated leishmaniasis; symptomatic HIV-associated nephropathy; symptomatic HIV-associated cardiomyopathy; reactivation of American trypanosomiasis (meningoencephalitis or myocarditis)

*CDC definition: wasting syndrome caused by HIV (involuntary weight loss > 10% of baseline body weight) associated with either chronic diarrhea (two or more loose stools per day for ≥ 1 month) or chronic weakness and documented fever for ≥ 1 month.

Source: World Health Organization. 2007. WHO case definitions of HIV for surveillance and revised clinical staging and immunological classification of HIV-related disease in adults and children.

nutritional support.[15,16,19] Approaches that can be used to monitor changes in body fat distribution include waist circumference, waist-to-hip ratio, skinfold measurements, dual-energy X-ray absorptiometry (DXA), and computed tomography. Somatic or skeletal muscle status can be assessed using midarm circumference, arm muscle area, the creatinine-height index, and computed tomography. Changes in body composition can be assessed using skinfold measurements, bioelectrical impedance analysis, DXA, and computed tomography.[15,16,19]

EATING DISORDERS

Anorexia nervosa and bulimia nervosa are conditions in which a disturbance in eating behavior and body dissatisfaction develop. Both have clinical signs aiding in their diagnosis. In the United States, 20 million women and 10 million men suffer from a clinically significant eating disorder at some time in their life, including anorexia nervosa, bulimia nervosa, binge eating disorder, or other specified feeding or eating disorder (OSFED)

TABLE 10.6	Causes of and Contributing Factors for HIV Wasting Syndrome

Causes	Contributing Factors
Decreased Food Intake	
Loss of appetite	Nausea, vomiting, medications, altered taste; anorexia caused by the effects of cytokines, such as tissue necrosis factor, interleukin-1, and interferon; the presence of undigested micronutrients in ileum and colon may also depress appetite
Difficulty chewing and swallowing	Mouth and throat sores from Kaposi sarcoma and opportunistic infections, such as candidiasis and herpes simplex; esophageal ulcers of viral, mycobacterial, and neoplastic origin; neurologic disease
Decreased interest in eating	Depression, ostracism, isolation, loneliness
Inability to prepare meals	Lack of access to food, poverty, profound weakness, AIDS-induced dementia
Increased Nutrient Requirements	
Hypermetabolism	Resting metabolic rate is generally increased in persons with AIDS unless severe wasting is present; loss of adipose tissue and negative nitrogen balance are exacerbated by near-normal serum levels of the thyroid hormone triiodothyronine (T_3) that ordinarily fall below normal in the presence of malnutrition and wasting
Fever	Opportunistic infections of viral, mycobacterial, and neoplastic origin
Nutrient Malabsorption	
Diarrhea	Occurs in > 50% of persons with AIDS; many cases apparently caused by protozoal infections
Inflammation of bowel mucosa	Protozoal infections (cryptosporidiosis and microsporidiosis) appear to result in malabsorption apart from diarrhea; deficiency of lactase and disaccharidase activity seen; HIV alone may affect the structure and function of the small bowel

Sources: Oster MH, Enders SR, Samuels SJ, Cone LA, Hooton TM, Browder HP, Flynn NM. 1994. Megestrol acetate in patients with AIDS and cachexia. _Annals of Internal Medicine_ 121:400–408; Von Roenn JH, Armstrong D, Kotler DP, Cohn DL, Klimas NG, Tchekmedyian NS, Cone L, Brennan PJ, Weitzman SA. 1994. Megestrol acetate in patients with AIDS-related cachexia. _Annals of Internal Medicine_ 121:393–399; Hecker LM, Kotler DP. 1990. Malnutrition in patients with AIDS. _Nutrition Reviews_ 48:393–401; Singer P, Katz DP, Dillon L, Kirvelä O, Lazarus T, Askanazi J. 1992. Nutritional aspects of the acquired immunodeficiency syndrome. _American Journal of Gastroenterology_ 87:265–273.

(www.nationaleatingdisorder.org). Anorexia nervosa is characterized by a refusal to maintain a minimally normal body weight, an intense fear of gaining weight that is not alleviated by losing weight, and a distorted perception of body shape or size in which a person feels overweight (either globally or in certain body areas) despite being markedly underweight.[20] Diagnostic criteria, signs and symptoms, and potential medical consequences for anorexia nervosa are shown in Box 10.4. A prominent clinical feature of persons with anorexia nervosa is marked weight loss, which in some instances can become extreme and life threatening. Figure 10.7 gives an example of the severe wasting commonly seen in persons with anorexia nervosa.

Bulimia nervosa is characterized by episodes of binging (eating unusually large amounts of food in a discrete period of time), followed by some behavior to prevent weight gain, such as purging (usually self-induced vomiting but also including misuse of laxatives, diuretics, enemas, or other medications), fasting, or excessive exercise.[20–23] Diagnostic criteria, signs and symptoms, and medical consequences for bulimia nervosa are shown in Box 10.5. Persons with bulimia nervosa are usually within the normal weight range, although some may be slightly underweight or overweight. Recurrent vomiting

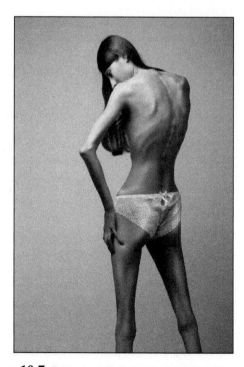

Figure 10.7 Severe wasting seen in a person with anorexia nervosa.
©Denis Putilov/Alamy Stock Photo RF

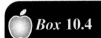

Box 10.4 | **Diagnostic Criteria, Signs and Symptoms, and Medical Complications for Anorexia Nervosa**

DIAGNOSTIC CRITERIA

A. Energy Intake Restriction

- Restriction of energy intake relative to requirement
- Leads to a significantly low body weight in the context of age, sex, developmental trajectory, and physical health

B. Fear of Weight Gain

- Intense fear of gaining weight or of becoming fat
- Or persistent behavior that interferes with weight gain, even though at a significantly low weight

C. Disturbed Self-evaluation of Body Weight or Shape

- Disturbance in the way in which one's body weight or shape is experienced
- Undue influence of body weight or shape on self-evaluation
- Or persistent lack of recognition of the seriousness of the current low body weight

SIGNS AND SYMPTOMS OF ANOREXIA NERVOSA

Weight and Shape Concerns

- Dramatic weight loss, or failure to make expected weight gains during periods of normal growth
- Excessive weighing and setting progressively lower and lower goal weights
- Body checking behaviors (looking in mirrors, assessing body parts, asking "do I look fat?")
- Changes in weight leading to significant impact on mood and self-evaluation
- Frequent comments about feeling "fat" and focus on "fat" body parts
- Excessive exercise
- Intense fear of weight gain
- Inability to appreciate the severity of the situation

Food and Eating Behaviors

- Denial of hunger, dieting, restricting food intake
- Rigid calorie and fat gram counting

- Refusal to eat certain foods and entire food categories
- Collecting or hoarding recipes
- Cooking but not eating elaborate meals
- Development of strange food rituals
- Possible use of laxatives, diet aids, or herbal weight loss products
- Consistent excuses to avoid mealtimes

Changes in Personality and Social Behavior

- Heightened tendency toward high achievement and perfectionism
- Increasing isolation and withdrawal from friends and enjoyable activities
- Symptoms of depression, anxiety, irritability, moodiness
- Interpersonal conflicts and defensive stance when confronted
- Low energy and fatigue
- Use of pro-Ana websites (which support anorexia)
- Wearing layers or baggy clothes to hide weight loss and keep warm

MEDICAL COMPLICATIONS OF ANOREXIA NERVOSA

- Abnormally slow heart rate and low blood pressure
- Heart damage with potential for heart failure and death (5–20% death rate)
- Reduction of bone density (osteopenia and osteoporosis)
- Muscle loss and weakness, fatigue, fainting
- Severe dehydration and potential for kidney failure
- Edema
- Dry skin and hair, brittle hair and nails, hair loss
- Anemia
- Severe constipation
- Children may have arrested sexual maturity and growth failure
- Drop in internal body temperature and growth of a downy layer of hair
- Amenorrhea and infertility
- Increased risk for suicide

Sources: https://www.nationaleatingdisorders.org and www.eatingdisorder.org.

may erode the teeth, especially the lingual surfaces of the front teeth, and increase the incidence of dental caries. There may also be noticeable enlargement of the salivary glands, particularly the parotid glands. Binge eating disorder is now a separate diagnosable eating disorder, and is characterized by large quantity eating episodes that occur at least once a week for three months. The binge eating episodes typically occur quickly and to the point of discomfort accompanied by feelings of a loss of control, shame, and distress or guilt afterwards.

Compensatory measures (e.g., purging) are usually not engaged in to counter the binge eating.

Another category of disordered eating is called Other Specified Feeding and Eating Disorders (OSFED) and is applied when an individual's symptoms cause significant distress but do not fit neatly within the strict criteria for anorexia or bulimia. OSFED includes atypical anorexia nervosa with weight loss but normal weight, bulimia nervosa of low frequency and duration, binge eating disorder of low frequency and duration, purging disorder, and night eating syndrome.

Box 10.5   Diagnostic Criteria, Signs, and Symptoms for Bulimia Nervosa

A. Recurrent episodes of binge eating. An episode of binge eating is characterized by both of the following:

   (1) Eating, in a discrete period (e.g., within any two-hour period), an amount of food that is definitely larger than most people would eat during a similar period of time and under similar circumstances

   (2) A sense of lack of control over eating during the episode

B. Recurrent inappropriate compensatory behavior (such as self-induced vomiting, misuse of laxatives, fasting, or excessive exercise) in order to prevent weight gain

C. The binge eating and inappropriate compensatory behaviors both occur, on average, at least once a week for three months

D. Self-evaluation is unduly influenced by body shape and weight

E. The disturbance does not occur exclusively during episodes of anorexia nervosa

SIGNS AND SYMPTOMS OF BULIMIA NERVOSA

Weight and Shape Concerns

- Preoccupation with weight and body shape; dramatic weight fluctuations up or down
- Frequently or excessively weighing oneself
- Changes in weight, even slight fluctuations, have a significant impact on mood, self-esteem, and self-evaluation; negative and self-critical comments about one's body/weight
- Excessive exercise despite weather, fatigue, illness, or injury

Food and Eating Behaviors

- Evidence of binge eating (food and medication disappearance and packaging).
- Eating until the point of discomfort or pain.
- Frequent trips to the bathroom immediately after meals; signs or smells of vomiting.

- Eating volume swings (fasting then binging).
- Avoiding mealtimes or social situations involving food; eating alone or in secret; hiding food.
- Unusual swelling of the cheeks or jaw area.
- Calluses on the back of the hands and knuckles from self-induced vomiting.

Changes in Personality and Social Behavior

- Changing rituals to make time for binge-and-purge sessions
- Withdrawal from usual friends and activities
- Behaviors that food control is a primary concern
- Symptoms of depression and anxiety; irritability or fluctuating moods
- Substance abuse
- Signs of self-injury
- Lying about food or making up excuses
- Interpersonal conflicts; defensive stance when confronted
- Low energy and fatigue

HEALTH CONSEQUENCES AND MEDICAL COMPLICATIONS

- Severe dehydration and electrolyte imbalances (can lead to irregular heartbeats, heart failure, and death)
- Chronically inflamed and sore throat; inflammation and possible rupture of the esophagus
- Potential for gastric rupture
- Decalcification of teeth, enamel loss, staining, severe tooth decay and gum disease
- Edema (swelling)
- Chronic irregular bowel movements, constipation and other gastrointestinal problems
- Peptic ulcers and pancreatitis
- Swollen, enlarged salivary glands in the neck and jaw area
- Acid reflux disorder
- Infertility, increased rates of miscarriage and other fetal complications

Note: Online eating disorders assessment tools are available at https://www.eatingdisorder.org/eating-disorder-information/online-self-assessment, http://www.mybodyscreening.org/, http://foodaddictioninstitute.org/Publications/Assessment-Acorn-Eating-Disorder-Inventory.pdf, http://www.eat-26.com/, http://ceed.org.au/wp-content/uploads/2012/05/scoffqairehandout.pdf.

Sources: https://www.nationaleatingdisorders.org and www.eatingdisorder.org

SUMMARY

1. The first step in the clinical assessment of nutritional status is obtaining a patient's history. This includes pertinent facts about past and current health and use of medications, as well as personal and household information. Sources include the patient's medical record and data obtained directly from the patient or those familiar with the patient.

2. A diet history is valuable in understanding a patient's nutritional status. This includes information about a patient's usual eating pattern, food likes and dislikes, and intolerances and allergies, as well as money available for purchasing food, ability to obtain and prepare food, eligibility for and access to food assistance programs, and use of vitamin, mineral, and other supplements.

3. Subjective Global Assessment is a clinical technique for assessing the nutritional status of a patient based on features of the patient's history and physical examination, rather than relying on more objective measures of nutritional status, such as anthropometric and biochemical data.

4. In severe PEM, the conditions known as kwashiorkor and marasmus are seen. Kwashiorkor is predominantly a protein deficiency characterized by a relatively normal weight, generally intact skeletal musculature, decreased concentrations of serum proteins, and edema. Marasmus is mainly an energy deficiency characterized by significant loss of body weight, skeletal muscle, and adipose tissue mass, but with serum protein concentrations relatively intact and no edema.

5. Severe cases of PEM and wasting can result from AIDS, certain cancers, some gastrointestinal diseases, and alcoholism and other drug abuse. The emaciation and general ill health seen in these diseases are sometimes called cachexia.

6. Growth failure and flag sign are two conditions seen in severe PEM. The flag sign is characterized by alternating bands of depigmented and normal-colored hair produced by alternating periods of poor and relatively good protein intake. Growth failure, a failure to gain weight and height at the expected rate, is the most common sign of malnutrition in children.

7. The severity of PEM in children and adolescents can be assessed by calculating weight as a percentage of reference median weight for height and by calculating height as a percentage of reference height for age. These two values can then be compared with published guidelines. The severity of PEM in an adult can be assessed by comparing body mass index (kg/m^2) with the reference values.

8. Prior to the development of HIV antiretroviral drugs for treating HIV infection, HIV wasting was a common feature of patients with AIDS. Although advances in HIV/AIDS drug treatment have led to decreased incidence of HIV wasting syndrome, altered metabolism and body fat distribution remain common in HIV patients, particularly those treated with protease inhibitors. Metabolic alterations include hyperlipidemia, insulin resistance, and diabetes mellitus. Changes in body fat distribution include fat accumulation in the abdominal region (truncal and visceral obesity) and in the dorsocervical pads of the neck ("buffalo hump" or "bull neck") and loss of fat in the arms, legs, and nasolabial and cheek pads (peripheral lipodystrophy).

9. Anorexia nervosa is characterized by a refusal to maintain a minimally normal body weight, an intense fear of gaining weight, and a distorted perception of body shape or size. Bulimia nervosa is characterized by episodes of binging, followed by some behavior to prevent weight gain, such as purging, fasting, or exercising excessively.

REFERENCES

1. Corish CA, Kennedy NP. 2000. Protein-energy undernutrition in hospital in-patients. *British Journal of Nutrition* 83:575–591.

2. Dwyer J. 2012. Nutrient requirements and dietary assessment. In Longo DL, Fauci AS, Kasper DL, Hauser SL, Jameson JL, Loscalzo J (eds.), *Harrison's principles of internal medicine,* 18th ed. New York: McGraw-Hill, 588–593.

3. Charney P, Malone AM. 2009. *ADA pocket guide to nutrition assessment,* 2nd ed. Chicago: American Dietetic Association.

4. Detsky AS, Smalley PS, Change J. 1994. Is this patient malnourished? *Journal of the American Medical Association* 271:54–58.

5. Gupta D, Lammersfeld CA, Vashi PG, Burrows J, Lis CG, Grutsch JF. 2005. Prognostic significance of Subjective Global Assessment (SGA) in advanced colorectal cancer. *European Journal of Clinical Nutrition* 59:35–40.

6. Makhija S, Baker J. 2008. The Subjective Global Assessment: A review of its use in clinical practice. *Nutrition in Clinical Practice* 23:405–409.

7. Keith JN. 2008. Bedside nutrition assessment past, present, and future: A review of the Subjective Global Assessment. *Nutrition in Clinical Practice* 23:410–416.

8. Torun B. 2006. Protein-energy malnutrition. In Shils ME, Shike M, Ross AC, Cabellero B, Cousins RJ (eds.), *Modern nutrition in health and disease,* 10th ed. Philadelphia: Lippincott Williams & Wilkins, 881–908.

9. Heimburger DC. 2012. Malnutrition and nutritional assessment. In Longo DL, Fauci AS, Kasper DL, Hauser SL, Jameson JL, Loscalzo J (eds.), *Harrison's principles of internal medicine,* 18th ed. New York: McGraw-Hill, 605–612.

10. McLaren DS. 1992. *A colour atlas and text of diet-related disorders,* 2nd ed. London: Mosby Europe.

11. Kotler DP. 2000. Nutritional alterations associated with HIV infection. *Journal of Acquired Immune Deficiency Syndromes* 25:S81–S87.

12. Semba RD. 2006. Nutrition and infection. In Shils ME, Shike M, Ross AC, Cabellero B, Cousins RJ (eds.), *Modern nutrition in health and disease,* 10th ed. Philadelphia: Lippincott Williams & Wilkins, 1401–1413.

13. Scevola D, DiMatteo A, Uberti F, Minoia G, Poletti F, Faga A. 2000. Reversal of cachexia in patients treated with potent antiretroviral therapy. *AIDS Reader* 10:365–369.

14. Fauci AS, Lane HC. 2012. Human immunodeficiency virus disease: AIDS and related disorders. In Longo DL, Fauci AS, Kasper DL, Hauser SL, Jameson JL, Loscalzo J (eds.), *Harrison's principles of internal medicine,* 18th ed. New York: McGraw-Hill, 1506–1587.

15. Thibault R, Cano N, Pichard C. 2011. Quantification of lean tissue losses during cancer and HIV infection/AIDS. *Current Opinion in Clinical Nutrition and Metabolic Care* 14:261–267.

16. Moreno S, Miralles C, Negredo E, Domingo P, Estrada V, Gutierrez F, Lozano F, Martinez E. 2009. Disorders of body fat distribution in HIV-1-infected patients. *AIDS Reviews* 11:126–134.

17. Engleson ES, Kotler DP, Tan YX, Agin D, Wang J, Pierson RN, Heymsfield SB. 1999. Fat distribution in HIV-infected patients reporting truncal enlargement quantified by whole-body magnetic resonance imaging. *American Journal of Clinical Nutrition* 69:1162–1169.

18. Peters W, Phillips A. 1999. Buffalo hump and HIV-1 infection: Current concepts and treatment of a patient with the use of suction-assisted lipectomy. *Canadian Journal of Plastic Surgery* 7:129–131.

19. Ruiz M, Kamerman LA. 2010. Nutritional screening tools for HIV-infected patients: Implications for elderly patients. *Journal of the International Association of Physicians in AIDS Care* 9:362–367.

20. American Psychiatric Association. 2013. *Diagnostic and statistical manual of mental disorders,* 5th ed. Arlington, VA: American Psychiatric Publishing.

21. American Psychiatric Association. 2006. *Practice guideline for the treatment of patients with eating disorders,* 3rd ed. Washington, DC: American Psychiatric Association.

22. Williams PM, Goodie J, Motsinger CD. 2008. Treating eating disorders in primary care. *American Family Physician* 77:187–195.

23. Weaver L, Liebman R. 2011. Assessment of anorexia nervosa in children and adolescents. *Current Psychiatry Reports* 13:93–98.

ASSESSMENT ACTIVITY 10.1

Using Subjective Global Assessment

This assessment activity gives you an opportunity to practice using Subjective Global Assessment (SGA), a clinical technique for assessing nutritional status using data from a patient's history and physical examination, both of which can be found in a patient's medical record. Begin by making two photocopies of the SGA rating form found in Figure 10.1. Then, using the information from each of the following two cases, complete the chart and arrive at an SGA rating of each patient's nutritional status. You may find it helpful to review the section "Subjective Global Assessment," which explains SGA.

The following cases are straightforward; you and your classmates should arrive at the same rating for each case. However, because of the subjective nature of this approach, there may be an occasional instance when two or more health professionals do not arrive at the same rating of one patient's nutritional status. This should not detract from the usefulness of SGA because clinicians generally arrive at decisions by carefully evaluating the available evidence in light of professional knowledge and past experiences. Thus, health care is not only a science but also an art.

Case 1

A 73-year-old female is admitted to the hospital complaining of loss of appetite and rapid onset of satiety for 6 weeks. For the past 3 days, she has vomited practically all food and beverages consumed. She is ambulatory but has felt weak and has been unable to carry out her activities of daily living for the past 2 weeks. On physical examination, the woman looks somewhat wasted with moderate loss of subcutaneous tissue in the upper arms, shoulders, and thoracic regions. There is moderate edema in the ankles but no ascites present. For the past 10 years or so, her body weight has been stable at approximately 147 lb (66.8 kg). However, in the past 4 months or so, she has steadily lost weight. Her current weight is 123 lb (55.9 kg). Using SGA, how would you rate her nutritional status?

Case 2

A 61-year-old male is admitted to the hospital for resection of his sigmoid colon and rectum, following discovery of a mass in the sigmoid colon by his physician during a flexible sigmoidoscopy. The patient originally complained of bright red blood in his bowel movements. He reported no significant gastrointestinal symptoms other than the bleeding. He denies any change in his functional capacity. His maximum weight was 167 lb (75.9 kg) at age 46 years. In his late 40s, he lost about 15 lb (6.8 kg) and for the past 12 years has maintained his weight at about 152 lb (69.1 kg). Between 2 and 6 months before admission, his appetite was less than normal and he gradually lost 13 lb (5.9 kg). In the past 2 months before admission, his appetite improved and he gained 5 lb (2.3 kg). On physical examination, there is no evidence of subcutaneous tissue loss, muscle wasting, edema, or ascites.

ASSESSMENT ACTIVITY 10.2

Assessment of Eating Disorders

As reviewed in this chapter, there are several online assessment tools for eating disorders. Go to each of the websites listed below, and enter your personal information. Prepare a one-page summary describing each assessment tool and which one you feel is best.

Online eating disorders assessment tools are available at https://www.eatingdisorder.org/eating-disorder-information/online-self-assessment

http://www.mybodyscreening.org/

http://foodaddictioninstitute.org/Publications/Assessment-Acorn-Eating-Disorder-Inventory.pdf

http://www.eat-26.com/

http://ceed.org.au/wp-content/uploads/2012/05/scoffqairehandout.pdf

Excellent clinical case histories are available online. Review this clinical case of an obese woman seeking treatment for binge eating. Bring notes to the class for discussion.

https://www.ncbi.nlm.nih.gov/pmc/articles/PMC2860740/

11 COUNSELING THEORY AND TECHNIQUE

STUDENT LEARNING OUTCOMES

After studying this chapter, the student will be able to:

1. Describe the communication model.
2. Name the six steps of listening.
3. Differentiate between open questions and closed questions.
4. Discuss the key concepts of the major counseling theories.
5. Name the characteristics of effective counselors.
6. Identify instances when a patient should be referred to someone else for counseling.

INTRODUCTION

Awareness of nutritional status and dietary practices obtained through nutritional assessment often is followed by attempts to change dietary behavior. This chapter provides a brief introduction to several counseling theories that provide a variety of useful techniques for initiating and maintaining dietary change.

The purpose of this chapter is *not* to teach you how to be a therapist. It is intended to briefly introduce you to those theories that are most pertinent to nutritional counseling and to acquaint you with some fundamental approaches to counseling your clients. The most effective counselors are those who adapt techniques from several counseling theories to suit their needs and those of their individual clients. As you study this chapter, note the different counseling theories and techniques. Then, based on your professional judgment, use those techniques you feel are best suited to you and the needs of your clients.

Because communication lies at the foundation of interviewing and counseling, the first part of this chapter deals with fundamentals of communication theory and basic skills necessary for effective listening and interviewing. The chapter ends with a practical plan for initiating and maintaining dietary change.

Finally, as important as good nutrition is to health, do not lose sight of the fact that other practices, such as cigarette smoking, physical inactivity, and excessive alcohol use, have a profound impact on health. Cigarette smoking, for example, has been called the "leading cause of preventable death in the United States" and is responsible for more than 480,000 deaths every year in the United States.[1] You should be a model of good health habits, not only those relating to diet but in all areas. By so doing, you will be most effective in helping your clients achieve better health.

COMMUNICATION

Communication is the process of sending and receiving messages. It lies at the foundation of all efforts to interview, counsel, educate, and change behavior. Although we all communicate (or at least attempt to) and have a basic idea of what it involves, communication is a complex process and is not easily defined. The simplified communication model in Figure 11.1 shows the major components of human communication: sender, receiver, message, and feedback.

The *sender* is the one initiating the communication, the first person to speak. The *message* is the communication. It contains components that are both verbal (what is spoken) and nonverbal (what is implied by the emotional tone of the sender's voice, facial expression, posture, diction, pronunciation, choice of words, dress, and the environment in which the communication occurs).[2] Verbal and nonverbal communication occur simultaneously. The *receiver* is the listener, the one to whom the message is sent. *Feedback* is the response the receiver gives to messages after interpreting them. Feedback distinguishes one-way communication from two-way communication.[2] The absence of feedback or making no provision for it will likely result in distorted communication because the sender is unable to determine how the message was received. As with the message, feedback is both verbal and nonverbal.

Interference is anything adversely affecting transmission or interpretation of the message. It can arise from the environment or the emotional or physiologic state of either the sender or the receiver. Noise, lack of privacy, interruptions, an office that is too hot or too cold, and uncomfortable seating are examples of environmental factors that may cause interference. Emotional factors leading to interference include fear of disease or death, loneliness, grief, prejudice, and bias. Physiologic factors such as pain, deficits of hearing or vision, and difficulty in speaking can often be sources of interference.

Verbal Communication

Dietary counseling generally involves some type of behavioral change on the receiver's part. The receiver may perceive attempts to change lifelong habits or practices he or she enjoys as a potential threat. Thus, the receiver may become defensive, which interferes with good communication. The receiver's defensive reactions can be prevented or minimized through the use of the guidelines to supportive communication outlined in Box 11.1 and the following paragraphs. The more supportive communication is, the less the receiver perceives it as a threat and the more he or she is able to concentrate on the structure, content, and meaning of the message.[2]

Describe behavior rather than evaluate it. Discussing a client's behavior in a judgmental or evaluative way will likely cause the client to become defensive. The client will then be thinking of ways to defend himself or herself rather than concentrating on the counselor's message. Evaluating or judging behavior can lead to an argument. Instead, the counselor can present the facts or seek information in objective, nonjudgmental ways that do not imply guilt or ask the client to change his or her behavior.

For example, in an attempt to raise awareness of the seriousness of the problem at hand, a counselor may accuse a client with poorly controlled diabetes of being "irresponsible" or "committing suicide." A better approach would be to objectively discuss the client's blood sugar levels and nonjudgmentally discuss factors that may be affecting them.

Use problem orientation rather than manipulation. Much of our speech is an attempt to persuade others to alter their behavior, attitudes, or activities. Often, when we want people to see things our way, we lead them through a series of questions until they arrive at the "correct conclusion." This is a form of manipulation and implies that the person being directed is inadequate or inferior. This is likely to result in a defensive response that interferes with communication. Problem orientation, on the other hand, is the antithesis of persuasion. The sender communicates a desire to work with the receiver

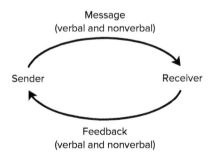

Message
(verbal and nonverbal)

Sender   Receiver

Feedback
(verbal and nonverbal)

Figure 11.1 A communication model.

 Box 11.1   Guidelines to More Supportive Communication

Description rather than evaluation
Problem orientation rather than manipulation
Equality rather than superiority

Empathy rather than neutrality
Provisionalism rather than certainty

in defining a mutual problem and seeking a workable solution. The sender implies that he or she has no prearranged answer or viewpoint and no hidden agenda to exert control over the receiver. Thus, the receiver arrives at his or her own conclusions and establishes goals and objectives to which there will be greater adherence.

Communicate equality rather than superiority. A sender can promote supportive communication by considering himself or herself a collaborator with or an equal to the receiver. When treated with respect and trust and involved in participative problem solving, the receiver will feel more obligated to the success of any agreed-on solution. If the sender communicates superiority, the receiver will likely become defensive. Although clients often need and appreciate the reassurance of a dietitian's nutritional expertise, dietitians should avoid urging a particular plan of action based primarily on their superior knowledge or ability.

Empathize rather than remain neutral. Communication conveying compassion and respect for others is supportive and defense-reducing. Particularly reassuring is a sender who identifies with the problems and shares in the feelings of the receiver. Communication conveying neutrality may indicate a lack of concern for the receiver's welfare. Attempts to reassure the receiver that he or she is overly anxious or need not feel rejected or bad deny the legitimacy of the receiver's emotions and suggest a lack of acceptance.

Be receptive rather than dogmatic. A willingness to hold one's own attitudes as provisional, to examine other ideas rather than take sides, and to solve problems rather than debate issues gives listeners a sense of participation in and control over the problem-solving process. On the other hand, persons who seem to know all the answers or who regard themselves as teachers rather than team players tend to put others on guard and stifle supportive communication.

Nonverbal Communication

As was shown in Figure 11.1, communication occurs simultaneously on two levels—verbal and nonverbal. Sometimes referred to as *body language,* nonverbal communication in the form of gestures, posture, facial expressions, and tone of voice is sometimes a more reliable indicator of the client's feelings and attitudes than are his or her words.[3] Verbal communication is generally under conscious control and is subject to censorship. It can be used to persuade, mislead, or cover facts a client wishes to hide. Nonverbal communication, on the other hand, is not as easily controlled by conscious thought and often can be a more reliable indicator of a person's dominant emotions than are his or her words.[2,4] Lack of congruence, or agreement, between verbal and nonverbal communication can be an important indicator that a client is consciously or unconsciously omitting something.

Facial expressions are an important source of nonverbal communication. Sadness often can be seen in the face of a distressed client through a downturned mouth or quivering lip. Unusually prolonged and intense eye contact may indicate anger. Guilt, insecurity, or fear may be indicated by failure to maintain eye contact, especially when this occurs during discussion of a particularly sensitive topic.[4]

Posture may indicate a person's feelings. A client seated with arms relaxed at the sides and slightly slouched in the chair can communicate openness, whereas a client may communicate a distrustful, defensive attitude by sitting up very straight with arms tightly crossed over the chest. A client who leans away from the counselor or moves her chair to distance herself may indicate defensiveness or distrust. One leaning closer to the counselor may express a desire for greater intimacy.[3,4] Cultural differences exist in what is considered to be a comfortable distance between two communicating persons. In general, people from Latin cultures prefer being closer, whereas those from North America and parts of Europe favor a somewhat greater distance.[4]

The tone of voice is an important indicator, as well. A client asked about his diet may warmly and pleasantly respond, "It's going well," and mean just that. The same words uttered in a mechanistic and toneless way may indicate a problem with the diet.

Nonverbal communication also facilitates the dietitian's communication to clients. Appropriate eye contact, gestures, facial expressions, and posture assure the client of the dietitian's attention, interest, acceptance, and support. The astute dietitian should carefully note the client's nonverbal cues and their possible significance and use nonverbal communication to respond to the client in a supportive way.[2]

Effective Communication

Effective communication requires consideration of several factors. It is important that messages and feedback be transmitted in ways that are understandable to both sender and receiver. When talking with clients or providing instruction, health professionals should use understandable language and minimize use of medical terminology. Feedback should be encouraged, and the receiver should be given ample opportunity to ask questions and clarify any potential misunderstandings. Both sender and receiver should be aware of their nonverbal communication, so that it supports, rather than interferes with, effective communication.

The environment in which communication takes place should be comfortable, conducive to good communication, and as free as possible of interferences that can adversely affect communication. Adequate time for counseling and client instruction is necessary before clients can even begin to change lifelong habits and adopt new ones. Awareness of the client's abilities, concerns, and fears is also important to effective communication. The dietitian also should be aware of his or her own concerns and limitations and should avoid allowing these to interfere with the communication process.

Consider a dietitian seated at the bedside of a patient in whom diabetes has been recently diagnosed. The dietitian is giving the patient some last-minute instructions on the diabetic exchange system before the patient is discharged. Environmental interference can come from the roommate's television, interruptions from a nurse or physician, a phone call, or the arrival of a visitor. The patient's fear about having diabetes, concerns about being able to manage a new diet, worries about hospitalization costs, and thoughts about what the future holds may preoccupy her mind and interfere with the instruction. The dietitian also may be preoccupied with concerns of his own, such as other patients needing assessment and instruction, and these can interfere with the communication process. This is obviously not an ideal situation for communication or instruction, but, unfortunately, it is one commonly encountered in real life. Awareness of these and other impediments to good communication, however, is necessary before they can be addressed and effectively dealt with.

Listening

Communication is a two-way process. It involves not only *sending* messages but *receiving* them as well. Listening, therefore, is essential to the interviewing and counseling process. In some instances, the best help a counselor can give a client is to simply listen attentively and nonjudgmentally. It is also an excellent way to establish good rapport with a client.[2,4] As important as listening is, most of us are not very good at it.[4] Listening is a highly active process demanding concentration and attention. It involves six steps (Table 11.1).[4]

A number of misconceptions exist about listening.[4] For example, some people believe that *hearing* and *listening* are the same activity. Listening is a process involving much more than simply hearing sounds, such as music or

TABLE 11.1	**The Six Steps of Listening**

1. Hearing: Receiving sound waves by the ear
2. Attending: Mentally focusing on a specific sound
3. Understanding: Interpreting the message and assignment of meaning by the brain
4. Remembering: Storing the message for later use
5. Evaluating: Making an evaluative judgment about the message
6. Responding: Making a verbal and/or nonverbal response to the message

Source: Samovar LA. 2000. *Oral communication: Speaking across cultures,* 11th ed. Los Angeles: Roxbury Publishing Company.

voices. It is mistakenly assumed that, when several people hear the same sound (for example, a person talking), they all receive the same message. Quite the opposite is true. Listening is a highly subjective experience, and the interpretations placed on what is heard can vary widely from person to person.

Some people believe that listening is a passive activity, when in reality it is an active process requiring concentration and specific skills that can be learned if one wants to be a better listener.[4,5] Listening skills can be grouped under four categories: openness, concentration, attention, and comprehension.[3,4]

Openness, or objectivity, involves a willingness to investigate new ideas and to interact with others with minimal internal distortion from personal prejudices. Openness does not necessarily mean acceptance or approval of another's ideas but simply a willingness to "hear a person out." It requires the listener to set aside his or her personal biases, which may interfere with effective listening.[4]

Concentration entails focusing the mind on what the speaker is saying. It is made easier when environmental distractions and interferences are minimized. Counseling should take place in a room that is quiet, comfortable, and private.

It is estimated that people with normal intelligence think about five times faster than they talk.[2] Thus, while listening to another person talk, our minds can simultaneously be thinking other things. Unfortunately, many people have allowed this to become a major barrier to effective listening. Rather than focusing the mind on critical and careful listening, we often take mental excursions ranging from thinking about the speaker's hair style to daydreaming.[4] A good listener uses this extra mental capacity to analyze and understand the speaker's verbal and nonverbal messages.

The counselor should indicate that the client has his or her full attention and acceptance by maintaining good eye contact with the client and having an empathic facial expression and relaxed posture. The counselor should give the client ample opportunity for expression without interruption while providing occasional, brief verbal and nonverbal responses indicating reception of the message. Appropriately timed nods or verbal responses such as "I understand" or "I see" will help assure the client of the counselor's attentive listening.

Comprehension involves not only attaching meaning to information but also correctly interpreting the meaning of the client's communication. The counselor's comprehension of the client's message can be enhanced through use of such techniques as reflection, paraphrasing, clarification, and probing. Reflection is restating the affective, or emotional, part of the client's words. This gives the client an opportunity to hear what she has just said and to elaborate on her emotions. A client may say, "I feel depressed about my lack of progress." The affective part of this message is the statement "I feel depressed." In reflection, the counselor simply restates the client's words: "You say you feel depressed." This gives the client an opportunity to elaborate on her feelings. In paraphrasing, the client's message is restated, or rephrased, in the counselor's own words. This helps ensure that the counselor has correctly interpreted the client's message. Clarification is simply asking the client to repeat or restate what was just said. Probing is asking the client to provide greater detail on some specific point. It is often used when collecting a 24-hour dietary recall.

INTERVIEWING

Interviewing can be defined as a guided communication process between two persons or parties with the predetermined purpose of obtaining or exchanging specific information through the asking and answering of questions.[2,5] The goal of the interview is obtaining specific information from the client while maintaining an interpersonal environment conducive to disclosure by the client.[2] Of the several types of interviews that exist, the nutrition counselor is primarily concerned with interviews to gather information from clients, give information to clients, and deal with client problems.[5]

Interviewing Skills

As in communication, there are several basic conditions or skills that increase a person's effectiveness as an interviewer. Among these are physical surroundings, freedom from interruption and interference, privacy, good rapport, attentiveness, openness, and the client's context.[2] Factors to consider in the physical surroundings are the comfort of both the client and the interviewer, the seating arrangement, the distance between the interviewer and client, and the presence of physical barriers separating them.

It is best to conduct an interview in a location free of interruptions and interferences. In an office setting, the counselor should arrange to have phone calls held. In a hospital, interviews should not be scheduled during the time of physicians' rounds, nursing or other care, or visiting hours. A convenient time should be arranged with nursing and other staff. When held in the patient's room, arrangements can be made with nursing staff to avoid unnecessary interruptions, the patient's door can be closed, televisions and radios can be turned down or off, and visitors can be kindly asked to step outside.[2,3,5] However, parents, spouses, partners, and siblings can be important sources of information about the patient. The counselor may want to have them present during the interview or available for questions later.

Early establishment of good rapport is essential to an effective interview. Establishing good client rapport will place the client at ease and make him or her more willing to share important information.[2] A counselor should begin the interview with a pleasant greeting. She should introduce herself and briefly give the reason for the interview. If the counselor is late, she should apologize for any inconvenience and explain why.[5]

Attentiveness, as in the context of listening, is also an important interviewing skill. Nonverbal and verbal expressions of attention, such as appropriate eye contact, posture, facial expressions, well-timed nods, or relevant verbal responses, will help assure the client of the counselor's interest and attention. Openness, or interviewer objectivity, as in listening, is an important interviewing skill.

The client's emotional context—his or her beliefs, attitudes, feelings, and values—is also an important consideration when interviewing. Fears about health, concerns about death, feelings of loneliness, or grief may preoccupy a client's thoughts and interfere with his or her ability to participate in the interview. Putting apprehensive clients at ease and allowing them to express their feelings can help alleviate their fears and facilitate the interviewing process.

Obtaining Information

Before the interview, the counselor should review the client's medical record for pertinent information. This provides the counselor with considerable background information on the client and allows the interview to be more directed and concise. Using the "funnel sequence" is suggested. This begins with more general, open questions and gradually narrows to more specific inquiries using closed questions.[5]

Open questions invite rather than demand answers and provide clients substantial freedom in determining the amount and type of information to give.[2,5] Open questions let the client talk and offer information that he or she feels is important. They are generally easy to answer and pose little threat to the client. They give the counselor the opportunity to listen and observe. However, they have the disadvantage of consuming large amounts of time if clients dwell on irrelevant information.[5] Examples of open questions are given in Box 11.2.

Closed questions, on the other hand, are restrictive; they allow the counselor to control answers and to ask for specific information. They often provide too little information and fail to reveal why a client has a particular attitude.[5] Examples of closed questions are given in Box 11.2.

Questions also can be classified as neutral or leading (Box 11.2).[5] *Neutral questions* allow the client to answer without pressure or direction from the counselor. In *leading questions,* the counselor makes implicit or explicit suggestions about the expected or desired answer. In answering leading questions, the client merely agrees with what the counselor is apparently suggesting. Counselors should avoid leading clients either by verbal or nonverbal means. When

Box 11.2 Examples of Different Types of Questions

OPEN QUESTIONS

"Tell me about yourself."

"Tell me about your eating habits."

"What have you been doing to lower your blood cholesterol level?"

CLOSED QUESTIONS

"Do you smoke?"

"Do you salt your food at the table?"

"Do you eat chicken with or without the skin?"

NEUTRAL QUESTIONS

"What is the first thing you have to eat or drink after waking up in the morning?"

"What kind of milk do you drink?"

"How many times a week do you eat ice cream?"

LEADING QUESTIONS

"What do you eat for breakfast?"

"You don't use whole milk, do you?"

"Do you eat ice cream *every* evening?"

---

clients respond to their questions, counselors must avoid such expressions as surprise, agreement, disagreement, or disgust, which can suggest expected or desired answers.[2]

When information is sought from or provided to clients, counselors should use understandable language. Health-care professionals often make the mistake of assuming that clients understand the technical language used daily in hospitals and other health-care organizations. Or they assume that if a client does not understand something, he or she will simply ask what a word means. Many clients are so overwhelmed by the unfamiliar or intimidated by the authority of health-care professionals that they fail to seek answers to their questions. Thus, a counselor should avoid using technical language with clients and should not assume that clients will understand medical terminology even if it is explained to them.

COUNSELING THEORIES

Several counseling theories and techniques have been developed and are currently in use. The purpose of this section is not to teach you how to be a therapist; that takes considerable professional training and practice. Rather, the purpose is to briefly introduce you to those theories that are most pertinent to nutritional counseling and to acquaint you with some fundamental approaches to counseling your clients.

Each counseling theory discussed in the following pages has something of value to offer the dietetic practitioner. Each also has certain limitations or drawbacks. An awareness of these theories and an ability to adapt their more fundamental and benign counseling techniques to suit each unique counseling situation will greatly enhance your ability as a helping professional.

Person-Centered Approach

The person-centered approach to counseling is based primarily on the work of psychologist Carl Rogers.[6–8] Rogers

taught that, if people could experience human relationships characterized by respect and trust, they would develop in a positive and constructive manner. He objected to the idea that people need to be instructed, punished, rewarded, and managed by others who are in a superior and "expert" position. He believed that people possess an innate ability to move away from maladjustment to psychologic health. The primary responsibility for this rests with the client, rather than with an authority who directs a passive client.[9]

Rogers advocated three qualities of counselors that create a growth-promoting climate in which persons advance to become what they are capable of becoming. These counselor qualities are genuineness, or realness; unconditional positive regard and acceptance of the client; and deep understanding of the client's feelings. According to Rogers, if a counselor communicates these attitudes, clients will become less defensive, more open to experiences within themselves and the world, and able to relate to others in social and constructive ways.[9] Rogers wrote, "If I can provide a certain type of relationship, the other person will discover within himself the capacity to use that relationship for growth and change, and personal development will occur."[6]

The client's personality change is brought about by the counselor's attitudes instead of by certain techniques, theories, or knowledge. The counselor's primary task is providing a therapeutic climate in which the client feels free to explore areas of his or her life that are currently distorted or denied to awareness. Within this climate, the client is then able to lose his or her "defenses and rigid perceptions and move to a higher level of personal functioning."[9]

The counselor's genuineness, or realness, is the congruence between what is expressed to the client and what is experienced within the counselor's mind. Through genuineness, the counselor serves as a model of a human struggling toward greater awareness and personal functioning.[9]

Unconditional positive regard and acceptance allow the client to be accepted as he or she is and to express feelings and attitudes without risk of losing the counselor's acceptance. Although the client's *feelings* are accepted, not all *overt behavior* is approved or accepted. According to Rogers, the greater the counselor's degree of positive regard and acceptance of the client, the greater will be the success of therapy.[9]

As the counselor develops a deep understanding of the client's feelings and experiences, he or she is able to sense the client's feelings as if they were his or her own. This permits the counselor to expand the client's awareness and understanding of these feelings and to help the client resolve internal conflicts and become more the person the client wishes to become.[9]

The person-centered approach has the advantage of being a safer approach to counseling than other models that place the counselor in a directive position of making interpretations, forming diagnoses, and attempting more drastic personality changes. Its core skills of listening, understanding, caring, and acceptance are needed by all counselors. No matter what counseling approach they use, counselors lacking in these core skills will not be effective in carrying out their treatment. These skills are also valuable for others in the helping professions. Although people in crisis do not necessarily need answers, they do need someone willing to really listen, care, and understand and on whom they can unload their feelings and experiences without fear of rejection. The presence of a caring, listening, understanding person can do much to promote healing.[9]

Counselors using the person-centered approach have been criticized for merely giving support to clients without challenging them. Rogers has suggested, therefore, that counselors include more "caring confrontations." Counselors using caring confrontation are more active in suggesting topics for exploration, interpreting behavior, helping clients set goals, and giving advice.[9]

Behavior Modification

Behavior modification (also known as behavior therapy) attempts to alter previously learned human behavior or to encourage the development of new behavior through a variety of action-oriented methods, as opposed to changing feelings or thoughts.[2,9,10] A major premise of behavior modification is that "all behavior, normal or abnormal, is acquired and maintained according to certain definable principles."[11] Behaviors resulting in positive consequences tend to be repeated, and those behaviors not followed by favorable consequences tend not to be repeated.

Early, or "radical," behaviorists viewed human behavior as almost totally the result of positive reinforcements (the addition of something, such as praise or money, as a consequence of behavior) or negative reinforcements (the removal of unpleasant stimuli once a certain behavior is performed). Currently, behaviorists view humans as both the *product* of environmental influences and the *producer* of their environment. Early behaviorists viewed humans as lacking freedom and self-determination. Modern behaviorists, on the other hand, acknowledge the presence of freedom and self-determination. They attempt to increase clients' freedom and control by assisting them in overcoming crippling behaviors and becoming freer to choose from options that were previously not available to them.[9]

Antecedents and Consequences

Behaviorists view actions as being preceded by antecedents and followed by consequences.[10,12] For example, eating is generally preceded by some antecedent or stimulus, such as smelling or seeing food, coming home from work or school, sitting down to study or watch television, seeing an advertisement for food on television or in a magazine, or experiencing anxiety, boredom, or loneliness. Behavior modification holds that, when antecedents to behaviors are recognized, they can be modified or controlled to decrease the occurrence of negative behaviors and increase the occurrence of positive behaviors. This is referred to as stimulus control. Examples of stimulus control include eating before grocery shopping, preparing a shopping list and purchasing only the items on the list, storing food out of sight, and avoiding the purchase of ready-to-eat foods.

Consequences reinforce the behavior they follow. They may be positive, negative, or neutral. When consequences are positive, behavior is more likely to be repeated. Behavior followed by negative consequences is less likely to be repeated. The delicious tastes and feelings of satiety accompanying a meal are examples of positive consequences that reinforce, or reward, the practice of eating. Behaviorists also believe that positive consequences are more effective in promoting behavioral change than are negative consequences.[10]

Self-monitoring

A valuable behavior modification technique is self-monitoring, or recordkeeping—the careful observation and accurate recording of the behavior to be controlled.[9,11,13] If the behavior is eating, for example, clients carefully observe their eating and record its occurrence, along with comments about relevant antecedents and consequences related to their eating. Self-monitoring has several functions:[13]

- It provides information about eating habits and the factors influencing them.
- It involves clients in observing and analyzing their dietary habits.
- It increases clients' awareness of their diets and behavior as it happens.
- It gives the counselor and client something to review objectively and impartially. For example,

they focus on specific problem behaviors in the record, not in the client.
- It increases the clients' skills in manipulating their diets to achieve desired results (for example, finding suitable low-fat entrees to replace others that are high in total fat and saturated fat or finding acceptable low-calorie snack foods to replace high-calorie snacks).
- It increases counselor-client interaction.
- It allows client and counselor to monitor behavior over time and track client progress.

Various forms have been developed for self-monitoring.[13] One example is shown in Appendix N. In general, forms for self-monitoring eating behavior should allow the recording of such information as the food eaten, how food was prepared, the amount eaten, where and when the food was eaten, what happened or how the client felt before eating, what happened or how the client felt after eating, and whether the food was eaten alone or with someone else and with whom.

For monitoring behaviors related to a specific goal (for example, substitution of high-calorie snacks with low-calorie snacks), the client can record the day, time, type of snack eaten, and amount eaten on a pocket-sized card, which he or she can carry.

To be successful, the self-monitoring method ought to be easy to use, convenient, and readily available when the behavior occurs; be clearly understood by the client; be relevant to the dietary problem; and be used for observational purposes rather than to judge the problem.

Goals and Self-contracts

Behaviorists believe that feelings result from behavior.[9] Consequently, the focus of attention in counseling is changing behavior, not altering feelings or delving into past experiences. Goals are of central importance in behavior modification and are expressed in terms of altering overt behavior in ways that are both specific and measurable. Therefore, the goals of therapy must be clear, specific, measurable, attainable, and agreed on by both the client and the counselor. The client selects counseling goals at the beginning of the counseling process.

For example, a client may want to decrease his elevated total cholesterol level to less than 200 mg/dL. Having been taught by the counselor that total cholesterol levels are related to saturated fat intake, the client, with the counselor's assistance, may decide to use soft tub margarine instead of butter at home and to remove the skin from chicken before eating it. The client's progress then can be evaluated objectively in terms of goal attainment and other measurable ways. For example, the client's self-monitoring records can demonstrate adherence to the goals, and measurements of total serum cholesterol may indicate overall progress in lowering serum cholesterol.

Once goals are identified, the counselor can help the client write a self-contract. This is an agreement the client enters into with himself or herself to help build commitment to the goal for change.[12,13] The contract should clearly state the goal in terms of a specific time frame and detail the reward for successfully achieving the goal. As an option, it may state the punishment, if any, for not reaching the goal. An example of a self-contract is shown in Figure 11.2.

Modeling

In addition to believing that learning occurs through positive or negative reinforcements, behaviorists hold that people learn through the process of modeling.[9,10,12,13] Also known as observational learning or imitation, modeling is "the process by which the behavior of an individual or a group (the model) acts as a stimulus for similar thoughts, attitudes, and behaviors on the part of observers."[9] Through modeling, clients develop new behaviors without trial-and-error learning. Clients, for example, can learn new behaviors by observing the success of other group members or through others' success stories shared by the counselor.[10]

Modeling can take place by observing a live model (for example, counselors demonstrate the behavior they hope clients will acquire), symbolic models (the client observes the desired behavior performed on videotape or film), or multiple models (new skills are learned as successful peers within the group demonstrate the desired behavior).[9] Modeling is more likely to be successful when the model is similar to the client in age, sex, race, and

Self-contract

____
Name

____
Period of time

____
Specific behavior goal

____
Reward when successful

Signature	Date
Signature	Date

Figure 11.2 A self-contract.

attitudes than when the model is unlike the client. The likelihood that behaviors will be imitated by clients is increased when models are competent in performing the behavior, exhibit warmth, and possess a realistic degree of prestige and status.

Reinforcers

According to behavior modification, behavior is maintained and strengthened when followed by positive reinforcers.[9,11,12] Thus, a positive reinforcer is any consequence that maintains and strengthens behavior by its presence; in other words, the positive reinforcer makes the behavior more likely to recur.[12] A negative reinforcer is an unpleasant consequence that maintains and strengthens behavior by its being removed from the situation.[12] Reinforcers are often referred to as rewards. Rewards that are effective in reinforcing behavior can take many forms and vary from client to client.

If rewards are used, the counselor must identify rewards likely to effectively reinforce desired behaviors and set up a reinforcement system. As an example, consider a client on a weight control program. The counselor and client can set up a system that allows the client to receive a reward for having lost a certain amount of weight. The weight loss goal may be set rather low to make it easily attainable at the beginning of counseling. As counseling progresses and the client develops skill in managing his behavior, successive goals can be somewhat more difficult to attain. Rewards can include money or material items (an amount of money or a certain purchase for each goal reached), activities (doing something the client especially enjoys each time a goal is reached), or social interaction (visiting someone special or making a phone call when a goal is attained).[10,12] Examples of rewards are shown in Box 11.3.

Behavior Modification Techniques Summarized

Behavior modification uses a number of techniques. The major ones employed in weight management are outlined in Table 11.2.[11] Some of these techniques were not originally developed by behaviorists but were adapted from other approaches or disciplines and incorporated into behavior modification programs to increase the success of behavioral change. Among these are nutrition education, physical activity, and cognitive restructuring. Cognitive

restructuring will be discussed in the section "Rational-Emotive Therapy."

Behavior modification has contributed a variety of specific behavioral techniques to nutritional counseling and the treatment of diet-related problems. Its emphasis on changing problem behaviors rather than merely talking about problems and gathering insights allows counselors to focus on assisting clients in formulating a specific plan of action. However, in its attempt to deal with problem solving and the changing of certain behaviors, it has been criticized for deemphasizing the role of feelings and emotions in counseling.[9]

Rational-Emotive Therapy

Unlike behavior modification, which primarily focuses on the relationship between our environment and behavior, rational-emotive therapy (RET) deals with the effects that our thoughts have on our behavior.[2] The major premise of RET is that emotional disturbances are largely the product of irrational thinking.[9] RET holds that our emotions are mainly the product of our beliefs, evaluations, interpretations, and reactions to life situations.[9]

RET views humans as having the potential for both rational thinking and irrational thinking. It views humans as engaging in considerable self-talk and self-evaluation, much of which is irrational and self-denigrating and can result in emotional disturbances. Rather than factors outside of ourselves being the main determinants of behavior, RET holds that our irrational beliefs about ourselves primarily determine our behavior, emotions, and the resulting consequences. In other words, people "are disturbed not by things, but by the view which they take of them."[9] Thus, RET focuses on disputing irrational beliefs and helping people change the irrational beliefs that directly result in disturbed emotions and dysfunctional behavior.[9]

A client's self-talk can be viewed as positive, neutral, or negative. Positive self-talk supports behavioral change, whereas negative self-talk opposes change. Consider a client beginning a weight management program. An example of positive self-talk is the client's silently observing, "I'm going to like this program." Negative self-talk is the thought "I don't think I can handle this" or "I'm no good at dieting; I'll never succeed at this program." According to RET, the likelihood of successful behavioral change is

 Box 11.3   **Examples of Rewards Used in Behavior Modification**

Spending money on appropriate things	Taking an afternoon or day off
Reading a book	Visiting a friend
Watching television	Spending time at a favorite hobby
Making a long-distance call	Relaxing or taking a nap

TABLE 11.2	**Examples of Behavior Modification Techniques Used in Weight Control Programs**

Stimulus Control

Shopping

Shop for food after eating.
Shop from a list.
Avoid ready-to-eat foods.
Do not carry more cash than needed for shopping.

Plans

Plan to limit food intake.
Substitute exercise for snacking.
Eat meals and snacks at scheduled times.
Do not accept food offered by others.

Activities

Store food out of sight.
Eat all food in the same place.
Remove food from inappropriate storage areas in the house.
Keep serving dishes off the table.
Use smaller dishes and utensils.
Avoid being the food server.
Leave the table immediately after eating.
Do not save leftovers.

Holidays and Parties

Drink fewer alcoholic beverages.
Plan eating habits before parties.
Eat a low-calorie snack before parties.
Practice polite ways to decline food.
Do not get discouraged by an occasional setback.

Eating Behavior

Put the fork down between mouthfuls.
Chew thoroughly before swallowing.
Prepare foods one portion at a time.
Leave some food on the plate.
Pause in the middle of the meal.
Do nothing else while eating (read, watch television).
Solicit help from family and friends.
Have family and friends provide help in the form of praise and material reward.
Use self-monitoring records as basis for rewards.
Plan specific rewards for specific behaviors (behavioral contracts).

Self-monitoring

Keep diet diary that includes time and place of eating, type and amount of food, who is present, and how you feel.

Nutrition Education

Use diet diary to identify problem areas.
Make small changes that you can continue.
Learn nutritional values of foods.
Decrease fat intake; increase intake of complex carbohydrates.

Physical Activity

Routine activity: increase routine activity, increase use of stairs, and keep record of distance walked daily.
Exercise: begin a very mild exercise program, keep a record of daily exercise, and increase the exercise very gradually.

Cognitive Restructuring

Avoid setting unreasonable goals.
Think about progress, not shortcomings.
Avoid imperatives, such as "always" and "never."
Counter negative thoughts with rational statements.
Set weight goals.

Source: Stunkard AJ, Berthold HC. 1985. What is behavior therapy? A very short description of behavioral weight control. *American Journal of Clinical Nutrition* 41:821–823.

considerably less when people view themselves as failing, as compared with when they see themselves succeeding. In addition, persons viewing themselves as failing at weight management are less likely to begin addressing their behavioral problems, and, when faced with difficult challenges (for example, the urging of friends to eat fattening food at a party), they are more likely to slip from their program and to give it up altogether.[9,10]

Although our irrational beliefs may have begun through early indoctrination by our parents or significant others ("You're never going to amount to anything!"), it is primarily our own repetition of these irrational thoughts that keeps these dysfunctional attitudes alive and operative within us. Thus, RET teaches that we are largely responsible for creating our own problems, that we have the ability to change, that we must identify our irrational beliefs, and that we must dispute these irrational beliefs using the process of cognitive restructuring.[9]

The first step in cognitive restructuring is becoming aware of negative self-talk.[2,9,14,15] One approach is asking the client to record his or her irrational and destructive internal messages on a form similar to the one shown in Table 11.3.[15] Once an irrational internal message is identified, it can be disputed by substituting it with a rational, self-defensive statement.

Clients can be led to dispute their irrational self-talk and beliefs by encouraging them to ask such questions as "What is the factual evidence in support of my thoughts?" "Why do I assume I am a rotten person because of the way I behave?" "Would it really be catastrophic if my worst fears were to come true?" and "What can I say in defense of myself?"[9,14] As clients learn to recognize and dispute their irrational self-criticisms, they then can be encouraged to substitute negative self-talk with positive, self-affirming statements.

Other RET techniques include the changing of one's language, cognitive rehearsal, and thought stopping.[2,9,12,14,15] An example of changing one's language is avoiding negative self-fulfilling statements ("I will fail, I will look like a pig, and no one will like me"). People telling themselves that they will fail may actually increase the probability of failure. Cognitive rehearsal (also known as rational-emotive imagery) involves clients' thinking, feeling, and behaving the way they would like to in real life. As clients see themselves overcoming in their thoughts, the likelihood of them overcoming in real life is increased. Thought stopping is a two-step process. First, whenever a negative thought enters the client's mind, he or she says, "Stop!" either out loud or very clearly within the mind. This is followed by substituting a positive, rational thought for the negative, irrational thought. Again, the basis of these exercises is that our language (either audible or silent) influences our thoughts, which in turn influence our emotions and behavior.

Reality Therapy

The central premises of reality therapy are that individuals are responsible for their behavior and that, if a person's current behavior is not meeting his or her needs, steps can be taken to change behavior so that personal needs are met.[9,16] Reality therapy is based primarily on the work of psychiatrist William Glasser, who abandoned traditional psychoanalysis early in his career and went on to develop his own counseling approach. According to Glasser, every person's behavior is an attempt to fulfill his or her basic human needs. "It is always what we want at the time that causes our behavior."[17] According to Glasser, rather than being determined by outside forces (as is taught by behaviorists), behavior is completely driven from within the person by the necessity to fulfill five innate needs: survival, love, power, fun, and freedom.[17] "All of our lives we must attempt to live in a way that will best satisfy one or more of these needs."[17]

Glasser teaches that each of us creates our own inner world from which we view the world outside of ourselves. Each person is responsible for the kind of inner world he or she creates. Instead of external factors depressing or angering us, we anger or depress ourselves. "Neurotic" and "psychotic" behavior does not just happen to us; it is something we choose in an attempt to control our world. If a client complains of anxiety, the counselor may ask what behavior is causing the anxiety. The focus is not on the anxiety but on whatever behavior is causing the anxiety. According to Glasser, once people acknowledge

TABLE 11.3	Identifying and Disputing Irrational and Destructive Thoughts
Irrational Thought	**Rational, Self-defensive Statement**
"I can't believe I ate six of those cookies! I've blown it. Oh well, I may as well go ahead and finish the rest of the bag."	"I *did* slip by eating those six cookies, but I *did not* blow my program. The best thing for me to do now is to stop eating them. I *can* do better."
"I ate half a bag of potato chips! I'm an absolute failure."	"My success or failure at anything is not based on one incident. I'm human. It's okay to make mistakes once in awhile. I don't have to be perfect."
"The way she's looking at me, she must think my idea is stupid."	"I can't read other people's minds. The way to find out what she thinks is to just ask. Besides, not everyone has to like my idea."

and act on the reality that their behavior is the result of their choices, change occurs.[9]

Reality therapy begins by the counselor's establishing an accepting and supportive relationship with the client. The client is then led to examine and evaluate his own behavior to determine if it is contributing to his problems. Once the client acknowledges he is not getting what he wants from his behavior, the counselor helps the client develop an action plan for changing his behavior so that it contributes to his success. The plan should have goals that are simple, specific, clear, and attainable and that involve something the client will do soon and on a daily basis. The counselor then helps the client make a commitment to follow through with the plan and to refuse to give up. The counselor makes it clear to the client that he will neither accept excuses nor use punishment to coerce the client.

Many people tend to blame other individuals or circumstances for their problems. Reality therapy asserts that people are responsible for their own behavior and attacks the excuses many people make for their actions in an attempt to evade responsibility.[18] A client who runs to the refrigerator every time she feels anxious, for example, may benefit from acknowledging that her behavior does not depend on an outside stimulus (in this case, the "anxiety") but on her own conscious choice. The client should be helped to recognize that she has a variety of options for dealing with her anxiety. Then, under the guidance of a counselor, the client can select from her options and develop a plan to deal with her problematic behavior in positive ways.[18]

INITIATING AND MAINTAINING DIETARY CHANGE: A PRACTICAL PLAN

A number of counselor characteristics and behavioral change techniques can be identified. These characteristics and techniques are effective in initiating and maintaining nutrition behavior, but their use does not guarantee success. Each nutrition counselor will want to integrate them into a total program with which he or she feels comfortable. The counselor will also want to consider clients' needs, resources, and social support, as well as the skill level of support staff.

No single counseling approach can be recommended for all clients. Rather, counselors are encouraged to use an eclectic approach—that is, one composed of elements drawn from a variety of approaches. An effective behavioral change program would selectively incorporate several techniques into a multicomponent program that is suitable to both the counselor and the client. However, it is neither necessary nor wise to use all the counseling techniques at one's disposal.

Motivation

No counselor can motivate a client. Motivation comes only from within the client. A counselor can only create a climate that will help clients motivate themselves. People tend to be motivated by challenge, growth, achievement, promotion, and recognition. Emphasis should be placed on providing a proper environment for self-growth by challenging clients, giving them responsibility and encouragement, and giving full range to individual strength.

Characteristics of Effective Counselors

From this discussion of counseling theories, it is possible to identify several characteristics of effective counselors. By practicing good communication, listening, and counseling skills, one of the first steps in initiating behavioral change can take place—establishing good rapport with the client. The following are characteristics of effective counselors:

- Empathy—the ability to climb into the world of the client and communicate back feelings of understanding
- Respect—a deep and genuine appreciation for the worth of a client, separate and apart from his or her behavior; the strength and ability of the client to overcome and adjust is appreciated
- Warmth—communication of concern and appropriate affection
- Genuineness—being freely and deeply oneself; one is congruent and not just playing a role
- Concreteness—essential ideas and elements are ferreted out
- Self-disclosure—information about self is revealed for the benefit of the client at the appropriate time
- Potency and self-actualization—one is dynamic, is in command, conveys feelings of trust and warmth, is competent, is inner-directed, is creative, is sensitive, is nonjudgmental, is productive, is serene, and is satisfied; this comes across to the client in a helpful way[19]

Initial Assessment

The initial assessment of the client serves several important functions:

- It makes the counselor and client aware of the client's dietary habits and health history, as well as related factors.
- It provides baseline information from which to gauge progress.
- It alerts the counselor and client to the various demands being placed on the client, so that realistic priorities can be set.
- It gives the counselor and client ideas for making dietary changes.
- It gives the counselor an opportunity to develop rapport and a sense of partnership with the client.
- It enables the counselor to develop a plan of gradual change suitable to the client's way of living.[13]

As discussed in Chapters 3 and 8, a variety of techniques can be used for obtaining dietary information. In addition to these data, however, information should be collected on the client's current health status, health history, and past and present health habits.

Initiating Dietary Change

Counselors and clients should have reasonable expectations about what changes should be undertaken, the extent of change, and the rate at which change is made. Clients should be carefully guided in what benefits they can reasonably expect from dietary change and the amount of change necessary to realize those benefits.[13,20,21]

Goals can be set by the client under the guidance of the counselor. Goals should be specific, measurable, reasonable, and attainable. Whatever the final behavioral goal is, most people will not be able to master it at the first effort or in one step. Behavioral change should be approached gradually, with a number of small, easily attained goals that collectively lead to the final goal. A client can never begin too low and the steps upward can never be too small.[12] Short-term goals spanning one to two weeks are more effective than long-term goals covering months.[20] Because obstacles and setbacks will be encountered, goals should have some flexibility. One approach to building a client's commitment to attaining goals can be through a written self-contract.

Reinforcers, or rewards, can help promote maintenance of behavioral change, especially at the beginning of a program. If they are used, counselors will need to work with each client (and possibly with a key individual providing social support for the client) to identify reinforcers providing ample incentive to goal attainment. At this time, the use of other behavior modification strategies can be discussed with the client. Serious consideration should be given to using stimulus control, self-monitoring, and cognitive restructuring in ways suitable to both counselor and client.

Maintaining Dietary Change

Although counselors can assist clients in making dietary changes (for example, in learning about nutrition, setting realistic goals, and managing the antecedents to behaviors), it is ultimately the client's responsibility to change dietary habits. To be permanently successful, clients will need to be guided toward self-sufficiency.[13]

A key element in self-sufficiency is the client's involvement in the change process.[13] The client should be asked, "What changes can *you* make?" "What can *you* say when someone offers you another serving of dessert?" "What steps can *you* take to avoid overeating at a party?" The more the client "owns" the program, the more successful he or she will be at maintaining dietary change.

Four areas where counselors can help clients increase self-control over eating habits are maintenance of commitment, recordkeeping, environmental restructuring,

and use of rewards.[13] At first, most clients are enthusiastic about behavioral change. After several days or weeks, however, this enthusiasm begins to wane. Some suggestions for strengthening commitment to dietary change include the following:

- Praise the client for his or her successful experiences and attribute success to the client's abilities.
- Encourage the client to tell family members and friends about his or her dietary goals. After making a public commitment to dietary change, adherence to the program is more likely.
- Ask the client to state the kinds of problems he or she will likely encounter. Problems will occur, but they will be less likely to derail the client's progress when they are anticipated and planned for.
- Concentrate on foods the client can eat, rather than those to be avoided. Help clients realize that healthy eating is not synonymous with deprivation.[13]

Recordkeeping provides information on the client's performance, aids the client in observing and analyzing his or her environment, and helps in recognizing the antecedents to eating behavior. Recordkeeping can range from marking a 3 × 5-inch card every time a between-meal snack is declined to keeping elaborate food records.[13]

Some researchers think that restructuring the environment is the most important technique in maintaining change. Counselors can ask clients to identify specific changes that can be made in their physical, social, and cognitive (mental) environments to promote long-term dietary change.

A client may associate an event—such as sitting in a favorite chair, reading the newspaper, or watching television—with eating high-calorie foods. The presence of inappropriate foods at home also can be a deterrent to successful change. Altering the arrangement of furniture in the room where television is watched or the newspaper is read can help promote and maintain change. Purchasing healthful foods to substitute for inappropriate items can be helpful as well.

The counselor should ask the client to identify social situations that promote poor eating habits. How is the client's eating behavior affected by various social functions or what family and friends say to the client? The counselor should explore with the client ways that social interactions can be supportive of dietary change. What could family and friends say to promote the client's success? Through role playing, the client can develop skill in asking for support from others.[13] In dealing with the mental environment, the client should be encouraged to use some of the cognitive restructuring techniques discussed in the "Rational-Emotive Therapy" section.

Relapse Prevention

For the purposes of behavioral change, a relapse can be defined as the resumption of an unwanted habit or behavior that one has, for a period of time, overcome or turned from.[12,22] Consider a man with the habit of eating a half-pint of premium butter-pecan ice cream every evening. For several weeks he has limited himself to only 1 cup of nonfat frozen dessert four evenings a week. When he returns to 2 cups of butter-pecan ice cream every evening for several weeks, he has relapsed. However, if he merely indulges once or twice in butter-pecan ice cream while spending a weekend with relatives and then returns to 1 cup of the nonfat variety four evenings a week, he has only experienced a lapse. A lapse can be defined as "a single event, a reemergence of a previous habit, which may or may not lead to a state of relapse."[21] Thus, a lapse is a temporary fall, a slip, or a mistake. When a lapse occurs, corrective action can be taken to prevent a relapse—a total loss of control—from occurring.[21]

A key to relapse prevention is to prepare clients for the occurrence of lapses and to help them cope in ways that prevent a relapse.[20] If counselors and clients have previously discussed the likelihood of lapses' occurring, clients will be better prepared when they do occur, and the risk of lapses' leading to full-blown relapses will be minimized. Clients should be taught to anticipate situations likely to produce lapses, such as illness, travel, live-in visitors, overwork, emotional distress, and schedule changes.[20]

Counselors should help clients view a lapse for what it really is—merely a temporary fall. A counselor and client can discuss what corrective actions the client can take to recover from the lapse and to prevent a relapse from occurring. Techniques such as modeling, role playing, cognitive rehearsal, and direct instruction can help in this.[2] A client needs to be assured that, if a lapse does occur, it is not the end of the world. The client has suffered a setback, but prompt action can limit the lapse to a temporary setback.

KNOWING ONE'S LIMITS

When working with clients, it is important that counselors know the limits of their abilities to help people and when they need to refer a client to more experienced help. Emotional problems are common, and from time to time nutrition counselors encounter individuals needing psychologic counseling. If a client indicates that she is having emotional problems, a nutrition counselor may very gently and tactfully ask if she would like assistance in getting psychologic counseling from a local mental health clinic or professional. The counselor may help her in calling and making an appointment with an appropriate agency or person.[9,20]

Some individuals may not be ready or willing to change certain habits. Circumstances in a person's life may not be conducive to change at the particular time he is seeing a counselor. It may be necessary to suggest that a client postpone weight loss or control of mildly elevated serum cholesterol until *after* he deals with a more pressing problem, such as separation, divorce, bankruptcy, or substance abuse.

This chapter has offered a very brief overview of dietary counseling. It is meant to be only an introduction to the topic. Readers interested in developing the skill of nutritional counseling are encouraged to take coursework and to study other sources for further information. Other excellent resources include the following:

Bauer KD, Liou D, Sokolik CA. 2012. *Nutrition counseling and education skill development,* 2nd ed. Belmont, CA: Wadsworth, Cengage Learning.

Holli BB, Maillet J, Beto JA, Calabrese RJ. 2009. *Communication and education skills for dietetics professionals,* 5th ed. Philadelphia: Wolters Kluwer Health/Lippincott Williams & Wilkins.

Watson DL, Tharp RG. 2007. *Self-directed behavior: Self-modification for personal adjustment,* 9th ed. Belmont, CA: Wadsworth/Thomson Learning.

SUMMARY

1. Communication, the process of sending and receiving messages, lies at the foundation of all efforts to interview, counsel, educate, and change diet. The basic components of human communication are the sender, receiver, message, feedback, and interference.

2. A counselor's attempts to help bring about dietary change may elicit a defensive reaction from the receiver or client. When this occurs, the receiver fails to concentrate on the structure, content, and meaning of the message. This is one source of interference to communication. When communication is supportive of the receiver, this defensive reaction can be prevented, and the interference to communication can be minimized.

3. Communication occurs simultaneously at both the verbal and nonverbal levels. Nonverbal communication involves gestures, posture, facial expressions, and tone of voice. It is sometimes a more reliable indicator of a person's true feelings than are words. Unlike verbal communication, which is generally under conscious control and subject to censorship, nonverbal communication is not as easily controlled by conscious thought. It is also an effective way for the counselor to communicate to the client.

4. Effective communication is promoted by proper use of feedback, language that is understandable to both counselor and client, an environment that is conducive to good communication, and awareness of the physical and psychologic barriers to communication.

5. Listening is an important part of interviewing and counseling and an excellent way to establish rapport. Despite its importance, most people are not good listeners. Listening involves six steps: hearing, attending, understanding, remembering, evaluating, and responding.

6. Rather than being a passive activity, listening is a highly active process demanding concentration and attention. It is also a skill that can be learned. Listening skills can be grouped under four categories: openness, concentration, attention, and comprehension.

7. Interviewing is a guided communication process between two persons for the purpose of obtaining or exchanging specific information through the asking and answering of questions. The goal of the interview is obtaining specific information from the client while maintaining an interpersonal environment conducive to disclosure by the client. Conditions that increase interviewing effectiveness include comfortable physical surroundings, freedom from interruption and interference, and privacy. Counselor qualities that contribute to a successful interview include the ability to establish good rapport, attentiveness, openness, and an understanding of the client's situation.

8. Several types of questions can be used in the interview. Open questions invite rather than demand answers and give the client substantial freedom in determining the amount and type of information to give. Closed questions are restrictive and allow the counselor to control answers and ask for specific information. Neutral questions allow the client to answer without pressure or direction from the counselor. Leading questions contain implicit or explicit suggestions about the expected or desired answer.

9. The person-centered approach to counseling is largely based on the idea that, if people experience human relationships characterized by respect and trust, they will develop in a positive and constructive manner. Three counselor qualities that create a growth-promoting climate for the client are genuineness, or realness; unconditional positive regard and acceptance of the client; and deep understanding of the client's feelings. Within this climate, the client is then able to lose his or her "defenses and rigid perceptions and move to a higher level of personal functioning."[10]

10. The main contribution of person-centered therapy is its core skills: listening, understanding, caring, and acceptance. Regardless of the approach used, counselors deficient in these skills will lack efficiency in carrying out their treatment. The presence of a caring, listening, understanding person can do much to promote healing in a person experiencing a crisis.

11. Behavior modification attempts to alter previously learned human behavior or encourage the learning of new behavior through a variety of action-oriented methods, as opposed to changing feelings or thoughts. Although early behaviorists viewed human behavior as almost totally the result of reinforcements, modern behaviorists view humans as both the product of environmental influences and the producer of their environment.

12. Behaviorists view actions as being preceded by antecedents and followed by consequences. The modification or control of antecedents to decrease the occurrence of negative behaviors and increase the occurrence of positive behaviors is referred to as stimulus control. Other techniques of behavior modification include self-monitoring, or recordkeeping; modeling; cognitive restructuring; education; physical activity; and the use of goals, self-contracts, and reinforcers.

13. The major premise of rational-emotive therapy (RET) is that emotional disturbances are largely the product of irrational thinking. RET holds that our emotions are mainly the product of our beliefs, evaluations, interpretations, and reactions to life situations. Rather than factors outside of ourselves being the main determinants of behavior, RET holds that our irrational beliefs about ourselves primarily determine our behavior, emotions, and the resulting consequences.

14. A major technique of RET is cognitive restructuring, which focuses on helping people dispute their irrational beliefs and change the thoughts that directly result in disturbed emotions and dysfunctional behavior. RET also uses such techniques as cognitive rehearsal and thought stopping.

15. Reality therapy views every person's behavior as an attempt to fulfill his or her basic human needs. Reality therapy views behavior as being driven not by outside forces but from within the person by the necessity to fulfill the need for survival, love, power, fun, and freedom. Each individual is responsible for his or her behavior, and, if current behavior is not meeting a person's needs, he or she can take steps to change behavior so that personal needs are met.

16. In reality therapy, the counselor begins by establishing an accepting and supportive

relationship with a client. The client is then led to examine and evaluate his behavior to determine if it is contributing to his problems. Once the client acknowledges he is not getting what he wants from his behavior, the counselor helps the client develop an action plan for changing his behavior, so that it contributes to his success.

17. No single counseling approach can be recommended for all clients. Counselors are encouraged to use an eclectic approach—one composed of elements drawn from a variety of methods. An effective behavioral change program would selectively incorporate several techniques into a multicomponent program that is suitable to both the counselor and the client.

18. In addition to having good communication and listening skills, effective counselors convey empathy, respect, warmth, genuineness, concreteness, openness, potency, and self-actualization.

19. It is important for counselors and clients to have reasonable expectations about what changes should be undertaken, the extent of change, and the rate at which change is made. Goals set by the client under the guidance of the counselor should be specific, measurable, reasonable, and attainable. Behavioral change will be more successful when achieved through a number of small steps. Short-term goals spanning one to two weeks are more effective than long-term goals covering months.

20. If rewards are used, counselors will need to work with each client to identify those providing ample incentive to goal attainment. Serious consideration also should be given to using stimulus control, self-monitoring, and cognitive restructuring in ways suitable to both counselor and client.

21. It is ultimately the client's responsibility to change dietary habits. To be permanently successful, clients need to be guided toward self-sufficiency. Four areas where counselors can help clients develop self-sufficiency in dietary change are maintenance of commitment, recordkeeping, environmental restructuring, and use of reinforcers.

22. A relapse can be defined as the resumption of an unwanted habit or behavior that one has, for a period of time, overcome or turned from. A lapse can be defined as a temporary fall, or a reemergence of a previous habit, which may or may not lead to a state of relapse. Counselors should prepare clients for the occurrence of lapses and help them cope in ways that will prevent a relapse. Clients should be taught to anticipate situations likely to produce lapses, such as illness, travel, live-in visitors, overwork, emotional distress, and schedule changes.

23. Counselors should know the limits of their abilities and when they need to refer clients needing psychologic counseling to more experienced help. Some individuals may not be ready or willing to change certain habits. It may be necessary to suggest that a client postpone dietary change until after his or her more pressing problems have been resolved.

REFERENCES

1. U.S. Department of Health and Human Services. 2014. *The health consequences of smoking—50 years of progress: A report of the surgeon general.* Atlanta, GA: U.S. Department of Health and Human Services, Centers for Disease Control and Prevention, National Center for Chronic Disease Prevention and Health Promotion, Office on Smoking and Health.

2. Holli BB, Maillet J, Beto JA, Calabrese RJ. 2009. *Communication and education skills for dietetics professionals,* 5th ed. Philadelphia: Wolters Kluwer Health/Lippincott Williams & Wilkins.

3. Bauer KD, Liou D, Sokolik CA. 2012. *Nutrition counseling and education skill development,* 2nd ed. Belmont, CA: Wadsworth, Cengage Learning.

4. Samovar LA. 2000. *Oral communication: Speaking across cultures,* 11th ed. Los Angeles: Roxbury.

5. Stewart CJ, Cash WB. 2006. *Interviewing: Principles and practices,* 11th ed. Boston: McGraw-Hill.

6. Rogers C. 1961. *On becoming a person.* Boston: Houghton Mifflin.

7. Rogers C. 1970. *Carl Rogers on encounter groups.* New York: Harper & Row.

8. Rogers C. 1977. *Carl Rogers on personal power: Inner strength and its revolutionary impact.* New York: Delacorte.

9. Corey G. 2009. *Theory and practice of counseling and psychotherapy,* 8th ed. Belmont, CA: Thomson Brooks/Cole.

10. Elder JA, Ayala GX, Harris S. 1999. Theories and intervention approaches to health-behavior change in primary care. *American Journal of Preventive Medicine* 17:275–284.

11. Stunkard AJ, Berthold HC. 1985. What is behavior therapy? A very short description of behavioral weight control. *American Journal of Clinical Nutrition* 41:821–823.

12. Watson DL, Tharp RG. 2007. *Self-directed behavior: Self-modification for personal adjustment,* 9th ed. Belmont, CA: Wadsworth/Thomson Learning.

13. Raab C, Tillotson JL. 1985. *Heart to heart: A manual on nutrition counseling for the reduction of cardiovascular disease risk factors.* Bethesda, MD: U.S. Department of Health and Human Services, Public Health Service; National Institutes of Health.

14. Bandura A. 1997. *Self-efficacy: The exercise of control.* New York: W. H. Freeman.

15. Burns DD. 2000. *Feeling good: The new mood therapy.* New York: Quill.

16. Burns DD. 1999. *The feeling good handbook.* New York: Plume.

17. Glasser W. 2001. *Reality therapy in action.* New York: Harper-Collins.

18. Glasser W. 1998. *The quality school: Managing students without coercion.* New York: Harper-Perennial.

19. Hoeltzel KE. 1986. Counseling methods for dietitians. *Topics in Clinical Nutrition* 1:33–42.

20. Nieman DC. 2011. *Exercise testing and prescription: A health-related approach,* 7th ed. New York: McGraw-Hill.

21. Thompson WR, Gordon NF, Pescatello LS. 2010. *ASCM's guidelines for exercise testing and prescription,* 8th ed. Philadelphia: Lippincott Williams & Wilkins.

22. Brownell KD, Marlatt GA, Lichtenstein E, Wilson GT. 1986. Understanding and preventing relapse. *American Psychologist* 41:765–782.

ASSESSMENT ACTIVITY 11.1

Counseling Practice

Becoming an effective counselor requires considerable skill and practice. This assessment activity is designed to help you get your feet wet.

Members of your class should divide into groups of two students each. You should take the three-day food record that you completed in Assessment Activity 3.2 and the result of the computerized analysis of that food record and give these to your partner.

Review your partner's food record and computerized analysis. Study the Competency Checklist for Nutrition Counselors shown in Appendix O. Use this as a guide for your counseling session and to evaluate yourself after you have counseled your partner.

Using techniques discussed in this chapter, assist your partner in identifying one specific, measurable, and attainable goal that will improve his or her diet. Guide your partner in developing a simple action plan for attaining the goal he or she has decided on.

Videotape (or audiotape) the counseling session and view (or listen to) it alone later to see how you did. Look for what you did right and note improvements you can make next time. Use the Competency Checklist for Nutrition Counselors in Appendix O to evaluate your counseling skills.

If time allows, repeat this exercise.

Food Record Recording Form

7 - Day Food Diary

Name _____ Age _____

Address _____ City _____

State _____ Zip _____ Phone _____

Height _____ Weight _____ Sex _____

Physician/Dietitian _____ Phone _____

For Females Only: Are you pregnant? _____

                       Are you breast-feeding? _____

Directions for Using the Food Diary

1. Keep your food diary current. List foods immediately after they are eaten. **Please print all entries**.
2. Record only one food item per line in this record booklet.
3. Be as specific as possible when describing the food item eaten: the way it was cooked (if it was cooked) and the amount that was eaten.
4. Include brand names whenever possible.
5. Report only the food portion that was actually eaten — for example: **T-bone steak, 4-oz broiled.** (Do not include the bones.)
6. Record amounts in household measures — for example: **ounces, tablespoons, cups, slices** or **units**, as in 1 cup nonfat milk, two slices of wheat toast, or one raw apple.
7. Include method that was used to prepare food item — for example: **fresh, frozen, stewed, fried, baked, canned, broiled, raw,** or **braised**.
8. For canned foods, include the liquid in which it was canned — for example: **sliced peaches in heavy syrup, fruit cocktail in light syrup,** or **tuna in water**.
9. Food items listed without specific amounts eaten will be analyzed using portion sizes.
10. Do not alter your normal diet during the period you keep this diary.
11. Remember to record the amounts of visible fats (oils, butter, salad dressings, margarine, and so on) you eat or use in cooking.

Time	Food Item and Method of Preparation	Amount Eaten
7 am	Apple, raw, fresh	1 medium
12 pm	Beef Stew	10 oz portion
12 pm	Bread, whole wheat, fresh	2 Slices
3 pm	Cereal, Corn Flakes	2 Cups
	with sugar	2 Tbs.
	with milk, non fat	½ cup
7 pm	Chicken, Fried	2 legs
7 pm	Coleslaw, with mayo	1 cup
7 pm	Eggs, Chicken (fried in butter)	2 large
7 pm	Fish, salmon, baked	10 oz

Name _____   Date _____

Time	Food Item and Method of Preparation	Amount Eaten

Fruit and Vegetable Screener Developed by the U.S. National Cancer Institute

From National Cancer Institute, National Institutes for Health, U.S. Department of Health and Human Services. See https://epi.grants.cancer.gov/diat/screeners/fruitveg/instrument.html for scoring instructions.

NATIONAL INSTITUTES OF HEALTH
EATING AT AMERICA'S TABLE STUDY
QUICK FOOD SCAN

- The person who completed the telephone interviews for the Eating at America's Table Study should fill out this questionnaire.

- Use only a No. 2 pencil.

- Be certain to completely blacken in each of the answers, and erase completely if you make any changes.

- Do not make any stray marks on this form.

- When you complete this questionnaire, please return it in the postage-paid envelope to:

    National Cancer Institute
    EPN, Room 313
    6130 Executive Blvd., MSC 7344
    Bethesda, MD 20892-7344

BAR
CODE
LABEL
HERE

PLEASE DO NOT WRITE IN THIS AREA

SERIAL

INSTRUCTIONS

- Think about what you usually ate last month.
- Please think about all the fruits and vegetables that you ate last month. Include those that were:
    - raw and cooked,
    - eaten as snacks and at meals,
    - eaten at home and away from home (restaurants, friends, take-out), and
    - eaten alone and mixed with other foods.
- Report how many times per month, week, or day you ate each food, and if you ate it, how much you usually had.
- If you mark "Never" for a question, follow the "Go to" instruction.
- Choose the best answer for each question. Mark only one response for each question.

1. Over the last month, how many times per month, week, or day did you drink **100% juice** such as orange, apple, grape, or grapefruit juice? **Do not count** fruit drinks like Kool-Aid, lemonade, Hi-C, cranberry juice drink, Tang, and Twister. Include juice you drank at all mealtimes and between meals.

Never (Go to Question 2)	1-3 times last month	1-2 times per week	3-4 times per week	5-6 times per week	1 time per day	2 times per day	3 times per day	4 times per day	5 or more times per day
○	○	○	○	○	○	○	○	○	○

1a. Each time you drank **100% juice**, how much did you usually drink?

○	○	○	○
Less than ¾ cup (less than 6 ounces)	¾ to 1¼ cup (6 to 10 ounces)	1¼ to 2 cups (10 to 16 ounces)	More than 2 cups (more than 16 ounces)

2. Over the last month, how many times per month, week, or day did you eat **fruit**? Count any kind of fruit—fresh, canned, and frozen. **Do not count** juices. Include fruit you ate at all mealtimes and for snacks.

Never (Go to Question 3)	1-3 times last month	1-2 times per week	3-4 times per week	5-6 times per week	1 time per day	2 times per day	3 times per day	4 times per day	5 or more times per day
○	○	○	○	○	○	○	○	○	○

2a. Each time you ate **fruit**, how much did you usually eat?

○	○	○	○
Less than 1 medium fruit	1 medium fruit	2 medium fruits	More than 2 medium fruits

OR

○	○	○	○
Less than ½ cup	About ½ cup	About 1 cup	More than 1 cup

3.   Over the last month, how often did you eat **lettuce salad (with or without other vegetables)**?

○	○	○	○	○	○	○	○	○	○
Never (Go to Question 4)	1-3 times last month	1-2 times per week	3-4 times per week	5-6 times per week	1 time per day	2 times per day	3 times per day	4 times per day	5 or more times per day

3a. Each time you ate **lettuce salad**, how much did you usually eat?

○	○	○	○
About ½ cup	About 1 cup	About 2 cups	More than 2 cups

4.   Over the last month, how often did you eat **French fries** or **fried potatoes**?

○	○	○	○	○	○	○	○	○	○
Never (Go to Question 5)	1-3 times last month	1-2 times per week	3-4 times per week	5-6 times per week	1 time per day	2 times per day	3 times per day	4 times per day	5 or more times per day

4a. Each time you ate **French fries** or **fried potatoes**, how much did you usually eat?

○	○	○	○
Small order or less (About 1 cup or less)	Medium order (About 1½ cups)	Large order (About 2 cups)	Super Size order or more (About 3 cups or more)

5.   Over the last month, how often did you eat **other white potatoes**? Count **baked, boiled**, and **mashed potatoes, potato salad**, and **white potatoes that were not fried.**

○	○	○	○	○	○	○	○	○	○
Never (Go to Question 6)	1-3 times last month	1-2 times per week	3-4 times per week	5-6 times per week	1 time per day	2 times per day	3 times per day	4 times per day	5 or more times per day

5a. Each time you ate **these potatoes**, how much did you usually eat?

○	○	○	○
1 small potato or less (½ cup or less)	1 medium potato (½ to 1 cup)	1 large potato (1 to 1½ cups)	2 medium potatoes or more (1½ cups or more)

6.   Over the last month, how often did you eat **cooked dried beans**? Count **baked beans, bean soup, refried beans, pork and beans** and **other bean dishes.**

○	○	○	○	○	○	○	○	○	○
Never (Go to Question 7)	1-3 times last month	1-2 times per week	3-4 times per week	5-6 times per week	1 time per day	2 times per day	3 times per day	4 times per day	5 or more times per day

6a. Each time you ate **these beans**, how much did you usually eat?

○	○	○	○
Less than ½ cup	½ to 1 cup	1 to 1½ cups	More than 1½ cups

7. Over the last month, how often did you eat **other vegetables**?

    DO NOT COUNT: • Lettuce salads
    • White potatoes
    • Cooked dried beans
    • Vegetables in mixtures, such as in sandwiches, omelets, casseroles, Mexican dishes, stews, stir-fry, soups, etc.
    • Rice

    COUNT: • All other vegetables—raw, cooked, canned, and frozen

○	○	○	○	○	○	○	○	○	○
Never	1-3	1-2	3-4	5-6	1	2	3	4	5 or more
(Go to	times	times	times	times	time	times	times	times	times
Question 8)	last month	per week	per week	per week	per day	per day	per day	per day	per day

7a. Each of these times that you ate **other vegetables**, how much did you usually eat?

○	○	○	○
Less than ½ cup	½ to 1 cup	1 to 2 cups	More than 2 cups

8. Over the last month, how often did you eat **tomato sauce**? Include tomato sauce on pasta or macaroni, rice, pizza and other dishes.

○	○	○	○	○	○	○	○	○	○
Never	1-3	1-2	3-4	5-6	1	2	3	4	5 or more
(Go to	times	times	times	times	time	times	times	times	times
Question 9)	last month	per week	per week	per week	per day	per day	per day	per day	per day

8a. Each time you ate **tomato sauce**, how much did you usually eat?

○	○	○	○
About ¼ cup	About ½ cup	About 1 cup	More than 1 cup

9. Over the last month, how often did you eat **vegetable soups**? Include tomato soup, gazpacho, beef with vegetable soup, minestrone soup, and other soups made with vegetables.

○	○	○	○	○	○	○	○	○	○
Never	1-3	1-2	3-4	5-6	1	2	3	4	5 or more
(Go to	times	times	times	times	time	times	times	times	times
Question 10)	last month	per week	per week	per week	per day	per day	per day	per day	per day

9a. Each time you ate **vegetable soup**, how much did you usually eat?

○	○	○	○
Less than 1 cup	1 to 2 cups	2 to 3 cups	More than 3 cups

10. Over the last month, how often did you eat **mixtures that included vegetables**? Count such foods as sandwiches, casseroles, stews, stir-fry, omelets, and tacos.

○	○	○	○	○	○	○	○	○	○
Never	1-3	1-2	3-4	5-6	1	2	3	4	5 or more
	times	times	times	times	time	times	times	times	times
	last month	per week	per week	per week	per day	per day	per day	per day	per day

DesignExpert™ by NCS   Printed in U.S.A.   Mark Reflex® EW-226427-1:654321   HC03

**Thank you very much for completing this questionnaire.
Please return it in the enclosed, postage-paid envelope or to the
address listed on the front page.**

MEDFICTS* Dietary Assessment Questionnaire

In each food category for both Group 1 and Group 2 foods check one box from the "Weekly Consumption" column (number of servings eaten per week) and then check one box from the "Serving Size" column. If you check Rarely/Never, do not check a serving size box. See next page for score.

Food Category	Weekly Consumption			Serving Size			Score
	Rarely/ never	3 or less	4 or more	Small < 5 oz/d 1 pt	Average 5 oz/d 2 pts	Large > 5 oz/d 3 pts	

Meats
- Recommended amount per day: ≤ 5 oz (equal in size to 2 decks of playing cards)
- Base your estimate on the food you consume most often.
- Beef and lamb selections are trimmed to 1/8" fat.

Food Category	Rarely/never	3 or less	4 or more		Small	Average	Large	Score
Group 1. 10 gm or more total fat in 3 oz cooked portion **Beef** – Ground beef, Ribs, Steak (T-bone, Flank, Porterhouse, Tenderloin), Chuck blade roast, Brisket, Meatloaf (w/ground beef), Corned beef **Processed meats** – ¼ lb burger or lg. sandwich, Bacon, Lunch meat, Sausage/knockwurst, Hot dogs, Ham (bone-end), Ground turkey **Other meats, Poultry, Seafood**—Pork chops (center loin), Pork roast (Blade, Boston, Sirloin), Pork spareribs, Ground pork, Lamb chops, Lamb (ribs), Organ meats[†], Chicken w/skin, Eel, Mackerel, Pompano	☐ 0 pts	☐ 3 pts	☐ 7pts	x	☐ 1 pt	☐ 2 pts	☐ 3 pts	_____
Group 2. Less than 10 gm total fat in 3 oz cooked portion **Lean beef** – Round steak (Eye of round, Top round), Sirloin[‡], Tip & bottom round[‡], Chuck arm pot roast[‡], Top Loin[‡] **Low-fat processed meats** – Low-fat lunch meat, Canadian bacon, "Lean" fast food sandwich, Boneless ham **Other meats, Poultry, Seafood** – Chicken, Turkey (w/o skin)[§], most Seafood[†], Lamb leg shank, Pork tenderloin, Sirloin top loin, Veal cutlets, Sirloin, Shoulder, Ground veal, Venison, Veal chops and ribs[‡], Lamb (whole leg, loin, fore-shank, sirloin)[‡]	☐	☐	☐	x	☐	☐	☐* 6 pts	_____

Eggs – Weekly consumption is the number of times you eat eggs each week | Check the number of eggs eaten each time

Food Category	Rarely/never	3 or less	4 or more		≤1	2	≥3	Score
Group 1. Whole eggs, Yolks	☐ 0 pts	☐ 3 pts	☐ 7 pts	x	☐ 1 pt	☐ 2 pts	☐ 3 pts	_____
Group 2. Egg whites, Egg substitutes (½ cup)	☐	☐	☐		☐	☐	☐	_____

Dairy

Food Category	Rarely/never	3 or less	4 or more		Small	Average	Large	Score
Milk – Average serving 1 cup **Group 1.** Whole milk, 2% milk, 2% buttermilk, Yogurt (whole milk)	☐ 0 pts	☐ 3 pts	☐ 7 pts	x	☐ 1 pt	☐ 2 pts	☐ 3 pts	_____
Group 2. Fat-free milk, 1% milk, Fat-free buttermilk, Yogurt (Fat-free, 1% low fat)	☐	☐	☐		☐	☐	☐	_____
Cheese – Average serving 1 oz **Group 1.** Cream cheese, Cheddar, Monterey Jack, Colby, Swiss, American processed, Blue cheese, Regular cottage cheese (½ cup), and Ricotta (¼ cup)	☐ 0 pts	☐ 3 pts	☐ 7 pts	x	☐ 1 pt	☐ 2 pts	☐ 3 pts	_____
Group 2. Low-fat & fat-free cheeses, Fat-free milk mozzarella, String cheese, Low-fat, Fat-free milk & Fat-free cottage cheese (½ cup) and Ricotta (¼ cup)	☐	☐	☐		☐	☐	☐	_____
Frozen Desserts – Average serving ½ cup **Group 1.** Ice cream, Milk shakes	☐ 0 pts	☐ 3 pts	☐ 7 pts	x	☐ 1 pt	☐ 2 pts	☐ 3 pts	_____
Group 2. Low-fat ice cream, Frozen yogurt	☐	☐	☐		☐	☐	☐	_____

Food Category	Weekly Consumption			Serving Size			Score
	Rarely/ never	3 or less	4 or more	Small < 5 oz/d 1 pt	Average 5 oz/d 2 pts	Large > 5 oz/d 3 pts	
Frying Foods – Average servings: see below. This section refers to method of prepartion for vegetables and meat.							
Group 1. French fries, Fried vegetables (½ cup), Fried chicken, fish, meat (3 oz)	☐ 0 pts	☐ 3 pts	☐ 7 pts	x ☐ 1 pt	☐ 2 pts	☐ 3 pts	_____
Group 2. Vegetables, not deep fried (½ cup), Meat, poultry, or fish—prepared by baking, broiling, grilling, poaching, roasting, stewing: (3 oz)	☐	☐	☐	☐	☐	☐	_____
In Baked Goods – 1 Average serving							
Group 1. Doughnuts, Biscuits, Butter rolls, Muffins, Croissants, Sweet rolls, Danish, Cakes, Pies, Coffee cakes, Cookies	☐ 0 pts	☐ 3 pts	☐ 7 pts	x ☐ 1 pt	☐ 2 pts	☐ 3 pts	_____
Group 2. Fruit bars, Low-fat cookies/cakes/pastries, Angel food cake, Homemade baked goods with vegetable oils, breads, bagels	☐	☐	☐	☐	☐	☐	_____
Convenience Foods							
Group 1. Canned, Packaged, or Frozen dinners: e.g., Pizza (1 slice), Macaroni & cheese (1 cup), Pot pie (1), Cream soups (1 cup), Potato, rice & pasta dishes with cream/cheese sauces (½ cup)	☐ 0 pts	☐ 3 pts	☐ 7 pts	x ☐ 1 pt	☐ 2 pts	☐ 3 pts	_____
Group 2. Diet/Reduced calorie or reduced fat dinners (1), Potato, rice & pasta dishes without cream/cheese sauces (½ cup)	☐	☐	☐	☐	☐	☐	_____
Table Fats – Average serving: 1 Tbsp							
Group 1. Butter, Stick margarine, Regular salad dressing, Mayonnaise, Sour cream (2 Tbsp)	☐ 0 pts	☐ 3 pts	☐ 7 pts	x ☐ 1 pt	☐ 2 pts	☐ 3 pts	_____
Group 2. Diet and tub margarine, Low-fat & fat-free salad dressing, Low-fat & fat-free mayonnaise	☐	☐	☐	☐	☐	☐	_____
Snacks							
Group 1. Chips (potato, corn, taco), Cheese puffs, Snack mix, Nuts (1 oz), Regular crackers (½ oz), Candy (milk chocolate, caramel, coconut) (about 1½ oz), Regular popcorn (3 cups)	☐ 0 pts	☐ 3 pts	☐ 7 pts	x ☐ 1 pt	☐ 2 pts	☐ 3 pts	_____
Group 2. Pretzels, Fat-free chips (1 oz), Low-fat crackers (1/2 oz), Fruit, Fruit rolls, Licorice, Hard candy (1 med piece), Bread sticks (1–2 pcs), Air-popped or low-fat popcorn (3 cups)	☐	☐	☐	☐	☐	☐	_____

† Organ meats, shrimp, abalone, and squid are low in fat but high in cholesterol.
‡ Only lean cuts with all visible fat trimmed. If not trimmed of all visible fat, score as if in Group 1.
¥ Score 6 pts if this box is checked.
§ All parts not listed in group 1 have < 10 gm total fat.

Total from page 1 _____

Total from page 2 _____

FINAL SCORE _____

To Score: For each food category, multiply points in weekly consumption box by points in serving size box and record total in score column. If Group 2 foods checked, no points are scored (except for Group 2 meats, large serving = 6 pts).

Example:

☐ 0 pts	☐ 3 pts	☑ 7 pts	x ☐ 1 pt	☐ 2 pts	☑ 3 pts	21

Add score on page 1 and page 2 to get final score.

Key:
≥ 70   Need to make some dietary changes
40–70   Heart-Healthy Diet
< 40   TLC Diet

From National Cholesterol Education Program. 2001. *Third report of the Expert Panel on Detection, Evaluation, and Treatment of High Blood Cholesterol in Adults.* Bethesda, MD: U.S. Department of Health and Human Services.
*MEDFICTS = Meats, Eggs, Dairy, Frying Foods, In baked goods, Convenience foods, Table fats, Snacks.

The National Institute of Health's
The Diet History Questionnaire II

From the National Cancer Institute, National Institutes of Health, U.S. Department of Health and Human Services.

*This appendix contains the first eight pages of the Diet History Questionnaire II. For the complete questionnaire go to: http://epi.grants.cancer.gov/dhq2.

NATIONAL INSTITUTES OF HEALTH

Diet History Questionnaire II

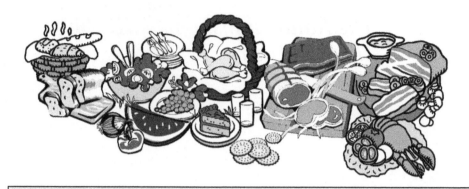

GENERAL INSTRUCTIONS

- Answer each question as best you can. Estimate if you are not sure. A guess is better than leaving a blank.

- Use only a black ball-point pen. Do not use a pencil or felt-tip pen. Do not fold, staple, or tear the pages.

- Put an X in the box next to your answer.

- If you make any changes, cross out the incorrect answer and put an X in the box next to the correct answer. Also draw a circle around the correct answer.

- If you mark NEVER, NO, or DON'T KNOW for a question, please follow any arrows or instructions that direct you to the next question.

BEFORE TURNING THE PAGE, PLEASE COMPLETE THE FOLLOWING QUESTIONS.

Today's date:

MONTH	DAY	YEAR
☐ Jan	|__|__|	☐ 2010
☐ Feb	☐0 ☐0	☐ 2011
☐ Mar	☐1 ☐1	☐ 2012
☐ Apr	☐2 ☐2	☐ 2013
☐ May	☐3 ☐3	☐ 2014
☐ Jun	☐4	☐ 2015
☐ Jul	☐5	☐ 2016
☐ Aug	☐6	☐ 2017
☐ Sep	☐7	☐ 2018
☐ Oct	☐8	☐ 2019
☐ Nov	☐9	☐ 2020
☐ Dec		

DHQ II PastYear

In what month were you born?

- ☐ Jan
- ☐ Feb
- ☐ Mar
- ☐ Apr
- ☐ May
- ☐ Jun
- ☐ Jul
- ☐ Aug
- ☐ Sep
- ☐ Oct
- ☐ Nov
- ☐ Dec

In what year were you born?

19 \|__\|__\|

☐0	☐0
☐1	☐1
☐2	☐2
☐3	☐3
☐4	☐4
☐5	☐5
☐6	☐6
☐7	☐7
☐8	☐8
☐9	☐9

Are you male or female?

- ☐ Male
- ☐ Female

BAR CODE LABEL OR SUBJECT ID HERE

\|__\|__\|__\|__\|__\|__\|__\|__\|__\|

1. Over the <u>past 12 months</u>, how often did you drink **carrot juice**?

    ☐ NEVER (GO TO QUESTION 2)

    ☐ 1 time per month or less   ☐ 1 time per day
    ☐ 2–3 times per month   ☐ 2–3 times per day
    ☐ 1–2 times per week   ☐ 4–5 times per day
    ☐ 3–4 times per week   ☐ 6 or more times per day
    ☐ 5–6 times per week

    1a. Each time you drank **carrot juice**, how much did you usually drink?

         ☐ Less than ½ cup (4 ounces)
         ☐ ½ to 1¼ cups (4 to 10 ounces)
         ☐ More than 1¼ cups (10 ounces)

2. Over the <u>past 12 months</u>, how often did you drink **tomato juice** or **other vegetable juice**? *(Please do not include carrot juice.)*

    ☐ NEVER (GO TO QUESTION 3)

    ☐ 1 time per month or less   ☐ 1 time per day
    ☐ 2–3 times per month   ☐ 2–3 times per day
    ☐ 1–2 times per week   ☐ 4–5 times per day
    ☐ 3–4 times per week   ☐ 6 or more times per day
    ☐ 5–6 times per week

    2a. Each time you drank **tomato juice** or **other vegetable juice**, how much did you usually drink?

         ☐ Less than ¾ cup (6 ounces)
         ☐ ¾ to 1¼ cups (6 to 10 ounces)
         ☐ More than 1¼ cups (10 ounces)

3. Over the <u>past 12 months</u>, how often did you drink **orange juice** or **grapefruit juice?**

    ☐ NEVER (GO TO QUESTION 4)

    ☐ 1 time per month or less   ☐ 1 time per day
    ☐ 2–3 times per month   ☐ 2–3 times per day
    ☐ 1–2 times per week   ☐ 4–5 times per day
    ☐ 3–4 times per week   ☐ 6 or more times per day
    ☐ 5–6 times per week

    3a. Each time you drank **orange juice** or **grapefruit juice**, how much did you usually drink?

         ☐ Less than ¾ cup (6 ounces)
         ☐ ¾ to 1¼ cups (6 to 10 ounces)
         ☐ More than 1¼ cups (10 ounces)

Question 4 appears in the next column

3b. How often was the orange juice or grapefruit juice you drank **calcium-fortified**?

     ☐ Almost never or never
     ☐ About ¼ of the time
     ☐ About ½ of the time
     ☐ About ¾ of the time
     ☐ Almost always or always

4. Over the <u>past 12 months</u>, how often did you drink **other 100% fruit juice** or **100% fruit juice mixtures** (such as apple, grape, pineapple, or others)?

    ☐ NEVER (GO TO QUESTION 5)

    ☐ 1 time per month or less   ☐ 1 time per day
    ☐ 2–3 times per month   ☐ 2–3 times per day
    ☐ 1–2 times per week   ☐ 4–5 times per day
    ☐ 3–4 times per week   ☐ 6 or more times per day
    ☐ 5–6 times per week

    4a. Each time you drank **other 100% fruit juice** or **100% fruit juice mixtures**, how much did you usually drink?

         ☐ Less than ¾ cup (6 ounces)
         ☐ ¾ to 1½ cups (6 to 12 ounces)
         ☐ More than 1½ cups (12 ounces)

    4b. How often were the other 100% fruit juice or 100% fruit juice mixtures you drank **calcium-fortified**?

         ☐ Almost never or never
         ☐ About ¼ of the time
         ☐ About ½ of the time
         ☐ About ¾ of the time
         ☐ Almost always or always

5. How often did you drink **other fruit drinks** (such as cranberry cocktail, Hi-C, lemonade, or Kool-Aid, diet or regular)?

    ☐ NEVER (GO TO QUESTION 6)

    ☐ 1 time per month or less   ☐ 1 time per day
    ☐ 2–3 times per month   ☐ 2–3 times per day
    ☐ 1–2 times per week   ☐ 4–5 times per day
    ☐ 3–4 times per week   ☐ 6 or more times per day
    ☐ 5–6 times per week

Question 6 appears on the next page

Over the <u>past 12 months</u>...

5a. Each time you drank **fruit drinks**, how much did you usually drink?

☐ Less than 1 cup (8 ounces)
☐ 1 to 2 cups (8 to 16 ounces)
☐ More than 2 cups (16 ounces)

5b. How often were your fruit drinks **diet** or **sugar-free**?

☐ Almost never or never
☐ About ¼ of the time
☐ About ½ of the time
☐ About ¾ of the time
☐ Almost always or always

6. How often did you drink **milk as a beverage** (NOT in coffee, NOT in cereal)? *(Please do not include chocolate milk and hot chocolate.)*

☐ NEVER (GO TO QUESTION 7)

☐ 1 time per month or less   ☐ 1 time per day
☐ 2–3 times per month   ☐ 2–3 times per day
☐ 1–2 times per week   ☐ 4–5 times per day
☐ 3–4 times per week   ☐ 6 or more times per day
☐ 5–6 times per week

6a. Each time you drank **milk as a beverage**, how much did you usually drink?

☐ Less than 1 cup (8 ounces)
☐ 1 to 1½ cups (8 to 12 ounces)
☐ More than 1½ cups (12 ounces)

6b. What kind of **milk** did you usually drink?

☐ Whole milk
☐ 2% fat milk
☐ 1 % fat milk
☐ Skim, nonfat, or ½% fat milk
☐ Soy milk
☐ Rice milk
☐ Other

7. How often did you drink **chocolate milk** (including hot chocolate)?

☐ NEVER (GO TO QUESTION 8)

☐ 1 time per month or less   ☐ 1 time per day
☐ 2–3 times per month   ☐ 2–3 times per day
☐ 1–2 times per week   ☐ 4–5 times per day
☐ 3–4 times per week   ☐ 6 or more times per day
☐ 5–6 times per week

Question 8 appears in the next column

7a. Each time you drank **chocolate milk**, how much did you usually drink?

☐ Less than 1 cup (8 ounces)
☐ 1 to 1½ cups (8 to 12 ounces)
☐ More than 1½ cups (12 ounces)

7b. How often was the chocolate milk **reduced-fat** or **fat-free**?

☐ Almost never or never
☐ About ¼ of the time
☐ About ½ of the time
☐ About ¾ of the time
☐ Almost always or always

8. How often did you drink **meal replacement** or **high-protein beverages** (such as Instant Breakfast, Ensure, SlimFast, Sustacal or others)?

☐ NEVER (GO TO QUESTION 9)

☐ 1 time per month or less   ☐ 1 time per day
☐ 2–3 times per month   ☐ 2–3 times per day
☐ 1–2 times per week   ☐ 4–5 times per day
☐ 3–4 times per week   ☐ 6 or more times per day
☐ 5–6 times per week

8a. Each time you drank **meal replacement** or **high-protein beverages**, how much did you usually drink?

☐ Less than 1 cup (8 ounces)
☐ 1 to 1½ cups (8 to 12 ounces)
☐ More than 1½ cups (12 ounces)

9. Over the <u>past 12 months</u>, did you drink **soda** or **pop**?

☐ NO (GO TO QUESTION 10)

☐ YES

9a. How often did you drink **soda** or **pop IN THE SUMMER**?

☐ NEVER

☐ 1 time per month or less   ☐ 1 time per day
☐ 2–3 times per month   ☐ 2–3 times per day
☐ 1–2 times per week   ☐ 4–5 times per day
☐ 3–4 times per week   ☐ 6 or more times
☐ 5–6 times per week   per day

Question 10 appears on the next page

Over the <u>past 12 months</u>…

9b. How often did you drink **soda** or **pop**
DURING THE REST OF THE YEAR?

☐ NEVER

☐ 1 time per month or less ☐ 1 time per day
☐ 2–3 times per month ☐ 2–3 times per day
☐ 1–2 times per week ☐ 4–5 times per day
☐ 3–4 times per week ☐ 6 or more times
☐ 5–6 times per week per day

9c. Each time you drank **soda** or **pop**, how
much did you usually drink?

☐ Less than 12 ounces or less than 1 can or bottle
☐ 12 to 16 ounces or 1 can or bottle
☐ More than 16 ounces or more than 1 can or bottle

9d. How often were these sodas or pop **diet** or
sugar-free?

☐ Almost never or never
☐ About ¼ of the time
☐ About ½ of the time
☐ About ¾ of the time
☐ Almost always or always

9e. How often were these sodas or pop
caffeine-free?

☐ Almost never or never
☐ About ¼ of the time
☐ About ½ of the time
☐ About ¾ of the time
☐ Almost always or always

10. Over the <u>past 12 months</u>, did you drink **sports
drinks** (such as Propel, PowerAde, or
Gatorade)?

☐ NO (GO TO QUESTION 11)

☐ YES

10a. How often did you drink **sports drinks IN
THE SUMMER**?

☐ NEVER

☐ 1 time per month or less ☐ 1 time per day
☐ 2–3 times per month ☐ 2–3 times per day
☐ 1–2 times per week ☐ 4–5 times per day
☐ 3–4 times per week ☐ 6 or more times
☐ 5–6 times per week per day

Question 11 appears in the next column

10b. How often did you drink **sports drinks
DURING THE REST OF THE YEAR**?

☐ NEVER

☐ 1 time per month or less ☐ 1 time per day
☐ 2–3 times per month ☐ 2–3 times per day
☐ 1–2 times per week ☐ 4–5 times per day
☐ 3–4 times per week ☐ 6 or more times
☐ 5–6 times per week per day

10c. Each time you drank **sports drinks**, how
much did you usually drink?

☐ Less than 12 ounces or less than 1 bottle
☐ 12 to 24 ounces or 1 to 2 bottles
☐ More than 24 ounces or more than 2 bottles

11. Over the <u>past 12 months</u>, did you drink **energy
drinks** (such as Red Bull or Jolt)?

☐ NO (GO TO QUESTION 12)

☐ YES

11a. How often did you drink **energy drinks IN
THE SUMMER**?

☐ NEVER

☐ 1 time per month or less ☐ 1 time per day
☐ 2–3 times per month ☐ 2–3 times per day
☐ 1–2 times per week ☐ 4–5 times per day
☐ 3–4 times per week ☐ 6 or more times
☐ 5–6 times per week per day

11b. How often did you drink **energy drinks
DURING THE REST OF THE YEAR**?

☐ NEVER

☐ 1 time per month or less ☐ 1 time per day
☐ 2–3 times per month ☐ 2–3 times per day
☐ 1–2 times per week ☐ 4–5 times per day
☐ 3–4 times per week ☐ 6 or more times
☐ 5–6 times per week per day

11c. Each time you drank **energy drinks**, how
much did you usually drink?

☐ Less than 8 ounces or less than 1 cup
☐ 8 to 16 ounces or 1 to 2 cups
☐ More than 16 ounces or more than 2 cups

Question 12 appears on the next page

Over the <u>past 12 months</u>…

12. Over the <u>past 12 months</u>, did you drink **beer**?

☐ NO (GO TO QUESTION 13)

☐ YES

12a. How often did you drink **beer IN THE SUMMER**?

☐ NEVER

☐ 1 time per month or less   ☐ 1 time per day
☐ 2–3 times per month   ☐ 2–3 times per day
☐ 1–2 times per week   ☐ 4–5 times per day
☐ 3–4 times per week   ☐ 6 or more times
☐ 5–6 times per week   per day

12b. How often did you drink **beer DURING THE REST OF THE YEAR**?

☐ NEVER

☐ 1 time per month or less   ☐ 1 time per day
☐ 2–3 times per month   ☐ 2–3 times per day
☐ 1–2 times per week   ☐ 4–5 times per day
☐ 3–4 times per week   ☐ 6 or more times
☐ 5–6 times per week   per day

12c. Each time you drank **beer**, how much did you usually drink?

☐ Less than a 12-ounce can or bottle
☐ 1 to 3 12-ounce cans or bottles
☐ More than 3 12-ounce cans or bottles

13. Over the <u>past 12 months</u>, did you drink **water** (including tap, bottled, and carbonated water)?

☐ NO (GO TO QUESTION 14)

☐ YES

13a. How often did you drink **water** (including tap, bottled, and carbonated water) **IN THE SUMMER**?

☐ NEVER

☐ 1 time per month or less   ☐ 1 time per day
☐ 2–3 times per month   ☐ 2–3 times per day
☐ 1–2 times per week   ☐ 4–5 times per day
☐ 3–4 times per week   ☐ 6 or more times
☐ 5–6 times per week   per day

Question 14 appears in the next column

13b. How often did you drink **water** (including tap, bottled, and carbonated water) **DURING THE REST OF THE YEAR**?

☐ NEVER

☐ 1 time per month or less   ☐ 1 time per day
☐ 2–3 times per month   ☐ 2–3 times per day
☐ 1–2 times per week   ☐ 4–5 times per day
☐ 3–4 times per week   ☐ 6 or more times
☐ 5–6 times per week   per day

13c. Each time you drank **water**, how much did you usually drink?

☐ Less than 12 ounces or less than 1 bottle
☐ 12 to 24 ounces or 1 to 2 bottles
☐ More than 24 ounces or more than 2 bottles

13d. How often was the water you drank **tap water**?

☐ Almost never or never
☐ About ¼ of the time
☐ About ½ of the time
☐ About ¾ of the time
☐ Almost always or always

13e. How often was the water you drank **bottled, sweetened water** (with low or no-calorie sweetener, including carbonated water)?

☐ Almost never or never
☐ About ¼ of the time
☐ About ½ of the time
☐ About ¾ of the time
☐ Almost always or always

13f. How often was the water you drank **bottled, unsweetened water** (including carbonated water)?

☐ Almost never or never
☐ About ¼ of the time
☐ About ½ of the time
☐ About ¾ of the time
☐ Almost always or always

14. How often did you drink **wine** or **wine coolers**?

☐ NEVER (GO TO QUESTION 15)

☐ 1 time per month or less   ☐ 1 time per day
☐ 2–3 times per month   ☐ 2–3 times per day
☐ 1–2 times per week   ☐ 4–5 times per day
☐ 3–4 times per week   ☐ 6 or more times per day
☐ 5–6 times per week

Question 15 appears on the next page

Over the <u>past 12 months</u>...

14a. Each time you drank **wine** or **wine coolers**, how much did you usually drink?

☐ Less than 5 ounces or less than 1 glass
☐ 5 to 12 ounces or 1 to 2 glasses
☐ More than 12 ounces or more than 2 glasses

15. How often did you drink **liquor** or **mixed drinks**?

☐ NEVER (GO TO QUESTION 16)

☐ 1 time per month or less   ☐ 1 time per day
☐ 2–3 times per month   ☐ 2–3 times per day
☐ 1–2 times per week   ☐ 4–5 times per day
☐ 3–4 times per week   ☐ 6 or more times per day
☐ 5–6 times per week

15a. Each time you drank **liquor** or **mixed drinks**, how much did you usually drink?

☐ Less than 1 shot of liquor
☐ 1 to 3 shots of liquor
☐ More than 3 shots of liquor

16. Over the <u>past 12 months</u>, did you eat **oatmeal, grits,** or **other cooked cereal?**

☐ NO (GO TO QUESTION 17)

☐ YES

16a. How often did you eat **oatmeal, grits,** or **other cooked cereal IN THE WINTER?**

☐ NEVER

☐ 1–6 times per winter   ☐ 2 times per week
☐ 7–11 times per winter   ☐ 3–4 times per week
☐ 1 time per month   ☐ 5–6 times per week
☐ 2–3 times per month   ☐ 1 time per day
☐ 1 time per week   ☐ 2 or more times
                              per day

16b. How often did you eat **oatmeal, grits,** or **other cooked cereal DURING THE REST OF THE YEAR?**

☐ NEVER

☐ 1–6 times per year   ☐ 2 times per week
☐ 7–11 times per year   ☐ 3–4 times per week
☐ 1 time per month   ☐ 5–6 times per week
☐ 2–3 times per month   ☐ 1 time per day
☐ 1 time per week   ☐ 2 or more times
                              per day

16c. Each time you ate **oatmeal, grits,** or **other cooked cereal,** how much did you usually eat?

☐ Less than ¾ cup
☐ ¾ to 1¼ cups
☐ More than 1¼ cups

16d. How often was **butter** or **margarine** added to your oatmeal, grits or other cooked cereal?

☐ Almost never or never
☐ About ¼ of the time
☐ About ½ of the time
☐ About ¾ of the time
☐ Almost always or always

17. How often did you eat **cold cereal**?

☐ NEVER (GO TO QUESTION 18)

☐ 1–6 times per year   ☐ 2 times per week
☐ 7–11 times per year   ☐ 3–4 times per week
☐ 1 time per month   ☐ 5–6 times per week
☐ 2–3 times per month   ☐ 1 time per day
☐ 1 time per week   ☐ 2 or more times per day

17a. Each time you ate **cold cereal,** how much did you usually eat?

☐ Less than 1 cup
☐ 1 to 2½ cups
☐ More than 2½ cups

17b. How often was the cold cereal you ate **Total Raisin Bran, Total Cereal,** or **Product 19**?

☐ Almost never or never
☐ About ¼ of the time
☐ About ½ of the time
☐ About ¾ of the time
☐ Almost always or always

17c. How often was the cold cereal you ate **All Bran, Fiber One, 100% Bran,** or **All-Bran Bran Buds**?

☐ Almost never or never
☐ About ¼ of the time
☐ About ½ of the time
☐ About ¾ of the time
☐ Almost always or always

Question 17 appears in the next column

Question 18 appears on the next page

Over the <u>past 12 months</u>...

17d. How often was the cold cereal you ate **some other bran** or **fiber cereal** (such as Cheerios, Shredded Wheat, Raisin Bran, Bran Flakes, Grape-Nuts, Granola, Wheaties, or Healthy Choice)?

☐ Almost never or never
☐ About ¼ of the time
☐ About ½ of the time
☐ About ¾ of the time
☐ Almost always or always

17e. How often was the cold cereal you ate any **other type of cold cereal** (such as Corn Flakes, Rice Krispies, Frosted Flakes, Special K, Froot Loops, Cap'n Crunch, or others)?

☐ Almost never or never
☐ About ¼ of the time
☐ About ½ of the time
☐ About ¾ of the time
☐ Almost always or always

17f. Was **milk** added to your cold cereal?

☐ NO (GO TO QUESTION 18)

☐ YES

17g. What kind of **milk** was usually added?

☐ Whole milk
☐ 2% fat milk
☐ 1% fat milk
☐ Skim, nonfat, or ½% fat milk
☐ Soy milk
☐ Rice milk
☐ Other

17h. Each time **milk was added to your cold cereal**, how much was usually added?

☐ Less than ½ cup
☐ ½ to 1 cup
☐ More than 1 cup

18. How often did you eat **applesauce**?

☐ NEVER (GO TO QUESTION 19)

☐ 1–6 times per year   ☐ 2 times per week
☐ 7–11 times per year   ☐ 3–4 times per week
☐ 1 time per month   ☐ 5–6 times per week
☐ 2–3 times per month   ☐ 1 time per day
☐ 1 time per week   ☐ 2 or more times per day

Question 19 appears in the next column

18a. Each time you ate **applesauce**, how much did you usually eat?

☐ Less than ½ cup
☐ ½ to 1 cup
☐ More than 1 cup

19. How often did you eat **apples**?

☐ NEVER (GO TO QUESTION 20)

☐ 1–6 times per year   ☐ 2 times per week
☐ 7–11 times per year   ☐ 3–4 times per week
☐ 1 time per month   ☐ 5–6 times per week
☐ 2–3 times per month   ☐ 1 time per day
☐ 1 time per week   ☐ 2 or more times per day

19a. Each time you ate **apples**, how many did you usually eat?

☐ Less than 1 apple
☐ 1 apple
☐ More than 1 apple

20. How often did you eat **pears** (fresh, canned, or frozen)?

☐ NEVER (GO TO QUESTION 21)

☐ 1–6 times per year   ☐ 2 times per week
☐ 7–11 times per year   ☐ 3–4 times per week
☐ 1 time per month   ☐ 5–6 times per week
☐ 2–3 times per month   ☐ 1 time per day
☐ 1 time per week   ☐ 2 or more times per day

20a. Each time you ate **pears**, how many did you usually eat?

☐ Less than 1 pear
☐ 1 pear
☐ More than 1 pear

21. How often did you eat **bananas?**

☐ NEVER (GO TO QUESTION 22)

☐ 1–6 times per year   ☐ 2 times per week
☐ 7–11 times per year   ☐ 3–4 times per week
☐ 1 time per month   ☐ 5–6 times per week
☐ 2–3 times per month   ☐ 1 time per day
☐ 1 time per week   ☐ 2 or more times per day

Question 22 appears on the next page

Over the <u>past 12 months</u>...

21a. Each time you ate **bananas**, how many did you usually eat?

- ☐ Less than 1 banana
- ☐ 1 banana
- ☐ More than 1 banana

22. How often did you eat **dried fruit** (such as prunes or raisins)? *(Please do not include dried apricots.)*

- ☐ NEVER (GO TO QUESTION 23)

☐ 1–6 times per year	☐ 2 times per week
☐ 7–11 times per year	☐ 3–4 times per week
☐ 1 time per month	☐ 5–6 times per week
☐ 2–3 times per month	☐ 1 time per day
☐ 1 time per week	☐ 2 or more times per day

22a. Each time you ate **dried fruit**, how much did you usually eat?

- ☐ Less than 2 tablespoons
- ☐ 2 to 5 tablespoons
- ☐ More than 5 tablespoons

23. Over the <u>past 12 months</u>, did you eat **peaches, nectarines, or plums**?

- ☐ NO (GO TO QUESTION 24)
- ☐ YES

23a. How often did you eat **fresh peaches, nectarines, or plums WHEN IN SEASON**?

- ☐ NEVER

☐ 1–6 times per season	☐ 2 times per week
☐ 7–11 times per season	☐ 3–4 times per week
☐ 1 time per month	☐ 5–6 times per week
☐ 2–3 times per month	☐ 1 time per day
☐ 1 time per week	☐ 2 or more times per day

23b. How often did you eat **peaches, nectarines, or plums** (fresh, canned, or frozen) **DURING THE REST OF THE YEAR**?

- ☐ NEVER

☐ 1–6 times per year	☐ 2 times per week
☐ 7–11 times per year	☐ 3–4 times per week
☐ 1 time per month	☐ 5–6 times per week
☐ 2–3 times per month	☐ 1 time per day
☐ 1 time per week	☐ 2 or more times per day

23c. Each time you ate **peaches, nectarines, or plums,** how much did you usually eat?

- ☐ Less than 1 fruit or less than ½ cup
- ☐ 1 to 2 fruits or ½ to ¾ cup
- ☐ More than 2 fruits or more than ¾ cup

24. How often did you eat **grapes**?

- ☐ NEVER (GO TO QUESTION 25)

☐ 1–6 times per year	☐ 2 times per week
☐ 7–11 times per year	☐ 3–4 times per week
☐ 1 time per month	☐ 5–6 times per week
☐ 2–3 times per month	☐ 1 time per day
☐ 1 time per week	☐ 2 or more times per day

24a. Each time you ate **grapes**, how much did you usually eat?

- ☐ Less than ½ cup or less than 10 grapes
- ☐ ½ to 1 cup or 10 to 30 grapes
- ☐ More than 1 cup or more than 30 grapes

25. Over the <u>past 12 months</u>, did you eat **cantaloupe**?

- ☐ NO (GO TO QUESTION 26)
- ☐ YES

25a. How often did you eat **fresh cantaloupe WHEN IN SEASON**?

- ☐ NEVER

☐ 1–6 times per season	☐ 2 times per week
☐ 7–11 times per season	☐ 3–4 times per week
☐ 1 time per month	☐ 5–6 times per week
☐ 2–3 times per month	☐ 1 time per day
☐ 1 time per week	☐ 2 or more times per day

25b. How often did you eat **cantaloupe** (fresh or frozen) **DURING THE REST OF THE YEAR**?

- ☐ NEVER

☐ 1–6 times per year	☐ 2 times per week
☐ 7–11 times per year	☐ 3–4 times per week
☐ 1 time per month	☐ 5–6 times per week
☐ 2–3 times per month	☐ 1 time per day
☐ 1 time per week	☐ 2 or more times per day

Question 24 appears in the next column

Question 26 appears on the next page

E

The NHANES Food Frequency Questionnaire

From the National Cancer Institute, National Institutes of Health, U.S. Department of Health and Human Services.

*This appendix contains the first eight pages of the NHANES Food Frequency Questionnaire. For the complete questionnaire, visit http://www.cdc.gov/nchs/data/nhanes/nhanes_03_04/tq_fpq_c.pdf

Note: this questionnaire was used in NHANES 2003–2004, and is archived by the CDC at: wwwn.cdc.gov/nchs/nhanes/

NHANES Food Questionnaire

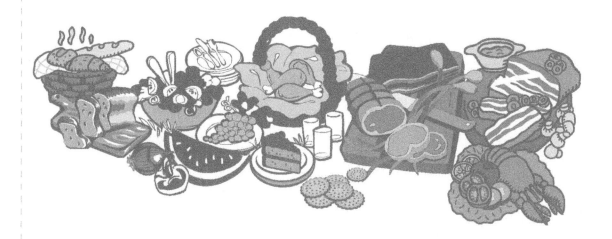

> *More than one member of your household may have received a questionnaire. Please make sure this is your booklet before answering any questions.*

LABEL HERE

GENERAL INSTRUCTIONS

- Answer each question as best you can. Estimate if you are not sure. A guess is better than leaving a blank.
- Use only a No. 2 pencil.
- Be certain to completely blacken in each of the answers.
- Erase completely if you make any changes.
- Do not make any stray marks on this form.
- If you blacken NEVER or NO for a question, please follow any arrows or instructions that direct you to the next question.

PLEASE DO NOT WRITE IN THIS AREA

SERIAL #

1. Over the <u>past 12 months</u>, how often did you drink **tomato juice** or **vegetable juice**?

○ NEVER

○ 1 time per month or less ○ 1 time per day
○ 2–3 times per month ○ 2–3 times per day
○ 1–2 times per week ○ 4–5 times per day
○ 3–4 times per week ○ 6 or more times per day
○ 5–6 times per week

2. How often did you drink **orange juice** or **grapefruit juice?**

○ NEVER

○ 1 time per month or less ○ 1 time per day
○ 2–3 times per month ○ 2–3 times per day
○ 1–2 times per week ○ 4–5 times per day
○ 3–4 times per week ○ 6 or more times per day
○ 5–6 times per week

3. How often did you drink **apple juice?**

○ NEVER

○ 1 time per month or less ○ 1 time per day
○ 2–3 times per month ○ 2–3 times per day
○ 1–2 times per week ○ 4–5 times per day
○ 3–4 times per week ○ 6 or more times per day
○ 5–6 times per week

4. How often did you drink **grape juice?**

○ NEVER

○ 1 time per month or less ○ 1 time per day
○ 2–3 times per month ○ 2–3 times per day
○ 1–2 times per week ○ 4–5 times per day
○ 3–4 times per week ○ 6 or more times per day
○ 5–6 times per week

5. How often did you drink **other 100% fruit juice** or **100% fruit juice mixtures** (such as pineapple, prune, or others)?

○ NEVER

○ 1 time per month or less ○ 1 time per day
○ 2–3 times per month ○ 2–3 times per day
○ 1–2 times per week ○ 4–5 times per day
○ 3–4 times per week ○ 6 or more times per day
○ 5–6 times per week

6. How often did you drink other **fruit drinks** (such as cranberry cocktail, Hi-C, lemonade, or Kool-Aid, diet or regular)?

○ NEVER (GO TO QUESTION 7)

○ 1 time per month or less ○ 1 time per day
○ 2–3 times per month ○ 2–3 times per day
○ 1–2 times per week ○ 4–5 times per day
○ 3–4 times per week ○ 6 or more times per day
○ 5–6 times per week

6a. How often were your fruit drinks **diet** or **sugar-free drinks**?

○ Almost never or never
○ About $1/4$ of the time
○ About $1/2$ of the time
○ About $3/4$ of the time
○ Almost always or always

7. How often did you drink **milk as a beverage** (NOT in coffee, NOT in cereal)? (Please include chocolate milk and hot chocolate.)

○ NEVER (GO TO QUESTION 8)

○ 1 time per month or less ○ 1 time per day
○ 2–3 times per month ○ 2–3 times per day
○ 1–2 times per week ○ 4–5 times per day
○ 3–4 times per week ○ 6 or more times per day
○ 5–6 times per week

7a. What kind of **milk** did you usually drink?

○ Whole milk
○ 2% fat milk
○ 1% fat milk
○ Skim, nonfat, or $1/2$% fat milk
○ Soy milk
○ Rice milk
○ Raw, unpasteurized milk
○ Other

BAR

CODE

LABEL

HERE

Question 8 appears on the next page.

Over the <u>past 12 months</u>...

8. How often did you drink **meal replacement, energy, or high-protein beverages** such as Instant Breakfast, Ensure, Slimfast, Sustacal or others?

○ NEVER

○ 1 time per month or less   ○ 1 time per day
○ 2–3 times per month   ○ 2–3 times per day
○ 1–2 times per week   ○ 4–5 times per day
○ 3–4 times per week   ○ 6 or more times per day
○ 5–6 times per week

9. Over the <u>past 12 months</u>, did you drink **soft drinks, soda,** or **pop**?

○ NO (GO TO QUESTION 10)

○ YES

9a. How often did you drink **soft drinks, soda,** or **pop IN THE SUMMER**?

○ NEVER

○ 1 time per month or less   ○ 1 time per day
○ 2–3 times per month   ○ 2–3 times per day
○ 1–2 times per week   ○ 4–5 times per day
○ 3–4 times per week   ○ 6 or more times
○ 5–6 times per week   per day

9b. How often did you drink **soft drinks, soda,** or **pop DURING THE REST OF THE YEAR**?

○ NEVER

○ 1 time per month or less   ○ 1 time per day
○ 2–3 times per month   ○ 2–3 times per day
○ 1–2 times per week   ○ 4–5 times per day
○ 3–4 times per week   ○ 6 or more times
○ 5–6 times per week   per day

9c. How often were these soft drinks, soda, or pop **diet** or **sugar-free**?

○ Almost never or never
○ About $1/4$ of the time
○ About $1/2$ of the time
○ About $3/4$ of the time
○ Almost always or always

9d. How often were these soft drinks, soda, or pop **caffeine-free**?

○ Almost never or never
○ About $1/4$ of the time
○ About $1/2$ of the time
○ About $3/4$ of the time
○ Almost always or always

Question 10 appears in the next column.

10. Over the <u>past 12 months</u>, did you drink **beer**?

○ NO (GO TO QUESTION 11)

○ YES

10a. How often did you drink **beer IN THE SUMMER**?

○ NEVER

○ 1 time per month or less   ○ 1 time per day
○ 2–3 times per month   ○ 2–3 times per day
○ 1–2 times per week   ○ 4–5 times per day
○ 3–4 times per week   ○ 6 or more times
○ 5–6 times per week   per day

10b. How often did you drink **beer DURING THE REST OF THE YEAR**?

○ NEVER

○ 1 time per month or less   ○ 1 time per day
○ 2–3 times per month   ○ 2–3 times per day
○ 1–2 times per week   ○ 4–5 times per day
○ 3–4 times per week   ○ 6 or more times
○ 5–6 times per week   per day

11. How often did you drink **wine** or **wine coolers**?

○ NEVER

○ 1 time per month or less   ○ 1 time per day
○ 2–3 times per month   ○ 2–3 times per day
○ 1–2 times per week   ○ 4–5 times per day
○ 3–4 times per week   ○ 6 or more times per day
○ 5–6 times per week

12. How often did you drink **liquor** or **mixed drinks**?

○ NEVER

○ 1 time per month or less   ○ 1 time per day
○ 2–3 times per month   ○ 2–3 times per day
○ 1–2 times per week   ○ 4–5 times per day
○ 3–4 times per week   ○ 6 or more times per day
○ 5–6 times per week

244004 - 2/6

Over the past 12 months...

13. Did you eat **oatmeal, grits,** or **other cooked cereal?**

○ NO (GO TO QUESTION 14)

○ YES

13a. How often did you eat **oatmeal, grits,** or **other cooked cereal IN THE WINTER?**

○ NEVER

○ 1–6 times per winter   ○ 2 times per week
○ 7–11 times per winter   ○ 3–4 times per week
○ 1 time per month   ○ 5–6 times per week
○ 2–3 times per month   ○ 1 time per day
○ 1 time per week   ○ 2 or more times
                               per day

13b. How often did you eat **oatmeal, grits,** or **other cooked cereal DURING THE REST OF THE YEAR?**

○ NEVER

○ 1–6 times per year   ○ 2 times per week
○ 7–11 times per year   ○ 3–4 times per week
○ 1 time per month   ○ 5–6 times per week
○ 2–3 times per month   ○ 1 time per day
○ 1 time per week   ○ 2 or more times
                               per day

13c. How often was the cooked cereal you ate **oatmeal?**

○ Almost never or never
○ About $1/4$ of the time
○ About $1/2$ of the time
○ About $3/4$ of the time
○ Almost always or always

14. How often did you eat **cold cereal?**

○ NEVER (GO TO QUESTION 15)

○ 1–6 times per year   ○ 2 times per week
○ 7–11 times per year   ○ 3–4 times per week
○ 1 time per month   ○ 5–6 times per week
○ 2–3 times per month   ○ 1 time per day
○ 1 time per week   ○ 2 or more times per day

Question 15 appears in the next column.

14a. How often was the cold cereal you ate a **whole grain type** (such as Shredded Wheat, Wheaties, Cheerios, Raisin Bran or other bran, oat, or whole wheat cereal)?

○ Almost never or never
○ About $1/4$ of the time
○ About $1/2$ of the time
○ About $3/4$ of the time
○ Almost always or always

14b. Was **milk** added to your cold cereal?

○ NO (GO TO QUESTION 15)

○ YES

14c. What kind of **milk** was usually added?

○ Whole milk
○ 2% fat milk
○ 1% fat milk
○ Skim, nonfat, or $1/2$% fat milk
○ Soy milk
○ Rice milk
○ Raw, unpasteurized milk
○ Other

15. How often did you eat **applesauce?**

○ NEVER

○ 1–6 times per year   ○ 2 times per week
○ 7–11 times per year   ○ 3–4 times per week
○ 1 time per month   ○ 5–6 times per week
○ 2–3 times per month   ○ 1 time per day
○ 1 time per week   ○ 2 or more times per day

16. How often did you eat **apples?**

○ NEVER

○ 1–6 times per year   ○ 2 times per week
○ 7–11 times per year   ○ 3–4 times per week
○ 1 time per month   ○ 5–6 times per week
○ 2–3 times per month   ○ 1 time per day
○ 1 time per week   ○ 2 or more times per day

17. How often did you eat **pears** (fresh, canned, or frozen)?

○ NEVER

○ 1–6 times per year   ○ 2 times per week
○ 7–11 times per year   ○ 3–4 times per week
○ 1 time per month   ○ 5–6 times per week
○ 2–3 times per month   ○ 1 time per day
○ 1 time per week   ○ 2 or more times per day

■ Over the <u>past 12 months</u>...

18. How often did you eat **bananas** ?

○ NEVER

○ 1–6 times per year	○ 2 times per week
○ 7–11 times per year	○ 3–4 times per week
○ 1 time per month	○ 5–6 times per week
○ 2–3 times per month	○ 1 time per day
○ 1 time per week	○ 2 or more times per day

19. How often did you eat **pineapple**?

○ NEVER

○ 1–6 times per year	○ 2 times per week
○ 7–11 times per year	○ 3–4 times per week
○ 1 time per month	○ 5–6 times per week
○ 2–3 times per month	○ 1 time per day
○ 1 time per week	○ 2 or more times per day

20. How often did you eat **dried fruit**, such as prunes or raisins?

○ NEVER

○ 1–6 times per year	○ 2 times per week
○ 7–11 times per year	○ 3–4 times per week
○ 1 time per month	○ 5–6 times per week
○ 2–3 times per month	○ 1 time per day
○ 1 time per week	○ 2 or more times per day

21. Over the <u>past 12 months</u>, did you eat **peaches, nectarines,** or **plums**?

○ NO (GO TO QUESTION 22)

○ YES

21a. How often did you eat **fresh peaches, nectarines,** or **plums WHEN IN SEASON**?

○ NEVER

○ 1–6 times per season	○ 2 times per week
○ 7–11 times per season	○ 3–4 times per week
○ 1 time per month	○ 5–6 times per week
○ 2–3 times per month	○ 1 time per day
○ 1 time per week	○ 2 or more times per day

Question 22 appears in the next column.

21b. How often did you eat **peaches, nectarines,** or **plums** (fresh, canned, or frozen) **DURING THE REST OF THE YEAR?**

○ NEVER

○ 1–6 times per year	○ 2 times per week
○ 7–11 times per year	○ 3–4 times per week
○ 1 time per month	○ 5–6 times per week
○ 2–3 times per month	○ 1 time per day
○ 1 time per week	○ 2 or more times per day

22. How often did you eat **grapes**?

○ NEVER

○ 1–6 times per year	○ 2 times per week
○ 7–11 times per year	○ 3–4 times per week
○ 1 time per month	○ 5–6 times per week
○ 2–3 times per month	○ 1 time per day
○ 1 time per week	○ 2 or more times per day

23. Over the <u>past 12 months</u>, did you eat **melons** (such as cantaloupe, watermelon, or honeydew)?

○ NO (GO TO QUESTION 24)

○ YES

23a. How often did you eat **fresh melons** (such as cantaloupe, watermelon, or honeydew) **WHEN IN SEASON**?

○ NEVER

○ 1–6 times per season	○ 2 times per week
○ 7–11 times per season	○ 3–4 times per week
○ 1 time per month	○ 5–6 times per week
○ 2–3 times per month	○ 1 time per day
○ 1 time per week	○ 2 or more times per day

23b. How often did you eat **fresh or frozen melons** (such as cantaloupe, watermelon, or honeydew) **DURING THE REST OF THE YEAR?**

○ NEVER

○ 1–6 times per year	○ 2 times per week
○ 7–11 times per year	○ 3–4 times per week
○ 1 time per month	○ 5–6 times per week
○ 2–3 times per month	○ 1 time per day
○ 1 time per week	○ 2 or more times per day

244004 - 3/6

Question 24 appears on the next page.

Over the past 12 months...

24. Did you eat **strawberries**?

○ NO (GO TO QUESTION 25)

○ YES

24a. How often did you eat **fresh strawberries WHEN IN SEASON**?

○ NEVER

○ 1–6 times per season   ○ 2 times per week
○ 7–11 times per season   ○ 3–4 times per week
○ 1 time per month   ○ 5–6 times per week
○ 2–3 times per month   ○ 1 time per day
○ 1 time per week   ○ 2 or more times
                            per day

24b. How often did you eat **fresh** or **frozen** strawberries **DURING THE REST OF THE YEAR**?

○ NEVER

○ 1–6 times per year   ○ 2 times per week
○ 7–11 times per year   ○ 3–4 times per week
○ 1 time per month   ○ 5–6 times per week
○ 2–3 times per month   ○ 1 time per day
○ 1 time per week   ○ 2 or more times
                            per day

25. Over the past 12 months, did you eat **oranges, tangerines, clementines,** or **tangelos**?

○ NO (GO TO QUESTION 26)

○ YES

25a. How often did you eat **fresh oranges, tangerines, clementines,** or **tangelos WHEN IN SEASON**?

○ NEVER

○ 1–6 times per season   ○ 2 times per week
○ 7–11 times per season   ○ 3–4 times per week
○ 1 time per month   ○ 5–6 times per week
○ 2–3 times per month   ○ 1 time per day
○ 1 time per week   ○ 2 or more times
                            per day

Question 26 appears in the next column.

25b. How often did you eat **oranges, tangerines, clementines,** or **tangelos** (fresh or canned) **DURING THE REST OF THE YEAR**?

○ NEVER

○ 1–6 times per year   ○ 2 times per week
○ 7–11 times per year   ○ 3–4 times per week
○ 1 time per month   ○ 5–6 times per week
○ 2–3 times per month   ○ 1 time per day
○ 1 time per week   ○ 2 or more times
                            per day

26. Over the past 12 months, did you eat **grapefruit**?

○ NO (GO TO QUESTION 27)

○ YES

26a. How often did you eat **fresh grapefruit WHEN IN SEASON**?

○ NEVER

○ 1–6 times per season   ○ 2 times per week
○ 7–11 times per season   ○ 3–4 times per week
○ 1 time per month   ○ 5–6 times per week
○ 2–3 times per month   ○ 1 time per day
○ 1 time per week   ○ 2 or more times
                            per day

26b. How often did you eat **grapefruit** (fresh or canned) **DURING THE REST OF THE YEAR**?

○ NEVER

○ 1–6 times per year   ○ 2 times per week
○ 7–11 times per year   ○ 3–4 times per week
○ 1 time per month   ○ 5–6 times per week
○ 2–3 times per month   ○ 1 time per day
○ 1 time per week   ○ 2 or more times
                            per day

27. How often did you eat **other kinds of fruit**?

○ NEVER

○ 1–6 times per year   ○ 2 times per week
○ 7–11 times per year   ○ 3–4 times per week
○ 1 time per month   ○ 5–6 times per week
○ 2–3 times per month   ○ 1 time per day
○ 1 time per week   ○ 2 or more times per day

3/8" SPINE PERF

■ Over the <u>past 12 months</u>...

28. How often did you eat **COOKED greens** (such as spinach, turnip, collard, mustard, chard, or kale)?

○ NEVER

○ 1–6 times per year	○ 2 times per week
○ 7–11 times per year	○ 3–4 times per week
○ 1 time per month	○ 5–6 times per week
○ 2–3 times per month	○ 1 time per day
○ 1 time per week	○ 2 or more times per day

29. How often did you eat **RAW greens** (such as spinach, turnip, collard, mustard, chard, or kale)? (*We will ask about lettuce later.*)

○ NEVER

○ 1–6 times per year	○ 2 times per week
○ 7–11 times per year	○ 3–4 times per week
○ 1 time per month	○ 5–6 times per week
○ 2–3 times per month	○ 1 time per day
○ 1 time per week	○ 2 or more times per day

30. How often did you eat **coleslaw**?

○ NEVER

○ 1–6 times per year	○ 2 times per week
○ 7–11 times per year	○ 3–4 times per week
○ 1 time per month	○ 5–6 times per week
○ 2–3 times per month	○ 1 time per day
○ 1 time per week	○ 2 or more times per day

31. How often did you eat **sauerkraut** or **cabbage** (other than coleslaw)?

○ NEVER

○ 1–6 times per year	○ 2 times per week
○ 7–11 times per year	○ 3–4 times per week
○ 1 time per month	○ 5–6 times per week
○ 2–3 times per month	○ 1 time per day
○ 1 time per week	○ 2 or more times per day

32. How often did you eat **carrots** (fresh, canned, or frozen)?

○ NEVER

○ 1–6 times per year	○ 2 times per week
○ 7–11 times per year	○ 3–4 times per week
○ 1 time per month	○ 5–6 times per week
○ 2–3 times per month	○ 1 time per day
○ 1 time per week	○ 2 or more times per day

33. How often did you eat **string beans** or **green beans** (fresh, canned, or frozen)?

○ NEVER

○ 1–6 times per year	○ 2 times per week
○ 7–11 times per year	○ 3–4 times per week
○ 1 time per month	○ 5–6 times per week
○ 2–3 times per month	○ 1 time per day
○ 1 time per week	○ 2 or more times per day

34. How often did you eat **peas** (fresh, canned, or frozen)?

○ NEVER

○ 1–6 times per year	○ 2 times per week
○ 7–11 times per year	○ 3–4 times per week
○ 1 time per month	○ 5–6 times per week
○ 2–3 times per month	○ 1 time per day
○ 1 time per week	○ 2 or more times per day

35. Over the <u>past 12 months</u>, did you eat **corn**?

○ NO (GO TO QUESTION 36)

○ YES

⇩

35a. How often did you eat **corn** (fresh, canned, or frozen) **WHEN IN SEASON**?

○ NEVER

○ 1–6 times per season	○ 2 times per week
○ 7–11 times per season	○ 3–4 times per week
○ 1 time per month	○ 5–6 times per week
○ 2–3 times per month	○ 1 time per day
○ 1 time per week	○ 2 or more times per day

35b. How often did you eat **corn** (fresh, canned, or frozen) **DURING THE REST OF THE YEAR**?

○ NEVER

○ 1–6 times per year	○ 2 times per week
○ 7–11 times per year	○ 3–4 times per week
○ 1 time per month	○ 5–6 times per week
○ 2–3 times per month	○ 1 time per day
○ 1 time per week	○ 2 or more times per day

Question 36 appears on the next page.

244004 - 4/6

F *2016 Behavioral Risk Factor Surveillance System Questionnaire*

The BRFSS questionnaire is designed by a working group of BRFSS state coordinators and CDC staff. The questionnaire has three parts: (1) the core component, consisting of the fixed core, rotating core, and emerging core, (2) optional modules, and (3) state-added questions.

All health departments must ask the core component questions without modification in wording; however, the modules are optional. The fixed core is a standard set of questions asked by all states that includes questions on demographic characteristics, plus queries on current health behaviors, such as tobacco use and seat belt use. The rotating core is made up of two distinct sets of questions, each asked in alternating years by all states, addressing different topics. In the years that rotating core topics are not used, they are supported as optional modules. The emerging core is a set of up to five questions that are added to the fixed and rotating cores. Emerging core questions typically focus on "late breaking" issues. These questions are part of the core for one year and are evaluated during, or soon after the year concludes to determine their potential value in future surveys.

Sample questions are included in this appendix, with the full BRFSS questionnaire available at https://www.cdc.gov/brfss/questionnaires/.

Source: Centers for Disease Control and Prevention. 2015.

BEHAVIORAL RISK FACTOR SURVEILLANCE SYSTEM 2016 QUESTIONNAIRE

Table of Contents

CORE SECTIONS

I will not ask for your last name, address, or other personal information that can identify you. You do not have to answer any question you do not want to, and you can end the interview at any time. Any information you give me will be confidential. If you have any questions about the survey, please call **(give appropriate state telephone number)**.

SECTION 1: HEALTH STATUS

1.1 Would you say that in general your health is— (90)

	Please read:
1	Excellent
2	Very good
3	Good
4	Fair
	Or
5	Poor
	Do not read:
7	Don't know / Not sure
9	Refused

SECTION 2: HEALTHY DAYS — HEALTH-RELATED QUALITY OF LIFE

2.1 Now thinking about your physical health, which includes physical illness and injury, for how many days during the past 30 days was your physical health not good? (91–92)

_ _	Number of days
8 8	None
7 7	Don't know / Not sure
9 9	Refused

2.2 Now thinking about your mental health, which includes stress, depression, and problems with emotions, for how many days during the past 30 days was your mental health not good? (93–94)

_ _	Number of days
8 8	None **[If Q2.1 and Q2.2 = 88 (None), go to next section]**
7 7	Don't know / Not sure
9 9	Refused

2.3 During the past 30 days, for about how many days did poor physical or mental health keep you from doing your usual activities, such as self-care, work, or recreation? (95–96)

_ _	Number of days
8 8	None
7 7	Don't know / Not sure
9 9	Refused

SECTION 3: HEALTH CARE ACCESS

3.1 Do you have any kind of health care coverage, including health insurance, prepaid plans such as HMOs, government plans such as Medicare, or Indian Health Service? (97)

1	Yes
2	No **[If using Health Care Access (HCA) Module go to Module 4, Q1, else continue]**
7	Don't know / Not sure
9	Refused

3.2 Do you have one person you think of as your personal doctor or health care provider?

If "No," ask: "Is there more than one, or is there no person who you think of as your personal doctor or health care provider?" (98)

1	Yes, only one
2	More than one
3	No
7	Don't know / Not sure
9	Refused

3.3 Was there a time in the past 12 months when you needed to see a doctor but could not because of cost? (99)

1	Yes
2	No
7	Don't know / Not sure
9	Refused

> **CATI NOTE: If using HCA Module, go to Module 4, Q3, else continue.**

3.4 About how long has it been since you last visited a doctor for a routine checkup? A routine checkup is a general physical exam, not an exam for a specific injury, illness, or condition. (100)

1	Within the past year (anytime less than 12 months ago)
2	Within the past 2 years (1 year but less than 2 years ago)
3	Within the past 5 years (2 years but less than 5 years ago)
4	5 or more years ago
7	Don't know / Not sure
8	Never
9	Refused

> **CATI NOTE: If using HCA Module and Q3.1 = 1 go to Module 4, Question 4a or if using HCA Module and Q3.1 = 2, 7, or 9 go to Module 4, Question 4b, or if not using HCA Module go to next section.**

SECTION 4: EXERCISE

4.1 During the past month, other than your regular job, did you participate in any physical activities or exercises such as running, calisthenics, golf, gardening, or walking for exercise? (101)

1	Yes
2	No
7	Don't know / Not sure
9	Refused

SECTION 5: INADEQUATE SLEEP

5.1 On average, how many hours of sleep do you get in a 24-hour period?

INTERVIEWER NOTE: Enter hours of sleep in whole numbers, rounding 30 minutes (1/2 hour) or more up to the next whole hour and dropping 29 or fewer minutes. (102–103)

_	_	Number of hours [01–24]
7	7	Don't know / Not sure
9	9	Refused

SECTION 6: CHRONIC HEALTH CONDITIONS

Has a doctor, nurse, or other health professional EVER told you that you had any of the following? For each, tell me "Yes," "No," or you're "Not sure."

6.1 (Ever told) you that you had a heart attack also called a myocardial infarction? (104)

1	Yes
2	No
7	Don't know / Not sure
9	Refused

6.2 (Ever told) you had angina or coronary heart disease? (105)

1	Yes
2	No
7	Don't know / Not sure
9	Refused

6.3 (Ever told) you had a stroke? (106)

1	Yes
2	No
7	Don't know / Not sure
9	Refused

6.4 (Ever told) you had asthma? (107)

1	Yes	
2	No	**[Go to Q6.6]**
7	Don't know / Not sure	**[Go to Q6.6]**
9	Refused	**[Go to Q6.6]**

6.5 Do you still have asthma? (108)

1	Yes
2	No
7	Don't know / Not sure
9	Refused

6.6 (Ever told) you had skin cancer? (109)

1	Yes
2	No
7	Don't know / Not sure
9	Refused

6.7 (Ever told) you had any other types of cancer? (110)

1	Yes
2	No
7	Don't know / Not sure
9	Refused

6.8 (Ever told) you have chronic obstructive pulmonary disease (COPD), emphysema or chronic bronchitis? (111)

1	Yes
2	No
7	Don't know / Not sure
9	Refused

6.9 (Ever told) you have some form of arthritis, rheumatoid arthritis, gout, lupus, or fibromyalgia? (112)

1	Yes
2	No
7	Don't know / Not sure
9	Refused

INTERVIEWER NOTE: Arthritis diagnoses include:

- rheumatism, polymyalgia rheumatica
- osteoarthritis (not osteoporosis)
- tendonitis, bursitis, bunion, tennis elbow
- carpal tunnel syndrome, tarsal tunnel syndrome
- joint infection, Reiter's syndrome
- ankylosing spondylitis; spondylosis
- rotator cuff syndrome
- connective tissue disease, scleroderma, polymyositis, Raynaud's syndrome
- vasculitis (giant cell arteritis, Henoch-Schonlein purpura, Wegener's granulomatosis, polyarteritis nodosa)

6.10 (Ever told) you have a depressive disorder (including depression, major depression, dysthymia, or minor depression)? (113)

1	Yes
2	No
7	Don't know / Not sure
9	Refused

6.11 (Ever told) you have kidney disease? Do NOT include kidney stones, bladder infection or incontinence.

INTERVIEWER NOTE: Incontinence is not being able to control urine flow. (114)

1	Yes
2	No
7	Don't know / Not sure
9	Refused

6.12 (Ever told) you have diabetes? (115)

If "Yes" and respondent is female, ask: "Was this only when you were pregnant?"

If respondent says pre-diabetes or borderline diabetes, use response code 4.

1	Yes
2	Yes, but female told only during pregnancy
3	No
4	No, pre-diabetes or borderline diabetes
7	Don't know / Not sure
9	Refused

> **CATI NOTE: If Q6.12 = 1 (Yes), go to next question. If any other response to Q6.12, go to Pre-Diabetes Optional Module (if used). Otherwise, go to next section.** (116–117)

6.13 How old were you when you were told you have diabetes?

_	_	Code age in years **[97 = 97 and older]**
9	8	Don't know / Not sure
9	9	Refused

SECTION 10: E-CIGARETTES

Read if necessary: Electronic cigarettes (e-cigarettes) and other electronic "vaping" products include electronic hookahs (e-hookahs), vape pens, e-cigars, and others. These products are battery-powered and usually contain nicotine and flavors such as fruit, mint, or candy.

10.1 Have you ever used an e-cigarette or other electronic "vaping" product, even just one time, in your entire life? (199)

1	Yes
2	No [Go to next section]
7	Don't know / Not sure
9	Refused [Go to next section]

10.2 Do you now use e-cigarettes or other electronic "vaping" products every day, some days, or not at all? (200)

1	Every day
2	Some days
3	Not at all
7	Don't know / Not sure
9	Refused

Section 11: Alcohol Consumption

11.1 During the past 30 days, how many days per week or per month did you have at least one drink of any alcoholic beverage such as beer, wine, a malt beverage, or liquor? (201–203)

1   _   _   Days per week

2   _   _   Days in past 30 days

8   8   8   No drinks in past 30 days   [Go to next section]

7   7   7   Don't know / Not sure   [Go to next section]

9   9   9   Refused   [Go to next section]

11.2 One drink is equivalent to a 12-ounce beer, a 5-ounce glass of wine, or a drink with one shot of liquor. During the past 30 days, on the days when you drank, about how many drinks did you drink on the average? (204–205)

NOTE: A 40 ounce beer would count as 3 drinks, or a cocktail drink with 2 shots would count as 2 drinks.

_   _   Number of drinks

7   7   Don't know / Not sure

9   9   Refused

11.3 Considering all types of alcoholic beverages, how many times during the past 30 days did you have **X [CATI X = 5 for men, X = 4 for women]** or more drinks on an occasion? (206–207)

_   _   Number of times

8   8   None

7   7   Don't know / Not sure

9   9   Refused

11.4 During the past 30 days, what is the largest number of drinks you had on any occasion? (208–209)

_   _   Number of drinks

7   7   Don't know / Not sure

9   9   Refused

Section 12: Immunization

Now I will ask you questions about the flu vaccine. There are two ways to get the flu vaccine; one is a shot in the arm and the other is a spray, mist, or drop in the nose called FluMist.™

12.1 During the past 12 months, have you had either a flu shot or a flu vaccine that was sprayed in your nose? (210)

Read if necessary: A new flu shot came out in 2011 that injects vaccine into the skin with a very small needle.

It is called Fluzone Intradermal vaccine. This is also considered a flu shot.

1   Yes

2   No   [Go to Q12.3]

7   Don't know / Not sure   [Go to Q12.3]

9   Refused   [Go to Q12.3]

12.2 During what month and year did you receive your most recent flu shot injected into your arm or flu vaccine that was sprayed in your nose? (211–216)

_ _ / _ _ _ _   Month / Year

7 7 / 7 7 7 7   Don't know / Not sure

9 9 / 9 9 9 9   Refused

12.3 A pneumonia shot or pneumococcal vaccine is usually given only once or twice in a person's lifetime and is different from the flu shot. Have you ever had a pneumonia shot? (217)

1   Yes

2   No

7   Don't know / Not sure

9   Refused

12.4 Since 2005, have you had a tetanus shot? (218)

If yes, ask: "Was this Tdap, the tetanus shot that also has pertussis or whooping cough vaccine?"

1   Yes, received Tdap

2   Yes, received tetanus shot, but not Tdap

3   Yes, received tetanus shot but not sure what type

4   No, did not receive any tetanus since 2005

7   Don't know/Not sure

9   Refused

Section 13: Falls

If respondent is 45 years or older continue, otherwise go to next section.

The next questions ask about recent falls. By a fall, we mean when a person unintentionally comes to rest on the ground or another lower level.

13.1 In the past 12 months, how many times have you fallen? (219–220)

_   _   Number of times   [76 = 76 or more]

8   8   None   [Go to next section]

7   7   Don't know / Not sure   [Go to next section]

9   9   Refused   [Go to next section]

13.2 [Fill in "Did this fall (from Q13.1) cause an injury?"] If only one fall from Q13.1 and response is "Yes" (caused an injury), code 01. If response is "No," code 88.

How many of these falls caused an injury? By an injury, we mean the fall caused you to limit your regular activities for at least a day or to go see a doctor. (221–222)

_ _	Number of falls	[76 = 76 or more]
8 8	None	
7 7	Don't know / Not sure	
9 9	Refused	

SECTION 14: SEATBELT USE

14.1 How often do you use seat belts when you drive or ride in a car? Would you say— (223)

Please read:

1   Always
2   Nearly always
3   Sometimes
4   Seldom
5   Never

Do not read:

7   Don't know / Not sure
8   Never drive or ride in a car
9   Refused

CATI note: If Q14.1 = 8 (Never drive or ride in a car), go to Section 16; otherwise continue.

SECTION 15: DRINKING AND DRIVING

CATI note: If Q11.1 = 888 (No drinks in the past 30 days), go to next section.

15.1 During the past 30 days, how many times have you driven when you've had perhaps too much to drink? (224–225)

_ _	Number of times	
8 8	None	
7 7	Don't know / Not sure	
9 9	Refused	

SECTION 16: BREAST AND CERVICAL CANCER SCREENING

CATI NOTE: If male go to the next section.

The next questions are about breast and cervical cancer.

16.1 A mammogram is an x-ray of each breast to look for breast cancer. Have you ever had a mammogram? (226)

1	Yes	
2	No	[Go to Q16.3]
7	Don't know / Not sure	[Go to Q16.3]
9	Refused	[Go to Q16.3]

16.2 How long has it been since you had your last mammogram? (227)

1   Within the past year (anytime less than 12 months ago)
2   Within the past 2 years (1 year but less than 2 years ago)
3   Within the past 3 years (2 years but less than 3 years ago)
4   Within the past 5 years (3 years but less than 5 years ago)
5   5 or more years ago
7   Don't know / Not sure
9   Refused

16.3 A Pap test is a test for cancer of the cervix. Have you ever had a Pap test? (228)

1	Yes	
2	No	[Go to Q16.5]
7	Don't know / Not sure	[Go to Q16.5]
9	Refused	[Go to Q16.5]

16.4 How long has it been since you had your last Pap test? (229)

1   Within the past year (anytime less than 12 months ago)
2   Within the past 2 years (1 year but less than 2 years ago)
3   Within the past 3 years (2 years but less than 3 years ago)
4   Within the past 5 years (3 years but less than 5 years ago)
5   5 or more years ago
7   Don't know / Not sure
9   Refused

Now, I would like to ask you about the Human Papillomavirus (**Pap·uh·loh·muh virus**) or HPV test.

16.5 An HPV test is sometimes given with the Pap test for cervical cancer screening.

Have you ever had an HPV test? (230)

1	Yes	
2	No	[Go to Q16.7]
7	Don't know/Not sure	[Go to Q16.7]
9	Refused	[Go to Q16.7]

16.6 How long has it been since you had your last HPV test? (231)

1   Within the past year (anytime less than 12 months ago)

2   Within the past 2 years (1 year but less than 2 years ago)

3   Within the past 3 years (2 years but less than 3 years ago)

4   Within the past 5 years (3 years but less than 5 years ago)

5   5 or more years ago

7   Don't know / Not sure

9   Refused

CATI NOTE: If response to Core Q8.21 = 1 (is pregnant), then go to next section.

16.7 Have you had a hysterectomy? (232)

Read only if necessary: A hysterectomy is an operation to remove the uterus (womb).

1   Yes

2   No

7   Don't know / Not sure

9   Refused

SECTION 17: PROSTATE CANCER SCREENING

CATI note: If respondent is ≤ 39 years of age, or is female, go to next section.

Now, I will ask you some questions about prostate cancer screening.

17.1 A Prostate-Specific Antigen test, also called a PSA test, is a blood test used to check men for prostate cancer. Has a doctor, nurse, or other health professional EVER talked with you about the advantages of the PSA test? (233)

1   Yes

2   No

7   Don't know / Not sure

9   Refused

17.2 Has a doctor, nurse, or other health professional EVER talked with you about the disadvantages of the PSA test? (234)

1   Yes

2   No

7   Don't know / Not sure

9   Refused

17.3 Has a doctor, nurse, or other health professional EVER recommended that you have a PSA test? (235)

1   Yes

2   No

7   Don't know / Not sure

9   Refused

17.4 Have you EVER HAD a PSA test? (236)

1	Yes	
2	No	[Go to next section]
7	Don't know / Not sure	[Go to next section]
9	Refused	[Go to next section]

17.5 How long has it been since you had your last PSA test? (237)

Read only if necessary:

1   Within the past year (anytime less than 12 months ago)

2   Within the past 2 years (1 year but less than 2 years)

3   Within the past 3 years (2 years but less than 3 years)

4   Within the past 5 years (3 years but less than 5 years)

5   5 or more years ago

Do not read:

7   Don't know / Not sure

9   Refused

17.6 What was the MAIN reason you had this PSA test—was it …? (238)

Please read:

1   Part of a routine exam

2   Because of a prostate problem

3 Because of a family history of prostate cancer

4 Because you were told you had prostate cancer

5 Some other reason

   Do not read:

7 Don't know / Not sure

9 Refused

Section 18: Colorectal Cancer Screening

> **CATI note: If respondent is ≤ 49 years of age, go to next section.**

The next questions are about colorectal cancer screening.

18.1 A blood stool test is a test that may use a special kit at home to determine whether the stool contains blood. Have you ever had this test using a home kit? (239)

1 Yes

2 No   **[Go to Q18.3]**

7 Don't know / Not sure **[Go to Q18.3]**

9 Refused   **[Go to Q18.3]**

18.2 How long has it been since you had your last blood stool test using a home kit? (240)

   Read only if necessary:

1 Within the past year (anytime less than 12 months ago)

2 Within the past 2 years (1 year but less than 2 years ago)

3 Within the past 3 years (2 years but less than 3 years ago)

4 Within the past 5 years (3 years but less than 5 years ago)

5 5 or more years ago

   Do not read:

7 Don't know / Not sure

9 Refused

18.3 Sigmoidoscopy and colonoscopy are exams in which a tube is inserted in the rectum to view the colon for signs of cancer or other health problems. Have you ever had either of these exams? (241)

1 Yes

2 No   **[Go to next section]**

7 Don't know / Not sure **[Go to next section]**

9 Refused   **[Go to next section]**

18.4 For a SIGMOIDOSCOPY, a flexible tube is inserted into the rectum to look for problems.

  A COLONOSCOPY is similar, but uses a longer tube, and you are usually given medication through a needle in your arm to make you sleepy and told to have someone else drive you home after the test. Was your MOST RECENT exam a sigmoidoscopy or a colonoscopy? (242)

1 Sigmoidoscopy

2 Colonoscopy

7 Don't know / Not sure

9 Refused

18.5 How long has it been since you had your last sigmoidoscopy or colonoscopy? (243)

   Read only if necessary:

1 Within the past year (anytime less than 12 months ago)

2 Within the past 2 years (1 year but less than 2 years ago)

3 Within the past 3 years (2 years but less than 3 years ago)

4 Within the past 5 years (3 years but less than 5 years ago)

5 Within the past 10 years (5 years but less than 10 years ago)

6 10 or more years ago

   Do not read:

7 Don't know / Not sure

9 Refused

Section 19: HIV/AIDS

The next few questions are about the national health problem of HIV, the virus that causes AIDS. Please remember that your answers are strictly confidential and that you don't have to answer every question if you do not want to. Although we will ask you about testing, we will not ask you about the results of any test you may have had.

19.1 Not counting tests you may have had as part of blood donation, have you ever been tested for HIV? Include testing fluid from your mouth. (244)

1 Yes

2 No   **[Go to Q19.3]**

7 Don't know / Not sure **[Go to Q19.3]**

9 Refused   **[Go to Q19.3]**

19.2 Not including blood donations, in what month and year was your last HIV test? (245–250)

NOTE: If response is before January 1985, code "Don't know."

> **CATI INSTRUCTION: If the respondent remembers the year but cannot remember the month, code the first two digits 77 and the last four digits for the year.**

_ _ / _ _ _ _	Code month and year
7 7 / 7 7 7 7	Don't know / Not sure
9 9 / 9 9 9 9	Refused / Not sure

19.3 I am going to read you a list. When I am done, please tell me if any of the situations apply to you. You do not need to tell me which one. (251)

You have used intravenous drugs in the past year.

You have been treated for a sexually transmitted or venereal disease in the past year.

You have given or received money or drugs in exchange for sex in the past year.

You had anal sex without a condom in the past year.

You had four or more sex partners in the past year.

Do any of these situations apply to you?

1	Yes
2	No
7	Don't know / Not sure
9	Refused

CDC Clinical Growth Charts* G

From National Center for Health Statistics, Centers for Disease Control and Prevention, U.S. Department of Health and Human Services.
*For additional information relating to the CDC Growth Charts, visit http://www.cdc.gov/growthcharts/

Birth to 24 months: Boys
Length-for-age and Weight-for-age percentiles

NAME _____

RECORD # _____

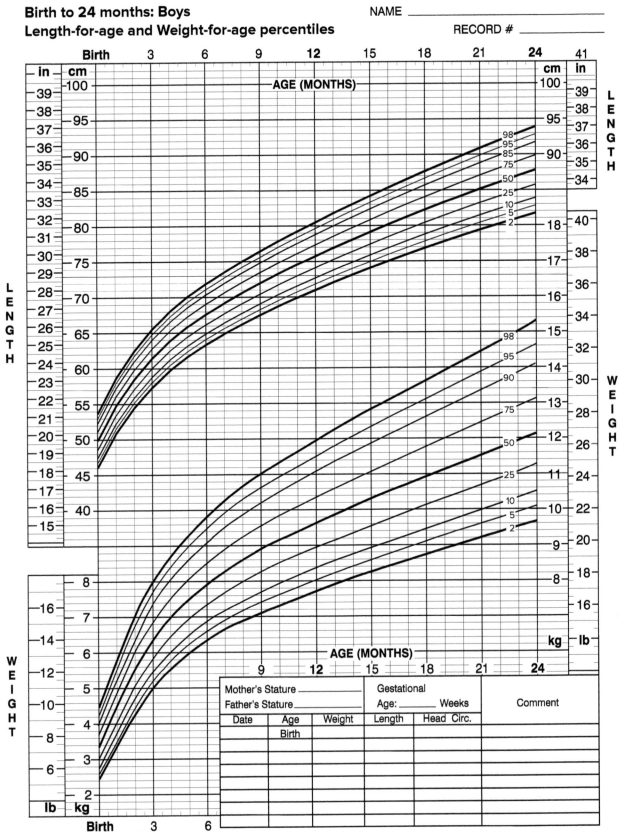

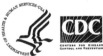

Birth to 24 months: Boys
Head circumference-for-age and
Weight-for-length percentiles

NAME _____

RECORD # _____

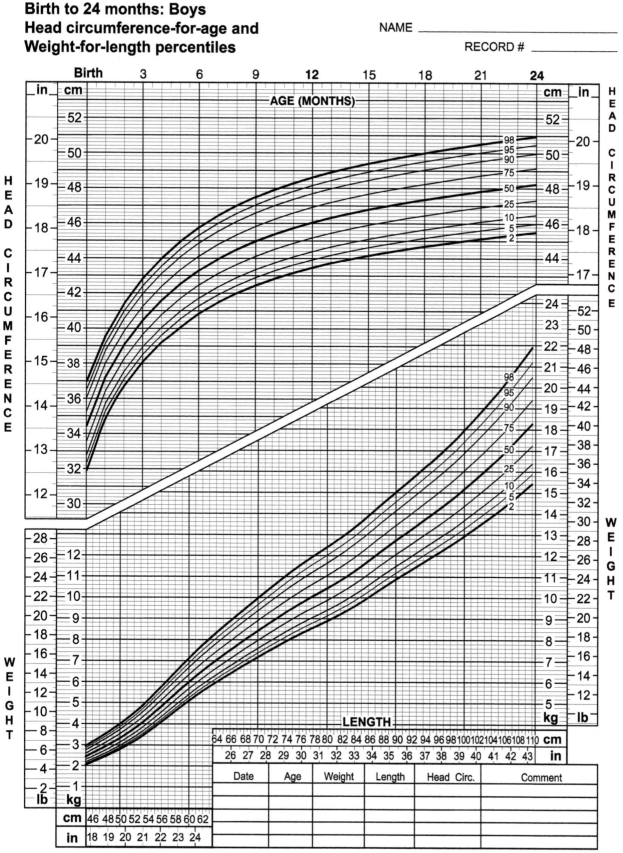

Date	Age	Weight	Length	Head Circ.	Comment

Published by the Centers for Disease Control and Prevention, November 1, 2009
SOURCE: WHO Child Growth Standards (http://www.who.int/childgrowth/en)

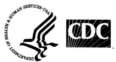

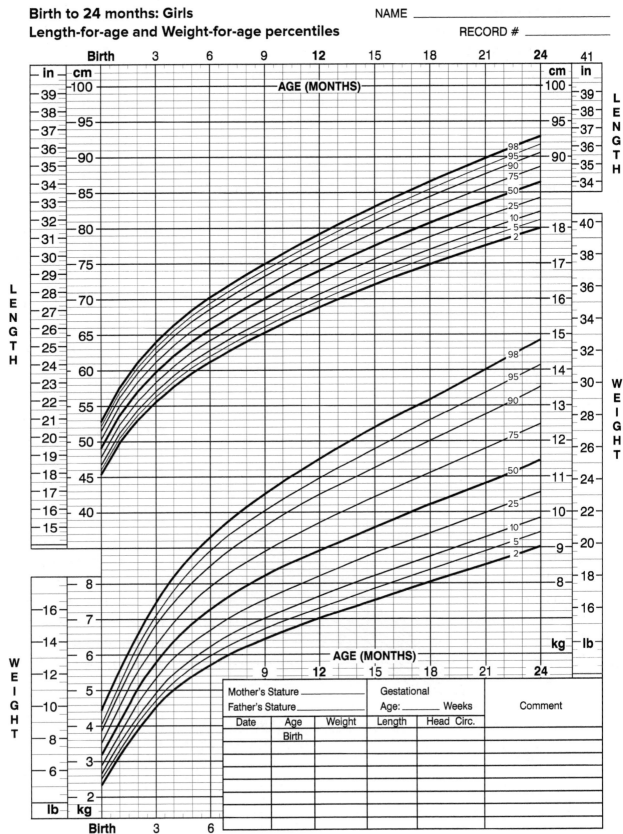

Birth to 24 months: Girls
Length-for-age and Weight-for-age percentiles

NAME _____

RECORD # _____

Published by the Centers for Disease Control and Prevention, November 1, 2009
SOURCE: WHO Child Growth Standards (http://www.who.int/childgrowth/en)

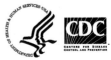

Birth to 24 months: Girls
Head circumference-for-age and
Weight-for-length percentiles

NAME _____

RECORD # _____

AGE (MONTHS)

Birth   3   6   9   12   15   18   21   24

HEAD CIRCUMFERENCE

98
95
90
75
50
25
10
5
2

WEIGHT

Date	Age	Weight	Length	Head Circ.	Comment

LENGTH

cm   64 66 68 70 72 74 76 78 80 82 84 86 88 90 92 94 96 98 100 102 104 106 108 110
in   26 27 28 29 30 31 32 33 34 35 36 37 38 39 40 41 42 43

cm   46 48 50 52 54 56 58 60 62
in   18 19 20 21 22 23 24

Published by the Centers for Disease Control and Prevention, November 1, 2009
SOURCE: WHO Child Growth Standards (http://www.who.int/childgrowth/en)

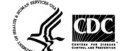

2 to 20 years: Boys
Stature-for-age and Weight-for-age percentiles

NAME _____

RECORD # _____

Mother's Stature _____		Father's Stature _____		
Date	Age	Weight	Stature	BMI*

*To Calculate BMI: Weight (kg) ÷ Stature (cm) ÷ Stature (cm) x 10,000
or Weight (lb) ÷ Stature (in) ÷ Stature (in) x 703

AGE (YEARS)

STATURE

WEIGHT

Revised and corrected November 21, 2000.
SOURCE: Developed by the National Center for Health Statistics in collaboration with
the National Center for Chronic Disease Prevention and Health Promotion (2000).
http://www.cdc.gov/growthcharts

2 to 20 years: Boys
Body mass index-for-age percentiles

NAME _____

RECORD # _____

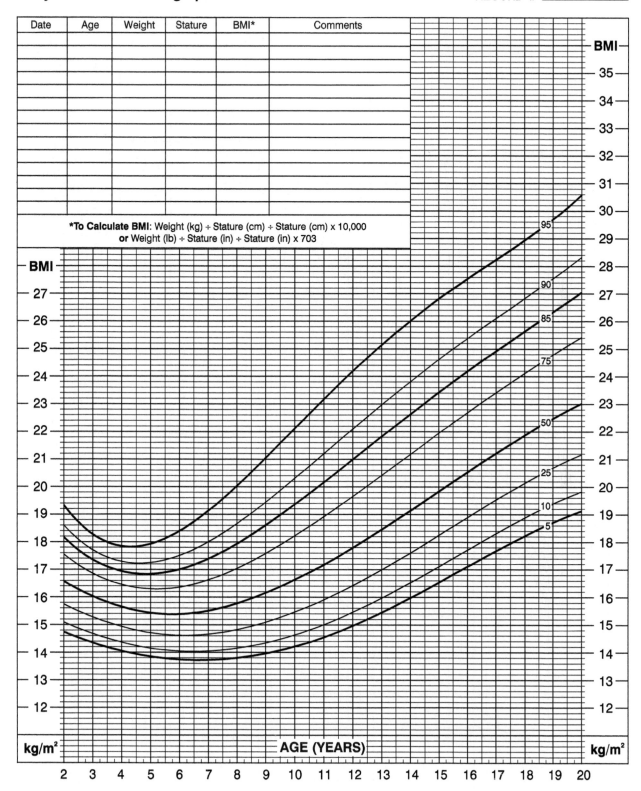

Date	Age	Weight	Stature	BMI*	Comments

*To Calculate BMI: Weight (kg) ÷ Stature (cm) ÷ Stature (cm) x 10,000
or Weight (lb) ÷ Stature (in) ÷ Stature (in) x 703

SOURCE: Developed by the National Center for Health Statistics in collaboration with
the National Center for Chronic Disease Prevention and Health Promotion (2000).
http://www.cdc.gov/growthcharts

2 to 20 years: Girls
Stature-for-age and Weight-for-age percentiles

NAME _____

RECORD # _____

Mother's Stature _____		Father's Stature _____		
Date	Age	Weight	Stature	BMI*

*To Calculate BMI: Weight (kg) ÷ Stature (cm) ÷ Stature (cm) x 10,000
or Weight (lb) ÷ Stature (in) ÷ Stature (in) x 703

AGE (YEARS)

12 13 14 15 16 17 18 19 20

STATURE

95
90
75
50
25
10
5

cm   in
190   76
185   74
180   72
175   70
170   68
165   66
160   64
155   62
150   60

in   cm   3 4 5 6 7 8 9 10 11

STATURE

in   cm
62   160
60   155
58   150
56   145
54   140
52   135
50   130
48   125
46   120
44   115
42   110
40   105
38   100
36   95
34   90
32   85
30   80

WEIGHT

95
90
75
50
25
10
5

cm   lb
105   230
100   220
95   210
90   200
85   190
80   180
75   170
70   160
65   150
60   140
55   130
50   120
45   100

WEIGHT

lb   kg
80   35
70   30
60   25
50   20
40   15
30
10

WEIGHT

kg   lb
35   80
30   70
25   60
20   50
15   30
10

AGE (YEARS)

2 3 4 5 6 7 8 9 10 11 12 13 14 15 16 17 18 19 20

Revised and corrected November 21, 2000.
SOURCE: Developed by the National Center for Health Statistics in collaboration with
the National Center for Chronic Disease Prevention and Health Promotion (2000).
http://www.cdc.gov/growthcharts

2 to 20 years: Girls
Body mass index-for-age percentiles

NAME _____

RECORD # _____

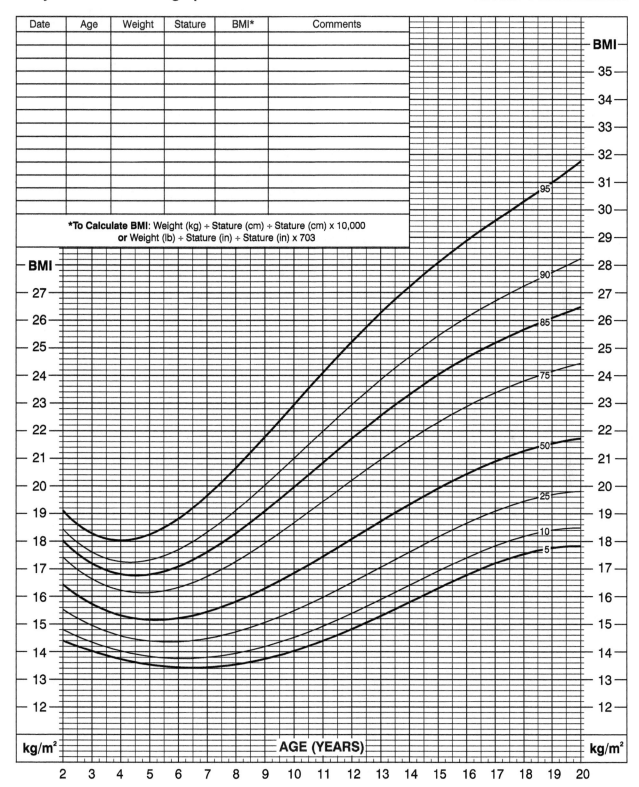

*To Calculate BMI: Weight (kg) ÷ Stature (cm) ÷ Stature (cm) x 10,000
or Weight (lb) ÷ Stature (in) ÷ Stature (in) x 703

Date	Age	Weight	Stature	BMI*	Comments

AGE (YEARS)

SOURCE: Developed by the National Center for Health Statistics in collaboration with
the National Center for Chronic Disease Prevention and Health Promotion (2000).
http://www.cdc.gov/growthcharts

Weight-for-stature percentiles: Boys

NAME _____

RECORD # _____

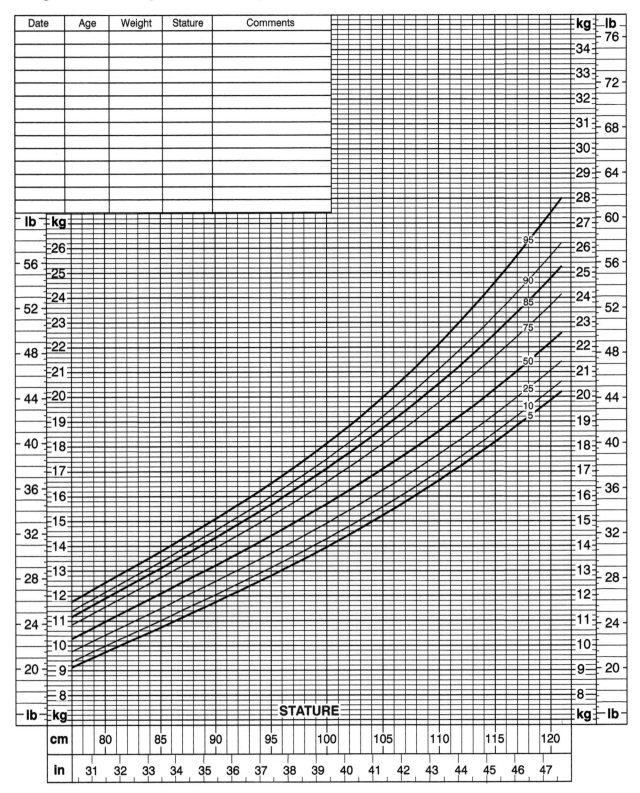

Date	Age	Weight	Stature	Comments

SOURCE: Developed by the National Center for Health Statistics in collaboration with
the National Center for Chronic Disease Prevention and Health Promotion (2000).
http://www.cdc.gov/growthcharts

NAME _____

Weight-for-stature percentiles: Girls

RECORD # _____

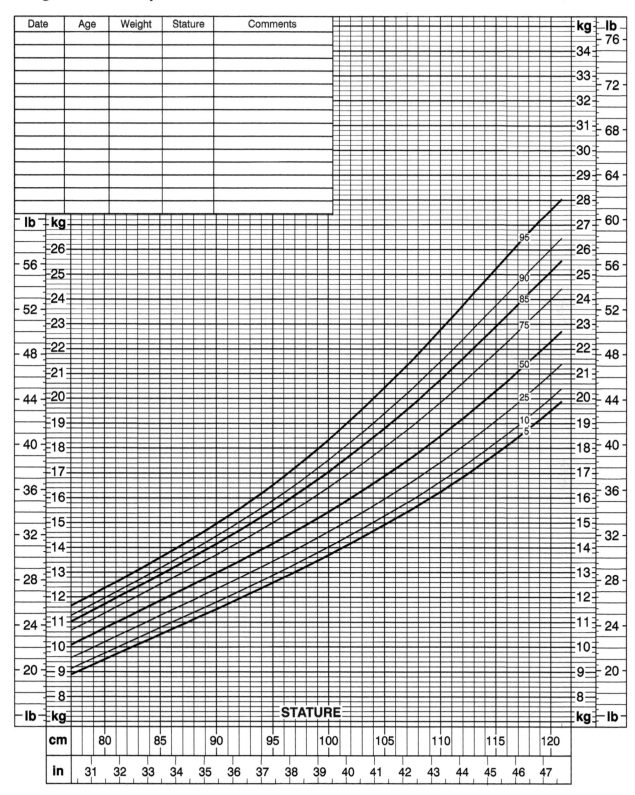

Date	Age	Weight	Stature	Comments

SOURCE: Developed by the National Center for Health Statistics in collaboration with
the National Center for Chronic Disease Prevention and Health Promotion (2000).
http://www.cdc.gov/growthcharts

H Anthropometric Reference Data for Children and Adults: United States, 2011–2014

(weight, height, body mass index, head circumference, recumbent length, waist circumference, sagittal abdominal diameter, midarm circumference)

Data from the National Health and Nutrition Examination Survey

Source: Fryar CD, Gu Q, Ogden CL, Flegal KM. Anthropometric reference data for children and adults: United States, 2011–2014. National Center for Health Statistics. 2016. *Vital and Health Statistics* 3(39). www.cdc.gov/nchs/

U.S. DEPARTMENT OF HEALTH AND HUMAN SERVICES
Centers for Disease Control and Prevention
National Center for Health Statistics

Hyattsville, Maryland
August 2016
DHHS Publication No. 2016–1604

CONTENTS

Detailed Tables

TABLE 1	Weight in pounds for children and adolescents from birth through age 19 years and number of examined persons, mean, standard error of the mean, and selected percentiles, by sex and age: United States, 2011–2014

Sex and age[1]	Number of examined persons	Mean	Standard error of the mean	Percentile								
				5th	10th	15th	25th	50th	75th	85th	90th	95th
Male				Pounds								
Birth–2 months	75	11.8	0.22	8.7	9.5	9.7	10.3	11.7	12.9	14.0	14.4	14.8
3–5 months	90	16.1	0.27	12.8	13.2	13.7	14.3	16.0	17.7	18.1	19.1	19.5
6–8 months	103	18.7	0.27	15.2	15.8	16.3	16.9	18.5	20.2	21.1	21.4	22.2
9–11 months	97	21.5	0.36	16.9	17.7	18.3	19.2	21.0	23.3	24.8	25.2	26.0
1 year	240	25.2	0.22	20.4	21.3	22.3	23.0	24.9	26.5	28.7	29.2	30.7
2 years	258	31.3	0.30	25.3	26.2	27.3	28.6	30.8	33.0	35.2	36.6	38.7
3 years	234	35.3	0.34	29.4	30.3	31.2	32.4	34.6	37.3	39.9	40.3	42.2
4 years	230	40.8	0.39	32.1	33.8	34.4	36.1	39.8	43.9	45.6	47.6	52.8
5 years	195	46.6	0.87	37.2	38.6	40.1	41.5	44.4	50.9	53.6	56.0	64.2
6 years	247	52.8	0.85	40.3	42.1	44.3	46.3	50.8	56.8	60.5	63.4	71.7
7 years	231	61.9	1.15	45.0	47.9	48.3	51.3	57.4	66.4	74.4	85.8	93.6
8 years	228	69.4	1.27	47.8	50.7	53.2	57.2	65.5	77.2	83.7	88.3	102.3
9 years	218	74.4	1.52	51.4	55.3	57.1	62.1	70.2	79.9	92.6	101.9	111.1
10 years	207	88.7	2.76	58.6	63.4	67.9	70.8	80.5	100.9	111.4	119.3	138.5
11 years	186	107.0	3.07	68.2	73.4	78.0	83.8	100.9	122.7	140.1	157.4	167.8
12 years	181	111.6	3.17	73.6	79.3	82.2	90.9	105.0	121.1	141.3	154.7	175.9
13 years	175	133.9	3.61	87.8	92.1	96.1	107.1	125.1	149.2	166.0	84.9	207.0
14 years	184	145.2	4.03	96.7	104.7	113.3	118.9	135.4	163.1	185.5	198.1	223.6
15 years	156	157.3	4.20	104.0	113.7	118.1	127.3	144.5	182.1	186.9	207.7	243.2
16 years	178	164.1	2.67	116.0	122.7	126.7	135.1	151.4	185.7	198.9	211.8	243.2
17 years	147	165.5	4.58	115.5	124.9	130.0	136.1	156.8	177.8	201.7	219.6	251.7
18 years	160	179.4	7.09	118.9	127.4	132.3	145.3	168.5	193.6	221.1	237.6	†
19 years	144	174.0	4.95	120.2	122.8	131.3	140.8	162.5	192.5	212.3	249.3	†
Female												
Birth–2 months	72	10.6	0.18	8.2	8.6	8.9	9.5	10.4	11.2	11.9	12.7	†
3–5 months	104	14.9	0.26	11.3	11.9	12.3	13.4	14.7	16.4	17.2	17.4	18.1
6–8 months	91	17.7	0.26	13.6	14.7	14.9	16.1	17.2	18.8	19.5	20.3	†
9–11 months	104	20.4	0.36	15.6	17.0	17.5	18.4	20.1	22.3	23.1	23.3	25.3
1 year	224	24.6	0.30	18.7	20.0	20.9	21.7	24.4	26.9	28.3	29.3	30.6
2 years	293	29.3	0.26	23.6	24.7	25.0	26.3	28.8	31.5	33.1	34.0	36.0
3 years	201	34.5	0.49	28.1	28.8	29.9	31.3	33.4	36.3	38.6	41.2	42.8
4 years	206	40.3	0.62	30.7	31.7	32.8	35.0	39.5	43.6	45.3	47.2	56.0
5 years	179	45.0	0.74	33.7	35.2	36.6	39.5	43.8	48.0	52.6	54.3	61.3
6 years	216	52.4	1.05	38.2	39.2	41.1	44.4	49.0	58.4	64.8	67.8	73.7
7 years	211	58.7	1.38	42.4	43.8	45.6	48.0	53.9	64.9	74.1	80.2	89.7
8 years	197	69.9	1.37	49.7	51.4	52.5	56.0	63.3	78.1	86.1	94.8	102.0
9 years	206	82.7	1.90	54.9	58.6	59.9	64.4	75.5	93.0	106.2	112.9	129.4
10 years	187	90.9	2.80	56.5	61.1	65.3	72.8	85.3	104.2	114.4	126.3	139.0
11 years	230	104.5	2.58	66.2	73.4	76.4	83.4	97.0	119.2	131.1	142.8	167.0
12 years	166	122.9	3.61	76.3	83.6	88.5	95.2	112.2	144.8	159.5	171.3	199.9
13 years	160	122.4	3.25	85.1	90.3	95.7	100.1	113.2	135.2	156.6	170.7	172.3
14 years	169	131.4	3.35	93.7	99.5	104.1	109.9	118.5	145.9	165.1	179.4	187.7
15 years	150	141.7	5.50	96.3	103.8	108.8	115.2	128.1	158.9	181.0	195.4	†
16 years	187	143.3	5.73	100.9	103.5	107.8	112.1	132.3	155.0	184.6	210.1	†
17 years	139	148.5	4.11	103.8	111.2	113.2	118.1	133.8	170.9	189.0	199.6	239.7
18 years	154	148.2	5.72	99.1	105.3	113.1	119.6	137.0	160.2	180.5	201.0	†
19 years	152	150.9	4.77	97.5	101.4	109.6	119.6	137.9	174.1	188.5	220.5	249.9

†Estimate not shown because the standard error could not be computed due to small sample size.

[1]Age at time of examination.

NOTE: Data exclude pregnant females.

SOURCE: NCHS, National Health and Nutrition Examination Survey.

TABLE 2	Weight in pounds for females aged 20 and over and number of examined persons, mean, standard error of the mean, and selected percentiles, by race and Hispanic origin and age: United States, 2011–2014

Race and Hispanic origin and age	Number of examined persons	Mean	Standard error of the mean	Percentile								
				5th	10th	15th	25th	50th	75th	85th	90th	95th
All racial and Hispanic-origin groups[1]				Pounds								
20 years and over	5425	168.5	0.92	110.5	119.8	126.8	136.0	159.1	191.1	212.2	229.3	256.8
20–29 years	853	161.8	1.88	107.2	113.9	119.7	128.8	149.8	184.6	212.8	228.7	255.2
30–39 years	915	172.9	1.92	114.9	124.0	128.7	137.7	160.5	195.9	218.1	237.7	269.2
40–49 years	979	173.1	2.21	115.6	124.8	130.7	138.8	164.0	196.8	217.7	237.2	261.3
50–59 years	923	174.4	2.31	115.2	124.9	129.2	141.0	167.4	197.2	219.4	239.4	271.3
60–69 years	889	168.8	1.98	107.9	122.5	129.6	140.3	164.4	191.2	206.8	224.8	245.6
70–79 years	527	165.8	2.08	108.2	120.2	128.1	138.6	158.5	188.5	205.8	216.5	238.2
80 years and over	339	141.9	1.64	96.9	103.8	110.7	121.7	141.0	160.6	172.4	180.4	190.6
Non-Hispanic white												
20 years and over	2157	168.4	1.19	112.2	122.2	127.7	137.4	158.7	190.3	209.1	226.5	256.1
20–39 years	649	167.9	1.90	112.6	119.8	126.1	134.0	155.9	189.0	215.0	230.8	256.7
40–59 years	686	173.4	2.12	118.0	127.0	131.3	140.9	166.1	195.4	217.8	237.5	265.0
60 years and over	822	162.9	1.83	105.7	117.0	125.9	136.2	157.0	183.4	201.1	215.3	236.2
Non-Hispanic black												
20 years and over	1264	190.2	1.52	121.0	131.6	140.4	154.0	183.1	217.8	240.3	256.8	283.7
20–39 years	380	190.0	2.76	115.2	129.6	137.0	151.0	183.1	219.0	243.4	263.3	284.8
40–59 years	481	196.5	2.47	128.6	140.0	148.4	159.2	187.3	223.5	246.2	259.6	286.5
60 years and over	403	179.9	2.39	111.0	126.0	134.8	147.2	174.7	208.9	226.6	235.1	260.7
Non-Hispanic Asian												
20 years and over	691	131.4	1.28	99.8	104.6	107.8	113.0	127.0	143.6	156.5	164.2	178.2
20–39 years	258	128.6	1.56	100.1	104.2	106.6	110.5	122.4	137.5	156.7	161.0	174.3
40–59 years	267	136.3	2.01	101.6	107.8	110.2	115.9	130.4	150.8	162.7	171.2	186.5
60 years and over	166	128.2	1.93	95.3	101.9	106.0	112.6	129.3	141.7	149.4	153.3	159.1
Hispanic[2]												
20 years and over	1166	164.7	1.39	113.1	121.3	125.4	135.5	157.4	186.2	205.7	219.2	241.0
20–39 years	408	163.5	2.66	112.3	120.7	125.0	134.8	152.9	182.5	206.6	220.7	245.5
40–59 years	417	169.1	2.11	116.8	122.7	127.7	138.6	163.6	191.8	209.8	221.7	241.1
60 years and over	341	158.3	1.76	106.4	114.4	122.5	132.5	154.0	179.9	195.0	204.8	219.7
Mexican American												
20 years and over	611	167.6	1.86	114.4	122.6	127.8	137.5	159.8	189.4	208.6	222.0	245.1
20–39 years	238	165.3	3.45	114.1	122.7	127.0	135.7	155.5	182.7	207.1	226.0	252.5
40–59 years	220	173.0	2.49	120.2	124.9	132.2	141.8	169.0	196.5	213.1	223.9	243.0
60 years and over	153	*161.9	2.42	*105.4	*113.0	*120.0	*138.0	*155.2	*188.3	*201.0	*209.3	*225.9

*Estimate does not meet standards of reliability or precision based on less than 12 degrees of freedom.

[1]Includes persons of other races.

[2]Includes Mexican-American persons.

NOTE: Data exclude pregnant females.

SOURCE: NCHS, National Health and Nutrition Examination Survey.

| TABLE 3 | Weight in pounds for males aged 20 and over and number of examined persons, mean, standard error of the mean, and selected percentiles, by race and Hispanic origin and age: United States, 2011–2014 |

Race and Hispanic origin and age	Number of examined persons	Mean	Standard error of the mean	Percentile								
				5th	10th	15th	25th	50th	75th	85th	90th	95th
All racial and Hispanic-origin groups[1]				**Pounds**								
20 years and over	5236	195.7	0.94	136.7	146.2	154.2	165.1	189.3	218.8	236.7	249.9	275.4
20–29 years	936	186.8	2.60	126.2	137.6	143.9	152.9	177.8	208.5	232.1	247.2	280.8
30–39 years	914	198.8	1.73	140.2	150.2	158.2	168.1	190.8	221.2	242.8	259.6	281.9
40–49 years	872	201.7	1.60	146.2	156.3	162.9	171.7	196.4	222.5	237.2	249.0	279.2
50–59 years	854	199.5	2.03	140.0	152.0	160.0	170.2	195.9	222.3	236.9	250.4	279.4
60–69 years	874	199.7	3.02	137.9	147.0	154.3	168.0	195.3	223.1	244.2	255.3	279.2
70–79 years	486	189.3	2.03	136.5	146.2	152.6	166.6	183.6	212.0	227.0	236.3	251.5
80 years and over	300	174.6	1.90	125.2	132.6	141.4	154.2	171.1	194.5	207.1	216.1	233.5
Non-Hispanic white												
20 years and over	2099	198.8	1.23	140.9	151.6	158.9	169.1	192.9	221.4	237.9	250.5	275.2
20–39 years	715	193.8	2.72	136.6	144.9	151.6	161.7	183.5	218.5	237.7	255.0	282.3
40–59 years	655	204.6	2.07	150.4	161.2	165.5	175.7	199.3	225.5	237.8	250.4	281.3
60 years and over	729	196.5	2.11	138.2	149.0	157.2	168.9	190.2	219.3	238.1	249.2	264.8
Non-Hispanic black												
20 years and over	1222	199.3	1.61	130.0	141.4	149.4	161.4	191.6	227.2	247.0	264.4	295.2
20–39 years	404	197.7	3.07	125.2	138.6	145.4	157.9	189.0	228.0	248.9	264.2	302.6
40–59 years	396	204.8	2.64	130.9	147.0	154.8	169.8	196.6	231.4	251.8	270.3	299.5
60 years and over	422	191.4	2.86	132.6	141.2	147.8	158.8	185.5	214.4	233.7	251.9	271.8
Non-Hispanic Asian												
20 years and over	665	161.0	1.09	118.5	129.1	133.6	142.1	157.2	175.9	188.8	197.0	215.8
20–39 years	260	165.0	2.15	117.1	129.6	133.5	140.9	159.6	181.6	197.8	211.5	222.2
40–59 years	247	161.3	1.23	122.0	131.7	137.0	146.6	158.9	178.6	183.2	192.0	198.8
60 years and over	158	151.1	1.89	106.8	124.6	128.0	135.7	150.1	163.2	171.2	176.6	†
Hispanic[2]												
20 years and over	1089	189.9	1.98	134.2	143.1	150.6	161.6	184.7	209.1	227.3	240.0	264.9
20–39 years	385	192.2	2.87	133.4	142.3	149.2	160.7	186.0	214.1	234.6	243.9	273.7
40–59 years	381	190.1	2.44	137.2	147.2	155.5	166.0	186.8	207.2	221.6	232.2	256.6
60 years and over	323	179.3	2.32	131.6	140.1	143.3	153.3	175.4	198.3	211.8	226.5	243.9
Mexican American												
20 years and over	628	192.1	2.06	137.1	144.9	153.8	162.7	186.9	211.1	231.2	242.1	270.6
20–39 years	233	194.6	3.40	137.3	143.8	153.0	162.1	190.8	216.5	237.2	245.8	284.4
40–59 years	228	190.5	3.01	134.8	145.8	156.1	167.1	186.8	207.5	222.0	236.8	257.1
60 years and over	167	185.1	2.90	131.8	143.3	148.6	160.6	178.6	204.4	218.8	234.0	245.8

† Estimate not shown because the standard error could not be computed due to small sample size.

[1] Includes persons of other races.

[2] Includes Mexican-American persons.

SOURCE: NCHS, National Health and Nutrition Examination Survey.

TABLE 4	Height in inches for children and adolescents aged 2–19 years and number of examined persons, mean, standard error of the mean, and selected percentiles, by sex and age: United States, 2011–2014

Sex and age[1]	Number of examined persons	Mean	Standard error of the mean	Percentile								
				5th	10th	15th	25th	50th	75th	85th	90th	95th
Male				Inches								
2 years	220	36.3	0.18	33.5	34.1	34.5	34.9	36.4	37.6	38.0	38.4	†
3 years	225	39.0	0.14	36.0	36.5	37.3	37.6	39.0	40.1	40.9	41.2	42.4
4 years	229	42.0	0.15	39.1	39.7	40.3	40.5	41.9	43.4	43.9	44.2	44.9
5 years	195	44.8	0.21	41.6	42.2	42.7	43.6	44.5	46.3	47.1	47.6	48.0
6 years	246	47.2	0.19	44.1	44.6	45.1	45.6	47.3	48.6	49.5	49.8	50.9
7 years	231	49.8	0.19	45.7	46.7	47.2	48.0	49.9	51.5	52.4	52.7	53.8
8 years	227	51.9	0.24	47.2	48.7	49.2	50.2	51.7	53.4	54.8	55.4	56.1
9 years	218	53.7	0.23	50.0	50.3	51.4	52.1	53.4	55.3	56.4	57.1	†
10 years	207	56.3	0.26	51.4	52.5	53.3	54.3	56.3	58.0	58.7	59.2	60.3
11 years	186	59.2	0.31	54.5	55.1	55.9	56.8	58.7	61.2	63.0	63.9	†
12 years	181	61.4	0.31	56.4	57.4	58.1	59.3	61.2	63.5	64.4	64.9	66.3
13 years	175	64.3	0.32	57.8	59.7	60.4	62.1	64.5	66.4	67.8	68.3	69.1
14 years	184	66.7	0.31	60.5	62.7	63.8	65.1	66.5	68.5	70.2	70.7	†
15 years	156	68.3	0.28	64.2	64.6	65.1	66.3	68.4	69.6	70.8	71.5	73.6
16 years	178	68.5	0.24	64.0	65.4	66.0	66.9	68.7	69.9	70.7	71.8	73.0
17 years	147	68.9	0.40	63.6	64.6	65.3	66.4	68.8	71.0	72.6	73.9	75.0
18 years	160	69.1	0.33	64.1	64.8	65.7	66.9	69.0	71.3	72.2	73.0	73.6
19 years	144	69.4	0.44	64.0	65.4	66.4	67.2	69.3	71.3	72.2	73.0	†
Female												
2 years	264	35.4	0.11	32.9	33.2	33.8	34.3	35.2	36.5	37.3	37.7	38.2
3 years	199	38.6	0.13	35.8	36.5	37.2	37.6	38.5	39.6	40.3	40.7	41.3
4 years	206	41.7	0.16	38.2	39.2	39.5	40.4	41.7	42.9	43.5	44.1	44.5
5 years	178	44.2	0.21	40.6	41.1	41.8	42.5	44.0	45.6	46.8	47.4	48.2
6 years	216	46.7	0.17	43.3	44.1	44.6	45.1	46.7	48.3	49.0	49.4	50.3
7 years	211	49.0	0.18	45.2	46.1	46.7	47.7	48.7	50.4	51.6	52.2	53.0
8 years	197	51.8	0.18	47.7	48.6	49.0	50.0	51.7	53.6	54.6	55.4	56.2
9 years	206	54.2	0.24	50.2	51.2	51.6	52.5	54.1	55.9	56.6	57.3	58.8
10 years	187	56.8	0.30	51.8	53.3	54.0	54.9	56.3	58.7	59.8	61.3	†
11 years	230	59.3	0.25	53.5	55.7	56.3	57.6	59.5	61.1	61.9	63.0	63.8
12 years	166	61.5	0.27	56.5	57.3	58.7	59.6	61.5	63.4	64.6	65.0	65.8
13 years	160	62.4	0.23	58.4	59.5	60.0	61.1	62.4	63.7	64.9	65.5	66.6
14 years	169	63.1	0.21	59.0	59.9	60.3	61.6	63.4	64.6	65.3	66.1	66.3
15 years	150	63.4	0.30	58.7	59.1	60.6	61.6	63.6	65.4	66.0	66.8	67.2
16 years	187	63.9	0.28	60.1	60.8	61.3	61.9	63.7	65.6	66.9	67.7	68.1
17 years	140	64.0	0.20	60.5	60.9	61.5	62.3	64.1	65.1	66.2	67.3	68.0
18 years	154	63.6	0.22	59.6	60.1	61.0	61.7	63.9	65.4	66.0	66.5	67.2
19 years	152	64.2	0.16	60.1	60.5	61.4	62.7	64.4	66.1	66.7	67.0	67.7

† Estimate not shown because the standard error could not be computed due to small sample size.

[1]Age at time of examination.

SOURCE: NCHS, National Health and Nutrition Examination Survey.

| TABLE 5 | Height in inches for females aged 20 and over and number of examined persons, mean, standard error of the mean, and selected percentiles, by race and Hispanic origin and age: United States, 2011–2014 |

Race and Hispanic origin and age	Number of examined persons	Mean	Standard error of the mean	Percentile									
				5th	10th	15th	25th	50th	75th	85th	90th	95th
All racial and Hispanic-origin groups[1]				Inches								
20 years and over	5547	63.7	0.08	59.0	60.1	60.7	61.7	63.7	65.5	66.5	67.2	68.3
20–29 years	928	64.1	0.12	59.8	60.8	61.4	62.3	64.1	65.8	66.6	67.4	68.6
30–39 years	957	64.3	0.12	59.5	60.5	61.3	62.3	64.4	66.4	67.3	67.9	69.0
40–49 years	987	64.1	0.12	59.4	60.5	61.2	62.2	64.2	65.9	66.8	67.6	68.7
50–59 years	924	63.7	0.15	59.4	60.2	60.9	61.8	63.9	65.3	66.3	67.1	68.2
60–69 years	888	63.2	0.15	59.0	60.1	60.5	61.5	63.2	64.9	65.8	66.5	67.7
70–79 years	527	62.7	0.14	58.1	59.2	59.8	60.8	63.0	64.5	65.4	66.1	67.1
80 years and over	336	61.3	0.15	56.9	57.7	58.3	59.6	61.3	63.1	63.7	64.3	65.5
Non-Hispanic white												
20 years and over	2199	64.1	0.09	59.7	60.6	61.3	62.3	64.1	65.8	66.8	67.5	68.6
20–39 years	689	64.9	0.08	60.7	61.7	62.2	63.2	64.9	66.6	67.5	68.2	69.5
40–59 years	692	64.4	0.15	60.2	61.1	61.6	62.8	64.4	66.0	67.0	67.8	68.8
60 years and over	818	63.0	0.12	58.6	59.7	60.3	61.1	63.0	64.7	65.6	66.3	67.2
Non-Hispanic black												
20 years and over	1302	64.2	0.10	59.6	60.7	61.3	62.5	64.2	65.9	66.8	67.4	68.3
20–39 years	418	64.4	0.15	60.1	60.9	61.5	62.9	64.4	66.0	66.9	67.5	68.8
40–59 years	482	64.5	0.14	60.1	61.1	61.9	62.9	64.6	66.1	67.1	67.7	68.5
60 years and over	402	63.1	0.16	58.8	59.6	60.3	61.4	63.2	64.9	65.8	66.4	67.3
Non-Hispanic Asian												
20 years and over	708	61.8	0.14	57.7	58.4	59.1	60.2	61.8	63.4	64.3	65.0	65.8
20–39 years	272	62.4	0.18	58.4	59.4	60.0	60.8	62.2	63.9	64.6	65.4	66.1
40–59 years	269	61.9	0.15	57.9	58.6	59.3	60.4	61.8	63.7	64.7	65.2	66.1
60 years and over	167	60.5	0.19	57.1	57.4	58.1	58.8	60.5	62.0	62.5	63.1	63.7
Hispanic[2]												
20 years and over	1186	62.0	0.09	57.8	58.7	59.3	60.3	61.9	63.7	64.8	65.3	66.3
20–39 years	428	62.6	0.13	58.2	59.2	59.9	60.8	62.6	64.2	65.0	65.5	66.6
40–59 years	417	61.9	0.11	57.9	58.7	59.3	60.1	61.6	63.5	64.8	65.4	66.3
60 years and over	341	60.6	0.11	56.7	57.5	58.1	59.1	60.6	62.1	63.1	63.6	64.5
Mexican American												
20 years and over	620	61.9	0.12	57.7	58.6	59.1	60.0	61.9	63.6	64.7	65.2	66.2
20–39 years	247	62.4	0.16	58.1	59.1	59.7	60.5	62.5	64.1	64.9	65.3	66.6
40–59 years	220	61.8	0.17	57.7	58.5	58.8	59.8	61.8	63.4	64.6	65.3	66.0
60 years and over	153	*60.5	0.16	*56.4	*57.6	*58.1	*59.1	*60.4	*61.9	*62.9	*63.2	*64.5

* Estimate does not meet standards of reliability or precision based on less than 12 degrees of freedom.

[1]Includes persons of other races.

[2]Includes Mexican-American persons.

SOURCE: NCHS, National Health and Nutrition Examination Survey.

TABLE 6	Height in inches for males aged 20 and over and number of examined persons, mean, standard error of the mean, and selected percentiles, by race and Hispanic origin and age: United States, 2011–2014

Race and Hispanic origin and age	Number of examined persons	Mean	Standard error of the mean	Percentile								
				5th	10th	15th	25th	50th	75th	85th	90th	95th
All racial and Hispanic-origin groups[1]				Inches								
20 years and over	5232	69.2	0.08	64.3	65.4	66.1	67.2	69.1	71.2	72.3	73.0	74.1
20–29 years	937	69.4	0.10	64.9	65.7	66.3	67.4	69.4	71.4	72.6	73.4	74.3
30–39 years	914	69.5	0.12	64.5	65.8	66.5	67.5	69.5	71.5	72.6	73.5	74.4
40–49 years	872	69.4	0.17	64.5	65.7	66.3	67.3	69.3	71.2	72.6	73.1	73.9
50–59 years	852	69.3	0.20	64.8	65.7	66.3	67.2	69.1	71.4	72.3	73.0	74.2
60–69 years	877	69.0	0.18	63.8	65.2	65.9	67.1	69.1	71.2	72.1	72.5	73.8
70–79 years	486	68.1	0.12	63.9	64.7	65.1	66.3	67.9	69.8	70.9	71.7	72.9
80 years and over	294	67.6	0.23	62.9	64.2	64.7	65.9	67.7	69.4	70.5	71.0	72.0
Non-Hispanic white												
20 years and over	2094	69.7	0.10	65.2	66.2	66.8	67.7	69.6	71.5	72.7	73.3	74.4
20–39 years	715	70.1	0.11	65.7	66.6	67.3	68.2	70.2	72.1	73.3	73.8	74.7
40–59 years	655	69.9	0.17	65.6	66.5	67.0	68.1	69.9	71.7	72.8	73.3	74.4
60 years and over	724	69.0	0.14	64.5	65.3	66.0	67.0	69.0	70.9	71.9	72.4	73.6
Non-Hispanic black												
20 years and over	1222	69.5	0.11	64.9	66.0	66.6	67.4	69.3	71.4	72.4	73.3	74.3
20–39 years	405	69.8	0.12	65.2	66.3	66.9	67.6	69.7	71.9	72.9	73.6	74.7
40–59 years	394	69.5	0.19	65.1	66.1	66.7	67.6	69.3	71.4	72.0	72.8	74.0
60 years and over	423	68.5	0.15	64.0	65.2	65.8	66.7	68.4	70.3	71.8	72.4	73.3
Non-Hispanic Asian												
20 years and over	666	67.0	0.16	62.5	63.4	64.2	65.2	67.0	68.8	69.9	70.5	71.4
20–39 years	260	67.8	0.15	63.4	64.5	65.4	66.2	67.8	69.5	70.4	71.0	72.0
40–59 years	247	67.0	0.22	62.7	63.7	64.3	65.3	66.9	68.7	69.6	70.4	71.2
60 years and over	159	65.2	0.24	61.0	62.1	62.6	63.6	65.1	66.7	67.7	68.3	69.7
Hispanic[2]												
20 years and over	1089	67.4	0.10	62.8	63.8	64.5	65.5	67.3	69.3	70.4	71.1	72.2
20–39 years	385	67.9	0.11	63.2	64.4	65.1	65.9	67.8	69.8	70.8	71.5	72.6
40–59 years	381	67.2	0.18	62.4	63.6	64.2	65.3	67.2	69.1	69.9	70.9	72.2
60 years and over	323	66.0	0.15	61.7	62.6	63.2	64.1	65.9	67.6	68.7	69.4	70.7
Mexican American												
20 years and over	627	67.3	0.12	62.6	63.8	64.5	65.4	67.1	69.2	70.2	71.1	72.0
20–39 years	233	67.8	0.17	63.0	64.4	65.0	66.0	67.8	69.7	70.9	71.5	72.2
40–59 years	227	66.9	0.21	62.2	63.4	63.9	64.9	66.8	68.6	69.7	70.3	71.8
60 years and over	167	66.3	0.15	62.3	62.9	63.7	64.7	66.2	67.9	69.2	69.7	70.4

[1]Includes persons of other races.
[2]Includes Mexican-American persons.
SOURCE: NCHS, National Health and Nutrition Examination Survey.

| TABLE 7 | Body mass index values for children and adolescents aged 2–19 years and number of examined persons, mean, standard error of the mean, and selected percentiles, by sex and age: United States, 2011–2014 |

Sex and age[1]	Number of examined persons	Mean	Standard error of the mean	Percentile								
				5th	10th	15th	25th	50th	75th	85th	90th	95th
Male				Body mass index								
2 years	220	16.8	0.13	14.7	15.1	15.4	15.9	16.7	17.6	18.1	18.3	18.9
3 years	223	16.3	0.12	14.4	14.7	15.1	15.4	16.0	17.1	17.4	17.7	18.8
4 years	229	16.2	0.11	14.1	14.5	14.6	14.9	15.8	16.7	17.4	17.8	19.7
5 years	195	16.3	0.17	13.9	14.3	14.6	15.0	16.1	16.9	17.4	18.3	20.6
6 years	246	16.5	0.18	14.1	14.3	14.6	15.1	16.0	17.1	18.0	18.8	20.5
7 years	231	17.4	0.24	13.9	14.4	14.7	15.2	16.2	18.3	20.4	22.8	25.0
8 years	227	17.9	0.24	14.1	14.7	15.1	15.5	16.6	19.3	21.3	22.5	24.2
9 years	218	18.0	0.28	†	14.2	14.8	15.5	17.1	19.1	21.5	22.9	25.6
10 years	207	19.5	0.47	14.4	14.8	15.5	16.2	17.9	21.8	23.7	25.2	28.0
11 years	186	21.2	0.46	15.2	15.7	16.0	17.1	20.5	23.8	26.3	27.8	30.3
12 years	181	20.6	0.45	15.2	16.1	16.8	17.6	19.2	22.3	25.3	27.9	29.7
13 years	175	22.6	0.56	16.3	17.0	17.4	18.7	21.0	25.4	27.4	29.7	31.6
14 years	184	22.8	0.48	16.8	17.7	18.6	19.4	21.2	24.2	28.1	30.0	33.7
15 years	156	23.6	0.58	17.1	17.9	18.3	19.5	22.0	26.0	28.4	30.7	36.5
16 years	178	24.5	0.40	18.3	18.8	19.1	20.4	22.9	26.9	30.4	31.3	36.7
17 years	147	24.5	0.58	18.1	18.8	19.1	20.4	23.6	26.2	29.1	31.8	36.2
18 years	160	26.3	0.86	18.8	19.7	20.0	21.6	24.6	28.8	32.5	33.4	38.8
19 years	144	25.4	0.71	17.0	17.8	19.5	21.8	23.7	27.6	31.2	36.1	40.2
Female												
2 years	264	16.6	0.11	14.4	14.8	15.3	15.7	16.3	17.2	17.8	18.3	18.9
3 years	199	16.3	0.17	14.3	14.6	14.9	15.3	15.9	16.7	17.6	18.0	19.2
4 years	206	16.2	0.18	13.5	14.1	14.3	14.7	15.9	17.2	17.7	18.0	20.4
5 years	178	16.1	0.18	13.7	14.1	14.4	14.8	15.6	16.8	17.6	18.2	20.8
6 years	216	16.7	0.26	13.6	14.0	14.3	14.7	15.9	18.1	19.6	20.4	22.3
7 years	211	17.0	0.30	13.4	13.6	14.1	14.7	16.1	18.3	20.5	21.9	23.4
8 years	197	18.1	0.28	14.1	14.5	14.7	15.5	17.1	19.7	21.5	22.4	25.2
9 years	206	19.6	0.34	14.4	15.1	15.4	16.2	18.3	21.4	24.1	25.5	29.2
10 years	187	19.5	0.45	13.9	14.6	15.1	16.4	19.1	21.6	24.2	25.1	26.8
11 years	230	20.7	0.47	14.5	15.4	16.1	17.0	19.3	23.3	25.8	28.1	31.8
12 years	166	22.6	0.64	15.5	16.6	17.0	18.0	21.0	26.1	27.7	30.3	35.9
13 years	160	22.0	0.59	16.0	16.5	17.1	18.1	20.5	24.3	27.0	30.4	31.6
14 years	169	23.2	0.58	16.9	18.3	18.6	19.1	21.5	26.6	28.3	29.4	32.7
15 years	150	24.6	0.86	17.4	18.8	19.1	20.4	23.2	27.2	30.8	32.6	37.3
16 years	187	24.6	0.76	17.7	18.6	19.1	20.0	22.5	26.1	31.9	35.4	40.0
17 years	139	25.4	0.68	18.4	19.1	19.6	20.3	22.9	29.4	33.0	34.6	38.8
18 years	154	25.7	1.12	18.3	19.5	20.4	20.9	23.5	27.5	30.3	35.5	43.4
19 years	152	25.8	0.84	17.0	18.4	18.9	20.2	23.4	29.5	32.7	37.6	42.5

† Estimate not shown because the standard error could not be computed due to small sample size.

[1] Age at time of examination.

NOTES: Data exclude pregnant females. Body mass index (BMI) is calculated as: BMI = weight(kilograms)/height(meters^2).

SOURCE: NCHS, National Health and Nutrition Examination Survey.

TABLE 8	Body mass index values for females aged 20 and over and number of examined persons, mean, standard error of the mean, and selected percentiles, by race and Hispanic origin and age: United States, 2011–2014

Race and Hispanic origin and age	Number of examined persons	Mean	Standard error of the mean	Percentile								
				5th	10th	15th	25th	50th	75th	85th	90th	95th
All racial and Hispanic-origin groups[1]				Body mass index								
20 years and over	5413	29.2	0.17	19.6	21.0	22.0	23.6	27.7	33.2	36.5	39.3	43.3
20–29 years	853	27.6	0.32	18.6	19.8	20.7	21.9	25.6	31.8	36.0	38.9	42.0
30–39 years	915	29.4	0.33	19.8	21.1	22.0	23.3	27.6	33.1	36.6	40.0	44.7
40–49 years	978	29.6	0.39	20.0	21.5	22.5	23.7	28.1	33.4	37.0	39.6	44.5
50–59 years	922	30.2	0.40	19.9	21.5	22.2	24.5	28.6	34.4	38.3	40.7	45.2
60–69 years	886	29.7	0.27	20.0	21.7	23.0	24.5	28.9	33.4	36.1	38.7	41.8
70–79 years	525	29.6	0.41	20.5	22.1	22.9	24.6	28.3	33.4	36.5	39.1	42.9
80 years and over	334	26.6	0.32	19.3	20.4	21.3	23.3	26.1	29.7	30.9	32.8	35.2
Non-Hispanic white												
20 years and over	2151	28.8	0.22	19.5	20.9	21.9	23.4	27.3	32.6	36.0	38.8	43.0
20–39 years	649	28.0	0.30	19.0	20.4	21.1	22.3	25.9	31.8	35.8	38.9	42.5
40–59 years	686	29.4	0.34	19.8	21.4	22.1	23.6	27.9	33.4	37.2	40.1	43.8
60 years and over	816	28.9	0.31	19.8	21.4	22.6	24.2	27.9	32.4	35.0	37.5	41.2
Non-Hispanic black												
20 years and over	1261	32.5	0.25	20.9	22.8	24.3	26.6	31.3	36.8	40.5	43.5	48.8
20–39 years	380	32.1	0.35	19.7	21.8	23.5	25.9	31.0	36.9	40.6	43.4	47.1
40–59 years	480	33.3	0.44	21.9	23.5	24.9	27.1	31.9	37.2	41.7	44.8	50.4
60 years and over	401	31.7	0.45	21.6	22.8	24.1	26.2	30.9	35.8	39.0	41.3	46.1
Non-Hispanic Asian												
20 years and over	691	24.2	0.22	18.4	19.1	19.8	20.8	23.3	26.7	28.8	30.5	32.6
20–39 years	258	23.3	0.31	17.9	18.6	19.0	19.9	22.4	25.0	28.3	30.0	31.8
40–59 years	267	24.9	0.30	19.1	19.9	20.4	21.5	23.9	27.2	29.1	31.6	34.2
60 years and over	166	24.7	0.34	18.9	19.9	20.5	21.7	24.1	27.2	29.2	30.2	31.4
Hispanic[2]												
20 years and over	1163	30.0	0.27	20.8	22.1	23.1	25.1	28.9	33.9	36.9	38.8	42.8
20–39 years	408	29.3	0.45	19.9	21.7	22.3	24.4	27.9	32.9	36.4	38.6	42.6
40–59 years	416	31.0	0.34	21.7	22.7	23.7	26.1	30.2	34.9	37.6	39.5	44.1
60 years and over	339	30.3	0.34	21.5	22.4	23.6	25.9	29.5	34.3	36.4	38.4	41.2
Mexican American												
20 years and over	609	30.7	0.35	21.4	22.5	23.8	25.8	29.6	34.8	37.5	39.5	43.8
20–39 years	238	29.8	0.55	20.3	21.9	23.0	24.9	28.8	32.9	36.5	38.7	42.7
40–59 years	219	31.8	0.40	22.6	23.8	25.0	26.4	30.8	35.8	38.0	40.5	44.1
60 years and over	152	*31.1	0.47	*21.3	*22.2	*23.9	*26.1	*30.2	*35.5	*38.2	*39.3	*41.6

* Estimate does not meet standards of reliability or precision based on less than 12 degrees of freedom.

[1]Includes persons of other races.

[2]Includes Mexican-American persons.

NOTES: Data exclude pregnant females. Body mass index (BMI) is calculated as: BMI = weight(kilograms)/height(meters^2).

SOURCE: NCHS, National Health and Nutrition Examination Survey.

TABLE 9	Body mass index values for males aged 20 and over and number of examined persons, mean, standard error of the mean, and selected percentiles, by race and Hispanic origin and age: United States, 2011–2014

Race and Hispanic origin and age	Number of examined persons	Mean	Standard error of the mean	Percentile								
				5th	10th	15th	25th	50th	75th	85th	90th	95th
All racial and Hispanic-origin groups[1]				**Body mass index**								
20 years and over	5223	28.7	0.13	20.7	22.2	23.0	24.6	27.7	31.6	34.0	36.1	39.8
20–29 years	936	27.2	0.38	19.3	20.5	21.2	22.5	25.5	30.5	33.1	35.1	39.2
30–39 years	914	28.9	0.24	21.1	22.4	23.3	24.8	27.5	31.9	35.1	36.5	39.3
40–49 years	871	29.4	0.20	21.9	23.4	24.3	25.7	28.5	31.9	34.4	36.5	40.0
50–59 years	852	29.1	0.24	21.6	22.7	23.6	25.4	28.3	32.0	34.0	35.2	40.3
60–69 years	873	29.4	0.41	21.6	22.7	23.6	25.3	28.0	32.4	35.3	36.9	41.2
70–79 years	484	28.6	0.30	21.5	23.2	23.9	25.4	27.8	30.9	33.1	34.9	38.9
80 years and over	293	26.7	0.25	20.0	21.5	22.5	24.1	26.3	29.0	31.1	32.3	33.8
Non-Hispanic white												
20 years and over	2091	28.7	0.16	20.9	22.3	23.2	24.8	27.7	31.6	34.0	36.0	39.5
20–39 years	715	27.7	0.37	20.1	21.1	21.9	23.2	26.4	30.6	33.4	35.9	38.5
40–59 years	655	29.4	0.25	22.0	23.2	24.1	25.7	28.5	32.2	34.2	36.0	40.0
60 years and over	721	29.0	0.30	21.4	22.8	23.7	25.3	27.9	31.6	34.1	36.0	39.4
Non-Hispanic black												
20 years and over	1218	28.9	0.20	20.0	21.1	22.4	24.0	27.9	32.2	35.2	37.7	41.9
20–39 years	404	28.4	0.38	19.5	20.5	21.4	23.3	26.4	32.5	35.4	37.2	41.3
40–59 years	394	29.7	0.33	20.2	21.9	22.9	25.1	28.7	32.4	35.5	39.2	42.5
60 years and over	420	28.6	0.37	20.4	22.1	22.7	24.2	27.7	31.6	33.6	36.5	40.4
Non-Hispanic Asian												
20 years and over	665	25.2	0.17	19.1	20.6	21.3	22.4	24.6	27.3	28.7	30.2	31.8
20–39 years	260	25.2	0.30	18.5	20.1	20.7	22.0	24.2	27.7	30.2	31.4	33.5
40–59 years	247	25.2	0.17	20.4	21.1	21.9	23.0	25.0	27.3	28.2	29.4	30.6
60 years and over	158	24.9	0.32	18.5	20.5	21.6	22.7	24.8	26.7	27.7	28.5	29.8
Hispanic[2]												
20 years and over	1088	29.3	0.26	21.4	22.9	23.9	25.5	28.6	32.0	33.9	36.4	39.9
20–39 years	385	29.3	0.39	20.7	22.1	23.4	24.9	28.6	32.4	34.8	37.3	40.1
40–59 years	380	29.5	0.28	22.6	23.8	24.7	26.4	28.8	31.7	33.5	35.3	38.9
60 years and over	323	28.8	0.31	22.4	23.7	24.2	25.5	27.9	31.6	33.0	34.5	37.5
Mexican American												
20 years and over	627	29.7	0.26	21.8	23.4	24.4	26.1	29.2	32.3	34.8	37.2	40.0
20–39 years	233	29.7	0.45	21.3	22.5	23.7	25.3	29.2	32.6	35.1	38.2	40.1
40–59 years	227	29.9	0.32	22.9	24.2	25.5	26.8	29.3	32.0	33.7	36.0	39.6
60 years and over	167	29.5	0.40	22.2	23.8	24.3	25.8	28.9	32.2	33.5	36.5	39.3

[1]Includes persons of other races.
[2]Includes Mexican-American persons.
NOTE: Body mass index (BMI) is calculated as: BMI = weight(kilograms)/height(meters^2).
SOURCE: NCHS, National Health and Nutrition Examination Survey.

TABLE 10	Head circumference in centimeters for infants from birth through age 6 months and number of examined persons, mean, standard error of the mean, and selected percentiles, by sex and age: United States, 2011–2014

Sex and age[1]	Number of examined persons	Mean	Standard error of the mean	Percentile								
				5th	10th	15th	25th	50th	75th	85th	90th	95th
Male				Centimeters								
Birth–2 months....................	75	39.4	0.20	36.3	36.7	37.3	38.3	39.4	40.4	41.2	41.6	41.9
3–5 months..........................	90	42.7	0.23	39.8	40.3	41.2	41.8	42.6	43.7	44.3	44.5	45.3
6 months..............................	35	*44.0	0.20	†	*42.3	*42.5	*43.4	*43.9	*44.7	*44.9	*45.4	†
Female												
Birth–2 months	72	38.0	0.16	35.7	36.2	36.4	37.0	38.0	38.7	39.4	39.9	40.2
3–5 months..........................	104	41.3	0.18	38.5	39.0	39.6	40.4	41.2	42.3	42.9	43.3	43.7
6 months..............................	38	*43.2	0.23	*41.3	*41.8	*42.0	*42.1	*42.7	*44.0	*44.4	*44.9	†

* Estimate does not meet standards of reliability or precision based on less than 12 degrees of freedom.

† Estimate not shown because the standard error could not be computed due to small sample size.

[1] Age at time of examination.

SOURCE: NCHS, National Health and Nutrition Examination Survey.

TABLE 11	Recumbent length in centimeters for children from birth through age 47 months and number of examined persons, mean, standard error of the mean, and selected percentiles, by sex and age: United States, 2011–2014

Sex and age[1]	Number of examined persons	Mean	Standard error of the mean	Percentile								
				5th	10th	15th	25th	50th	75th	85th	90th	95th
Male				Centimeters								
Birth–2 months	75	57.5	0.41	51.6	52.9	54.7	55.1	57.7	59.5	60.6	61.3	†
3–5 months	90	64.0	0.35	58.9	59.5	60.8	61.9	64.2	66.3	67.5	68.0	68.5
6–8 months	103	68.9	0.28	64.5	65.8	66.4	67.1	68.7	70.6	71.1	71.6	72.7
9–11 months	96	73.5	0.28	68.8	69.7	70.2	71.6	73.3	75.1	76.6	77.1	77.9
1 year	239	81.6	0.28	74.8	76.0	76.9	78.6	81.3	84.4	86.5	87.2	89.1
2 years	238	92.4	0.41	85.4	86.9	87.9	89.5	92.4	95.4	96.7	97.6	99.3
3 years	219	100.0	0.38	92.4	93.6	95.2	96.9	99.8	102.7	104.7	105.4	108.6
Female												
Birth–2 months	71	55.7	0.24	51.0	53.0	53.5	54.0	55.5	57.5	58.4	59.4	60.1
3–5 months	104	62.9	0.39	57.9	58.7	59.4	60.1	62.5	65.8	66.5	66.8	67.0
6–8 months	91	67.3	0.29	63.1	63.8	64.3	65.1	67.0	69.3	70.3	70.8	71.6
9–11 months	104	71.5	0.24	67.6	68.5	68.8	69.8	71.6	72.9	73.6	74.4	75.1
1 year	221	80.8	0.43	71.9	73.7	75.3	76.8	80.9	84.5	86.3	87.1	88.7
2 years	276	90.4	0.31	83.8	85.4	85.9	87.6	90.1	93.2	95.3	96.5	97.6
3 years	192	99.2	0.35	91.9	93.5	95.4	96.6	99.2	101.7	103.6	104.4	106.1

† Estimate not shown because the standard error could not be computed due to small sample size.

[1] Age at time of examination.

SOURCE: NCHS, National Health and Nutrition Examination Survey.

TABLE 12	Waist circumference in centimeters for children and adolescents aged 2–19 years and number of examined persons, mean, standard error of the mean, and selected percentiles, by sex and age: United States, 2011–2014

Sex and age[1]	Number of examined persons	Mean	Standard error of the mean	Percentile									
				5th	10th	15th	25th	50th	75th	85th	90th	95th
Male				Centimeters								
2 years	200	48.7	0.23	43.5	44.7	45.7	47.1	48.3	50.2	51.5	52.4	53.3
3 years	203	50.3	0.23	45.4	46.2	46.9	48.5	50.1	51.6	52.7	53.4	54.8
4 years	217	52.9	0.32	47.2	47.7	48.3	49.3	52.1	55.3	56.5	57.2	63.0
5 years	182	55.0	0.50	48.5	49.7	50.4	51.9	54.1	56.4	59.4	60.8	63.9
6 years	239	57.0	0.48	49.8	50.9	51.9	53.0	55.6	59.3	61.4	63.3	67.7
7 years	226	60.6	0.66	51.3	52.6	53.3	55.0	57.9	62.3	68.6	75.2	81.0
8 years	219	62.8	0.61	52.5	54.4	55.2	56.4	59.9	66.6	72.0	74.1	80.8
9 years	213	64.4	0.80	52.2	54.9	56.6	58.1	61.5	67.5	72.3	78.8	86.5
10 years	199	69.1	1.25	55.2	56.5	58.2	59.9	64.2	76.3	81.0	86.2	90.8
11 years	182	74.9	1.40	57.7	60.3	61.6	64.0	71.5	82.4	90.3	95.2	101.1
12 years	172	73.9	1.37	58.6	61.4	63.1	65.8	70.1	77.5	87.6	89.9	98.6
13 years	169	79.5	1.56	62.0	64.1	65.7	68.9	74.8	89.5	93.9	100.7	†
14 years	176	79.8	1.26	64.3	65.8	67.6	70.3	75.4	84.5	95.8	102.0	111.4
15 years	152	82.3	1.53	†	68.0	69.0	71.3	77.4	88.0	94.4	103.4	114.9
16 years	174	84.8	1.09	68.8	70.7	71.5	74.1	78.6	92.3	101.7	104.7	117.1
17 years	143	84.4	1.66	69.5	71.8	73.0	74.2	80.0	88.1	95.8	105.8	120.9
18 years	156	87.9	1.55	†	71.6	73.7	76.9	85.0	95.8	101.2	105.5	119.0
19 years	142	87.0	1.90	69.9	72.0	73.6	76.6	82.5	90.7	102.2	†	†
Female												
2 years	241	48.3	0.33	43.0	43.9	44.5	45.7	48.2	50.4	51.5	52.0	54.3
3 years	182	51.1	0.48	45.0	46.0	46.4	47.6	50.1	53.4	55.4	56.9	59.1
4 years	194	53.1	0.49	46.2	47.8	48.4	49.5	51.8	55.2	57.7	58.4	64.6
5 years	170	54.7	0.44	47.2	48.5	49.3	51.4	54.0	56.2	58.8	62.1	66.6
6 years	210	57.5	0.66	49.5	50.3	51.6	52.5	55.3	60.5	65.5	68.4	73.2
7 years	204	59.1	0.78	49.3	50.0	51.2	52.5	57.0	63.3	68.5	70.3	76.8
8 years	190	63.7	0.85	52.1	53.4	54.3	56.3	59.9	69.2	73.9	75.6	83.3
9 years	198	68.0	1.05	54.3	55.4	56.5	58.8	65.6	74.5	81.3	85.6	91.8
10 years	182	69.5	1.29	54.8	56.4	57.4	60.1	66.9	77.7	82.9	87.5	89.4
11 years	223	73.5	1.16	58.9	59.8	61.0	63.9	70.1	79.9	87.0	92.5	98.6
12 years	163	78.0	1.58	59.2	62.0	64.9	67.0	74.4	86.3	92.0	98.7	108.0
13 years	155	77.1	1.32	61.9	64.6	66.6	69.6	73.6	82.1	87.9	97.6	100.1
14 years	163	79.6	1.30	66.0	67.7	68.8	70.3	76.1	85.9	93.9	97.2	101.3
15 years	146	82.2	1.79	67.1	69.4	70.0	73.0	77.2	89.0	98.5	104.4	108.4
16 years	180	83.5	2.28	65.7	68.1	69.7	72.1	78.6	87.2	101.8	108.8	†
17 years	133	85.0	1.61	67.5	70.1	72.2	73.4	80.1	95.7	101.3	102.2	114.5
18 years	153	84.7	2.18	67.0	69.3	70.6	72.8	79.9	89.6	97.6	112.2	†
19 years	145	86.7	1.76	67.4	68.5	69.7	74.9	82.0	92.3	101.0	117.2	123.2

† Estimate not shown because the standard error could not be computed due to small sample size.

[1] Age at time of examination.

NOTE: Data exclude pregnant females.

SOURCE: NCHS, National Health and Nutrition Examination Survey.

TABLE 13	Waist circumference in centimeters for females aged 20 and over and number of examined persons, mean, standard error of the mean, and selected percentiles, by race and Hispanic origin and age: United States, 2011–2014

Race and Hispanic origin and age	Number of examined persons	Mean	Standard error of the mean	Percentile									
				5th	10th	15th	25th	50th	75th	85th	90th	95th
All racial and Hispanic-origin groups[1]								Centimeters				
20 years and over	5116	96.9	0.38	73.8	77.3	79.9	84.4	94.8	106.5	113.9	119.2	127.9
20–29 years	812	91.0	0.88	70.5	72.9	74.4	78.0	86.9	100.4	109.9	115.8	125.6
30–39 years	885	96.0	0.74	74.0	76.5	78.8	82.6	92.7	104.8	113.2	120.3	128.7
40–49 years	935	97.1	0.79	74.7	77.8	80.1	84.2	95.7	107.2	113.8	119.0	128.1
50–59 years	887	99.7	0.85	76.5	80.1	82.8	86.6	97.5	109.1	116.1	124.8	134.0
60–69 years	856	99.7	0.71	77.9	81.2	84.8	88.9	99.0	108.0	115.3	119.6	127.1
70–79 years	471	100.3	0.87	77.5	82.5	86.3	91.1	99.2	109.2	115.2	119.1	125.0
80 years and over	270	94.3	0.84	76.0	79.2	81.3	85.3	93.5	102.1	106.7	109.2	115.4
Non-Hispanic white												
20 years and over	2032	96.8	0.45	74.0	77.6	79.9	84.3	94.8	106.2	113.4	119.0	128.0
20–39 years	631	92.9	0.79	72.1	74.4	76.9	79.7	89.3	102.7	111.5	117.9	126.7
40–59 years	665	98.1	0.73	74.9	78.6	81.4	85.0	95.9	107.5	114.9	121.2	132.9
60 years and over	736	98.8	0.71	77.6	80.5	84.5	88.7	97.8	107.2	113.3	117.8	124.6
Non-Hispanic black												
20 years and over	1177	102.5	0.48	76.1	80.5	84.2	89.9	100.9	113.5	120.2	126.3	133.5
20–39 years	359	100.0	1.02	71.4	77.1	80.2	86.3	97.7	111.6	119.3	125.7	134.4
40–59 years	455	104.3	0.87	78.5	83.2	87.2	90.9	102.6	114.9	122.2	127.4	134.5
60 years and over	363	103.4	0.96	80.5	84.2	87.3	92.7	102.3	113.0	119.2	123.2	130.1
Non-Hispanic Asian												
20 years and over	652	85.3	0.56	69.5	72.0	73.5	77.1	83.5	92.4	97.3	101.2	106.3
20–39 years	246	81.6	0.73	66.2	69.5	70.9	73.6	79.8	87.1	92.5	96.4	102.2
40–59 years	248	87.3	0.71	71.9	73.8	75.8	79.2	85.3	93.4	99.1	102.9	108.5
60 years and over	158	88.5	0.94	71.4	76.1	78.6	81.5	86.9	95.0	99.2	103.6	106.8
Hispanic[2]												
20 years and over	1115	97.3	0.77	75.0	78.7	81.9	86.2	95.5	106.8	112.7	117.0	126.0
20–39 years	390	95.0	1.16	73.7	76.1	78.6	83.7	92.0	104.2	109.8	116.9	127.0
40–59 years	406	99.0	0.83	78.4	81.2	83.5	88.8	97.3	108.5	113.2	116.6	125.0
60 years and over	319	100.7	0.84	80.5	84.0	86.3	91.3	99.0	108.9	115.2	119.8	125.1
Mexican American												
20 years and over	585	98.7	0.96	75.9	80.3	83.5	87.5	96.7	108.4	113.9	119.5	126.7
20–39 years	230	96.4	1.47	74.1	77.4	80.4	85.0	93.9	106.0	111.0	119.4	127.7
40–59 years	213	100.7	0.93	80.5	83.7	86.4	90.4	98.8	110.2	113.7	116.5	123.3
60 years and over	142	*102.1	1.41	*78.5	*83.5	*85.2	*90.5	*101.5	*112.3	*120.0	*122.9	*126.4

* Estimate does not meet standards of reliability or precision based on less than 12 degrees of freedom.
[1] Includes persons of other races.
[2] Includes Mexican-American persons.
NOTE: Data exclude pregnant females.
SOURCE: NCHS, National Health and Nutrition Examination Survey.

TABLE 14	Waist circumference in centimeters for males aged 20 and over and number of examined persons, mean, standard error of the mean, and selected percentiles, by race and Hispanic origin and age: United States, 2011–2014

Race and Hispanic origin and age	Number of examined persons	Mean	Standard error of the mean	Percentile								
				5th	10th	15th	25th	50th	75th	85th	90th	95th
All racial and Hispanic-origin groups[1]				**Centimeters**								
20 years and over	5018	101.5	0.39	78.2	82.3	85.6	90.4	100.3	110.5	116.8	121.2	129.5
20–29 years	914	93.6	1.03	73.5	75.8	77.8	81.3	89.5	102.4	110.5	115.3	126.0
30–39 years	889	99.5	0.57	79.4	82.5	85.3	89.1	97.0	107.2	114.7	118.9	127.5
40–49 years	842	102.8	0.48	83.0	87.0	89.4	92.8	101.1	109.5	115.4	120.9	128.6
50–59 years	832	104.3	0.60	82.8	87.3	90.3	94.3	103.5	113.0	117.9	121.4	131.3
60–69 years	840	106.8	1.01	83.7	87.6	90.8	96.0	105.6	116.4	122.5	127.5	133.2
70–79 years	453	106.2	0.75	85.6	91.5	93.6	98.3	105.3	113.8	118.2	122.1	127.3
80 years and over	248	103.6	0.74	83.1	88.5	92.6	97.0	103.0	110.3	115.3	118.0	122.6
Non-Hispanic white												
20 years and over	2010	102.8	0.47	79.7	84.3	87.1	92.1	101.4	111.9	118.0	121.9	129.7
20–39 years	701	96.6	1.10	76.7	79.3	81.3	85.0	93.5	104.8	113.3	118.4	125.8
40–59 years	639	104.9	0.59	85.4	89.2	91.7	95.5	103.7	112.5	118.4	121.4	129.9
60 years and over	670	107.3	0.75	85.0	90.5	93.7	98.5	106.5	115.7	121.0	125.8	131.3
Non-Hispanic black												
20 years and over	1164	98.7	0.57	73.7	76.6	79.5	85.0	97.0	109.4	115.7	121.5	132.2
20–39 years	390	93.7	0.95	72.2	73.9	75.5	79.0	90.8	105.5	112.0	116.1	125.5
40–59 years	381	101.9	0.99	75.3	80.6	83.9	89.5	100.1	111.1	118.5	125.5	136.2
60 years and over	393	103.0	1.01	79.4	85.3	87.3	92.7	102.1	111.1	119.1	123.2	132.3
Non-Hispanic Asian												
20 years and over	636	90.4	0.47	73.9	76.7	79.1	82.9	90.2	97.0	101.2	103.9	107.6
20–39 years	250	88.7	0.87	70.6	74.6	76.3	79.4	87.2	96.0	102.5	104.8	110.3
40–59 years	236	91.4	0.41	77.2	79.7	82.2	85.6	91.1	96.5	100.2	101.7	105.9
60 years and over	150	92.7	0.71	74.3	81.2	84.0	86.2	93.4	98.3	101.8	102.9	107.4
Hispanic[2]												
20 years and over	1051	100.8	0.76	79.1	83.9	86.9	90.8	100.0	108.4	114.5	118.8	127.6
20–39 years	377	99.2	1.09	76.9	81.4	84.0	88.6	97.3	107.6	114.4	117.4	128.9
40–59 years	373	102.3	0.87	83.5	87.2	89.6	93.2	101.3	108.9	114.3	118.5	126.1
60 years and over	301	103.8	0.88	86.6	89.6	91.8	95.1	101.6	110.4	116.6	120.3	125.6
Mexican American												
20 years and over	604	101.9	0.85	79.7	85.2	87.9	92.0	100.8	109.2	116.3	120.1	128.1
20–39 years	228	100.5	1.33	77.8	82.5	85.2	89.9	99.0	108.8	115.9	120.1	128.9
40–59 years	223	103.0	0.96	85.3	88.6	90.9	93.8	101.9	108.9	115.9	119.5	125.9
60 years and over	153	105.5	1.07	85.1	89.7	93.7	97.0	102.5	112.8	118.5	120.7	127.1

[1]Includes persons of other races.
[2]Includes Mexican-American persons.
SOURCE: NCHS, National Health and Nutrition Examination Survey.

TABLE 15	Sagittal abdominal diameter in centimeters for children and adolescents aged 8–19 years and number of examined persons, mean, standard error of the mean, and selected percentiles, by sex and age: United States, 2011–2014

Sex and age[1]	Number of examined persons	Mean	Standard error of the mean	Percentile								
				5th	10th	15th	25th	50th	75th	85th	90th	95th
Male				Centimeters								
8 years	197	14.2	0.18	11.6	12.0	12.4	12.7	13.4	15.2	16.3	17.0	18.4
9 years	211	14.4	0.18	11.7	12.1	12.4	12.9	14.0	15.0	16.3	17.8	19.6
10 years	199	15.4	0.31	12.1	12.4	12.7	13.1	14.5	17.6	18.4	19.7	20.8
11 years	182	16.7	0.31	12.6	13.1	13.5	14.1	15.8	18.6	19.7	21.3	22.9
12 years	169	16.3	0.31	12.3	13.3	13.6	14.2	15.7	17.2	19.2	20.6	21.9
13 years	169	17.5	0.34	13.6	14.1	14.4	15.1	16.8	19.4	20.4	21.2	23.6
14 years	175	17.7	0.30	14.1	14.3	14.7	15.3	16.8	19.0	21.7	22.1	25.0
15 years	152	18.3	0.34	†	14.7	15.3	16.0	17.3	19.7	21.0	22.3	26.9
16 years	173	18.8	0.24	15.1	15.4	15.7	16.3	17.4	20.9	21.8	23.1	25.8
17 years	143	18.8	0.41	14.9	15.4	15.6	16.3	18.0	19.9	21.5	23.9	26.2
18 years	156	19.6	0.41	†	15.8	16.1	16.9	18.7	21.4	22.6	23.8	26.3
19 years	142	19.4	0.41	15.6	15.9	16.2	16.9	18.4	20.4	23.4	24.6	27.6
Female												
8 years	177	14.4	0.21	11.3	11.9	12.0	12.5	13.8	15.3	17.2	17.5	18.9
9 years	198	15.5	0.28	11.8	12.2	12.5	12.9	14.8	17.2	18.6	19.8	21.7
10 years	182	15.5	0.28	11.5	12.4	12.7	13.5	14.9	17.0	18.2	18.7	21.1
11 years	221	16.4	0.28	12.5	13.1	13.3	13.8	15.5	18.3	19.9	20.8	22.7
12 years	163	17.2	0.32	13.2	13.9	14.2	14.5	16.5	19.0	20.8	21.9	23.3
13 years	156	17.1	0.33	13.7	13.9	14.6	14.9	16.0	18.1	20.5	21.5	22.8
14 years	162	17.4	0.30	13.9	14.5	14.9	15.3	16.5	19.0	20.9	21.4	22.5
15 years	145	18.1	0.45	13.4	14.6	15.0	15.6	17.1	20.0	22.2	23.1	24.4
16 years	179	18.6	0.49	14.4	14.6	14.9	15.9	17.6	20.2	22.5	24.7	28.1
17 years	132	18.9	0.34	14.8	15.0	15.4	16.0	17.7	21.7	23.1	23.5	25.1
18 years	150	18.7	0.46	14.6	15.0	15.6	16.2	17.7	19.9	22.1	23.0	26.5
19 years	143	19.1	0.38	14.6	15.0	15.4	16.1	18.2	20.6	23.1	25.4	28.3

† Estimate not shown because the standard error could not be computed due to small sample size.

[1] Age at time of examination.

NOTE: Data exclude pregnant females.

SOURCE: NCHS, National Health and Nutrition Examination Survey.

TABLE 16	Sagittal abdominal diameter in centimeters for females aged 20 and over and number of examined persons, mean, standard error of the mean, and selected percentiles, by race and Hispanic origin and age: United States, 2011–2014

Race and Hispanic origin and age	Number of examined persons	Mean	Standard error of the mean	Percentile								
				5th	10th	15th	25th	50th	75th	85th	90th	95th
All racial and Hispanic-origin groups[1]				Centimeters								
20 years and over	4954	21.9	0.10	15.8	16.6	17.2	18.4	21.2	24.7	26.7	28.1	30.3
20–29 years	788	20.2	0.21	15.0	15.7	16.1	16.9	19.1	22.7	25.2	26.6	28.6
30–39 years	862	21.4	0.17	15.5	16.4	16.9	17.7	20.4	24.3	26.2	27.4	29.9
40–49 years	927	22.0	0.24	15.8	16.5	16.9	18.4	21.2	24.9	26.8	28.0	30.9
50–59 years	870	22.9	0.23	16.5	17.4	18.1	19.3	22.4	25.7	27.9	29.8	31.9
60–69 years	827	22.7	0.16	17.1	17.9	18.4	19.5	22.3	25.3	27.1	28.6	30.0
70–79 years	443	23.1	0.23	16.9	18.4	19.1	20.0	23.1	25.7	27.3	28.4	29.8
80 years and over	237	21.6	0.25	16.5	17.5	17.9	19.2	21.3	23.7	24.8	26.2	27.5
Non-Hispanic white												
20 years and over	1971	21.8	0.13	15.8	16.6	17.1	18.2	21.1	24.4	26.6	27.9	30.1
20–39 years	622	20.5	0.19	15.2	15.9	16.4	17.0	19.2	22.7	25.5	26.8	29.1
40–59 years	655	22.2	0.22	16.1	16.6	17.1	18.5	21.5	24.9	27.1	28.9	31.8
60 years and over	694	22.5	0.16	17.0	17.9	18.4	19.6	22.1	24.8	26.7	27.7	29.4
Non-Hispanic black												
20 years and over	1140	24.1	0.13	17.4	18.8	19.5	20.8	23.8	26.8	28.5	29.9	31.6
20–39 years	349	23.2	0.23	16.6	17.8	18.6	19.9	22.6	26.1	27.9	28.7	30.8
40–59 years	450	24.6	0.23	18.0	19.3	20.1	21.1	24.3	27.4	29.3	30.8	32.0
60 years and over	341	24.6	0.24	18.4	19.3	20.0	21.6	24.5	27.2	28.8	29.9	31.6
Non-Hispanic Asian												
20 years and over	634	18.9	0.17	14.6	15.1	15.7	16.5	18.2	20.6	22.1	23.6	24.9
20–39 years	235	18.0	0.18	14.2	14.7	15.1	15.8	17.4	19.5	20.9	21.7	22.7
40–59 years	248	19.3	0.27	15.0	15.6	15.9	16.8	18.5	21.0	23.2	24.1	25.5
60 years and over	151	20.0	0.28	15.1	16.2	16.9	18.0	19.3	21.6	23.3	24.2	26.3
Hispanic[2]												
20 years and over	1075	22.0	0.20	16.1	16.9	17.7	18.9	21.4	24.7	26.4	27.6	29.4
20–39 years	376	21.1	0.29	15.5	16.3	16.9	17.9	20.4	23.9	25.5	26.5	28.3
40–59 years	397	22.7	0.24	17.0	17.7	18.6	19.8	22.0	25.4	27.1	28.3	30.0
60 years and over	302	23.2	0.26	17.6	18.6	19.1	20.0	22.8	25.9	27.3	28.8	30.0
Mexican American												
20 years and over	567	22.3	0.26	16.2	17.2	17.9	19.2	21.7	24.9	26.7	27.7	29.7
20–39 years	221	21.4	0.37	15.5	16.4	17.0	18.3	20.7	24.3	25.6	26.6	28.4
40–59 years	210	23.1	0.26	17.4	17.9	19.1	20.2	22.5	25.7	27.4	28.2	29.8
60 years and over	136	*23.6	0.40	*17.4	*18.6	*19.3	*20.2	*23.0	*26.8	*28.8	*29.3	*30.5

* Estimate does not meet standards of reliability or precision based on less than 12 degrees of freedom.
[1]Includes persons of other races.
[2]Includes Mexican-American persons.
NOTE: Data exclude pregnant females.
SOURCE: NCHS, National Health and Nutrition Examination Survey.

TABLE 17	Sagittal abdominal diameter in centimeters for males aged 20 and over and number of examined persons, mean, standard error of the mean, and selected percentiles, by race and Hispanic origin and age: United States, 2011–2014

Race and Hispanic origin and age	Number of examined persons	Mean	Standard error of the mean	Percentile									
				5th	10th	15th	25th	50th	75th	85th	90th	95th
All racial and Hispanic-origin groups[1]				**Centimeters**								
20 years and over	4962	23.3	0.11	17.3	18.1	18.8	20.1	22.8	25.9	27.6	29.0	31.1
20–29 years	912	21.2	0.26	16.0	16.8	17.3	17.9	19.9	23.3	25.7	26.8	29.2
30–39 years	886	22.7	0.15	17.4	18.2	18.7	19.8	22.0	24.9	27.1	28.2	30.0
40–49 years	836	23.8	0.15	18.4	19.1	19.9	20.9	23.3	25.9	28.0	29.5	31.3
50–59 years	821	24.1	0.17	18.2	19.1	19.8	21.2	23.6	26.7	28.1	29.7	31.7
60–69 years	831	24.6	0.30	17.9	19.1	20.0	21.4	24.2	27.1	29.3	30.8	32.9
70–79 years	442	24.6	0.22	18.5	19.9	20.8	22.0	24.5	26.8	28.4	29.7	31.3
80 years and over	234	23.8	0.24	18.5	19.7	20.3	21.4	23.4	25.8	27.2	28.2	29.3
Non-Hispanic white												
20 years and over	1981	23.5	0.14	17.4	18.4	19.0	20.3	23.0	26.1	27.9	29.2	31.2
20–39 years	700	21.8	0.28	16.5	17.4	17.8	18.7	21.1	23.9	26.2	27.7	29.7
40–59 years	632	24.2	0.17	18.5	19.3	20.2	21.3	23.6	26.5	28.3	29.7	31.5
60 years and over	649	24.7	0.22	18.2	19.5	20.3	21.6	24.5	26.9	28.8	30.1	32.1
Non-Hispanic black												
20 years and over	1150	23.5	0.14	17.0	17.7	18.5	19.6	22.8	26.3	28.3	29.8	32.4
20–39 years	388	22.0	0.21	16.5	17.1	17.4	18.5	21.0	25.1	26.4	28.1	30.3
40–59 years	374	24.4	0.26	17.7	18.8	19.5	20.7	23.7	27.1	29.5	30.5	33.2
60 years and over	388	24.8	0.28	17.9	19.6	20.5	21.7	24.3	27.7	29.1	30.7	32.8
Non-Hispanic Asian												
20 years and over	635	20.5	0.15	16.0	16.7	17.3	18.2	20.3	22.4	23.6	24.4	25.6
20–39 years	250	19.9	0.24	15.4	16.3	16.7	17.4	19.1	21.9	23.6	24.5	25.8
40–59 years	236	20.7	0.14	16.4	17.4	17.8	18.9	20.7	22.3	23.3	23.9	25.1
60 years and over	149	21.5	0.22	16.1	17.5	18.6	19.6	21.8	23.0	24.3	24.9	25.7
Hispanic[2]												
20 years and over	1041	23.1	0.20	17.1	18.2	19.1	20.3	22.8	25.4	27.0	28.1	30.3
20–39 years	376	22.6	0.30	16.7	17.7	18.3	19.6	22.1	25.1	26.6	27.9	29.5
40–59 years	369	23.6	0.21	17.8	19.1	20.0	21.1	23.3	25.6	27.1	28.2	30.4
60 years and over	296	24.1	0.25	18.9	19.6	20.2	21.5	23.5	26.3	27.9	28.7	30.7
Mexican American												
20 years and over	600	23.4	0.23	17.4	18.5	19.5	20.6	23.0	25.6	27.5	28.7	30.5
20–39 years	227	22.9	0.39	16.7	17.9	18.8	19.8	22.5	25.4	27.0	28.3	29.5
40–59 years	221	23.9	0.22	18.4	19.8	20.5	21.5	23.5	25.7	27.5	29.0	30.7
60 years and over	152	24.5	0.31	18.4	19.7	20.3	21.6	24.2	27.2	28.2	29.1	31.6

[1]Includes persons of other races.
[2]Includes Mexican-American persons.
SOURCE: NCHS, National Health and Nutrition Examination Survey.

TABLE 18	Midarm circumference in centimeters for children and adolescents aged 2 months through 19 years and number of examined persons, mean, standard error of the mean, and selected percentiles, by sex and age: United States, 2011–2014

Sex and age[1]	Number of examined persons	Mean	Standard error of the mean	Percentile								
				5th	10th	15th	25th	50th	75th	85th	90th	95th
Male				Centimeters								
2–5 months	93	14.1	0.11	12.1	12.4	12.8	13.2	14.1	14.9	15.3	15.6	16.5
6–8 months	103	14.8	0.12	13.1	13.2	13.3	13.9	14.8	15.5	16.1	16.2	16.4
9–11 months	95	15.4	0.15	13.3	13.8	14.2	14.5	15.3	16.2	16.5	16.7	17.3
1 year	228	15.5	0.08	13.6	14.2	14.4	14.9	15.4	16.1	16.7	16.9	17.3
2 years	227	16.2	0.09	14.5	14.8	15.1	15.4	16.1	16.7	17.1	17.5	18.6
3 years	214	16.6	0.11	14.9	15.2	15.5	15.9	16.4	17.4	17.9	18.1	18.4
4 years	217	17.3	0.10	15.2	15.5	15.8	16.1	16.9	18.1	18.9	19.2	20.8
5 years	184	18.1	0.21	15.4	15.8	16.3	16.8	17.6	18.9	19.7	20.3	22.6
6 years	238	18.8	0.20	15.7	16.5	16.8	17.4	18.3	19.5	20.8	21.2	22.7
7 years	228	20.0	0.21	16.5	16.9	17.1	18.0	19.1	21.0	22.9	24.8	26.4
8 years	223	20.9	0.23	16.9	17.4	17.9	18.4	20.3	22.8	24.2	25.2	26.6
9 years	216	21.4	0.30	17.1	17.7	17.8	18.9	20.6	22.9	24.8	26.2	28.2
10 years	199	22.9	0.45	17.6	18.7	19.1	19.9	21.9	25.4	27.2	28.7	29.9
11 years	182	25.2	0.42	19.2	20.0	20.4	21.7	24.9	27.9	29.6	30.6	32.6
12 years	173	25.4	0.45	20.0	20.7	21.4	22.2	24.7	27.5	29.5	31.4	34.1
13 years	170	27.5	0.42	21.2	22.0	22.8	24.0	26.6	30.4	32.2	34.0	35.1
14 years	177	28.3	0.33	21.8	23.8	24.0	25.2	27.6	29.8	33.2	35.0	37.3
15 years	153	29.7	0.50	22.4	23.8	24.5	26.0	28.7	33.1	35.2	35.7	39.8
16 years	174	30.8	0.33	24.6	25.7	26.0	27.1	30.2	33.8	35.6	36.4	39.3
17 years	144	30.7	0.47	24.3	25.1	26.2	27.5	30.4	32.9	34.6	37.1	38.3
18 years	157	32.8	0.70	26.0	26.5	27.5	28.9	32.0	34.9	37.8	39.5	42.1
19 years	142	32.1	0.53	25.4	25.9	27.2	28.6	31.3	34.7	37.0	39.4	42.9
Female												
2–5 months	113	13.6	0.10	11.5	12.1	12.3	12.9	13.5	14.3	14.7	14.9	15.2
6–8 months	90	14.5	0.13	12.8	13.1	13.2	13.7	14.4	15.0	15.5	15.8	†
9–11 months	104	15.3	0.19	13.2	13.8	13.9	14.4	15.2	16.3	16.7	16.9	†
1 year	215	15.6	0.10	13.5	14.0	14.3	14.7	15.6	16.3	16.7	17.0	17.6
2 years	267	16.2	0.10	14.4	14.6	14.8	15.2	16.1	16.9	17.4	17.7	18.3
3 years	184	16.8	0.15	14.6	15.0	15.3	15.8	16.5	17.4	18.1	18.7	19.4
4 years	196	17.5	0.19	15.0	15.4	15.7	16.2	17.3	18.5	19.0	19.5	21.3
5 years	171	18.1	0.17	15.5	15.9	16.2	16.8	17.7	18.9	19.4	20.8	22.6
6 years	211	19.1	0.26	15.7	16.2	16.7	17.3	18.6	20.2	22.1	23.0	23.6
7 years	204	19.9	0.30	16.0	16.7	17.1	17.7	19.0	21.5	22.6	24.8	26.0
8 years	192	21.3	0.24	17.4	17.9	18.1	18.8	20.5	23.4	24.4	25.0	26.8
9 years	201	23.0	0.31	17.8	18.7	19.3	20.0	22.0	25.0	27.2	28.3	30.2
10 years	182	23.5	0.41	17.5	18.6	19.4	20.6	23.2	25.7	27.7	28.5	29.7
11 years	226	24.6	0.37	18.9	19.4	20.3	21.5	23.7	27.1	28.9	30.6	32.2
12 years	164	26.5	0.50	19.9	21.0	21.6	22.8	25.5	29.5	31.7	33.0	36.5
13 years	157	26.0	0.52	20.4	21.1	21.7	23.1	25.2	28.7	30.5	31.8	34.0
14 years	164	27.3	0.54	21.2	22.0	22.7	24.2	25.7	30.4	32.7	34.0	34.9
15 years	148	28.5	0.70	22.1	23.9	24.3	24.8	27.6	30.4	34.0	35.1	37.9
16 years	180	28.8	0.53	23.0	24.3	24.8	25.4	27.1	31.0	34.4	37.0	39.6
17 years	134	29.4	0.48	22.9	24.1	24.4	25.9	27.8	32.5	34.3	35.8	36.6
18 years	153	29.4	0.80	21.8	24.2	25.2	25.6	28.1	31.2	34.1	36.7	†
19 years	149	30.0	0.63	23.1	24.1	24.8	25.8	28.3	32.6	36.4	38.8	42.6

† Estimate not shown because the standard error could not be computed due to small sample size.

[1]Age at time of examination.

NOTE: Data exclude pregnant females.

SOURCE: NCHS, National Health and Nutrition Examination Survey.

TABLE 19	Midarm circumference in centimeters for females aged 20 and over and number of examined persons, mean, standard error of the mean, and selected percentiles, by race and Hispanic origin and age: United States, 2011–2014

Race and Hispanic origin and age	Number of examined persons	Mean	Standard error of the mean	Percentile								
				5th	10th	15th	25th	50th	75th	85th	90th	95th
All racial and Hispanic-origin groups[1]				Centimeters								
20 years and over	5191	32.2	0.12	24.6	25.9	26.9	28.3	31.4	35.4	37.7	39.6	42.3
20–29 years	821	31.4	0.26	24.1	24.9	26.0	27.2	30.4	34.5	37.5	39.4	41.6
30–39 years	892	32.7	0.24	25.1	26.5	27.4	28.6	31.6	35.6	38.2	40.3	43.4
40–49 years	952	32.7	0.25	25.4	26.5	27.4	28.5	32.0	36.0	38.0	39.7	43.1
50–59 years	898	32.8	0.28	25.2	26.1	27.3	28.8	31.9	36.0	38.9	40.7	42.8
60–69 years	863	32.4	0.23	24.7	26.4	27.6	28.7	31.9	35.4	37.4	38.7	41.3
70–79 years	484	32.1	0.31	24.8	26.3	27.3	28.4	31.5	35.1	37.2	39.4	42.1
80 years and over	281	29.1	0.27	22.5	23.7	24.5	26.0	29.1	31.9	33.3	34.1	34.9
Non-Hispanic white												
20 years and over	2070	32.0	0.16	24.6	25.9	26.8	28.3	31.2	35.0	37.4	39.3	41.9
20–39 years	640	31.9	0.22	24.6	25.8	26.5	28.0	30.7	34.8	37.7	39.4	42.2
40–59 years	676	32.4	0.25	25.2	26.2	27.1	28.5	31.6	35.5	38.0	40.0	42.5
60 years and over	754	31.6	0.25	23.9	25.6	26.7	28.3	31.1	34.6	36.2	38.0	40.3
Non-Hispanic black												
20 years and over	1193	34.8	0.15	25.6	27.5	28.7	30.6	34.2	38.1	40.9	42.6	45.6
20–39 years	360	34.6	0.29	24.5	26.6	28.0	30.3	34.2	38.1	40.9	42.3	45.4
40–59 years	465	35.4	0.24	26.7	28.2	29.3	31.3	34.8	38.7	41.7	43.8	46.3
60 years and over	368	34.0	0.31	25.8	27.3	28.5	30.0	33.5	36.9	39.7	41.3	44.0
Non-Hispanic Asian												
20 years and over	657	28.4	0.18	23.2	24.0	24.6	25.5	27.9	30.6	32.4	33.2	35.0
20–39 years	247	27.7	0.26	22.7	23.5	24.0	25.0	27.0	29.8	32.1	33.0	34.3
40–59 years	250	29.2	0.30	24.0	24.8	25.3	26.5	28.5	31.1	33.1	34.1	36.8
60 years and over	160	28.5	0.27	23.3	24.3	24.8	26.0	28.2	30.6	31.6	32.4	34.1
Hispanic[2]												
20 years and over	1129	32.6	0.21	25.4	26.7	27.7	29.1	31.9	35.5	37.6	39.0	41.4
20–39 years	395	32.2	0.38	24.9	26.4	27.3	28.7	31.4	34.9	37.4	39.2	41.2
40–59 years	409	33.1	0.27	25.8	27.3	28.1	29.3	32.4	36.3	37.9	39.0	41.9
60 years and over	325	32.5	0.25	24.9	26.6	27.5	29.2	32.1	35.0	37.0	38.6	40.9
Mexican American												
20 years and over	592	33.0	0.29	25.7	27.2	28.1	29.4	32.1	36.0	38.4	39.8	41.7
20–39 years	231	32.5	0.50	25.4	26.6	27.7	29.0	31.6	34.9	38.5	39.8	41.3
40–59 years	215	33.8	0.28	27.1	28.0	28.8	29.7	33.3	36.7	38.4	39.5	42.4
60 years and over	146	*33.0	0.36	*24.7	*26.1	*27.9	*29.5	*32.8	*36.2	*37.8	*39.7	*41.5

* Estimate does not meet standards of reliability or precision based on less than 12 degrees of freedom.

[1] Includes persons of other races.

[2] Includes Mexican-American persons.

NOTE: Data exclude pregnant females.

SOURCE: NCHS, National Health and Nutrition Examination Survey.

TABLE 20	Midarm circumference in centimeters for males aged 20 and over and number of examined persons, mean, standard error of the mean, and selected percentiles, by race and Hispanic origin and age: United States, 2011–2014

Race and Hispanic origin and age	Number of examined persons	Mean	Standard error of the mean	Percentile									
				5th	10th	15th	25th	50th	75th	85th	90th	95th
All racial and Hispanic-origin groups[1]				Centimeters								
20 years and over	5059	34.3	0.08	27.7	28.9	29.8	31.2	33.9	36.8	38.3	39.5	41.7
20–29 years	917	33.7	0.28	26.8	28.0	28.7	30.2	33.2	36.7	38.4	39.5	42.4
30–39 years	892	35.0	0.16	28.5	29.8	30.5	31.9	34.6	37.4	39.2	40.3	42.4
40–49 years	849	35.3	0.15	29.0	30.5	31.2	32.6	35.1	37.4	38.9	40.0	42.2
50–59 years	836	34.4	0.19	28.1	29.3	30.0	31.7	34.2	37.0	38.2	39.5	41.7
60–69 years	850	34.0	0.25	28.1	29.2	29.9	31.0	33.8	36.1	38.0	39.4	41.7
70–79 years	460	32.8	0.17	26.7	27.9	29.1	30.5	32.7	35.0	36.4	37.7	39.1
80 years and over	255	30.9	0.24	24.9	26.9	27.5	28.7	30.7	33.0	34.3	35.6	36.7
Non-Hispanic white												
20 years and over	2030	34.3	0.10	27.9	29.1	29.9	31.4	34.0	36.8	38.2	39.4	41.6
20–39 years	703	34.2	0.26	27.7	28.6	29.5	30.9	33.7	36.9	38.5	39.7	42.1
40–59 years	645	35.0	0.19	28.6	29.8	31.0	32.4	34.9	37.2	38.6	39.5	41.6
60 years and over	682	33.5	0.19	27.4	28.6	29.5	30.7	33.0	35.6	37.4	38.4	40.4
Non-Hispanic black												
20 years and over	1174	35.2	0.16	27.0	28.5	29.8	31.4	35.0	38.5	40.3	41.8	44.1
20–39 years	390	35.1	0.35	26.9	28.2	29.3	31.2	34.8	38.7	40.4	41.7	44.2
40–59 years	383	36.0	0.25	27.5	29.5	30.6	32.1	35.5	39.3	41.1	42.7	44.7
60 years and over	401	33.7	0.32	26.0	27.9	29.1	30.4	33.4	36.5	38.4	39.9	41.7
Non-Hispanic Asian												
20 years and over	641	31.3	0.17	25.7	27.1	27.9	29.0	30.9	33.5	34.8	35.9	37.4
20–39 years	251	31.9	0.32	25.5	26.7	27.6	28.9	31.4	34.5	36.1	37.0	38.5
40–59 years	238	31.3	0.20	26.8	28.0	28.6	29.5	30.9	33.0	34.0	34.8	36.3
60 years and over	152	29.9	0.23	25.2	26.2	26.8	28.2	29.6	31.6	32.6	33.6	35.0
Hispanic[2]												
20 years and over	1053	34.4	0.18	28.3	29.6	30.5	31.7	34.2	36.7	38.1	39.2	41.1
20–39 years	378	34.7	0.28	28.0	29.6	30.8	31.9	34.5	37.2	38.7	39.8	41.7
40–59 years	373	34.5	0.19	29.1	30.3	31.0	32.1	34.3	36.3	37.7	38.3	40.8
60 years and over	302	32.6	0.23	27.2	28.4	29.2	30.3	32.2	34.7	36.0	37.2	39.1
Mexican American												
20 years and over	606	34.5	0.16	28.5	30.1	30.9	32.0	34.3	36.7	38.1	39.0	41.1
20–39 years	229	34.9	0.28	28.6	30.3	31.1	32.2	34.7	37.2	38.7	39.8	41.7
40–59 years	223	34.4	0.25	29.1	30.4	31.1	32.2	34.3	36.2	37.7	38.2	39.9
60 years and over	154	33.0	0.28	27.1	28.5	29.4	30.5	32.7	35.2	36.5	38.0	39.5

[1]Includes persons of other races.
[2]Includes Mexican-American persons.
SOURCE: NCHS, National Health and Nutrition Examination Survey.

Triceps and Subscapular Skinfold Reference Data for Children and Adults: United States, 2007–2010

Data From the National Health and Nutrition Examination Survey

Source: Fryar CD, Gu Q, Ogden CL. 2012. Anthropometric reference data for children and adults: United States, 2007–2010. *Vital and Health Statistics* 11(252):1–48.

U.S. DEPARTMENT OF HEALTH AND HUMAN SERVICES
Centers for Disease Control and Prevention
National Center for Health Statistics

Hyattsville, Maryland
October 2012
DHHS Publication No. (PHS) 2013–1602

TABLE 1	Triceps skinfold thickness in millimeters for children and adolescents aged 2 months to 19 years and number of examined persons, mean, standard error of the mean, and selected percentiles, by sex and age: United States, 2007–2010

Sex and age[1]	Number of examined persons	Mean	Standard error of the mean	Percentile								
				5th	10th	15th	25th	50th	75th	85th	90th	95th
Male				Millimeters								
2–5 months	122	10.4	0.27	6.8	7.7	8.0	8.9	10.1	11.9	13.3	13.7	14.6
6–8 months	97	10.1	0.24	6.3	7.7	8.2	8.8	9.7	11.1	11.7	12.4	13.2
9–11 months	106	9.6	0.37	6.4	6.9	7.4	7.8	8.9	10.8	11.4	12.4	14.1
1 year	304	9.4	0.16	6.2	6.9	7.1	7.8	8.9	10.4	11.8	12.8	13.4
2 years	295	9.3	0.18	6.2	6.8	7.1	7.8	9.0	10.6	11.3	12.0	13.1
3 years	182	9.5	0.25	6.1	6.8	7.2	7.8	8.9	10.3	11.2	13.1	14.9
4 years	228	9.2	0.24	5.6	6.2	6.6	7.2	8.4	10.4	12.0	12.7	14.6
5 years	194	9.3	0.23	5.5	6.2	6.7	7.3	8.5	10.4	11.8	12.6	15.3
6 years	189	9.9	0.41	5.7	5.9	6.2	6.9	8.2	11.4	14.6	17.0	21.1
7 years	209	10.3	0.39	5.6	5.9	6.1	6.9	8.6	12.1	16.3	17.1	19.1
8 years	205	11.9	0.43	5.6	6.0	6.7	7.6	10.1	15.1	18.2	19.6	22.3
9 years	182	12.9	0.57	5.6	6.3	6.8	7.7	10.3	17.0	20.6	23.0	25.8
10 years	194	14.7	0.63	6.6	7.3	7.7	8.8	12.9	20.0	22.6	24.3	27.1
11 years	205	14.8	0.45	6.3	7.1	7.5	9.1	12.9	20.6	23.2	25.5	28.1
12 years	154	15.7	0.76	6.4	7.0	7.4	8.8	14.0	21.1	24.1	27.5	29.7
13 years	142	13.7	0.80	5.6	6.4	7.1	8.1	11.1	17.8	21.8	25.2	29.2
14 years	173	12.9	0.83	5.3	5.9	6.2	7.2	9.9	15.7	20.5	25.5	29.0
15 years	155	12.6	0.69	4.9	5.9	6.5	7.3	10.2	16.9	20.1	22.9	27.3
16 years	168	12.7	0.60	5.9	6.6	6.9	7.8	10.5	14.8	18.3	21.7	29.8
17 years	180	13.2	0.91	4.8	5.8	6.3	7.6	9.9	16.0	22.9	25.3	31.8
18 years	135	14.0	0.71	6.3	6.9	7.4	8.3	12.4	17.9	20.4	22.9	28.4
19 years	174	12.6	0.70	5.2	6.1	6.5	7.4	10.5	14.1	21.6	23.0	27.0
Female												
2–5 months	111	10.2	0.16	7.3	7.5	7.9	8.5	9.9	11.6	12.1	12.8	13.6
6–8 months	103	10.3	0.22	6.7	7.5	8.1	8.6	10.1	11.8	12.8	13.6	†
9–11 months	118	10.2	0.31	6.8	7.7	8.1	8.5	10.0	11.6	11.9	12.6	†
1 year	284	9.6	0.19	6.1	6.9	7.4	8.0	9.2	10.8	11.9	12.9	13.8
2 years	254	10.0	0.26	6.5	7.0	7.4	8.3	9.6	11.1	11.9	12.6	15.0
3 years	182	9.9	0.24	6.2	6.8	7.2	8.0	9.6	11.3	12.1	13.0	13.6
4 years	190	10.5	0.18	6.2	7.8	8.1	8.7	10.0	11.8	13.0	13.8	15.0
5 years	169	11.1	0.32	7.0	7.5	7.9	8.6	10.2	12.4	14.3	15.8	18.2
6 years	173	10.9	0.40	6.3	6.9	7.3	8.0	10.0	12.2	13.8	15.5	18.0
7 years	201	12.2	0.42	6.1	6.9	7.6	8.5	10.7	13.9	16.9	19.5	23.7
8 years	199	14.3	0.58	7.1	7.8	8.5	9.5	13.1	18.5	20.5	23.2	23.9
9 years	200	15.0	0.73	6.9	7.7	8.9	9.8	13.6	17.9	23.2	25.3	28.7
10 years	175	15.4	0.49	7.2	7.9	9.0	10.1	14.9	19.4	22.6	24.0	26.2
11 years	210	15.9	0.71	8.3	9.0	9.2	10.3	13.6	20.5	24.8	26.4	29.1
12 years	162	16.2	0.62	7.6	8.9	9.2	10.6	15.0	20.2	23.3	24.9	27.6
13 years	130	17.8	0.71	8.2	9.5	9.8	11.5	16.8	21.5	25.9	29.0	30.4
14 years	163	19.3	0.58	9.2	11.0	11.7	14.1	18.2	23.9	27.1	28.2	30.7
15 years	132	19.1	0.78	8.9	10.8	11.7	13.2	17.0	24.2	27.5	29.9	31.8
16 years	150	19.4	0.53	10.4	11.7	12.9	14.6	18.2	23.0	26.0	26.9	33.0
17 years	137	19.7	0.87	10.1	11.5	12.6	14.4	18.3	23.0	27.2	29.3	33.2
18 years	124	18.4	0.71	10.1	11.1	11.9	13.6	16.6	22.5	26.6	28.0	28.7
19 years	113	20.6	0.90	9.1	10.5	11.5	14.3	20.7	24.2	30.5	31.7	33.4

† Standard error not calculated by SUDAAN.
[1]Refers to age at time of examination.
NOTE: Pregnant females were excluded.
SOURCE: CDC/NCHS, National Health and Nutrition Examination Survey.

TABLE 2	Triceps skinfold thickness in millimeters for females aged 20 and over and number of examined persons, mean, standard error of the mean, and selected percentiles, by race and ethnicity and age: United States, 2007–2010

Race and ethnicity and age	Number of examined persons	Mean	Standard error of the mean	5th	10th	15th	25th	50th	75th	85th	90th	95th
All racial and ethnic groups[1]				Millimeters								
20 years and over	5198	23.7	0.17	11.9	14.0	15.8	18.0	23.5	29.0	31.9	33.7	35.9
20–29 years	815	22.2	0.44	11.0	13.2	14.0	16.5	21.3	27.7	31.1	32.6	35.1
30–39 years	858	24.2	0.40	12.1	14.7	16.2	18.6	24.1	30.0	32.2	33.8	36.0
40–49 years	943	24.2	0.26	11.5	14.1	15.9	18.7	24.7	29.5	32.1	33.9	35.8
50–59 years	769	24.6	0.30	12.9	15.6	16.8	19.2	24.5	29.8	32.2	34.0	36.3
60–69 years	845	24.7	0.34	13.0	15.8	17.2	20.2	24.9	29.4	31.9	33.8	35.9
70–79 years	613	23.4	0.33	11.5	14.3	16.3	18.9	22.9	28.0	31.0	32.8	35.2
80 years and over	355	19.4	0.34	9.4	11.2	12.4	14.7	19.0	23.2	25.9	27.8	31.7
Non-Hispanic white												
20 years and over	2470	23.4	0.24	11.7	13.9	15.6	17.9	23.0	28.7	31.3	33.0	35.4
20–39 years	711	22.8	0.41	11.6	13.4	14.4	17.0	22.1	28.6	31.4	32.7	35.0
40–59 years	780	24.0	0.30	12.0	14.2	16.2	18.5	24.3	29.2	31.8	33.8	35.8
60 years and over	979	23.1	0.22	11.4	13.9	15.8	18.1	22.5	27.9	30.9	32.5	34.9
Non-Hispanic black												
20 years and over	934	25.7	0.34	11.1	14.7	16.7	20.4	26.2	31.9	34.2	35.2	37.5
20–39 years	307	25.6	0.50	11.0	13.8	15.7	20.0	25.9	32.0	34.2	35.2	37.2
40–59 years	313	26.5	0.39	12.8	15.2	18.0	21.7	27.5	31.9	34.2	35.2	37.9
60 years and over	314	24.6	0.70	10.9	14.7	16.1	19.7	24.9	30.0	33.1	35.0	37.1
Hispanic[2]												
20 years and over	1546	24.4	0.22	13.4	15.7	16.9	19.2	24.3	29.1	31.9	33.8	35.8
20–39 years	561	23.7	0.35	13.3	15.1	16.4	18.7	23.5	28.0	31.0	33.0	35.7
40–59 years	526	25.8	0.36	15.0	17.0	18.3	21.0	25.7	30.8	33.1	34.4	36.1
60 years and over	459	23.4	0.24	12.1	13.9	15.6	18.0	23.1	28.5	31.0	32.9	35.1
Mexican American												
20 years and over	948	24.6	0.30	13.4	15.8	17.1	19.4	24.7	29.4	32.2	33.9	36.0
20–39 years	353	24.1	0.43	13.5	15.5	16.6	19.0	24.0	28.5	31.8	33.4	36.0
40–59 years	320	26.1	0.55	15.0	17.2	19.1	21.8	25.9	30.9	33.3	34.9	36.5
60 years and over	275	23.0	0.26	11.3	13.1	15.3	17.9	23.0	28.1	30.7	31.9	34.2

[1]Persons of other races and ethnicities are included.
[2]Mexican-American persons are included in the Hispanic group.
NOTE: Pregnant females were excluded.
SOURCE: CDC/NCHS, National Health and Nutrition Examination Survey.

| TABLE 3 | Triceps skinfold thickness in millimeters for males aged 20 and over and number of examined persons, mean, standard error of the mean, and selected percentiles, by race and ethnicity and age: United States, 2007–2010 |

Race and ethnicity and age	Number of examined persons	Mean	Standard error of the mean	Percentile								
				5th	10th	15th	25th	50th	75th	85th	90th	95th
All racial and ethnic groups[1]				Millimeters								
20 years and over	5307	14.9	0.17	6.2	7.5	8.4	9.9	13.4	18.6	22.0	24.3	27.8
20–29 years	846	14.0	0.28	5.5	6.6	7.2	8.5	12.5	17.9	21.9	23.3	26.4
30–39 years	875	15.1	0.26	5.9	7.7	8.5	9.9	13.9	18.8	22.2	24.8	28.3
40–49 years	885	14.7	0.33	6.3	7.9	8.4	9.5	12.9	18.2	22.0	24.5	28.0
50–59 years	880	15.1	0.37	7.0	8.2	9.0	10.5	13.3	18.8	21.8	24.2	28.4
60–69 years	880	15.9	0.31	7.2	8.4	9.3	10.8	14.9	19.8	23.2	24.9	27.9
70–79 years	606	15.7	0.41	7.6	8.6	9.4	10.9	14.6	19.2	22.1	24.9	27.7
80 years and over	335	14.4	0.25	7.0	8.5	8.9	9.9	13.2	16.9	20.2	22.0	25.4
Non-Hispanic white												
20 years and over	2588	15.1	0.22	6.5	7.8	8.7	10.1	13.4	19.0	22.1	24.4	27.6
20–39 years	747	14.5	0.28	5.7	7.0	7.6	9.3	13.1	18.6	21.9	23.8	26.5
40–59 years	792	15.1	0.31	7.0	8.3	8.8	10.2	13.2	18.8	22.2	24.6	28.0
60 years and over	1049	15.8	0.28	7.4	8.7	9.5	11.0	14.8	19.5	22.6	24.8	27.4
Non-Hispanic black												
20 years and over	984	14.5	0.26	4.9	6.0	7.0	8.4	12.6	18.8	23.1	25.4	30.1
20–39 years	316	14.2	0.39	4.5	5.6	6.6	7.8	12.0	18.3	23.5	25.9	31.5
40–59 years	335	14.5	0.46	4.6	6.3	7.1	9.0	12.6	18.9	22.7	24.7	29.7
60 years and over	333	15.4	0.37	5.6	6.8	7.8	9.5	14.4	19.3	23.7	25.8	29.2
Hispanic[2]												
20 years and over	1475	14.4	0.27	6.7	7.8	8.6	9.9	13.3	17.1	20.1	22.6	27.7
20–39 years	547	14.5	0.32	6.1	7.5	8.5	9.9	13.6	17.1	20.3	22.9	28.1
40–59 years	559	14.2	0.34	7.0	7.9	8.4	9.8	12.9	16.9	19.5	21.8	26.8
60 years and over	369	14.6	0.33	7.0	8.3	9.1	10.0	13.1	17.5	20.8	22.8	27.9
Mexican American												
20 years and over	949	14.4	0.30	6.8	7.9	8.7	10.0	13.3	17.0	20.0	21.9	27.0
20–39 years	366	14.7	0.37	6.2	7.8	8.7	10.1	13.8	17.2	20.3	22.8	28.1
40–59 years	364	13.8	0.36	6.9	7.8	8.4	9.6	12.4	16.4	19.3	21.2	25.0
60 years and over	219	14.4	0.42	7.4	8.3	9.1	10.0	12.9	17.4	19.7	21.8	27.3

[1]Persons of other races and ethnicities are included.
[2]Mexican-American persons are included in the Hispanic group.
SOURCE: CDC/NCHS, National Health and Nutrition Examination Survey.

TABLE 4	Subscapular skinfold thickness in millimeters for children and adolescents aged 2 months to 19 years and number of examined persons, mean, standard error of the mean, and selected percentiles, by sex and age: United States, 2007–2010

Sex and age[1]	Number of examined persons	Mean	Standard error of the mean	Percentile 5th	10th	15th	25th	50th	75th	85th	90th	95th
Male				Millimeters								
2–5 months	121	7.9	0.17	5.5	5.8	6.2	6.5	7.7	8.8	9.9	10.0	11.2
6–8 months	98	7.9	0.26	†	5.4	5.9	6.5	7.7	9.1	9.9	10.1	10.3
9–11 months	106	7.5	0.22	†	5.3	5.5	5.9	7.0	8.3	9.0	10.2	11.5
1 year	305	6.9	0.11	4.7	5.0	5.2	5.7	6.5	7.7	8.4	9.0	9.8
2 years	289	6.5	0.18	4.4	4.8	5.0	5.2	6.2	7.1	7.9	8.4	9.6
3 years	179	6.4	0.17	†	4.5	4.7	5.1	5.9	6.8	7.9	9.0	10.5
4 years	226	6.3	0.17	4.0	4.2	4.5	4.9	5.7	6.9	7.6	8.4	10.1
5 years	190	6.3	0.16	4.0	4.2	4.4	4.7	5.7	6.9	7.9	8.7	11.0
6 years	187	7.0	0.31	4.0	4.3	4.5	4.8	5.4	6.8	8.9	13.4	17.2
7 years	207	7.6	0.36	4.0	4.3	4.5	4.9	5.6	8.1	11.8	13.1	18.1
8 years	201	8.9	0.49	4.1	4.2	4.9	5.1	6.6	9.8	13.9	15.6	21.0
9 years	177	9.6	0.57	4.2	4.5	4.7	5.2	6.7	11.1	15.7	20.5	23.2
10 years	192	11.0	0.62	4.2	4.9	5.2	5.7	7.9	14.2	17.4	19.9	25.9
11 years	200	10.9	0.52	4.9	5.0	5.2	5.9	8.0	14.5	18.2	20.6	23.7
12 years	151	12.0	0.50	4.6	4.9	5.4	5.9	8.9	16.1	19.8	24.6	26.8
13 years	140	11.4	0.84	5.1	5.9	6.1	6.7	8.2	13.5	19.8	22.0	26.3
14 years	169	11.0	0.68	4.9	5.7	6.0	6.3	8.2	12.9	18.2	22.0	25.5
15 years	152	11.8	0.55	5.7	6.3	6.8	7.4	9.1	14.0	16.6	20.4	27.7
16 years	165	12.8	0.59	†	6.9	7.4	8.2	10.0	15.3	19.2	22.0	28.3
17 years	176	13.0	0.70	6.3	7.0	7.7	8.4	10.1	15.2	20.6	23.4	25.9
18 years	130	14.8	0.71	7.3	7.6	8.5	9.3	13.2	19.0	21.2	24.7	27.5
19 years	167	13.6	0.60	6.6	7.0	7.9	9.0	11.3	16.4	19.9	23.0	26.5
Female												
2–5 months	111	8.2	0.19	5.2	5.4	5.8	6.7	8.0	9.2	10.4	11.1	11.8
6–8 months	103	7.5	0.17	†	5.4	5.7	6.5	7.4	8.2	9.0	9.3	†
9–11 months	118	7.8	0.23	5.0	5.3	5.8	6.6	7.5	8.9	9.2	9.7	11.1
1 year	284	7.2	0.14	4.8	5.2	5.4	5.8	6.8	8.0	8.7	9.2	10.4
2 years	253	6.8	0.19	4.5	4.9	5.0	5.5	6.4	7.5	8.2	9.0	10.5
3 years	179	6.7	0.19	4.6	4.9	5.0	5.3	6.2	7.5	8.8	9.3	9.8
4 years	188	6.9	0.14	4.6	4.8	4.9	5.2	6.1	7.5	8.2	9.3	12.1
5 years	166	7.9	0.39	4.4	4.6	4.9	5.2	6.3	8.6	11.1	13.4	17.2
6 years	172	7.5	0.31	4.3	4.7	4.8	5.2	6.2	8.3	10.4	11.7	14.3
7 years	200	9.0	0.47	4.3	4.7	4.9	5.5	6.5	10.2	13.9	16.6	20.0
8 years	192	10.6	0.67	4.5	5.1	5.3	6.1	7.8	14.0	17.4	19.7	24.3
9 years	190	11.3	0.77	4.3	5.1	5.6	6.0	7.8	15.5	19.7	22.6	27.5
10 years	169	12.0	0.55	5.6	6.0	6.5	7.1	9.7	15.2	18.6	21.7	23.0
11 years	196	12.9	0.64	4.9	5.7	6.3	7.0	10.2	17.5	21.3	25.4	27.2
12 years	156	13.1	0.75	5.5	5.9	6.4	7.5	10.7	16.8	20.5	24.7	28.0
13 years	122	14.2	0.81	†	6.8	7.7	8.3	11.0	17.4	24.0	25.4	31.3
14 years	155	15.1	0.60	6.3	7.2	8.2	9.8	13.6	18.4	21.9	24.9	30.3
15 years	129	16.7	0.97	6.9	8.1	9.1	10.0	14.2	22.7	25.8	30.0	31.8
16 years	138	15.6	0.85	†	7.9	8.7	10.2	12.7	20.1	23.2	25.7	29.0
17 years	132	15.6	0.70	7.2	8.6	9.3	11.0	13.0	19.1	24.0	26.1	28.5
18 years	118	16.0	0.91	8.1	8.6	8.8	9.5	12.7	21.8	24.4	28.6	30.9
19 years	108	18.3	0.85	†	9.3	10.6	12.7	16.8	22.1	27.2	31.1	33.6

†Standard error not calculated by SUDAAN.

[1]Refers to age at time of examination.

NOTE: Pregnant females were excluded.

SOURCE: CDC/NCHS, National Health and Nutrition Examination Survey.

TABLE 5	Subscapular skinfold thickness in millimeters for females aged 20 and over and number of examined persons, mean, standard error of the mean, and selected percentiles, by race and ethnicity and age: United States, 2007–2010

Race and ethnicity and age	Number of examined persons	Mean	Standard error of the mean	Percentile								
				5th	10th	15th	25th	50th	75th	85th	90th	95th
All racial and ethnic groups[1]				Millimeters								
20 years and over	4723	21.7	0.17	8.6	10.3	11.9	14.5	21.2	28.1	31.6	33.9	36.0
20–29 years	740	20.0	0.53	8.5	9.6	10.9	13.0	18.9	25.9	30.7	33.6	35.9
30–39 years	762	22.2	0.46	8.9	10.4	11.9	15.3	22.2	29.1	32.0	33.9	36.6
40–49 years	844	22.4	0.37	8.7	10.9	12.2	15.5	22.6	28.4	32.0	33.9	36.5
50–59 years	676	22.9	0.38	9.2	11.0	12.9	16.4	22.8	29.6	32.9	35.0	36.8
60–69 years	782	23.3	0.36	9.6	12.3	14.2	17.7	23.1	29.4	31.9	33.7	35.5
70–79 years	586	21.5	0.36	8.8	10.1	11.8	14.7	21.1	27.9	30.9	32.8	35.1
80 years and over	333	15.4	0.29	5.6	7.2	8.4	10.3	14.4	19.9	22.3	23.9	27.1
Non-Hispanic white												
20 years and over	2325	20.7	0.22	8.2	9.6	11.1	13.6	20.1	27.0	30.8	32.8	35.3
20–39 years	659	19.8	0.52	8.1	9.3	10.5	12.6	18.4	26.1	30.6	32.7	35.4
40–59 years	725	21.6	0.31	8.6	10.2	11.9	14.6	21.1	27.3	31.1	33.6	35.9
60 years and over	941	20.5	0.24	7.5	9.3	11.1	13.9	20.0	26.8	30.1	31.8	34.6
Non-Hispanic black												
20 years and over	773	26.1	0.39	10.3	13.2	16.4	19.9	27.1	32.9	35.3	36.7	38.0
20–39 years	250	25.1	0.49	10.0	11.9	15.1	18.4	25.5	32.7	35.0	36.3	37.4
40–59 years	256	27.3	0.48	11.1	14.9	17.7	21.2	28.6	34.3	36.2	37.2	38.6
60 years and over	267	25.4	0.54	10.1	13.2	17.0	20.3	26.2	31.8	33.0	35.3	37.8
Hispanic[2]												
20 years and over	1397	23.7	0.27	10.6	13.2	15.2	18.0	23.5	29.5	32.3	34.2	36.6
20–39 years	501	23.0	0.39	10.5	12.3	14.0	17.3	22.7	28.9	31.8	34.4	36.7
40–59 years	458	25.1	0.47	12.9	15.4	17.1	19.8	25.2	30.8	32.9	34.5	36.7
60 years and over	438	22.4	0.40	8.9	11.5	13.8	16.8	22.3	27.9	31.0	32.9	35.9
Mexican American												
20 years and over	841	23.9	0.34	10.7	13.7	15.5	18.3	23.8	29.8	32.4	34.1	36.6
20–39 years	307	23.7	0.48	10.9	13.5	15.3	17.9	23.3	29.2	32.3	34.6	36.9
40–59 years	276	25.2	0.60	12.7	15.3	16.8	20.1	25.3	30.9	32.8	33.6	36.2
60 years and over	258	21.6	0.59	8.2	10.5	12.8	16.3	21.3	26.9	30.4	32.6	35.4

[1]Persons of other races and ethnicities are included.
[2]Mexican-American persons are included in the Hispanic group.
NOTE: Pregnant females were excluded.
SOURCE: CDC/NCHS, National Health and Nutrition Examination Survey.

TABLE 6	Subscapular skinfold thickness in millimeters for males aged 20 and over and number of examined persons, mean, standard error of the mean, and selected percentiles, by race and ethnicity and age: United States, 2007–2010

Race and ethnicity and age	Number of examined persons	Mean	Standard error of the mean	Percentile									
				5th	10th	15th	25th	50th	75th	85th	90th	95th
All racial and ethnic groups[1]				Millimeters								
20 years and over	4645	20.2	0.21	8.9	10.3	11.5	14.2	19.6	25.2	28.6	30.5	33.3
20–29 years	792	17.8	0.40	7.6	8.8	9.5	11.0	16.5	23.2	27.0	28.9	31.4
30–39 years	758	20.5	0.42	8.9	10.6	11.4	14.7	20.0	25.8	29.0	31.1	33.8
40–49 years	764	21.0	0.37	9.6	11.0	12.6	15.3	20.4	26.1	28.9	30.9	33.8
50–59 years	755	21.2	0.32	10.2	11.9	13.4	15.5	20.5	26.1	29.0	31.2	34.0
60–69 years	752	21.5	0.35	9.6	11.3	13.1	15.8	21.2	26.3	29.9	31.4	35.0
70–79 years	522	20.6	0.33	9.8	11.8	13.0	15.0	20.1	25.4	27.8	29.9	33.8
80 years and over	302	17.9	0.41	9.4	10.3	11.1	13.0	17.0	21.9	24.3	26.3	29.7
Non-Hispanic white												
20 years and over	2302	20.0	0.26	8.8	10.2	11.3	14.0	19.4	25.0	28.3	30.1	33.0
20–39 years	695	18.6	0.46	7.8	9.0	9.8	11.8	17.9	24.3	27.9	29.0	32.4
40–59 years	690	20.9	0.30	10.1	11.4	13.0	15.2	20.1	25.8	28.8	30.9	33.7
60 years and over	917	20.6	0.26	9.5	11.0	12.4	14.9	20.1	25.3	28.5	30.3	33.8
Non-Hispanic black												
20 years and over	832	20.2	0.38	7.9	9.6	10.6	13.1	19.1	26.4	29.6	31.7	35.8
20–39 years	274	18.7	0.52	7.4	9.1	9.9	11.3	17.0	24.4	28.9	30.7	34.5
40–59 years	282	21.2	0.55	7.9	9.7	11.3	14.3	20.9	27.0	30.6	32.6	36.3
60 years and over	276	22.0	0.52	9.3	11.0	13.0	15.6	22.0	27.5	30.2	32.3	36.3
Hispanic[2]												
20 years and over	1283	21.0	0.31	9.6	11.3	13.1	15.4	20.5	26.0	28.7	30.6	33.5
20–39 years	481	20.1	0.39	8.9	10.5	11.8	14.2	19.7	25.1	28.0	29.7	33.2
40–59 years	482	22.4	0.48	11.0	13.2	15.0	17.1	21.9	27.2	30.0	31.8	34.9
60 years and over	320	20.8	0.35	11.0	12.8	14.1	15.4	20.1	25.6	27.2	29.4	32.1
Mexican American												
20 years and over	825	21.0	0.37	9.8	11.5	13.1	15.6	20.5	25.9	28.6	30.6	33.5
20–39 years	316	20.6	0.46	9.1	10.6	12.2	14.9	20.1	25.7	28.6	30.8	33.6
40–59 years	316	21.7	0.50	10.6	12.7	14.5	16.5	21.6	26.0	28.8	30.7	33.7
60 years and over	193	20.4	0.49	11.0	12.8	14.0	15.4	19.8	24.9	26.9	28.5	31.0

[1]Persons of other races and ethnicities are included.
[2]Mexican-American persons are included in the Hispanic group.
SOURCE: CDC/NCHS, National Health and Nutrition Examination Survey.

J

Percent Body Fat Reference Data for Children and Adults: United States, 1999–2004

Data From the Continuous National Health and Nutrition Examination Survey (NHANES)

Source: Borrud LG, Flegal KM, Looker AC, Everhart JE, et al. 2010. Body composition data for individuals 8 years of age and older: U.S. population, 1999–2004. National Center for Health Statistics. *Vital and Health Statistics* 11(250).

U.S. DEPARTMENT OF HEALTH AND HUMAN SERVICES
Centers for Disease Control and Prevention
National Center for Health Statistics

Hyattsville, Maryland
April 2010
DHHS Publication No. (PHS) 2010–1600

TABLE 1	Total percentage body fat for examined persons 8 years of age and older, by sex, race and ethnicity, and age: United States, 1999–2004

Sex, race and ethnicity, and age	Sample size	Mean	Standard error of the mean	Percentile								
				5th	10th	15th	25th	50th	75th	85th	90th	95th
Male				Percent								
All race and ethnicity:												
Age 20 years and older, age adjusted...........	6559	28.1	0.1	...	...	...	...	...	...	...	...	...
Age 20 years and older, crude.....................	6559	28.0	0.1	17.4	19.5	21.4	24.1	28.0	32.1	34.3	35.9	38.0
Age:												
8–11 years...	1067	28.0	0.4	18.2	19.6	20.6	22.1	25.9	33.2	37.5	39.6	42.9
12–15 years...	1726	25.2	0.3	15.1	16.1	16.9	18.6	23.0	31.1	34.3	37.7	40.6
16–19 years...	1751	22.9	0.3	14.0	14.9	15.6	17.0	20.7	27.5	31.3	33.6	37.3
20–39 years...	2183	26.1	0.1	15.5	17.4	18.9	21.2	26.1	30.4	32.8	34.6	37.2
40–59 years...	2024	28.6	0.2	19.3	21.5	23.0	25.2	28.5	32.2	34.1	35.5	37.7
60–79 years...	1851	30.8	0.1	22.0	24.2	25.3	27.3	30.7	34.4	36.4	37.7	39.6
80 years and older.................................	501	30.7	0.2	21.9	24.2	25.4	27.3	30.8	33.9	36.1	37.3	38.8
Mexican American:												
Age 20 years and older, age adjusted...........	1488	28.7	0.1	...	...	...	...	...	...	...	...	...
Age 20 years and older, crude.....................	1488	28.0	0.3	18.4	20.9	22.7	24.5	27.9	31.5	33.1	34.8	37.2
Age:												
8–11 years...	348	30.7	0.5	19.2	20.9	22.1	23.9	29.7	37.2	40.0	41.9	44.8
12–15 years...	599	26.9	0.4	15.9	17.1	18.1	20.0	25.8	32.7	36.4	38.3	40.7
16–19 years...	611	24.9	0.3	15.1	16.1	17.2	19.1	23.2	29.4	33.1	35.7	39.2
20–39 years...	570	27.4	0.3	17.7	19.6	21.6	23.7	27.0	30.8	32.7	34.2	36.9
40–59 years...	427	28.8	0.3	20.3	22.6	24.1	25.5	28.7	31.8	33.6	35.1	37.4
60–79 years...	443	30.5	0.2	22.6	24.4	25.5	27.4	30.8	33.5	35.5	36.6	38.3
80 years and older.................................	48	30.3	1.0	21.3	22.8	23.7	27.8	31.0	33.3	34.8	35.6	†
Non-Hispanic white:												
Age 20 years and older, age adjusted...........	3320	28.3	0.1	...	...	...	...	...	...	...		
Age 20 years and older, crude.....................	3320	28.5	0.1	18.0	20.2	22.1	24.6	28.4	32.4	34.7	36.2	38.4
Age:												
8–11 years...	280	28.1	0.6	19.2	20.4	21.1	22.9	25.8	32.3	37.0	39.5	42.8
12–15 years...	438	25.4	0.5	15.5	16.4	17.5	19.1	23.0	31.3	33.9	37.7	40.8
16–19 years...	447	23.1	0.4	14.3	15.2	16.0	17.3	21.0	27.9	31.2	33.5	36.4
20–39 years...	934	26.2	0.2	16.0	17.6	19.1	21.1	26.1	30.4	33.1	35.0	37.3
40–59 years...	1013	29.0	0.2	20.0	22.2	23.5	25.5	28.7	32.4	34.3	35.7	37.9
60–79 years...	975	31.2	0.2	22.5	24.6	25.7	27.5	31.1	34.7	36.7	37.9	39.7
80 years and older.................................	398	30.8	0.3	22.0	24.4	25.4	27.3	30.9	34.1	36.1	37.4	38.9
Non-Hispanic black:												
Age 20 years and older, age adjusted...........	1245	25.9	0.2	...	...	...	...	...	...	...	...	...
Age 20 years and older, crude.....................	1245	25.5	0.2	14.1	15.7	17.6	20.2	25.8	30.1	32.9	34.5	37.0
Age:												
8–11 years...	359	25.3	0.4	16.1	16.8	18.0	18.9	22.9	30.1	34.5	37.7	41.5
12–15 years...	566	23.1	0.3	13.8	14.7	15.1	16.3	20.3	27.5	32.9	36.8	40.7
16–19 years...	551	20.4	0.4	12.7	13.3	13.8	14.7	17.3	24.5	29.4	33.5	37.6
20–39 years...	450	24.0	0.3	13.4	14.3	15.3	18.3	23.6	28.8	32.1	33.9	36.2
40–59 years...	435	26.1	0.3	15.4	17.5	19.1	21.7	26.4	30.0	32.5	34.4	36.7
60–79 years...	324	28.6	0.3	17.7	20.1	22.2	24.9	28.7	32.7	34.8	36.4	38.7
80 years and older.................................	36	29.4	1.1	†	21.5	22.6	24.7	29.3	32.8	36.0	36.7	†
Female												
All race and ethnicity:												
Age 20 years and older, age adjusted...........	6532	39.8	0.1	...	...	...	...	...	...	...	...	...
Age 20 years and older, crude.....................	6532	39.9	0.2	27.6	30.5	32.4	35.4	40.5	44.7	46.8	48.4	50.4
Age:												
8–11 years...	1082	31.9	0.3	21.7	22.9	24.3	26.3	31.2	37.1	40.3	41.9	43.9
12–15 years...	1780	32.5	0.3	21.7	23.4	24.9	27.4	31.9	37.3	40.1	42.0	44.9
16–19 years...	1513	34.8	0.3	24.2	26.3	27.6	30.0	34.0	39.2	42.9	44.8	47.7
20–39 years...	2043	37.8	0.2	25.8	28.4	29.9	32.5	37.8	42.9	45.6	47.4	49.8
40–59 years...	2049	40.5	0.2	28.5	31.8	33.6	36.4	41.0	45.1	47.1	48.6	50.7
60–79 years...	1846	42.4	0.1	32.3	34.9	36.4	38.9	42.8	46.2	48.0	49.1	50.7
80 years and older.................................	594	40.4	0.3	29.8	32.7	34.3	36.9	41.0	44.4	46.3	47.5	48.9

| TABLE 1 | Total percentage body fat for examined persons 8 years of age and older, by sex, race and ethnicity, and age: United States, 1999–2004—Con. |

Sex, race and ethnicity, and age	Sample size	Mean	Standard error of the mean	Percentile								
				5th	10th	15th	25th	50th	75th	85th	90th	95th
Female—Con.				Percent								
Mexican American:												
Age 20 years and older, age adjusted..........	1438	41.4	0.2	...	...	...	...	...	...	...	...	...
Age 20 years and older, crude.....................	1438	40.9	0.3	30.6	33.1	34.7	36.9	41.1	45.0	46.8	47.9	50.1
Age:												
8–11 years...	342	33.0	0.5	23.2	24.6	25.5	27.7	32.0	37.7	40.6	43.0	45.2
12–15 years...	632	34.5	0.2	23.7	26.0	27.3	29.9	34.6	38.5	41.4	43.1	45.8
16–19 years...	533	36.7	0.3	26.9	28.6	30.4	32.2	36.3	40.9	43.8	45.3	47.0
20–39 years...	492	39.6	0.4	29.5	31.7	33.1	35.3	39.7	43.9	45.8	47.1	48.8
40–59 years...	442	42.3	0.3	34.3	36.0	36.7	39.1	42.3	45.8	47.1	48.5	50.6
60–79 years...	457	43.2	0.3	34.6	36.4	37.6	40.1	43.4	46.8	48.4	49.6	51.3
80 years and older......................................	47	40.6	1.3	†	†	32.6	35.8	41.6	46.0	47.6	48.0	†
Non-Hispanic white:												
Age 20 years and older, age adjusted..........	3250	39.4	0.1	...	...	...	...	...	...	...	...	...
Age 20 years and older, crude.....................	3250	39.7	0.2	27.1	30.1	32.0	35.0	40.4	44.8	46.9	48.5	50.3
Age:												
8–11 years...	281	32.0	0.4	22.3	23.6	25.0	26.5	31.1	36.9	40.1	41.5	43.6
12–15 years...	448	32.2	0.5	21.6	22.8	24.4	27.1	31.4	36.9	40.1	41.9	44.8
16–19 years...	409	34.6	0.4	24.1	26.2	27.6	29.9	33.4	38.4	42.2	44.5	47.9
20–39 years...	907	37.3	0.3	24.8	27.8	29.4	31.8	37.0	42.2	45.3	47.0	49.7
40–59 years...	964	40.1	0.3	27.5	30.8	32.7	35.7	40.8	45.1	47.2	48.6	50.6
60–79 years...	922	42.5	0.2	32.6	35.0	36.6	39.2	42.9	46.2	48.1	49.1	50.8
80 years and older......................................	457	40.6	0.3	29.8	32.7	34.3	37.1	41.1	44.7	46.5	47.7	49.0
Non-Hispanic black:												
Age 20 years and older, age adjusted..........	1312	40.6	0.2	...	...	...	...	...	...	...	...	...
Age 20 years and older, crude.....................	1312	40.6	0.2	27.5	30.9	33.1	36.5	41.1	45.3	47.5	49.0	50.9
Age:												
8–11 years...	373	30.7	0.5	19.6	21.2	22.3	24.3	30.0	36.4	40.0	42.0	43.6
12–15 years...	558	31.6	0.3	20.6	22.6	23.7	25.9	30.8	36.8	40.1	42.4	44.8
16–19 years...	435	34.3	0.4	21.6	24.6	26.1	28.3	33.5	40.0	44.0	45.8	48.7
20–39 years...	455	38.8	0.4	25.7	28.3	30.6	33.9	39.5	44.1	46.5	48.1	50.2
40–59 years...	453	41.8	0.3	30.6	33.5	35.6	38.2	42.3	45.8	48.2	49.8	51.7
60–79 years...	346	42.3	0.4	30.2	34.6	36.3	38.4	43.1	47.1	48.8	49.8	51.2
80 years and older......................................	58	39.3	0.8	28.4	30.7	33.6	36.0	39.9	42.6	44.8	45.5	†

. . . Category not applicable.

†Standard error not calculated by SUDAAN.

Total Lumbar Spine Bone Mineral Density (gm/cm³)

Data from the National Health and Nutrition Examination Survey (NHANES)

Source: Looker AC, Borrud LG, Hughes JP, Fan B, Shepherd JA, Melton LJ. 2012. Lumbar spine and proximal femur bone mineral density, bone mineral content, and bone area: United States, 2005–2008. *Vital and Health Statistics* 11(251):1–132.

U.S. DEPARTMENT OF HEALTH AND HUMAN SERVICES
Centers for Disease Control and Prevention
National Center for Health Statistics

Hyattsville, Maryland
March 2012
DHHS Publication No. (PHS) 2012–1601

TABLE 1	Total lumbar spine (L1–L4) bone mineral density (gm/cm²) of persons aged 8 years and over, by sex, race and ethnicity, and age: United States, 2005–2008

Sex, race and ethnicity, and age	Sample size	Mean	Standard deviation	Percentile								
				5th	10th	15th	25th	50th	75th	85th	90th	95th
Male												
All race and ethnicity:												
8–11 years	712	0.622	0.086	0.488	0.518	0.530	0.562	0.612	0.681	0.716	0.735	0.769
12–15 years	783	0.815	0.148	0.576	0.622	0.645	0.701	0.805	0.922	0.978	1.017	1.071
16–19 years	773	1.026	0.127	0.813	0.865	0.898	0.939	1.026	1.106	1.161	1.187	1.241
20–29 years	704	1.061	0.115	0.884	0.919	0.947	0.982	1.051	1.134	1.175	1.212	1.257
30–39 years	714	1.045	0.121	0.848	0.888	0.914	0.958	1.046	1.123	1.169	1.190	1.250
40–49 years	665	1.051	0.133	0.844	0.879	0.911	0.950	1.044	1.141	1.188	1.223	1.271
50–59 years	583	1.052	0.147	0.814	0.854	0.894	0.954	1.049	1.150	1.199	1.245	1.306
60–69 years	527	1.068	0.148	0.820	0.872	0.912	0.979	1.060	1.161	1.212	1.254	1.311
70–79 years	326	1.075	0.176	0.809	0.852	0.886	0.966	1.064	1.175	1.261	1.310	1.395
80 years and over	161	1.087	0.205	0.800	0.859	0.888	0.947	1.058	1.170	1.274	1.370	†
20 years and over, age adjusted	3680	1.057	...	...	...	...	...	...	...	...	...	...
Mexican American:												
8–11 years	210	0.607	0.080	0.477	0.504	0.519	0.555	0.600	0.657	0.685	0.707	0.753
12–15 years	231	0.828	0.147	0.581	0.631	0.678	0.732	0.820	0.923	0.989	1.013	1.059
16–19 years	216	0.989	0.116	0.800	0.830	0.869	0.906	0.989	1.068	1.106	1.135	1.176
20–29 years	191	1.033	0.100	0.881	0.907	0.927	0.954	1.017	1.097	1.140	1.165	1.206
30–39 years	149	1.026	0.124	0.801	0.869	0.897	0.956	1.017	1.104	1.134	1.172	1.253
40–49 years	140	0.990	0.117	0.809	0.835	0.858	0.909	0.985	1.064	1.102	1.155	1.196
50–59 years	98	1.000	0.148	0.763	0.803	0.838	0.889	1.004	1.090	1.140	1.195	1.271
60–69 years	94	*1.033	0.164	*0.812	*0.820	*0.859	*0.905	*1.011	*1.127	*1.166	*1.218	†
70–79 years	31	*1.012	0.162	†	†	*0.839	*0.864	*1.006	*1.137	*1.150	*1.224	†
80 years and over	12	*0.992	0.139	†	†	†	*0.915	*0.979	*1.056	*1.093	†	†
20 years and over, age adjusted	715	1.013	...	...	...	...	...	...	...	...	...	...
Non-Hispanic white:												
8–11 years	206	0.621	0.084	0.483	0.515	0.528	0.562	0.610	0.683	0.714	0.731	0.762
12–15 years	220	0.813	0.146	0.590	0.622	0.636	0.701	0.798	0.912	0.974	0.988	1.072
16–19 years	225	1.020	0.124	0.796	0.851	0.891	0.940	1.026	1.095	1.150	1.182	1.229
20–29 years	281	1.057	0.110	0.883	0.918	0.947	0.979	1.051	1.128	1.169	1.206	1.247
30–39 years	329	1.042	0.117	0.851	0.888	0.914	0.956	1.049	1.114	1.162	1.182	1.230
40–49 years	300	1.051	0.129	0.848	0.879	0.912	0.948	1.042	1.138	1.178	1.219	1.267
50–59 years	305	1.053	0.143	0.814	0.855	0.895	0.959	1.051	1.152	1.194	1.232	1.294
60–69 years	228	1.070	0.142	0.821	0.878	0.919	0.983	1.068	1.163	1.208	1.241	1.297
70–79 years	208	1.068	0.177	0.804	0.834	0.882	0.951	1.052	1.169	1.246	1.308	1.392
80 years and over	126	1.093	0.208	0.817	0.862	0.892	0.952	1.060	1.175	1.284	1.385	1.470
20 years and over, age adjusted	1777	1.056	...	...	...	...	...	...	...	...	...	...
Non-Hispanic black:												
8–11 years	197	0.659	0.091	0.523	0.558	0.571	0.595	0.651	0.717	0.750	0.767	0.808
12–15 years	231	0.832	0.148	0.578	0.639	0.667	0.732	0.835	0.933	0.987	1.017	1.073
16–19 years	255	1.069	0.128	0.881	0.915	0.934	0.971	1.058	1.144	1.218	1.239	1.288
20–29 years	157	1.124	0.138	0.911	0.943	0.990	1.039	1.115	1.189	1.258	1.316	1.348
30–39 years	139	1.113	0.130	0.903	0.958	0.975	1.021	1.120	1.183	1.236	1.286	†
40–49 years	140	1.107	0.142	0.887	0.952	0.982	1.013	1.086	1.188	1.251	1.280	1.387
50–59 years	108	1.125	0.162	0.882	0.921	0.948	1.000	1.108	1.233	1.307	1.353	1.406
60–69 years	139	1.117	0.171	0.832	0.887	0.936	1.014	1.116	1.224	1.305	1.337	1.385
70–79 years	62	*1.174	0.162	*0.872	*0.973	*0.988	*1.054	*1.172	*1.278	*1.355	*1.398	*1.432
80 years and over	13	*1.126	0.209	†	†	†	*0.947	*1.064	†	†	†	†
20 years and over, age adjusted	758	1.121	...	...	...	...	...	...	...	...	...	...
Female												
All race and ethnicity:												
8–11 years	741	0.660	0.120	0.501	0.527	0.543	0.570	0.638	0.731	0.783	0.823	0.881
12–15 years	707	0.928	0.139	0.698	0.745	0.782	0.836	0.933	1.014	1.062	1.092	1.161
16–19 years	631	1.010	0.114	0.832	0.864	0.891	0.927	1.005	1.082	1.125	1.153	1.216
20–29 years	591	1.063	0.115	0.884	0.923	0.944	0.979	1.059	1.150	1.179	1.201	1.251
30–39 years	641	1.068	0.118	0.875	0.916	0.949	0.991	1.069	1.144	1.190	1.213	1.252
40–49 years	744	1.058	0.135	0.851	0.906	0.932	0.965	1.051	1.144	1.190	1.229	1.274
50–59 years	588	0.989	0.144	0.772	0.808	0.834	0.886	0.975	1.085	1.150	1.180	1.232
60–69 years	578	0.953	0.145	0.736	0.786	0.813	0.851	0.939	1.046	1.110	1.149	1.219
70–79 years	313	0.904	0.166	0.646	0.711	0.740	0.787	0.892	1.003	1.067	1.107	1.176
80 years and over	154	0.931	0.151	0.684	0.737	0.781	0.813	0.919	1.038	1.103	1.126	1.157
20 years and over, age adjusted	3609	1.021	...	...	...	...	...	...	...	...	...	...

See footnotes at end of table.

TABLE 1	Total lumbar spine (L1–L4) bone mineral density (gm/cm²) of persons aged 8 years and over, by sex, race and ethnicity, and age: United States, 2005–2008—Con.

| | | | | Percentile | | | | | | | | |
Sex, race and ethnicity, and age	Sample size	Mean	Standard deviation	5th	10th	15th	25th	50th	75th	85th	90th	95th
Female—Con.												
Mexican American:												
8–11 years	236	0.657	0.120	0.501	0.515	0.527	0.561	0.644	0.734	0.772	0.811	0.874
12–15 years	228	0.913	0.118	0.721	0.757	0.781	0.842	0.912	0.980	1.019	1.056	1.101
16–19 years	178	0.983	0.112	0.815	0.830	0.853	0.891	0.982	1.055	1.091	1.111	1.140
20–29 years	144	1.024	0.110	0.845	0.881	0.908	0.948	1.010	1.106	1.155	1.179	1.197
30–39 years	149	1.056	0.133	0.844	0.896	0.928	0.965	1.056	1.124	1.177	1.207	†
40–49 years	136	1.036	0.110	0.855	0.893	0.926	0.948	1.044	1.108	1.150	1.167	1.208
50–59 years	99	*0.960	0.171	*0.701	*0.742	*0.797	*0.840	*0.955	*1.055	*1.110	*1.140	*1.249
60–69 years	126	*0.895	0.138	*0.686	*0.713	*0.735	*0.780	*0.909	*0.981	*1.011	*1.066	*1.116
70–79 years	40	*0.825	0.150	†	*0.628	*0.663	*0.698	*0.829	*0.915	*0.961	*1.036	†
80 years and over	6	*0.791	0.218	†	†	†	†	*0.719	†	†	†	†
20 years and over, age adjusted	700	0.983	…	…	…	…	…	…	…	…	…	…
Non-Hispanic white:												
8–11 years	198	0.651	0.111	0.497	0.529	0.546	0.568	0.627	0.710	0.772	0.798	0.864
12–15 years	178	0.920	0.138	0.692	0.741	0.770	0.829	0.926	1.008	1.056	1.080	1.138
16–19 years	172	1.004	0.107	0.832	0.861	0.892	0.923	1.001	1.075	1.106	1.139	1.172
20–29 years	236	1.064	0.106	0.888	0.932	0.947	0.980	1.060	1.148	1.176	1.189	1.242
30–39 years	258	1.065	0.110	0.886	0.921	0.947	0.991	1.070	1.133	1.168	1.207	1.233
40–49 years	348	1.056	0.134	0.850	0.908	0.932	0.962	1.049	1.140	1.185	1.218	1.263
50–59 years	281	0.993	0.141	0.781	0.813	0.832	0.889	0.978	1.090	1.151	1.179	1.230
60–69 years	245	0.952	0.142	0.738	0.792	0.814	0.847	0.935	1.047	1.107	1.148	1.211
70–79 years	197	0.902	0.167	0.637	0.712	0.738	0.777	0.891	0.994	1.060	1.107	1.178
80 years and over	117	0.932	0.141	0.690	0.738	0.784	0.820	0.927	1.034	1.094	1.126	1.155
20 years and over, age adjusted	1682	1.020	…	…	…	…	…	…	……	…	…	…
Non-Hispanic black:												
8–11 years	202	0.713	0.134	0.523	0.558	0.587	0.613	0.692	0.810	0.844	0.864	0.948
12–15 years	225	0.986	0.135	0.734	0.803	0.851	0.894	0.996	1.083	1.134	1.171	1.197
16–19 years	202	1.077	0.115	0.898	0.936	0.952	0.996	1.062	1.148	1.201	1.239	†
20–29 years	127	1.118	0.131	0.864	0.937	0.979	1.026	1.139	1.201	1.246	1.287	1.320
30–39 years	142	1.130	0.119	0.933	1.008	1.019	1.054	1.119	1.201	1.241	1.256	1.303
40–49 years	164	1.108	0.150	0.873	0.922	0.947	1.006	1.096	1.199	1.245	1.285	1.337
50–59 years	131	1.039	0.132	0.839	0.867	0.899	0.934	1.035	1.144	1.167	1.212	1.248
60–69 years	139	1.029	0.163	0.766	0.826	0.872	0.933	1.018	1.121	1.191	1.235	†
70–79 years	52	*0.997	0.143	*0.753	*0.808	*0.857	*0.914	*1.009	*1.074	*1.115	*1.166	†
80 years and over	22	*0.948	0.222	†	†	*0.768	*0.792	*0.844	*1.079	†	†	†
20 years and over, age adjusted	777	1.079	…	…	…	…	…	…	…	…	…	…

†Standard error not calculated by SUDAAN.

. . . Category not applicable.

*Figure does not meet standards of reliability or precision; relative standard error (standard error/estimate) is 30%–39% or estimate is based on less than 12 degrees of freedom.

APPENDIX

L   *Total Femur Bone Mineral Density (gm/cm³)*

Data from the National Health and Nutrition Examination Survey (NHANES)

Source: Looker AC, Borrud LG, Hughes JP, Fan B, Shepherd JA, Melton LJ. 2012. Lumbar spine and proximal femur bone mineral density, bone mineral content, and bone area: United States, 2005–2008. *Vital and Health Statistics* 11(251):1–132.

U.S. DEPARTMENT OF HEALTH AND HUMAN SERVICES
Centers for Disease Control and Prevention
National Center for Health Statistics

Hyattsville, Maryland
March 2012
DHHS Publication No. (PHS) 2012–1601

TABLE 1	Total proximal femur bone mineral density (gm/cm²) of persons aged 8 years and over, by sex, race and ethnicity, and age: United States, 2005–2008

| | | | | Percentile | | | | | | | | |
Sex, race and ethnicity, and age	Sample size	Mean	Standard deviation	5th	10th	15th	25th	50th	75th	85th	90th	95th
Male												
All race and ethnicity:												
8–11 years	704	0.747	0.098	0.594	0.626	0.646	0.679	0.738	0.806	0.836	0.871	0.929
12–15 years	778	0.924	0.152	0.689	0.731	0.765	0.817	0.914	1.021	1.085	1.132	1.192
16–19 years	762	1.086	0.148	0.850	0.907	0.941	0.982	1.069	1.181	1.240	1.284	1.345
20–29 years	722	1.081	0.130	0.870	0.919	0.955	0.990	1.078	1.163	1.215	1.248	1.292
30–39 years	736	1.045	0.136	0.826	0.878	0.909	0.953	1.039	1.125	1.178	1.222	1.290
40–49 years	721	1.046	0.131	0.833	0.882	0.914	0.966	1.045	1.130	1.175	1.196	1.243
50–59 years	670	1.020	0.144	0.790	0.836	0.877	0.923	1.013	1.113	1.169	1.203	1.273
60–69 years	689	1.001	0.143	0.770	0.822	0.857	0.904	0.999	1.087	1.144	1.194	1.254
70–79 years	487	0.966	0.142	0.731	0.790	0.818	0.873	0.960	1.049	1.095	1.138	1.210
80 years and over	265	0.919	0.155	0.667	0.742	0.766	0.813	0.896	1.019	1.075	1.124	1.190
20 years and over, age adjusted	4290	1.031	...	...	...	...	...	...	...	...	...	...
Mexican American:												
8–11 years	206	0.739	0.091	0.603	0.624	0.643	0.674	0.730	0.796	0.834	0.859	0.912
12–15 years	232	0.937	0.157	0.683	0.723	0.778	0.830	0.938	1.040	1.111	1.137	1.205
16–19 years	212	1.063	0.144	0.839	0.899	0.923	0.955	1.044	1.147	1.225	1.268	1.327
20–29 years	200	1.078	0.114	0.904	0.939	0.960	0.996	1.076	1.159	1.193	1.217	1.249
30–39 years	153	1.065	0.111	0.880	0.919	0.947	0.986	1.057	1.146	1.183	1.211	1.258
40–49 years	154	1.033	0.125	0.830	0.874	0.892	0.949	1.029	1.112	1.162	1.206	1.239
50–59 years	111	1.006	0.151	0.760	0.817	0.847	0.917	0.999	1.112	1.160	1.209	1.257
60–69 years	118	1.013	0.139	0.788	0.859	0.877	0.915	0.999	1.099	1.152	1.171	1.218
70–79 years	47	*0.952	0.129	†	*0.781	*0.821	*0.868	*0.931	*1.023	*1.099	*1.154	†
80 years and over	14	*0.878	0.146	†	†	†	*0.761	*0.815	*0.979	*1.082	†	†
20 years and over, age adjusted	797	1.028	...	...	...	...	...	...	...	...	...	...
Non-Hispanic white:												
8–11 years	205	0.739	0.096	0.589	0.613	0.640	0.671	0.732	0.792	0.828	0.846	0.899
12–15 years	218	0.915	0.146	0.691	0.720	0.759	0.804	0.912	1.008	1.068	1.123	1.165
16–19 years	223	1.071	0.141	0.836	0.897	0.938	0.979	1.061	1.160	1.224	1.244	1.300
20–29 years	285	1.067	0.120	0.868	0.916	0.951	0.983	1.059	1.153	1.194	1.228	1.272
30–39 years	337	1.029	0.134	0.804	0.857	0.894	0.942	1.028	1.113	1.151	1.201	1.258
40–49 years	329	1.040	0.130	0.821	0.869	0.914	0.966	1.040	1.123	1.167	1.193	1.227
50–59 years	341	1.015	0.142	0.766	0.830	0.875	0.920	1.007	1.109	1.161	1.195	1.257
60–69 years	309	0.997	0.137	0.776	0.822	0.859	0.903	0.994	1.078	1.138	1.175	1.243
70–79 years	330	0.961	0.143	0.727	0.782	0.815	0.868	0.960	1.047	1.089	1.129	1.200
80 years and over	214	0.917	0.157	0.660	0.738	0.766	0.812	0.886	1.016	1.075	1.123	1.190
20 years and over, age adjusted	2145	1.022	...	...	...	...	...	...	...	...	...	...
Non-Hispanic black:												
8–11 years	197	0.808	0.099	0.647	0.688	0.718	0.739	0.806	0.863	0.915	0.938	0.968
12–15 years	227	0.964	0.162	0.732	0.751	0.783	0.844	0.959	1.054	1.136	1.192	1.261
16–19 years	251	1.163	0.164	0.884	0.965	0.990	1.053	1.153	1.280	1.352	1.392	1.442
20–29 years	160	1.155	0.156	0.907	0.964	0.990	1.069	1.145	1.242	1.304	1.353	1.429
30–39 years	145	1.136	0.146	0.893	0.956	0.979	1.039	1.126	1.242	1.289	1.304	1.359
40–49 years	151	1.094	0.150	0.862	0.907	0.935	0.985	1.106	1.182	1.221	1.275	1.355
50–59 years	126	1.100	0.157	0.851	0.920	0.941	0.994	1.076	1.187	1.286	1.323	1.369
60–69 years	185	1.066	0.169	0.787	0.841	0.904	0.966	1.047	1.191	1.231	1.273	1.349
70–79 years	75	*1.033	0.147	*0.812	*0.848	*0.863	*0.928	*1.030	*1.162	*1.208	*1.218	*1.239
80 years and over	22	*0.959	0.143	†	*0.776	*0.815	*0.837	*0.914	*1.046	*1.092	†	†
20 years and over, age adjusted	864	1.101	...	...	...	...	...	...	...	...	...	...
Female												
All race and ethnicity:												
8–11 years	741	0.704	0.111	0.550	0.579	0.602	0.625	0.683	0.768	0.823	0.862	0.905
12–15 years	715	0.909	0.136	0.696	0.736	0.771	0.811	0.904	0.998	1.051	1.082	1.147
16–19 years	673	0.971	0.129	0.762	0.798	0.832	0.891	0.969	1.062	1.104	1.130	1.188
20–29 years	635	0.973	0.124	0.786	0.822	0.841	0.888	0.960	1.055	1.110	1.135	1.178
30–39 years	639	0.960	0.127	0.748	0.788	0.821	0.874	0.963	1.043	1.081	1.115	1.190
40–49 years	750	0.954	0.133	0.743	0.783	0.816	0.864	0.943	1.035	1.088	1.119	1.171
50–59 years	595	0.898	0.136	0.712	0.735	0.763	0.800	0.889	0.983	1.032	1.063	1.139
60–69 years	633	0.855	0.126	0.648	0.703	0.724	0.768	0.854	0.938	0.975	1.011	1.072
70–79 years	425	0.803	0.139	0.572	0.634	0.661	0.713	0.800	0.885	0.930	0.981	1.045
80 years and over	253	0.745	0.131	0.520	0.585	0.608	0.644	0.752	0.831	0.869	0.906	0.934
20 years and over, age adjusted	3930	0.918	...	...	...	...	...	...	...	...	...	...

See footnotes at end of table.

TABLE 1	Total proximal femur bone mineral density (gm/cm^2) of persons aged 8 years and over, by sex, race and ethnicity, and age: United States, 2005–2008—Con.

Sex, race and ethnicity, and age	Sample size	Mean	Standard deviation	5th	10th	15th	25th	50th	75th	85th	90th	95th
Female—Con.												
Mexican American:												
8–11 years	234	0.716	0.113	0.546	0.593	0.610	0.640	0.702	0.772	0.840	0.873	0.933
12–15 years	227	0.902	0.121	0.715	0.742	0.762	0.807	0.901	0.983	1.032	1.058	1.109
16–19 years	186	0.945	0.120	0.765	0.798	0.811	0.860	0.945	1.017	1.062	1.091	1.116
20–29 years	148	0.956	0.126	0.756	0.792	0.821	0.867	0.939	1.040	1.095	1.126	1.179
30–39 years	137	0.968	0.115	0.785	0.810	0.821	0.891	0.968	1.046	1.084	1.106	1.146
40–49 years	133	0.976	0.136	0.766	0.807	0.845	0.889	0.956	1.052	1.114	1.132	1.215
50–59 years	97	*0.926	0.171	*0.691	*0.753	*0.782	*0.827	*0.901	*0.995	*1.062	*1.097	*1.117
60–69 years	130	*0.856	0.124	*0.633	*0.669	*0.746	*0.781	*0.852	*0.929	*0.971	*0.996	*1.042
70–79 years	49	*0.772	0.152	†	*0.569	*0.597	*0.653	*0.777	*0.878	*0.930	*0.986	†
80 years and over	12	*0.708	0.158	†	†	†	†	*0.661	†	†	†	†
20 years and over, age adjusted	706	0.921	...	...	...	...	...	...	...	...	...	...
Non-Hispanic white:												
8–11 years	199	0.691	0.103	0.553	0.578	0.600	0.621	0.668	0.736	0.797	0.833	0.883
12–15 years	185	0.902	0.133	0.692	0.736	0.772	0.804	0.898	0.990	1.043	1.059	1.129
16–19 years	198	0.967	0.125	0.761	0.795	0.824	0.891	0.967	1.050	1.097	1.121	1.172
20–29 years	262	0.971	0.114	0.800	0.828	0.849	0.889	0.961	1.050	1.099	1.125	1.152
30–39 years	267	0.955	0.125	0.744	0.783	0.824	0.875	0.962	1.036	1.072	1.106	1.187
40–49 years	357	0.944	0.131	0.740	0.777	0.809	0.854	0.931	1.028	1.084	1.107	1.149
50–59 years	291	0.893	0.133	0.714	0.731	0.758	0.794	0.885	0.973	1.031	1.060	1.128
60–69 years	286	0.852	0.120	0.653	0.705	0.722	0.766	0.853	0.933	0.971	0.999	1.042
70–79 years	274	0.802	0.139	0.566	0.630	0.658	0.714	0.796	0.883	0.929	0.948	1.040
80 years and over	191	0.743	0.125	0.527	0.592	0.611	0.646	0.747	0.820	0.865	0.893	0.920
20 years and over, age adjusted	1928	0.913	...	...	...	...	...	...	...	...	...	...
Non-Hispanic black:												
8–11 years	202	0.771	0.113	0.600	0.633	0.651	0.686	0.761	0.845	0.893	0.920	0.974
12–15 years	226	0.974	0.137	0.759	0.803	0.837	0.872	0.966	1.060	1.117	1.152	1.204
16–19 years	206	1.035	0.128	0.821	0.853	0.898	0.946	1.026	1.125	1.172	1.211	1.232
20–29 years	136	1.036	0.147	0.798	0.828	0.884	0.941	1.025	1.133	1.184	1.230	1.283
30–39 years	140	1.010	0.130	0.788	0.850	0.875	0.918	1.005	1.083	1.140	1.196	1.229
40–49 years	160	1.012	0.141	0.777	0.818	0.857	0.917	1.016	1.102	1.153	1.184	1.224
50–59 years	134	0.949	0.140	0.727	0.776	0.802	0.829	0.957	1.036	1.099	1.123	1.183
60–69 years	141	0.911	0.170	0.616	0.693	0.738	0.803	0.909	1.015	1.078	1.111	†
70–79 years	66	*0.856	0.137	*0.604	*0.688	*0.712	*0.770	*0.855	*0.935	*0.999	*1.045	*1.089
80 years and over	31	*0.745	0.178	†	*0.519	*0.541	*0.592	*0.720	*0.881	†	†	†
20 years and over, age adjusted	808	0.970	...	...	...	...	...	...	...	...	...	...

... Category not applicable.

*Figure does not meet standards of reliability or precision; relative standard error (standard error/estimate) is 30%–39% or estimate is based on less than 12 degrees of freedom.

†Standard error not calculated by SUDAAN.

| TABLE 2 | Femur neck bone mineral density (gm/cm²) of persons aged 8 years and over, by sex, race and ethnicity, and age: United States, 2005–2008 |

Sex, race and ethnicity, and age	Sample size	Mean	Standard deviation	Percentile								
				5th	10th	15th	25th	50th	75th	85th	90th	95th
Male												
All race and ethnicity:												
8–11 years	704	0.710	0.094	0.566	0.595	0.613	0.637	0.703	0.763	0.802	0.835	0.886
12–15 years	778	0.853	0.133	0.647	0.682	0.712	0.761	0.846	0.934	0.995	1.029	1.085
16–19 years	762	0.994	0.152	0.758	0.805	0.845	0.887	0.984	1.083	1.148	1.192	1.260
20–29 years	722	0.963	0.132	0.748	0.810	0.841	0.872	0.949	1.047	1.103	1.136	1.187
30–39 years	736	0.900	0.131	0.699	0.745	0.771	0.805	0.894	0.971	1.034	1.081	1.132
40–49 years	721	0.879	0.123	0.688	0.727	0.755	0.788	0.878	0.948	0.992	1.021	1.108
50–59 years	670	0.839	0.128	0.640	0.688	0.707	0.753	0.828	0.914	0.971	1.002	1.062
60–69 years	689	0.812	0.129	0.614	0.655	0.674	0.723	0.803	0.888	0.939	0.973	1.042
70–79 years	487	0.776	0.131	0.591	0.625	0.648	0.692	0.762	0.839	0.892	0.938	1.020
80 years and over	265	0.735	0.132	0.546	0.580	0.602	0.647	0.719	0.807	0.878	0.902	0.974
20 years and over, age adjusted	4290	0.870	...	...	...	...	...	...	...	...	...	...
Mexican American:												
8–11 years	206	0.709	0.088	0.575	0.601	0.616	0.634	0.704	0.771	0.797	0.827	0.859
12–15 years	232	0.872	0.146	0.644	0.694	0.720	0.769	0.864	0.962	1.016	1.067	1.135
16–19 years	212	0.978	0.147	0.756	0.790	0.829	0.866	0.959	1.064	1.134	1.202	1.238
20–29 years	200	0.967	0.111	0.784	0.825	0.863	0.890	0.959	1.048	1.088	1.116	1.135
30–39 years	153	0.920	0.115	0.740	0.769	0.798	0.826	0.913	1.003	1.054	1.074	1.107
40–49 years	154	0.875	0.121	0.684	0.727	0.749	0.791	0.865	0.955	0.998	1.039	1.089
50–59 years	111	0.829	0.128	0.644	0.675	0.701	0.735	0.816	0.918	0.979	1.025	1.047
60–69 years	118	0.832	0.125	0.671	0.711	0.723	0.746	0.804	0.906	0.940	0.945	1.035
70–79 years	47	*0.772	0.106	†	*0.651	*0.675	*0.697	*0.770	*0.825	*0.873	*0.886	†
80 years and over	14	*0.694	0.128	†	†	†	†	*0.674	*0.725	*0.782	†	†
20 years and over, age adjusted	797	0.873	...	...	...	...	...	...	...	...	...	...
Non-Hispanic white:												
8–11 years	205	0.701	0.090	0.563	0.584	0.605	0.634	0.697	0.755	0.784	0.817	0.853
12–15 years	218	0.844	0.123	0.649	0.676	0.714	0.761	0.845	0.915	0.973	1.010	1.044
16–19 years	223	0.980	0.147	0.754	0.803	0.842	0.881	0.959	1.073	1.119	1.161	1.212
20–29 years	285	0.948	0.124	0.740	0.810	0.835	0.864	0.935	1.019	1.082	1.116	1.168
30–39 years	337	0.884	0.127	0.675	0.744	0.765	0.795	0.872	0.954	1.014	1.063	1.113
40–49 years	329	0.871	0.121	0.682	0.719	0.752	0.781	0.874	0.938	0.983	1.002	1.102
50–59 years	341	0.832	0.123	0.630	0.688	0.707	0.751	0.819	0.899	0.949	0.989	1.041
60–69 years	309	0.807	0.123	0.615	0.654	0.674	0.718	0.799	0.881	0.932	0.965	1.026
70–79 years	330	0.770	0.130	0.583	0.618	0.642	0.683	0.756	0.834	0.886	0.931	0.998
80 years and over	214	0.734	0.134	0.546	0.576	0.602	0.644	0.716	0.806	0.877	0.902	1.002
20 years and over, age adjusted	2145	0.861	...	...	...	...	...	...	...	...	...	...
Non-Hispanic black:												
8–11 years	197	0.773	0.096	0.628	0.647	0.676	0.709	0.761	0.835	0.862	0.894	0.939
12–15 years	227	0.885	0.148	0.658	0.696	0.740	0.783	0.879	0.971	1.045	1.079	1.125
16–19 years	251	1.064	0.159	0.803	0.860	0.881	0.955	1.053	1.173	1.255	1.291	1.320
20–29 years	160	1.038	0.157	0.796	0.849	0.878	0.918	1.024	1.128	1.188	1.244	1.310
30–39 years	145	0.982	0.143	0.730	0.821	0.845	0.885	0.965	1.081	1.146	1.162	1.210
40–49 years	151	0.938	0.140	0.726	0.770	0.791	0.831	0.938	1.024	1.073	1.109	1.166
50–59 years	126	0.916	0.154	0.678	0.705	0.766	0.816	0.891	1.012	1.082	1.122	1.167
60–69 years	185	0.888	0.154	0.655	0.688	0.727	0.785	0.873	0.985	1.052	1.095	1.159
70–79 years	75	*0.864	0.140	*0.648	*0.681	*0.714	*0.766	*0.853	*0.916	*1.030	*1.060	*1.103
80 years and over	22	*0.781	0.115	†	†	*0.659	*0.715	*0.747	*0.862	†	†	†
20 years and over, age adjusted	864	0.944	...	...	...	...	...	...	...	...	...	...
Female												
All race and ethnicity:												
8–11 years	741	0.667	0.103	0.524	0.554	0.569	0.592	0.647	0.729	0.781	0.815	0.862
12–15 years	715	0.848	0.134	0.646	0.680	0.707	0.759	0.841	0.928	0.983	1.025	1.094
16–19 years	673	0.900	0.130	0.686	0.743	0.766	0.812	0.900	0.984	1.036	1.069	1.121
20–29 years	635	0.889	0.125	0.711	0.739	0.764	0.801	0.881	0.964	1.015	1.046	1.108
30–39 years	639	0.856	0.123	0.664	0.694	0.727	0.774	0.843	0.935	0.976	1.013	1.072
40–49 years	750	0.835	0.129	0.644	0.673	0.701	0.743	0.822	0.913	0.967	0.999	1.059
50–59 years	595	0.772	0.125	0.588	0.619	0.637	0.683	0.762	0.839	0.896	0.932	1.014
60–69 years	633	0.728	0.115	0.565	0.592	0.610	0.646	0.711	0.803	0.850	0.883	0.923
70–79 years	425	0.682	0.121	0.502	0.537	0.556	0.594	0.670	0.758	0.800	0.832	0.906
80 years and over	253	0.633	0.120	0.445	0.495	0.514	0.545	0.628	0.703	0.741	0.770	0.833
20 years and over, age adjusted	3930	0.806	...	...	...	...	...	...	...	...	...	...

See footnotes at end of table.

TABLE 2	Femur neck bone mineral density (gm/cm²) of persons aged 8 years and over, by sex, race and ethnicity, and age: United States, 2005–2008—Con.

Sex, race and ethnicity, and age	Sample size	Mean	Standard deviation	Percentile								
				5th	10th	15th	25th	50th	75th	85th	90th	95th
Females—Con.												
Mexican American:												
8–11 years	234	0.681	0.106	0.522	0.556	0.586	0.606	0.669	0.732	0.787	0.833	0.886
12–15 years	227	0.847	0.123	0.651	0.691	0.710	0.756	0.835	0.917	0.986	0.999	1.063
16–19 years	186	0.875	0.122	0.703	0.731	0.751	0.784	0.870	0.945	0.988	1.012	1.071
20–29 years	148	0.870	0.116	0.692	0.721	0.746	0.783	0.861	0.940	0.993	1.017	1.074
30–39 years	137	0.867	0.108	0.692	0.716	0.753	0.790	0.869	0.933	0.962	0.984	1.061
40–49 years	133	0.848	0.125	0.659	0.698	0.726	0.764	0.833	0.925	0.955	0.987	1.042
50–59 years	97	*0.801	0.144	*0.600	*0.641	*0.669	*0.709	*0.788	*0.859	*0.925	*0.967	*1.014
60–69 years	130	*0.731	0.106	*0.582	*0.602	*0.620	*0.663	*0.715	*0.790	*0.821	*0.866	*0.904
70–79 years	49	*0.665	0.125	†	*0.480	*0.512	*0.576	*0.668	*0.755	*0.792	*0.828	*0.850
80 years and over	12	*0.596	0.102	†	†	†	†	*0.554	*0.677	†	†	†
20 years and over, age adjusted	706	0.810	...	...	...	...	...	...	...	...	...	...
Non-Hispanic white:												
8–11 years	199	0.652	0.094	0.523	0.545	0.569	0.585	0.631	0.698	0.749	0.782	0.845
12–15 years	185	0.840	0.130	0.633	0.665	0.703	0.754	0.836	0.918	0.962	1.018	1.076
16–19 years	198	0.896	0.122	0.683	0.746	0.766	0.812	0.904	0.974	1.023	1.050	1.108
20–29 years	262	0.884	0.113	0.718	0.742	0.771	0.805	0.880	0.952	0.995	1.022	1.078
30–39 years	267	0.849	0.119	0.663	0.693	0.727	0.774	0.835	0.924	0.967	0.997	1.060
40–49 years	357	0.821	0.124	0.643	0.665	0.692	0.736	0.805	0.903	0.951	0.986	1.021
50–59 years	291	0.763	0.122	0.583	0.616	0.634	0.674	0.752	0.833	0.875	0.906	1.014
60–69 years	286	0.723	0.106	0.565	0.597	0.614	0.647	0.710	0.789	0.845	0.867	0.915
70–79 years	274	0.676	0.117	0.501	0.532	0.551	0.594	0.667	0.751	0.787	0.825	0.896
80 years and over	191	0.629	0.115	0.445	0.499	0.515	0.546	0.627	0.692	0.729	0.759	0.802
20 years and over, age adjusted	1928	0.799	...	...	...	...	...	...	...	...	...	...
Non-Hispanic black:												
8–11 years	202	0.730	0.108	0.573	0.596	0.617	0.650	0.727	0.798	0.834	0.863	0.888
12–15 years	226	0.909	0.140	0.702	0.740	0.768	0.808	0.903	0.985	1.051	1.100	1.164
16–19 years	206	0.964	0.136	0.730	0.776	0.819	0.865	0.971	1.051	1.112	1.146	1.179
20–29 years	136	0.962	0.151	0.711	0.757	0.804	0.848	0.951	1.061	1.119	1.158	1.226
30–39 years	140	0.908	0.140	0.689	0.722	0.748	0.800	0.896	1.005	1.057	1.095	1.133
40–49 years	160	0.917	0.148	0.689	0.746	0.768	0.809	0.899	1.001	1.067	1.106	1.179
50–59 years	134	0.839	0.135	0.644	0.666	0.685	0.727	0.831	0.935	0.998	1.017	†
60–69 years	141	0.805	0.156	0.575	0.617	0.637	0.697	0.790	0.882	0.960	1.012	†
70–79 years	66	*0.761	0.136	*0.543	*0.571	*0.629	*0.659	*0.748	*0.841	*0.929	*0.958	†
80 years and over	31	*0.676	0.149	†	*0.479	*0.496	*0.520	*0.675	*0.787	†	†	†
20 years and over, age adjusted	808	0.876	...	...	...	...	...	...	...	...	...	...

... Category not applicable.

*Figure does not meet standards of reliability or precision; relative standard error (standard error/estimate) is 30%–39% or estimate is based on less than 12 degrees of freedom.

†Standard error not calculated by SUDAAN.

TABLE 3	Trochanter bone mineral density (gm/cm²) of persons aged 8 years and over, by sex, race and ethnicity, and age: United States, 2005–2008

Sex, race and ethnicity, and age	Sample size	Mean	Standard deviation	Percentile								
				5th	10th	15th	25th	50th	75th	85th	90th	95th
Male												
All race and ethnicity:												
8–11 years	704	0.585	0.081	0.464	0.490	0.506	0.528	0.581	0.629	0.662	0.692	0.735
12–15 years	778	0.740	0.134	0.538	0.569	0.598	0.647	0.731	0.824	0.885	0.916	0.991
16–19 years	762	0.845	0.136	0.622	0.679	0.708	0.741	0.841	0.942	0.990	1.030	1.078
20–29 years	722	0.811	0.117	0.636	0.669	0.698	0.724	0.804	0.882	0.931	0.969	1.008
30–39 years	736	0.780	0.115	0.601	0.637	0.657	0.696	0.773	0.854	0.896	0.926	0.980
40–49 years	721	0.791	0.114	0.614	0.640	0.665	0.711	0.789	0.863	0.909	0.933	0.972
50–59 years	670	0.777	0.128	0.574	0.613	0.643	0.685	0.775	0.859	0.913	0.938	0.999
60–69 years	689	0.772	0.126	0.569	0.619	0.643	0.683	0.765	0.857	0.901	0.932	0.986
70–79 years	487	0.751	0.133	0.534	0.583	0.625	0.670	0.742	0.825	0.882	0.914	0.977
80 years and over	265	0.725	0.143	0.523	0.563	0.584	0.620	0.703	0.804	0.877	0.932	0.984
20 years and over, age adjusted ...	4290	0.782	...	...	...	...	...	...	...	...	...	...
Mexican American:												
8–11 years	206	0.581	0.078	0.467	0.489	0.503	0.525	0.574	0.621	0.658	0.684	0.728
12–15 years	232	0.748	0.134	0.545	0.574	0.605	0.647	0.734	0.833	0.896	0.926	0.966
16–19 years	212	0.815	0.128	0.613	0.670	0.692	0.723	0.802	0.900	0.964	0.997	1.048
20–29 years	200	0.797	0.099	0.649	0.675	0.695	0.722	0.794	0.856	0.893	0.915	0.957
30–39 years	153	0.778	0.093	0.617	0.659	0.687	0.707	0.774	0.847	0.875	0.895	0.936
40–49 years	154	0.764	0.104	0.598	0.624	0.660	0.694	0.761	0.828	0.860	0.884	0.929
50–59 years	111	0.746	0.125	0.561	0.574	0.604	0.661	0.733	0.830	0.880	0.896	0.934
60–69 years	118	0.754	0.120	0.581	0.610	0.636	0.667	0.745	0.816	0.856	0.918	0.956
70–79 years	47	*0.714	0.112	†	*0.575	*0.595	*0.642	*0.708	*0.780	*0.825	*0.888	†
80 years and over	14	*0.671	0.121	†	†	†	*0.564	*0.626	*0.719	*0.782	†	†
20 years and over, age adjusted ...	797	0.761	...	...	...	...	...	...	...	...	...	...
Non-Hispanic white:												
8–11 years	205	0.580	0.078	0.463	0.481	0.493	0.522	0.579	0.624	0.656	0.679	0.727
12–15 years	218	0.735	0.133	0.536	0.559	0.590	0.641	0.729	0.820	0.872	0.913	0.982
16–19 years	223	0.835	0.131	0.615	0.672	0.693	0.737	0.838	0.919	0.974	0.994	1.053
20–29 years	285	0.804	0.111	0.625	0.669	0.700	0.719	0.795	0.875	0.924	0.958	1.003
30–39 years	337	0.775	0.115	0.591	0.637	0.656	0.694	0.765	0.843	0.882	0.918	0.972
40–49 years	329	0.790	0.113	0.614	0.637	0.662	0.710	0.790	0.858	0.908	0.932	0.972
50–59 years	341	0.776	0.126	0.576	0.614	0.642	0.686	0.777	0.855	0.912	0.933	0.989
60–69 years	309	0.774	0.122	0.579	0.627	0.648	0.683	0.764	0.859	0.901	0.927	0.985
70–79 years	330	0.750	0.134	0.533	0.582	0.622	0.670	0.741	0.822	0.878	0.902	0.973
80 years and over	214	0.727	0.146	0.523	0.564	0.583	0.625	0.704	0.806	0.885	0.938	0.988
20 years and over, age adjusted ...	2145	0.779	...	...	...	...	...	...	...	...	...	...
Non-Hispanic black:												
8–11 years	197	0.629	0.084	0.509	0.527	0.552	0.572	0.621	0.669	0.707	0.722	0.763
12–15 years	227	0.770	0.137	0.560	0.617	0.635	0.674	0.749	0.838	0.914	0.972	1.030
16–19 years	251	0.906	0.151	0.679	0.714	0.734	0.791	0.892	1.016	1.077	1.105	1.170
20–29 years	160	0.865	0.141	0.662	0.694	0.731	0.783	0.840	0.941	0.997	1.058	1.134
30–39 years	145	0.845	0.121	0.668	0.694	0.722	0.762	0.848	0.916	0.964	1.009	1.051
40–49 years	151	0.819	0.130	0.634	0.667	0.688	0.720	0.816	0.890	0.926	0.963	1.074
50–59 years	126	0.841	0.141	0.608	0.671	0.703	0.761	0.830	0.918	0.980	1.024	1.064
60–69 years	185	0.808	0.148	0.570	0.617	0.644	0.699	0.812	0.893	0.946	1.001	1.065
70–79 years	75	*0.803	0.140	*0.555	*0.649	*0.662	*0.690	*0.780	*0.915	*0.969	*0.989	*1.026
80 years and over	22	*0.731	0.126	†	*0.573	*0.593	*0.621	*0.713	*0.800	*0.877	†	†
20 years and over, age adjusted ...	864	0.830	...	...	...	...	...	...	...	...	...	...
Female												
All race and ethnicity:												
8–11 years	741	0.555	0.095	0.424	0.443	0.468	0.489	0.537	0.612	0.653	0.685	0.734
12–15 years	715	0.713	0.120	0.535	0.566	0.589	0.626	0.705	0.789	0.836	0.865	0.916
16–19 years	673	0.742	0.112	0.562	0.593	0.617	0.662	0.739	0.820	0.858	0.881	0.930
20–29 years	635	0.724	0.108	0.558	0.597	0.617	0.649	0.708	0.800	0.836	0.864	0.908
30–39 years	639	0.714	0.109	0.536	0.577	0.600	0.637	0.715	0.778	0.819	0.852	0.906
40–49 years	750	0.719	0.114	0.550	0.577	0.607	0.641	0.708	0.793	0.826	0.861	0.915
50–59 years	595	0.671	0.115	0.506	0.536	0.558	0.589	0.663	0.734	0.776	0.817	0.874
60–69 years	633	0.645	0.110	0.471	0.506	0.535	0.563	0.637	0.712	0.754	0.786	0.846
70–79 years	425	0.605	0.119	0.418	0.463	0.491	0.522	0.594	0.674	0.711	0.756	0.811
80 years and over	253	0.567	0.110	0.394	0.433	0.442	0.491	0.562	0.641	0.681	0.708	0.758
20 years and over, age adjusted ...	3930	0.687	...	...	...	...	...	...	...	...	...	...

See footnotes at end of table.

TABLE 3	Trochanter bone mineral density (gm/cm²) of persons aged 8 years and over, by sex, race and ethnicity, and age: United States, 2005–2008—Con.

Sex, race and ethnicity, and age	Sample size	Mean	Standard deviation	Percentile								
				5th	10th	15th	25th	50th	75th	85th	90th	95th
Female—Con.												
Mexican American:												
8–11 years	234	0.565	0.095	0.427	0.461	0.475	0.503	0.550	0.619	0.663	0.698	0.738
12–15 years	227	0.698	0.105	0.545	0.565	0.580	0.619	0.692	0.772	0.799	0.818	0.884
16–19 years	186	0.708	0.108	0.552	0.579	0.602	0.634	0.701	0.769	0.803	0.819	0.859
20–29 years	148	0.704	0.110	0.544	0.572	0.587	0.623	0.682	0.779	0.818	0.846	0.902
30–39 years	137	0.709	0.100	0.536	0.574	0.592	0.634	0.697	0.777	0.809	0.832	0.883
40–49 years	133	0.721	0.113	0.541	0.581	0.607	0.641	0.708	0.784	0.825	0.856	0.914
50–59 years	97	*0.684	0.157	*0.489	*0.542	*0.566	*0.583	*0.657	*0.757	*0.789	*0.803	*0.849
60–69 years	130	*0.630	0.105	*0.444	*0.476	*0.522	*0.564	*0.627	*0.692	*0.738	*0.755	*0.778
70–79 years	49	*0.561	0.117	†	*0.405	*0.445	*0.469	*0.552	*0.643	*0.679	*0.714	†
80 years and over	12	*0.539	0.133	†	†	†	†	*0.497	†	†	†	†
20 years and over, age adjusted	706	0.678	...	...	...	...	...	......	...	...	...	...
Non-Hispanic white:												
8–11 years	199	0.544	0.089	0.431	0.441	0.461	0.487	0.525	0.597	0.634	0.661	0.705
12–15 years	185	0.712	0.119	0.535	0.562	0.589	0.629	0.706	0.778	0.832	0.860	0.902
16–19 years	198	0.745	0.109	0.562	0.597	0.623	0.666	0.744	0.820	0.866	0.881	0.926
20–29 years	262	0.725	0.102	0.558	0.604	0.627	0.653	0.711	0.804	0.836	0.848	0.903
30–39 years	267	0.713	0.107	0.538	0.577	0.599	0.637	0.716	0.776	0.812	0.847	0.899
40–49 years	357	0.716	0.114	0.548	0.574	0.604	0.635	0.705	0.793	0.823	0.845	0.908
50–59 years	291	0.668	0.112	0.507	0.537	0.557	0.586	0.663	0.728	0.767	0.813	0.875
60–69 years	286	0.644	0.105	0.473	0.509	0.536	0.563	0.641	0.710	0.747	0.776	0.834
70–79 years	274	0.606	0.121	0.416	0.463	0.492	0.523	0.596	0.675	0.711	0.759	0.808
80 years and over	191	0.568	0.105	0.401	0.436	0.450	0.496	0.564	0.637	0.672	0.692	0.743
20 years and over, age adjusted	1928	0.686	...	...	...	...	...	...	...	...	...	...
Non-Hispanic black:												
8–11 years	202	0.608	0.098	0.472	0.497	0.512	0.530	0.603	0.669	0.714	0.744	0.780
12–15 years	226	0.763	0.118	0.573	0.604	0.645	0.676	0.761	0.834	0.891	0.920	0.972
16–19 years	206	0.786	0.112	0.592	0.631	0.671	0.704	0.784	0.869	0.919	0.945	0.969
20–29 years	136	0.762	0.120	0.572	0.607	0.637	0.669	0.755	0.834	0.892	0.908	0.975
30–39 years	140	0.749	0.112	0.584	0.603	0.620	0.664	0.749	0.812	0.866	0.897	0.948
40–49 years	160	0.756	0.122	0.561	0.592	0.618	0.668	0.752	0.838	0.890	0.916	0.946
50–59 years	134	0.707	0.120	0.522	0.560	0.589	0.615	0.696	0.769	0.836	0.871	0.938
60–69 years	141	0.686	0.147	0.452	0.514	0.537	0.588	0.688	0.784	0.838	0.864	0.946
70–79 years	66	*0.637	0.118	*0.433	*0.497	*0.515	*0.545	*0.627	*0.711	*0.748	*0.782	†
80 years and over	31	*0.547	0.132	†	†	*0.414	*0.432	*0.529	*0.660	*0.696	*0.740	†
20 years and over, age adjusted	808	0.721	...	...	...	...	...	...	...	...	...	...

... Category not applicable.

*Figure does not meet standards of reliability or precision; relative standard error (standard error/estimate) is 30%–39% or estimate is based on less than 12 degrees of freedom.

†Standard error not calculated by SUDAAN.

| TABLE 4 | Intertrochanter bone mineral density (gm/cm²) of persons aged 8 years and over, by sex, race and ethnicity, and age: United States, 2005–2008 |

Sex, race and ethnicity, and age	Sample size	Mean	Standard deviation	Percentile 5th	10th	15th	25th	50th	75th	85th	90th	95th
Male												
All race and ethnicity:												
8–11 years	704	0.830	0.117	0.647	0.680	0.715	0.747	0.824	0.900	0.941	0.973	1.044
12–15 years	778	1.044	0.176	0.761	0.816	0.865	0.919	1.031	1.165	1.236	1.278	1.344
16–19 years	762	1.251	0.163	0.987	1.044	1.092	1.146	1.238	1.357	1.422	1.470	1.522
20–29 years	722	1.267	0.150	1.027	1.075	1.114	1.163	1.265	1.361	1.417	1.444	1.509
30–39 years	736	1.233	0.160	0.980	1.035	1.074	1.128	1.226	1.325	1.393	1.442	1.507
40–49 years	721	1.231	0.155	0.973	1.042	1.085	1.136	1.229	1.329	1.386	1.410	1.491
50–59 years	670	1.205	0.171	0.913	0.997	1.035	1.093	1.201	1.317	1.381	1.425	1.499
60–69 years	689	1.181	0.170	0.896	0.971	1.004	1.070	1.169	1.287	1.360	1.410	1.484
70–79 years	487	1.136	0.165	0.869	0.924	0.967	1.018	1.127	1.243	1.293	1.348	1.421
80 years and over	265	1.075	0.185	0.774	0.869	0.897	0.946	1.049	1.190	1.266	1.333	1.403
20 years and over, age adjusted	4290	1.214	…	…	…	…	…	…	…	…	…	…
Mexican American:												
8–11 years	206	0.818	0.107	0.658	0.678	0.702	0.739	0.813	0.887	0.927	0.960	1.002
12–15 years	232	1.057	0.183	0.748	0.806	0.865	0.931	1.053	1.180	1.261	1.285	1.364
16–19 years	212	1.225	0.164	0.973	1.028	1.060	1.108	1.208	1.319	1.410	1.461	1.512
20–29 years	200	1.266	0.138	1.048	1.098	1.126	1.168	1.255	1.357	1.411	1.422	1.473
30–39 years	153	1.264	0.135	1.055	1.099	1.124	1.162	1.256	1.360	1.398	1.434	1.512
40–49 years	154	1.224	0.150	0.992	1.033	1.057	1.113	1.226	1.318	1.372	1.435	†
50–59 years	111	1.197	0.180	0.901	0.971	1.009	1.073	1.191	1.317	1.382	1.423	1.536
60–69 years	118	1.206	0.161	†	1.024	1.035	1.094	1.195	1.315	1.357	1.398	1.474
70–79 years	47	*1.133	0.161	†	*0.928	*0.949	*1.012	*1.108	*1.205	*1.310	*1.394	†
80 years and over	14	*1.043	0.183	†	†	†	*0.883	*0.976	†	†	†	†
20 years and over, age adjusted	797	1.218	…	…	…	…	…	…	…	…	…	…
Non-Hispanic white:												
8–11 years	205	0.821	0.116	0.643	0.670	0.703	0.744	0.820	0.888	0.931	0.953	1.013
12–15 years	218	1.033	0.168	0.762	0.811	0.862	0.909	1.025	1.147	1.203	1.259	1.326
16–19 years	223	1.233	0.152	0.981	1.040	1.082	1.135	1.223	1.335	1.382	1.422	1.505
20–29 years	285	1.248	0.138	1.018	1.063	1.107	1.154	1.250	1.347	1.387	1.423	1.462
30–39 years	337	1.210	0.157	0.949	1.013	1.050	1.106	1.202	1.308	1.357	1.409	1.496
40–49 years	329	1.222	0.153	0.965	1.036	1.082	1.135	1.220	1.314	1.369	1.398	1.456
50–59 years	341	1.199	0.170	0.895	0.979	1.033	1.091	1.196	1.308	1.371	1.417	1.492
60–69 years	309	1.172	0.163	0.900	0.971	1.002	1.065	1.156	1.269	1.335	1.389	1.453
70–79 years	330	1.131	0.166	0.865	0.917	0.959	1.015	1.126	1.238	1.285	1.323	1.419
80 years and over	214	1.070	0.187	0.769	0.861	0.896	0.945	1.048	1.188	1.257	1.323	1.403
20 years and over, age adjusted	2145	1.201	…	…	…	…	…	…	…	…	…	…
Non-Hispanic black:												
8–11 years	197	0.901	0.116	0.711	0.772	0.787	0.817	0.900	0.965	1.024	1.055	1.088
12–15 years	227	1.094	0.191	0.802	0.835	0.881	0.960	1.082	1.210	1.282	1.359	1.446
16–19 years	251	1.340	0.183	1.039	1.118	1.146	1.206	1.325	1.462	1.522	1.595	1.664
20–29 years	160	1.354	0.172	1.085	1.138	1.169	1.247	1.356	1.445	1.514	1.578	1.645
30–39 years	145	1.340	0.172	1.059	1.117	1.169	1.217	1.337	1.465	1.521	1.564	1.627
40–49 years	151	1.291	0.176	0.993	1.082	1.103	1.174	1.287	1.405	1.468	1.497	1.580
50–59 years	126	1.293	0.180	1.014	1.054	1.115	1.163	1.273	1.397	1.510	1.572	1.611
60–69 years	185	1.258	0.197	0.942	1.019	1.058	1.140	1.237	1.398	1.472	1.498	1.565
70–79 years	75	*1.208	0.170	*0.959	*0.990	*1.015	*1.080	*1.206	*1.336	*1.390	*1.421	*1.448
80 years and over	22	*1.126	0.172	†	†	†	*1.018	*1.062	*1.257	†	†	†
20 years and over, age adjusted	864	1.295	…	…	…	…	…	…	…	…	…	…
Female												
All race and ethnicity:												
8–11 years	741	0.789	0.131	0.613	0.643	0.669	0.699	0.763	0.866	0.929	0.974	1.035
12–15 years	715	1.040	0.155	0.794	0.851	0.886	0.929	1.037	1.148	1.199	1.229	1.306
16–19 years	673	1.126	0.148	0.868	0.931	0.973	1.032	1.126	1.220	1.278	1.301	1.358
20–29 years	635	1.141	0.142	0.934	0.969	0.989	1.046	1.128	1.241	1.296	1.326	1.371
30–39 years	639	1.130	0.149	0.882	0.920	0.974	1.024	1.136	1.226	1.284	1.324	1.395
40–49 years	750	1.123	0.157	0.868	0.916	0.964	1.018	1.117	1.222	1.279	1.319	1.373
50–59 years	595	1.067	0.162	0.833	0.879	0.897	0.943	1.060	1.184	1.235	1.268	1.347
60–69 years	633	1.013	0.151	0.766	0.829	0.856	0.908	1.008	1.113	1.153	1.192	1.258
70–79 years	425	0.957	0.171	0.678	0.745	0.776	0.852	0.947	1.069	1.129	1.185	1.248
80 years and over	253	0.882	0.163	0.613	0.666	0.705	0.755	0.882	0.987	1.037	1.071	1.143
20 years and over, age adjusted	3930	1.083	…	…	…	…	…	…	…	…	…	…

See footnotes at end of table.

| TABLE 4 | Intertrochanter bone mineral density (gm/cm^2) of persons aged 8 years and over, by sex, race and ethnicity, and age: United States, 2005–2008—Con. |

Sex, race and ethnicity, and age	Sample size	Mean	Standard deviation	Percentile								
				5th	10th	15th	25th	50th	75th	85th	90th	95th
Female—Con.												
Mexican American:												
8–11 years	234	0.802	0.134	0.601	0.650	0.678	0.713	0.776	0.876	0.947	0.988	1.053
12–15 years	227	1.032	0.140	0.806	0.856	0.875	0.927	1.034	1.126	1.174	1.219	1.273
16–19 years	186	1.105	0.134	0.886	0.930	0.965	1.013	1.095	1.190	1.238	1.272	1.300
20–29 years	148	1.125	0.143	0.895	0.938	0.966	1.027	1.113	1.218	1.285	1.317	1.390
30–39 years	137	1.145	0.138	0.918	0.961	0.987	1.050	1.137	1.243	1.281	1.324	1.379
40–49 years	133	1.162	0.163	0.873	0.965	0.997	1.058	1.162	1.248	1.333	1.362	1.419
50–59 years	97	*1.108	0.200	*0.799	*0.865	*0.936	*0.989	*1.082	*1.197	*1.254	*1.327	*1.361
60–69 years	130	*1.024	0.155	*0.768	*0.819	*0.857	*0.925	*1.011	*1.129	*1.165	*1.216	*1.241
70–79 years	49	*0.928	0.192	†	*0.666	*0.700	*0.765	*0.929	*1.062	*1.152	*1.190	*1.211
80 years and over	12	*0.837	0.186	†	†	†	†	*0.780	*0.991	†	†	†
20 years and over, age adjusted	706	1.094	...	...	...	...	...	...	...	...	...	...
Non-Hispanic white:												
8–11 years	199	0.775	0.122	0.617	0.644	0.666	0.696	0.749	0.835	0.904	0.937	1.013
12–15 years	185	1.030	0.151	0.787	0.837	0.882	0.924	1.024	1.136	1.184	1.214	1.280
16–19 years	198	1.119	0.145	0.855	0.916	0.968	1.030	1.125	1.210	1.261	1.298	1.328
20–29 years	262	1.138	0.131	0.942	0.974	0.994	1.048	1.127	1.231	1.291	1.312	1.349
30–39 years	267	1.124	0.146	0.881	0.919	0.975	1.021	1.135	1.214	1.270	1.294	1.379
40–49 years	357	1.112	0.156	0.863	0.900	0.948	1.002	1.106	1.206	1.266	1.306	1.356
50–59 years	291	1.059	0.159	0.834	0.877	0.895	0.937	1.051	1.177	1.229	1.258	1.335
60–69 years	286	1.008	0.144	0.769	0.831	0.852	0.906	1.006	1.112	1.149	1.189	1.220
70–79 years	274	0.955	0.172	0.674	0.745	0.772	0.852	0.944	1.064	1.127	1.181	1.240
80 years and over	191	0.880	0.157	0.614	0.668	0.710	0.759	0.880	0.978	1.035	1.061	1.135
20 years and over, age adjusted	1928	1.077	...	...	...	...	...	...	...	...	...	...
Non-Hispanic black:												
8–11 years	202	0.866	0.135	0.647	0.699	0.729	0.765	0.860	0.960	1.004	1.047	1.108
12–15 years	226	1.116	0.160	0.860	0.910	0.942	1.008	1.111	1.221	1.277	1.338	1.380
16–19 years	206	1.200	0.146	0.969	0.999	1.046	1.102	1.187	1.298	1.353	1.396	1.440
20–29 years	136	1.210	0.171	0.937	0.992	1.038	1.096	1.202	1.322	1.374	1.431	1.510
30–39 years	140	1.189	0.147	0.944	0.998	1.032	1.087	1.179	1.272	1.353	1.397	1.446
40–49 years	160	1.188	0.167	0.910	0.960	1.002	1.075	1.186	1.288	1.344	1.379	1.415
50–59 years	134	1.124	0.163	0.870	0.919	0.942	0.993	1.133	1.234	1.286	1.333	1.364
60–69 years	141	1.076	0.200	0.721	0.827	0.891	0.950	1.049	1.200	1.272	1.327	†
70–79 years	66	*1.010	0.160	†	*0.797	*0.844	*0.908	*1.006	*1.098	*1.187	*1.211	†
80 years and over	31	*0.878	0.230	†	*0.598	*0.627	*0.697	*0.857	*1.013	†	†	†
20 years and over, age adjusted	808	1.141	...	...	...	...	...	...	...	...	...	...

... Category not applicable.

†Standard error not calculated by SUDAAN.

*Figure does not meet standards of reliability or precision; relative standard error (standard error/estimate) is 30%–39% or estimate is based on less than 12 degrees of freedom.

TABLE 5	Ward's triangle bone mineral density (gm/cm²) of persons aged 8 years and over, by sex, race and ethnicity, and age: United States, 2005–2008

Sex, race and ethnicity, and age	Sample size	Mean	Standard deviation	Percentile								
				5th	10th	15th	25th	50th	75th	85th	90th	95th
Male												
All race and ethnicity:												
8–11 years	704	0.689	0.117	0.517	0.543	0.572	0.608	0.674	0.765	0.810	0.842	0.899
12–15 years	778	0.826	0.158	0.589	0.622	0.655	0.712	0.811	0.924	0.995	1.022	1.100
16–19 years	762	0.941	0.175	0.672	0.714	0.757	0.824	0.925	1.042	1.112	1.175	1.262
20–29 years	722	0.874	0.159	0.651	0.681	0.717	0.769	0.854	0.970	1.035	1.090	1.157
30–39 years	736	0.764	0.158	0.534	0.574	0.599	0.647	0.753	0.868	0.922	0.962	1.006
40–49 years	721	0.693	0.146	0.483	0.527	0.546	0.594	0.683	0.774	0.842	0.880	0.947
50–59 years	670	0.634	0.146	0.412	0.458	0.490	0.531	0.624	0.715	0.785	0.832	0.902
60–69 years	689	0.574	0.149	0.363	0.401	0.419	0.461	0.562	0.658	0.720	0.782	0.844
70–79 years	487	0.524	0.148	0.329	0.358	0.388	0.422	0.508	0.590	0.665	0.715	0.803
80 years and over	265	0.477	0.149	0.252	0.310	0.343	0.375	0.452	0.560	0.616	0.673	0.726
20 years and over, age adjusted	4290	0.696	…	…	…	…	…	…	…	…	…	…
Mexican American:												
8–11 years	206	0.683	0.111	0.504	0.529	0.552	0.602	0.683	0.760	0.809	0.828	0.863
12–15 years	232	0.849	0.174	0.589	0.627	0.677	0.733	0.832	0.958	1.018	1.091	1.148
16–19 years	212	0.931	0.161	0.697	0.735	0.759	0.814	0.927	1.036	1.098	1.175	1.224
20–29 years	200	0.876	0.134	0.671	0.705	0.741	0.776	0.860	0.969	1.013	1.042	1.112
30–39 years	153	0.787	0.144	0.556	0.603	0.639	0.682	0.785	0.871	0.937	0.977	1.033
40–49 years	154	0.702	0.132	0.491	0.541	0.568	0.604	0.701	0.798	0.826	0.859	0.916
50–59 years	111	0.621	0.144	0.411	0.442	0.476	0.523	0.604	0.711	0.792	0.822	0.877
60–69 years	118	0.607	0.138	0.434	0.465	0.474	0.502	0.575	0.692	0.731	0.759	0.829
70–79 years	47	*0.516	0.117	†	*0.403	*0.414	*0.422	*0.492	*0.572	*0.647	*0.693	†
80 years and over	14	*0.422	0.130	†	†	†	*0.311	*0.394	*0.484	*0.527	†	†
20 years and over, age adjusted	797	0.701	…	…	…	…	…	…	…	…	…	…
Non-Hispanic white:												
8–11 years	205	0.684	0.112	0.509	0.544	0.571	0.607	0.666	0.763	0.796	0.834	0.886
12–15 years	218	0.816	0.146	0.594	0.622	0.651	0.711	0.802	0.912	0.975	1.015	1.071
16–19 years	223	0.928	0.172	0.670	0.710	0.745	0.821	0.907	1.025	1.090	1.138	1.214
20–29 years	285	0.859	0.152	0.624	0.676	0.705	0.758	0.839	0.958	1.032	1.061	1.116
30–39 years	337	0.741	0.148	0.526	0.558	0.587	0.629	0.722	0.848	0.902	0.937	0.990
40–49 years	329	0.684	0.146	0.464	0.522	0.541	0.583	0.676	0.768	0.837	0.874	0.936
50–59 years	341	0.629	0.139	0.412	0.460	0.490	0.530	0.623	0.709	0.765	0.811	0.864
60–69 years	309	0.564	0.145	0.357	0.396	0.417	0.454	0.545	0.648	0.711	0.755	0.838
70–79 years	330	0.518	0.149	0.313	0.350	0.381	0.416	0.500	0.578	0.651	0.697	0.799
80 years and over	214	0.476	0.150	0.240	0.310	0.344	0.375	0.452	0.552	0.612	0.674	0.727
20 years and over, age adjusted	2145	0.684	…	…	…	…	…	…	…	…	…	…
Non-Hispanic black:												
8–11 years	197	0.752	0.130	0.563	0.585	0.618	0.658	0.746	0.838	0.884	0.931	0.967
12–15 years	227	0.856	0.171	0.554	0.630	0.694	0.737	0.851	0.961	1.010	1.054	1.145
16–19 years	251	1.001	0.184	0.713	0.767	0.797	0.870	0.989	1.119	1.199	1.261	1.326
20–29 years	160	0.952	0.190	0.681	0.720	0.775	0.827	0.932	1.074	1.148	1.218	1.274
30–39 years	145	0.858	0.188	0.577	0.652	0.697	0.730	0.844	0.948	1.046	1.105	1.190
40–49 years	151	0.752	0.171	0.508	0.556	0.575	0.620	0.733	0.860	0.936	0.989	1.046
50–59 years	126	0.708	0.183	0.450	0.495	0.530	0.577	0.690	0.821	0.910	0.943	1.053
60–69 years	185	0.660	0.182	0.415	0.444	0.469	0.526	0.627	0.777	0.864	0.904	0.981
70–79 years	75	*0.605	0.144	*0.379	*0.413	*0.480	*0.509	*0.593	*0.677	*0.752	*0.781	*0.863
80 years and over	22	*0.515	0.155	†	†	*0.368	*0.424	*0.452	*0.590	†	†	†
20 years and over, age adjusted	864	0.772	…	…	…	…	…	…	…	…	…	…
Female												
All race and ethnicity:												
8–11 years	741	0.627	0.124	0.461	0.487	0.509	0.538	0.607	0.699	0.755	0.794	0.870
12–15 years	715	0.830	0.159	0.594	0.635	0.669	0.719	0.823	0.921	0.994	1.028	1.111
16–19 years	673	0.871	0.150	0.637	0.678	0.701	0.765	0.863	0.965	1.029	1.076	1.136
20–29 years	635	0.839	0.149	0.612	0.659	0.696	0.741	0.831	0.927	0.986	1.030	1.107
30–39 years	639	0.767	0.143	0.546	0.590	0.623	0.666	0.754	0.857	0.918	0.959	1.007
40–49 years	750	0.706	0.150	0.487	0.525	0.557	0.595	0.697	0.793	0.857	0.908	0.968
50–59 years	595	0.617	0.151	0.402	0.443	0.471	0.513	0.605	0.699	0.776	0.820	0.902
60–69 years	633	0.541	0.139	0.355	0.384	0.405	0.449	0.519	0.616	0.677	0.732	0.807
70–79 years	425	0.484	0.134	0.294	0.332	0.355	0.394	0.455	0.565	0.614	0.654	0.743
80 years and over	253	0.426	0.133	0.230	0.282	0.309	0.341	0.403	0.495	0.532	0.591	0.676
20 years and over, age adjusted	3930	0.681	…	…	…	…	…	…	…	…	…	…

See footnotes at end of table.

				Percentile								

TABLE 5 | Ward's triangle bone mineral density (gm/cm^2) of persons aged 8 years and over, by sex, race and ethnicity, and age: United States, 2005–2008—Con.

Sex, race and ethnicity, and age	Sample size	Mean	Standard deviation	5th	10th	15th	25th	50th	75th	85th	90th	95th
Female—Con.												
Mexican American:												
8–11 years	234	0.642	0.127	0.471	0.490	0.515	0.546	0.629	0.717	0.773	0.810	0.874
12–15 years	227	0.834	0.157	0.600	0.627	0.662	0.708	0.843	0.932	0.999	1.038	1.101
16–19 years	186	0.854	0.141	0.643	0.683	0.700	0.761	0.838	0.944	1.002	1.026	1.089
20–29 years	148	0.825	0.143	0.614	0.639	0.677	0.716	0.813	0.910	0.962	1.013	1.073
30–39 years	137	0.789	0.125	0.580	0.630	0.657	0.702	0.775	0.880	0.938	0.963	†
40–49 years	133	0.741	0.147	0.515	0.563	0.581	0.652	0.727	0.829	0.871	0.908	0.982
50–59 years	97	*0.647	0.176	*0.416	*0.478	*0.496	*0.530	*0.617	*0.737	*0.809	*0.831	*0.900
60–69 years	130	*0.542	0.128	*0.330	*0.380	*0.416	*0.458	*0.541	*0.610	*0.655	*0.677	*0.740
70–79 years	49	*0.460	0.129	†	*0.277	*0.285	*0.351	*0.451	*0.559	*0.583	*0.598	†
80 years and over	12	*0.394	0.130	†	†	†	†	*0.352	†	†	†	†
20 years and over, age adjusted	706	0.692	...	...	...	...	...	...	...	...	...	...
Non-Hispanic white:												
8–11 years	199	0.615	0.118	0.436	0.485	0.506	0.537	0.595	0.683	0.731	0.776	0.853
12–15 years	185	0.826	0.158	0.592	0.634	0.666	0.722	0.821	0.904	0.969	1.006	1.111
16–19 years	198	0.864	0.143	0.634	0.677	0.700	0.764	0.861	0.944	1.017	1.064	1.105
20–29 years	262	0.834	0.137	0.611	0.670	0.704	0.746	0.828	0.914	0.966	1.004	1.040
30–39 years	267	0.759	0.141	0.534	0.592	0.618	0.658	0.748	0.844	0.895	0.948	1.005
40–49 years	357	0.695	0.148	0.483	0.517	0.548	0.585	0.684	0.787	0.843	0.894	0.957
50–59 years	291	0.609	0.148	0.392	0.438	0.465	0.511	0.592	0.688	0.757	0.807	0.893
60–69 years	286	0.536	0.130	0.355	0.386	0.408	0.445	0.512	0.615	0.671	0.725	0.797
70–79 years	274	0.483	0.133	0.297	0.338	0.365	0.394	0.453	0.564	0.609	0.652	0.745
80 years and over	191	0.425	0.126	0.235	0.292	0.310	0.341	0.402	0.492	0.523	0.588	0.675
20 years and over, age adjusted	1928	0.674	...	...	...	...	...	...	...	...	...	...
Non-Hispanic black:												
8–11 years	202	0.688	0.129	0.496	0.525	0.555	0.586	0.685	0.766	0.831	0.858	0.905
12–15 years	226	0.878	0.164	0.644	0.681	0.711	0.756	0.859	0.981	1.035	1.081	1.161
16–19 years	206	0.932	0.165	0.662	0.716	0.752	0.815	0.909	1.041	1.124	1.159	1.217
20–29 years	136	0.905	0.186	0.589	0.648	0.718	0.779	0.88	1.044	1.1	1.128	1.24
30–39 years	140	0.81	0.16	0.562	0.578	0.655	0.698	0.801	0.92	0.99	1.042	1.089
40–49 years	160	0.765	0.162	0.524	0.562	0.599	0.643	0.751	0.883	0.945	0.985	1.032
50–59 years	134	0.669	0.166	0.43	0.473	0.49	0.53	0.647	0.769	0.847	0.905	0.94
60–69 years	141	0.601	0.195	0.35	0.379	0.414	0.468	0.571	0.683	0.788	0.822	†
70–79 years	66	*0.517	0.149	*0.278	*0.305	*0.364	*0.412	*0.498	*0.609	*0.655	*0.696	†
80 years and over	31	*0.433	0.183	†	†	*0.249	*0.341	*0.406	*0.514	†	†	†
20 years and over, age adjusted	808	0.732	...	...	...	...	...	...	...	...	...	...

... Category not applicable.

*Figure does not meet standards of reliability or precision; relative standard error (standard error/estimate) is 30%–39% or estimate is based on less than 12 degrees of freedom.

†Standard error not calculated by SUDAAN.

Reference Data and Trends in Serum Total Cholesterol and High Blood Cholesterol Percentages, U.S. Adults

Source: National Center for Health Statistics. 2016. *Health, United States, 2015: With special feature on racial and ethnic health disparities.* Hyattsville, MD: National Center for Health Statistics.

Note: Similar detailed and current tables for HDL-C, LDL-C, and triglycerides have not been released by the NCHS. However, trend data for mean lipid and lipoprotein values are available in these publications (with graphs included in this appendix):

1. Rosinger A, Carroll MD, Lacher D, Ogden C. 2017. Trends in total cholesterol, triglycerides, and low-density lipoprotein in US adults, 1999–2014. *Journal of the American Medical Association Cardiology* 2:339–341.
2. Carroll MD, Kit BK, Lacher DA, Shero ST, Mussolino ME. 2012. Trends in lipids and lipoproteins in US adults, 1988–2010. *Journal of the American Medical Association* 308:1545–1554.
3. Kit BK, Carroll MD, Lacher DA, Sorlie PD, DeJesus JM, Ogden C. 2012. Trends in serum lipids among US youths aged 6 to 19 years, 1988–2010. *Journal of the American Medical Association* 308:591–600.

TABLE 1	Cholesterol among adults aged 20 and over, by selected characteristics: United States, selected years 1988–1994 through 2011–2014

[Data are based on interviews and laboratory data of a sample of the civilian noninstitutionalized population]

Sex, age, race and Hispanic origin[1], and percent of poverty level	1988–1994	1999–2002	2003–2006	2007–2010	2011–2014
20 years and over, age-adjusted[2]	Percent of population with hypercholesterolemia (serum total cholesterol greater than or equal to 240 mg/dL or taking cholesterol-lowering medications)[3]				
Both sexes[4]	22.8	25.0	27.7	27.4	27.8
Male	21.1	25.3	27.7	28.0	28.4
Female	24.0	24.3	27.4	26.7	27.3
Not Hispanic or Latino:					
White only	22.9	25.8	28.5	27.8	28.7
White only, male	21.1	26.0	28.7	28.1	29.4
White only, female	24.2	25.1	28.2	27.4	28.0
Black or African American only	21.3	21.3	23.2	25.6	25.2
Black or African American only, male	18.6	20.1	22.8	25.4	24.5
Black or African American only, female	23.1	22.0	23.3	25.6	25.7
Asian only	---	---	---	---	26.0
Asian only, male	---	---	---	---	27.4
Asian only, female	---	---	---	---	24.6
Hispanic or Latino	---	---	---	27.3	26.3
Hispanic or Latino, male	---	---	---	29.1	26.6
Hispanic or Latina, female	---	---	---	25.2	25.8
Mexican origin	20.0	20.6	24.2	27.4	24.8
Mexican origin, male	19.9	21.6	24.2	28.6	26.6
Mexican origin, female	19.8	19.3	24.1	25.5	22.7
Percent of poverty level:[5]					
Below 100%	23.0	25.0	27.9	26.5	29.2
100%–199%	22.1	25.9	27.6	27.6	25.4
200%–399%	23.1	26.5	27.5	28.9	29.0
400% or more	21.7	23.1	27.9	26.6	28.1
20 years and over, crude					
Both sexes[4]	21.5	25.0	28.0	28.7	29.8
Male	19.6	25.1	27.5	28.7	29.5
Female	23.2	24.8	28.5	28.7	30.1
Not Hispanic or Latino:					
White only	22.3	26.9	30.3	30.9	33.1
White only, male	20.0	26.8	29.7	30.4	32.6
White only, female	24.5	27.0	30.8	31.4	33.5
Black or African American only	18.1	19.3	21.7	24.4	24.8
Black or African American only, male	16.0	18.5	21.3	24.1	24.0
Black or African American only, female	19.7	19.9	21.9	24.7	25.4
Asian only	---	---	---	---	24.7
Asian only, male	---	---	---	---	25.9
Asian only, female	---	---	---	---	23.7
Hispanic or Latino	---	---	---	22.3	21.2
Hispanic or Latino, male	---	---	---	23.7	21.3
Hispanic or Latina, female	---	---	---	20.7	21.1
Mexican origin	15.6	15.5	19.0	22.4	19.1
Mexican origin, male	16.2	17.0	19.3	23.7	21.2
Mexican origin, female	14.9	13.8	18.7	21.0	16.8
Percent of poverty level:[5]					
Below 100%	19.4	21.6	24.1	22.3	25.3
100%–199%	21.3	25.4	28.3	28.7	27.4
200%–399%	21.3	26.2	28.1	30.6	31.6
400% or more	21.9	24.2	28.7	29.6	32.2
Male					
20–44 years	13.1	16.1	16.5	14.3	12.3
20–34 years	8.2	10.4	10.2	8.5	6.7
35–44 years	21.0	23.1	25.2	22.5	21.1
45–64 years	30.1	36.0	35.7	39.0	39.3
45–54 years	29.6	34.1	32.4	34.0	32.9
55–64 years	30.8	39.1	41.6	46.2	46.0
65–74 years	27.4	36.3	49.4	48.9	55.8
75 years and over	24.4	29.0	37.1	45.2	54.4

See footnotes at end of table.

TABLE 1	Cholesterol among adults aged 20 and over, by selected characteristics: United States, selected years 1988–1994 through 2011–2014—Con.

Sex, age, race and Hispanic origin[1], and percent of poverty level	1988–1994	1999–2002	2003–2006	2007–2010	2011–2014
Female	Percent of population with hypercholesterolemia (serum total cholesterol greater than or equal to 240 mg/dL or taking cholesterol-lowering medications)[3]				
20–44 years	9.9	11.4	12.9	10.6	9.0
20–34 years	7.3	9.1	10.8	6.8	6.1
35–44 years	13.5	14.4	15.8	15.7	13.2
45–64 years	36.4	31.7	37.3	39.1	40.6
45–54 years	28.2	27.2	29.6	29.1	31.2
55–64 years	45.8	39.2	49.2	51.4	51.2
65–74 years	46.9	51.9	55.3	53.3	58.1
75 years and over	41.2	44.0	47.3	52.5	59.1
20 years and over, age-adjusted[2]	Percent of population with high cholesterol (serum total cholesterol greater than or equal to 240 mg/dL)[6]				
Both sexes[4]	20.8	17.3	16.3	13.7	11.9
Male	19.0	16.4	15.1	12.6	10.8
Female	22.0	17.8	17.1	14.4	12.7
Not Hispanic or Latino:					
White only	20.8	17.5	16.9	13.9	12.4
White only, male	18.8	16.5	15.5	12.2	11.2
White only, female	22.2	18.1	18.0	15.3	13.3
Black or African American only	19.5	15.5	12.2	11.3	8.6
Black or African American only, male	16.9	12.4	10.9	10.8	7.7
Black or African American only, female	21.4	17.7	13.3	11.5	9.4
Asian only	---	---	---	---	10.9
Asian only, male	---	---	---	---	10.6
Asian only, female	---	---	---	---	11.0
Hispanic or Latino	---	---	---	14.7	13.0
Hispanic or Latino, male	---	---	---	15.5	13.1
Hispanic or Latina, female	---	---	---	13.7	12.7
Mexican origin	18.7	15.8	16.1	14.6	11.2
Mexican origin, male	18.5	17.4	17.6	15.1	12.8
Mexican origin, female	18.7	13.8	14.4	13.6	9.3
Percent of poverty level:[5]					
Below 100%	20.6	18.3	18.1	14.4	12.3
100%–199%	20.6	19.1	16.7	15.0	11.3
200%–399%	20.8	18.9	15.8	14.4	13.0
400% or more	19.5	14.4	15.9	12.3	11.5
20 years and over, crude					
Both sexes[4]	19.6	17.3	16.4	14.1	12.1
Male	17.7	16.5	15.2	12.9	10.7
Female	21.3	18.0	17.5	15.2	13.5
Not Hispanic or Latino:					
White only	20.3	18.0	17.4	14.7	12.9
White only, male	18.0	16.9	15.7	12.6	10.8
White only, female	22.5	19.1	18.9	16.7	14.9
Black or African American only	16.7	14.4	11.7	11.1	8.6
Black or African American only, male	14.7	12.2	10.8	10.9	7.4
Black or African American only, female	18.2	16.1	12.5	11.3	9.5
Asian only	---	---	---	---	10.9
Asian only, male	---	---	---	---	10.9
Asian only, female	---	---	---	---	10.9
Hispanic or Latino	---	---	---	13.5	12.1
Hispanic or Latina, male	---	---	---	14.7	12.7
Hispanic or Latina, female	---	---	---	12.2	11.6
Mexican origin	14.9	12.9	14.2	13.6	10.6
Mexican origin, male	15.4	15.0	15.7	14.7	12.3
Mexican origin, female	14.3	10.7	12.6	12.3	8.8
Percent of poverty level:[5]					
Below 100%	17.6	16.4	16.8	12.8	11.3
100%–199%	19.8	18.2	16.0	14.6	11.1
200%–399%	19.3	18.7	15.8	14.6	13.4
400% or more	19.9	15.5	17.1	13.7	12.5

See footnotes at end of table.

TABLE 1	Cholesterol among adults aged 20 and over, by selected characteristics: United States, selected years 1988–1994 through 2011–2014—Con.

Sex, age, race and Hispanic origin[1], and percent of poverty level	1988–1994	1999–2002	2003–2006	2007–2010	2011–2014
	Percent of population with high cholesterol (serum total cholesterol greater than or equal to 240 mg/dL)[6]				
Male					
20–44 years	12.5	14.2	14.1	11.1	10.0
20–34 years	8.2	9.8	9.5	7.6	6.0
35–44 years	19.4	19.7	20.5	16.2	16.2
45–64 years	27.2	22.2	19.1	17.7	13.6
45–54 years	26.6	23.6	20.8	18.7	15.7
55–64 years	28.0	19.9	16.0	16.3	11.5
65–74 years	21.9	13.7	10.9	7.5	7.6
75 years and over	20.4	10.2	9.6	6.8	*3.6
Female					
20–44 years	9.4	10.4	11.3	8.4	7.2
20–34 years	7.3	8.9	10.3	5.8	5.4
35–44 years	12.3	12.4	12.7	11.9	9.8
45–64 years	33.4	23.0	23.9	21.3	19.9
45–54 years	26.7	21.4	19.7	17.7	18.0
55–64 years	40.9	25.6	30.5	25.6	22.1
65–74 years	41.3	32.3	24.2	20.6	15.8
75 years and over	38.2	26.5	18.6	20.2	16.1
20 years and over, age-adjusted[2]	Mean serum total cholesterol level, mg/dL				
Both sexes[4]	206	203	200	196	192
Male	204	202	198	194	189
Female	207	204	202	198	195
Not Hispanic or Latino:					
White only	206	204	201	196	193
White only, male	205	202	198	193	189
White only, female	208	205	203	199	196
Black or African American only	205	199	194	192	186
Black or African American only, male	202	195	193	191	183
Black or African American only, female	207	202	195	192	189
Asian only	---	---	---	---	191
Asian only, male	---	---	---	---	189
Asian only, female	---	---	---	---	192
Hispanic or Latino	---	---	---	198	194
Hispanic or Latino, male	---	---	---	199	193
Hispanic or Latina, female	---	---	---	197	195
Mexican origin	206	202	202	198	192
Mexican origin, male	206	204	203	200	194
Mexican origin, female	206	199	200	196	191
Percent of poverty level:[5]					
Below 100%	205	201	203	196	191
100%–199%	205	204	201	198	191
200%–399%	207	205	199	196	193
400% or more	205	202	201	195	194

See footnotes at end of table.

TABLE 1	Cholesterol among adults aged 20 and over, by selected characteristics: United States, selected years 1988–1994 through 2011–2014—Con.

Sex, age, race and Hispanic origin[1], and percent of poverty level	1988–1994	1999–2002	2003–2006	2007–2010	2011–2014
20 years and over, crude	Mean serum total cholesterol level, mg/dL				
Both sexes[4]	204	203	200	197	192
Male	202	202	198	194	188
Female	206	204	202	199	196
Not Hispanic or Latino:					
White only	206	205	202	198	194
White only, male	203	203	198	193	188
White only, female	208	206	205	201	199
Black or African American only	200	197	193	191	186
Black or African American only, male	198	194	192	191	183
Black or African American only, female	201	199	194	191	189
Asian only	---	---	---	---	191
Asian only, male	---	---	---	---	190
Asian only, female	---	---	---	---	192
Hispanic or Latino	---	---	---	197	193
Hispanic or Latina, male	---	---	---	199	193
Hispanic or Latina, female	---	---	---	194	193
Mexican origin	199	197	198	198	192
Mexican origin, male	199	200	200	200	194
Mexican origin, female	198	194	196	195	189
Percent of poverty level:[5]					
Below 100%	200	198	200	194	189
100%–199%	202	202	199	197	190
200%–399%	205	204	199	197	193
400% or more	206	204	203	198	196
Male					
20–44 years	194	196	196	194	188
20–34 years	186	188	186	186	179
35–44 years	206	207	209	205	202
45–64 years	216	213	206	202	196
45–54 years	216	215	208	204	200
55–64 years	216	212	202	199	192
65–74 years	212	202	191	182	180
75 years and over	205	195	187	176	168
Female					
20–44 years	189	191	192	187	184
20–34 years	184	185	188	181	179
35–44 years	195	198	197	195	193
45–64 years	225	215	213	211	209
45–54 years	217	211	208	208	207
55–64 years	235	221	219	214	210
65–74 years	233	224	214	207	200
75 years and over	229	217	206	203	199

- - - Data not available.

[1]Persons of Hispanic and Mexican origin may be of any race. Starting with 1999 data, race-specific estimates are tabulated according to the 1997 *Revisions to the Standards for the Classification of Federal Data on Race and Ethnicity* and are not strictly comparable with estimates for earlier years. The non-Hispanic race categories shown in the table conform to the 1997 Standards. Starting with 1999 data, race-specific estimates are for persons who reported only one racial group. Prior to data year 1999, estimates were tabulated according to the 1977 Standards. Estimates for single-race categories prior to 1999 included persons who reported one race or, if they reported more than one race, identified one race as best representing their race. See Appendix II, Hispanic origin; Race.

[2]Estimates are age-adjusted to the year 2000 standard population using five age groups: 20–34 years, 35–44 years, 45–54 years, 55–64 years, and 65 years and over. Age-adjusted estimates may differ from other age-adjusted estimates based on the same data and presented elsewhere if different age groups are used in the adjustment procedure. See Appendix II, Age adjustment.

[3]Hypercholesterolemia is defined as measured serum total cholesterol greater than or equal to 240 mg/dL or reporting taking cholesterol-lowering medications. Respondents were asked, ''Are you now following this advice [from a doctor or health professional] to take prescribed medicine [to lower your cholesterol]?''

[4]Includes persons of all races and Hispanic origins, not just those shown separately.

[5]Percent of poverty level was calculated by dividing family income by the U.S. Department of Health and Human Services' poverty guideline specific to family size, as well as the appropriate year, and state. Persons with unknown percent of poverty level are excluded (6% in 2011–2014). See Appendix II, Family income; Poverty.

[6]High cholesterol is defined as serum total cholesterol greater than or equal to 240 mg/dL (6.20 mmol/L), regardless of whether the respondent reported taking cholesterol-lowering medications.

NOTES: See Appendix II, Cholesterol. Standard errors for selected years are available in the spreadsheet version of this table. Available from: http://www.cdc.gov/nchs/hus.htm. Data for additional years are available. See the Excel spreadsheet on the *Health, United States* website at: http://www.cdc.gov/nchs/hus.htm.

SOURCE: CDC/NCHS, National Health and Nutrition Examination Survey. See Appendix I, National Health and Nutrition Examination Survey (NHANES).

TRENDS IN TOTAL SERUM CHOLESTEROL, LDL-C, AND TRIGLYCERIDES, U.S. ADULTS

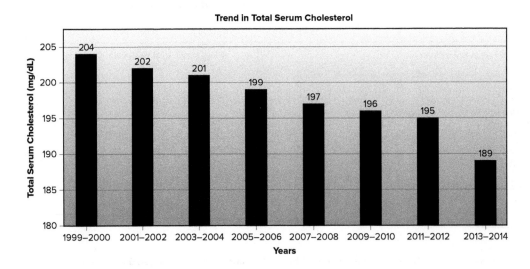

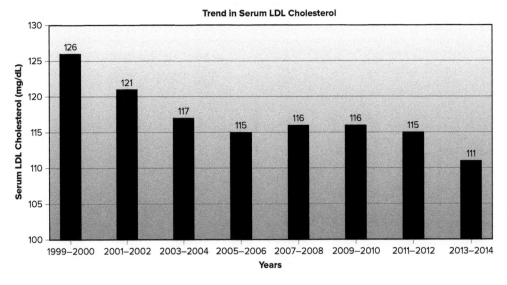

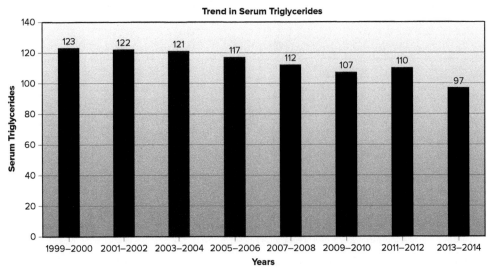

Source: Data for graphs from Rosinger A, Carroll MD, Lacher D, Ogden C. 2017. Trends in total cholesterol, triglycerides, and low-density lipoprotein in US adults, 1999–2014. *Journal of the American Medical Association Cardiology* 2:339–341.

Trends in Total Serum Cholesterol Among U.S. Children and Adolescents, Aged 6 to 19 Years, 1988–2010

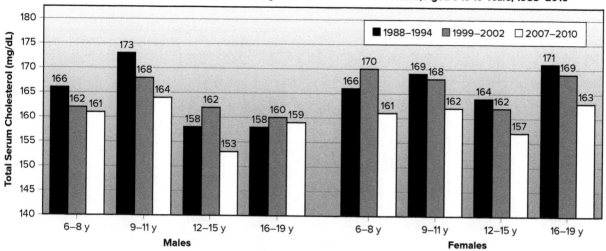

Trends in Serum HDL Cholesterol Among U.S. Children and Adolescents, Aged 6 to 19 Years, 1988–2010

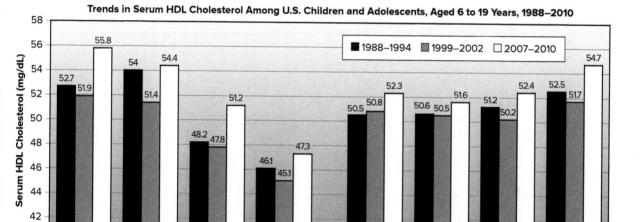

Source: Data for graphs: Kit BK, Carroll MD, Lacher DA, Sorlie PD, DeJesus JM, Ogden C. 2012. Trends in serum lipids among US youths aged 6 to 19 years, 1988–2010. *Journal of the American Medical Association* 308:591–600.

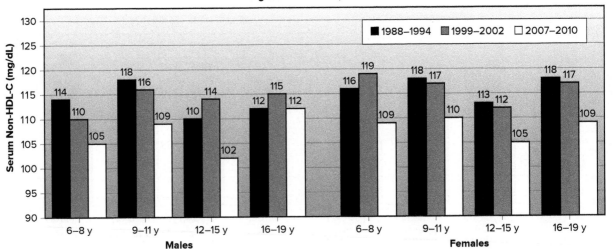

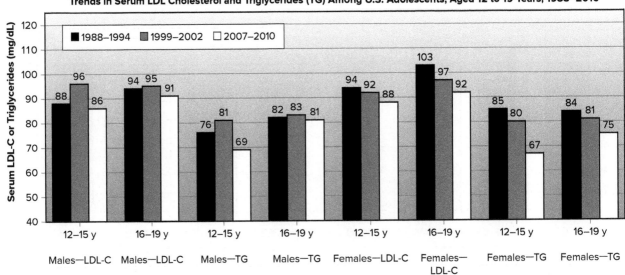

Source: Data for graphs: Kit BK, Carroll MD, Lacher DA, Sorlie PD, DeJesus JM, Ogden C. 2012. Trends in serum lipids among US youths aged 6 to 19 years, 1988–2010. *Journal of the American Medical Association* 308:591–600.

Example of a Form That Can Be Used for Self-Monitoring Eating Behavior

Food Record

Name _____ Day of week _____ Date _____

Time	Time Spent	Food Eaten—How Prepared	Amount	Place, Person(s) with Whom Food Was Eaten, Other Activities, Mood/Feelings

Remember: Do not alter your normal diet while keeping this record. For the requested information, provide responses that are as accurate as possible.

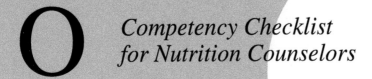

O *Competency Checklist for Nutrition Counselors*

This can be used by counselors to identify the competencies they already possess and those they want to develop.

From Raab C, and Tillotson JL. 1985. *Heart to heart: A manual on nutrition counseling for the reduction of cardiovascular disease risk factors.* Bethesda, MD: U.S. Department of Health and Human Services: Public Health Service; National Institutes of Health.

Nutrition Information for Particular Patient	Performance Objectives	Needs More Work	Not Attempted Yet	Good
1. Counselor knows the essential elements and rationale behind patient's prescribed diet (e.g., low-fat, low-sodium, etc.).	1a. Is familiar with all the food categories of the diet	_____	_____	_____
	1b. Is comfortable with substitutions and rationale for selection of food	_____	_____	_____
	1c. Is prepared to help patient adapt diet to his or her needs	_____	_____	_____
2. Counselor has knowledge of local eating patterns.	2a. Has some grasp of regional customs and of what foods are available in area	_____	_____	_____
	2b. Is familiar with frequently patronized restaurants and food chains and will ask patient his or her favorites	_____	_____	_____
3. At the outset, counselor makes reasonably sure that patient's knowledge of prescribed diet is adequate.	3a. Takes a history to find out patient's dietary background	_____	_____	_____
	3b. At first session, discusses long-term goals and explains diet thoroughly, making sure patient understands	_____	_____	_____
	3c. Eliminates patient's knowledge gaps (by discussing diet further, giving examples, using visuals, etc.) so following sessions can concentrate on goal setting	_____	_____	_____
	3d. Initially, asks patient for food diary; analyzes with patient to assess current diet and eating behavior	_____	_____	_____
Communication Skills				
4. Counselor sets appropriate tone for counseling sessions through preparation, manner, and physical setting.	4a. Makes appointment with patient, allowing enough time for comfortable, thorough discussion	_____	_____	_____
	4b. Arranges for private, quiet setting	_____	_____	_____

Nutrition Information for Particular Patient	Performance Objectives	Needs More Work	Not Attempted Yet	Good

Communication Skills—(cont'd)

	4c. Establishes patient's ability to see and to read and speak English; adapts counseling if necessary	_____	_____	_____
	4d. Shows interest in patient as an individual, looks for his or her particular needs and preferences	_____	_____	_____
	4e. Maintains relaxed, comfortable manner; makes patient feel at ease	_____	_____	_____
	4f. Indicates intentions to talk and to listen	_____	_____	_____
5. Counselor prepares self and patient for continuing relationship over a specified period.	5a. Explains initially the necessity of follow-up over time	_____	_____	_____
	5b. Outlines plans for working with patient—a certain number of sessions over a certain period of time with occasional contact by phone and mail	_____	_____	_____
6. Counselor uses principles of good communication.	6a. Uses primarily open-ended questions (rather than those answered by yes or no)	_____	_____	_____
	6b. Guards against doing most of the talking; shows ability to listen	_____	_____	_____
	6c. Is able to tolerate periods of silence	_____	_____	_____
	6d. Shows nonjudgmental, noncritical attitude toward patient's eating pattern and chosen lifestyle	_____	_____	_____
	6e. Uses words patient can understand	_____	_____	_____
7. Counselor communicates interest and confidence both nonverbally and verbally.	7a. Shows poise and interest through posture and "body language"	_____	_____	_____
	7b. Has frequent eye contact with patient	_____	_____	_____
	7c. Uses gestures and words to encourage patient to communicate freely, without putting words in patient's mouth	_____	_____	_____

Counseling Approaches

		_____	_____	_____
8. Counselor is aware that the change process is the responsibility of the patient.	8a. Does not assume responsibility for changes or consequences	_____	_____	_____
	8b. Does not become too ego-involved in patient's eventual success or failure	_____	_____	_____
9. Counselor is aware of need for patient to recognize manageable goals.	9a. Helps patient choose an initial goal that is easily achieved	_____	_____	_____
	9b. Helps patient set specific and short-term goals that are progressively more challenging	_____	_____	_____
	9c. Is able to help patient evaluate goals	_____	_____	_____
	9d. Helps patient avoid failure through too large or too many goals	_____	_____	_____
10. Counselor is able to help patient set up recordkeeping and/or tally systems.	10a. Can help patient verbalize a method appropriate to the task	_____	_____	_____
	10b. Can suggest alternate methods for patient's consideration without dictating choice	_____	_____	_____
	10c. Emphasizes need for accurate records	_____	_____	_____

continued

Nutrition Information for Particular Patient	Performance Objectives	Needs More Work	Not Attempted Yet	Good
Counseling Approaches—(cont'd)				
	10d. Is able to help patient review food records patient can understand	_____	_____	_____
11. Counselor is aware of the need to examine and anticipate obstacles that will interfere with progress.	11a. Can review with patient potential obstacles in social, personal, and physical environments	_____	_____	_____
	11b. Can help patient identify actual or potential problems and deal with these by encouraging patient to restructure environment and by role playing problem situations with him or her	_____	_____	_____
	11c. Discusses how patient will deal with possible failure	_____	_____	_____
12. Counselor is able to define own role in giving support and feedback.	12a. Can avoid taking the major responsibility	_____	_____	_____
	12b. Can place the responsibility for change on patient	_____	_____	_____
	12c. Is aware of own biases and belief systems and is able to ignore them	_____	_____	_____
13. Counselor is able to evaluate progress toward the stated goal.	13a. Is able to give patient feedback about progress	_____	_____	_____
	13b. Keeps notes in sufficient detail to depict patient's responsibilities and progress	_____	_____	_____
	13c. Measures progress by a combination of biological measures, food intake evaluation, and subjective judgments, with an emphasis on changing behavior	_____	_____	_____
14. Counselor encourages patient to get family and friends involved.	14a. Helps patient recognize their strong influence on him or her, suggests that patient ask openly for their support	_____	_____	_____
	14b. Suggests that patient ask them to participate in some way: sharing new tastes and habits, helping with food selection, limiting inappropriate foods	_____	_____	_____
	14c. Can help patient cope with negative feedback through anticipating and rehearsing problem situations	_____	_____	_____
	14d. Can evaluate whether they are potentially supportive or destructive	_____	_____	_____
	14e. Can utilize them as a support without losing sight of the primary responsibility resting with patient	_____	_____	_____
15. Counselor is able to understand that his or her role is not simply that of information-giver or instructor.	15a. Acts as facilitator for patient	_____	_____	_____
	15b. Is appropriately assertive	_____	_____	_____
	15c. Is able to resist "lecturing"	_____	_____	_____
16. Counselor is aware of the need to keep patient task-oriented.	16a. Recognizes delaying tactics and distractions	_____	_____	_____
	16b. Is able to redirect the session toward specifics	_____	_____	_____
	16c. Responds pleasantly but professionally to patient's attempts at humor	_____	_____	_____

GLOSSARY

absorptiometry A measurement approach based on the uptake of energy from radiation (e.g., photons or X rays) by the tissue or medium being measured (e.g., bone mineral content).

Acceptable Macronutrient Distribution Ranges Recommended levels of intake for total fat, n-6 polyunsaturated fatty acids (linolenic acid), n-3 polyunsaturated fatty acids (α-linolenic acid), carbohydrate, and protein to ensure adequate intake and to decrease risk of chronic disease.

accuracy The degree to which a measured value represents the real, or true, value.

acromion process The spine of the scapula (shoulder blade) extending toward the outside of the body. The acromion process, or tip, is used as an anatomic landmark in arm anthropometric measurements (e.g., midarm circumference and triceps skinfold measurement).

actuarial data Statistical information relating to life expectancy, collected by the insurance industry and used, for example, to develop height-weight charts.

Adequate Intake The recommended daily dietary intake level assumed to be adequate and based on experimentally determined approximations of nutrient intake by a group of healthy people. It is an observational standard used when there are insufficient data available to determine a Recommended Dietary Allowance. One of four nutrient reference intakes included in the Dietary Reference Intakes.

age-adjusted death rate The number of deaths in a specific age group for a given calendar year, divided by the population of the same age group as of July 1 of that year. (The quotient being multiplied by 1000.) Also known as "age-specific" death rate.

air displacement plethysmography An approach to measuring body volume that is based on the difference between the volume of air within an empty chamber of known volume and the volume of air when a subject is inside the chamber. The volume of air the subject displaces when inside the chamber is equivalent to the subject's volume, from which body density and percent body fat can then be calculated.

albumin A serum protein, produced by the liver, used as an indicator of nutritional status.

AMDR see Acceptable Macronutrient Distribution Ranges.

anabolism The process by which body cells convert simple biological substances into more complex compounds.

android obesity Excess body fat that is predominantly within the abdomen and upper body, as opposed to the hips and thighs. This is the typical pattern of male obesity.

anemia A hemoglobin level below the normal reference range for individuals of the same sex and age.

anergy A less than expected or absent immune reaction in response to the injection of antigens within the skin.

angina pectoris Chest pain caused by lack of oxygen supply (known as ischemia) within the heart muscle or myocardium.

anorexia nervosa A condition of disturbed or disordered eating behavior characterized by a refusal to maintain a minimally normal body weight, an intense fear of gaining weight (not alleviated by losing weight), and a distorted perception of body shape or size in which a person feels overweight (either globally or in certain body areas), despite being markedly underweight.

antecedent A preceding event, condition, or cause. Behaviorists regard an action as being preceded by an antecedent. Behavior modification theory holds that, when antecedents to behaviors are recognized, the antecedents can be modified or controlled to decrease the occurrence of negative behaviors and increase the occurrence of positive behaviors. This is referred to as stimulus control.

anthropometry Measurement of the body (stature, weight, circumferences, and skinfold thickness).

apoproteins Special proteins, found in lipoproteins, that control the interaction and metabolic fate of lipoproteins. Apoproteins activate enzymes that modify the composition and structure of lipoproteins, are involved in the binding and ingestion of lipoproteins by cells, and participate in the exchange of lipids between lipoproteins of different classes.

appendicular skeleton The portion of the skeleton that contains the bones of the limbs, pelvis, clavicles, and scapulae.

Archimedes' principle The fact that an object's volume, when submerged in water, equals the volume of water the object displaces. Thus, if the mass and the volume of a body are known, the density of that body can be calculated.

This principle is used to determine whole-body density in hydrostatic weighing.

arm muscle area An indicator of total body muscle calculated from the triceps skinfold thickness and midarm circumference.

arteriography A radiographic study of an artery or arterial system in which contrast medium is injected into an artery to determine the condition of the artery (e.g., narrowing due to atherosclerosis).

atherogenic Atherosclerosis-producing.

atherosclerosis A progressive disorder beginning in childhood with the appearance of lesions in the form of fatty streaks in the lining of the coronary arteries or aorta. These may eventually progress to fatty and fibrous plaques or even larger, more complicated lesions. As the lesions develop, the progressive narrowing of the vessels reduces blood flow to the tissues supplied by the affected vessels.

attenuate To decrease the amount, force, or value of something. In dual-energy X-ray absorptiometry (DXA), for example, minerals in bone oppose the transmission of X rays through bones, thus attenuating X rays. The degree to which bones attenuate (i.e., oppose the transmission of) X rays is used to determine bone mineral density in DXA.

auscultation The act of listening for sounds arising from organs (e.g., heart and lungs), typically using a stethoscope.

axial skeleton The part of the skeleton composed of the skull, vertebral column, sternum, and ribs.

balance sheet approach The most common method of estimating per capita food availability at the national level. Food exports, nonfood use (e.g., livestock feed, seed, and industrial use), and year-end inventories are subtracted from data on beginning-year inventories, total food production, and imports to arrive at an estimate of per capita food availability.

balloon angioplasty A surgical procedure in which a balloon catheter is inserted through the skin into a narrowed blood vessel and inflated to enlarge its interior opening, or lumen, in order to increase blood flow through the affected vessel.

basal metabolic rate (BMR) An individual's energy expenditure measured in the postabsorptive state (no food consumed during the previous 12 hours) after resting quietly for 30 minutes in a thermally neutral environment. (Room temperature is perceived as neither hot nor cold.)

behavior modification A behavioral change theory that attempts to alter previously learned behavior or to encourage the learning of new behavior through a variety of action-oriented methods, as opposed to changing feelings or thoughts.

Behavior Risk Factor Surveillance System An ongoing data-collection program administered by the U.S. Centers for Disease Control and Prevention to monitor state-level prevalence of the major behavioral risks associated with the leading causes of premature morbidity and mortality. It provides state-specific data on personal health behavior and disease risk factors, which allow states to better target their resources for disease risk factor intervention and health promotion activities.

beriberi A disease resulting from thiamin deficiency and characterized by nervous tingling throughout the body, poor arm-leg coordination, deep calf muscle pain, heart enlargement, and occasional edema.

bias A measure of inaccuracy or departure from accuracy.

binge eating The practice of eating an unusually large amount of food in a discrete period of time.

bioelectrical impedance The measure of resistance to an alternating current in an organism. Used to estimate total body water from which percent body fat and lean body mass can be calculated using various equations.

biological marker A nutrient, food component, or metabolite that can be objectively measured and used to represent dietary or nutrient intake.

biopsy The removal and examination of tissue samples to determine the presence or concentration of certain nutrients (or the presence or absence of disease).

BMI Body mass index. *See* Quetelet's index.

body cell mass The metabolically active, energy-requiring mass of the body.

body composition The proportions of various tissues (fat, muscle, and bone) or elements (e.g., hydrogen, potassium, carbon, calcium, nitrogen) making up the body, usually expressed as percent body fat and percent lean body mass.

body density The mass of the body per unit volume, generally measured by hydrostatic weighing. Percent body fat can then be estimated from body density using the Siri or Brozek equations.

body mass index *See* Quetelet's index.

bone mineral density The amount of mineral (primarily calcium and phosphorus) in bone per volume or per area. For example, dual-energy X-ray absorptiometry (DXA) provides an areal measurement of bone mineral density (BMD) in grams of bone mineral per cubic centimeter (g/cm^2).

bulimia nervosa An eating disorder characterized by episodes of binge eating followed by some behavior to prevent weight gain, such as purging, fasting, or exercising excessively.

bypass surgery A surgical procedure creating an auxiliary flow, a shunt, or a pathway around a diseased or malfunctioning body area to restore normal or nearly normal body function (e.g., coronary bypass, intestinal bypass).

cachexia Profound physical wasting and malnutrition usually associated with chronic disease, advanced acquired immune deficiency syndrome, alcoholism, or drug abuse.

cadaver A dead body used for anatomic, anthropometric, or other study. Only by analyzing cadavers can direct measurement of human body composition be made.

calorie count Calculation of the energy and nutrient value of foods eaten by a subject, such as a hospitalized patient.

calorimetry Measurement of a subject's energy expenditure.

cancer A group of diseases characterized by abnormal growth of cells that, when uncontrolled, invade other tissues or organs, interfering with their normal function and nutrition.

cardiovascular disease A variety of pathologic processes pertaining to the heart and blood vessels (coronary artery disease and hypertension).

case-control study Comparison of current disease status with the level of past exposure to some factor of interest (e.g., some nutrient or dietary component) in two groups of subjects (cases and controls), in an attempt to determine how past exposure to the factor relates to currently existing disease.

catabolism The breaking down of more complex compounds into simple biological substances, generally resulting in energy release.

cerebrovascular disease A group of disorders, characterized by decreased blood supply to the brain, resulting from hemorrhage of or atherosclerosis within the cerebral arteries.

CHD Coronary heart disease.

CHI Creatinine-height index.

cholesterol A fatlike sterol found in animal products and normally produced by the body. It serves as a precursor for bile acids and steroid hormones and is an essential component of the plasma membrane and the myelin sheaths of nerves. Serum cholesterol levels are causally related to risk for coronary artery disease.

chronic disease A disease progressing over a long period of time, such as coronary heart disease, certain cancers, stroke, diabetes mellitus, and atherosclerosis.

chylomicrons Lipoproteins synthesized in the small intestine that transport dietary triglycerides from the small intestine to adipose tissue, muscle, and the liver. They are 90% triglyceride by weight and are naturally found in serum shortly after meals, but they are not normally present in fasting serum.

cirrhosis Inflammation of the interstitial tissue of an organ, especially the liver.

closed questions Questions that are restrictive and allow an interviewer to control answers and ask for specific information. They are often answered by a simple yes or no response.

coding Assigning a number to each food item recorded in a 24-hour recall or food record that identifies the food for purposes of computerized nutrient analysis.

coefficient of variation (CV) A measure of precision calculated by dividing the standard deviation by the mean and multiplying by 100 ($CV = SD \div mean \times 100$).

cognitive restructuring Elimination of negative, irrational thoughts through increasing awareness of one's self-talk, disputing and changing negative self-talk, and using cognitive rehearsal and thought stopping.

cohort study *See* longitudinal study.

computed tomography (CT) An imaging technique producing highly detailed cross-sectional body images from computerized processing of X-ray beam transmission through body tissues of differing density.

computer hardware The physical components of a computer (e.g., the monitor, disc drives, central processing unit, and keyboard).

conjunctival impression cytology Microscopic examination of the conjunctival epithelial cells used to detect early morphologic changes indicative of vitamin A deficiency.

consequences Events that follow and are causally linked to certain behaviors. Consequences reinforce, or reward, the behavior they follow, and they may be positive, negative, or neutral. When consequences are positive, behavior is more likely to be repeated. Behavior followed by negative consequences is less likely to be repeated.

Continuing Survey of Food Intakes by Individuals (CSFII) A nationally representative survey of individual dietary intake by Americans that was conducted periodically by the U.S. Department of Agriculture between 1985 and 1998.

coronary heart disease (CHD) A disease of the heart resulting from inadequate circulation of blood to local areas of the heart muscle. The disease is almost always a consequence of focal narrowing of the coronary arteries by atherosclerosis and is known as ischemic heart disease or coronary artery disease.

correlational study A research design in which the occurrence of one variable is compared with the occurrence of another variable within the same population. The study is useful for generating hypotheses regarding the associations between suspected risk factors and disease risk.

creatine A nitrogen-containing compound, 98% of which is found in muscle in the form of creatine phosphate. Creatine spontaneously dehydrates to form creatinine, which is then excreted unaltered in the urine.

creatinine The end product of creatine metabolism. Twenty-four-hour urinary creatinine excretion is used as an index of body muscle mass.

creatinine-height index (CHI) An index or a ratio sometimes used to assess body protein status. CHI = 24-hour urinary creatinine excretion ÷ expected creatinine excretion of a reference adult of the same sex and stature × 100.

cross-sectional survey A study design in which disease and various factors of interest are simultaneously examined in groups at a specific period of time.

CSFII Continuing Survey of Food Intakes by Individuals.

CT Computed tomography.

CV Coefficient of variation.

Daily Reference Value (DRV) A dietary reference value serving as a basis for the Daily Values. DRVs are for nutrients (e.g., total fat, cholesterol, total carbohydrate, and dietary fiber) for which no set of standards existed before passage of the Nutrition Labeling and Education Act of 1990.

Daily Value (DV) A dietary reference value appearing on the nutrition labels of foods regulated by the FDA and the USDA as part of the Nutrition Labeling and Education Act of 1990. It is derived from the Daily Reference Values (DRVs) and the Reference Daily Intakes (RDIs). The daily value on food labels shows the percent of the DRVs or RDIs that a serving of food provides.

deciliter (dL) A unit of volume in the metric system. One deciliter equals 10^{-1} liter, 1/10 of a liter, or 100 milliliters.

deficiency diseases Diseases caused by a lack of adequate dietary nutrients, vitamins, or minerals (e.g., rickets, pellagra, beriberi, xerophthalmia, and goiter).

densitometry Measurement of body density.

density *See* body density.

deuterium A radioactive hydrogen isotope having twice the mass of common light hydrogen atoms. Known as "heavy hydrogen."

deuterium oxide "Heavy water" composed of oxygen and deuterium (D_2O or ^2H_2O). Used in the determination of total body water.

DHHS United States Department of Health and Human Services.

diabetes mellitus A metabolic disorder characterized by inadequate insulin secretion by the pancreas or the inability of certain cells to use insulin and resulting in abnormally high serum glucose levels. Diabetes mellitus can be classified as type 1 diabetes, type 2 diabetes, or gestational diabetes mellitus (GDM).

dietary fiber Nondigestible carbohydrates and lignin that are naturally present in plant foods and that are consumed in their natural, intact state as part of an unrefined food.

Dietary Goals for the United States Seven dietary goals established by the U.S. Senate Select Committee on Nutrition and Human Needs in 1977 for improving the quality of the American diet.

Dietary Reference Intakes Reference values that are quantitative estimates of nutrient intakes to be used for planning and assessing diets for apparently healthy people in various life-stage and gender groups in the United States and Canada. The Dietary Reference Intakes include the Estimated Average Requirement, the Recommended Dietary Allowance, the Adequate Intake, and the Tolerable Upper Intake Level.

diet history An approach to assessing an individual's usual dietary intake over an extended period of time (e.g., past month or year). This typically involves Burke's four assessment steps: collecting general information about the subject's health habits, questioning the subject about his or her usual eating pattern, performing a "cross check" on the data given in step 2, and having the subject complete a 3-day food record.

dilution techniques An approach to indirectly measure total body water (TBW). A known concentration and volume of a tracer is given to a subject orally or parenterally, time is allowed for the tracer to equilibrate with the subject's body water, and the concentration of the tracer is analyzed in a sample of the subject's blood, urine, or saliva.

direct calorimetry Measurement of the body's heat output using an airtight, thermally insulated living chamber.

distal Away from the center of the body.

diurnal variations Cyclical changes occurring throughout the day.

dL Deciliter.

DPA Dual-photon absorptiometry.

DRV Daily Reference Value.

dual-energy X-ray absorptiometry (DXA) An approach for measuring bone mineral content in the appendicular skeleton, axial skeleton, or whole body using an X-ray source operating at two energy levels.

dual-photon absorptiometry (DPA) An approach for measuring bone mineral content using photons at two different energy levels derived from a radioisotopic source (gadolinium-153).

duplicate food collections A direct method of calculating nutrient intake in which subjects place an identical portion of all foods and beverages consumed during a specified period in collection containers. This is then chemically analyzed at a laboratory for nutrient content, which provides a potentially more accurate determination of actual nutrient intake; it is compared with calculations based on food composition data.

DV Daily Value.

DXA Dual-energy X-ray absorptiometry.

electrolyte An electrically charged particle (anion or cation), present in solution within the body, that is capable of conducting an electrical charge. Sodium, chloride, potassium, and bicarbonate are electrolytes commonly found in the body.

endemic In epidemiology, a disease or condition that persistently occurs at low to moderate levels over a relatively long period of time.

enrichment The addition of certain nutrients lost in food during processing according to some standard stipulated by law.

enteral nutrition The delivery of food or nutrients into the esophagus, stomach, or small intestine through tubes to improve nutritional status.

epidemic In epidemiology, a disease or condition that occurs at a higher rate than is normally expected based on past experience.

epidemiology The study of the distribution and determinants of disease and health outcomes in human populations in order to generate evidence that contributes to the prevention of disease and adverse health outcomes and the promotion of health.

erythrocyte Red blood cell, or RBC.

essential lipid The small amount of lipid (constituting about 1.5% to 3% of lean body weight), serving as a structural component of cell membranes and the nervous system, that is necessary for life.

Estimated Average Requirement The daily dietary intake level estimated to meet the nutrient requirement of 50% of healthy individuals in a particular life stage and gender group. One of four nutrient reference intakes included in the Dietary Reference Intakes.

estimated food record A method of recording individual food intake in which the amounts and types of all food and beverages are recorded for a specific period of time, usually ranging from 1 to 7 days. Portion sizes are estimated using household measures (e.g., cups, tablespoons, teaspoons), a ruler, or containers (e.g., coffee cups, bowls, glasses). Certain items (e.g., eggs, apples, 12-ounce cans of soda) are counted as units.

Estimated Energy Requirement The average dietary energy intake that is predicted to maintain energy balance in a healthy adult of a defined age, gender, weight, height, and level of physical activity, consistent with good health. In children and pregnant and lactating women, it includes the needs associated with the deposition of tissues or the secretion of milk consistent with good health.

etiology The cause of a disease or an abnormal condition.

euglycemia A condition in which the plasma glucose level is considered within normal limits.

false negative Nutrient intake misclassified as adequate when it is actually inadequate.

false positive Nutrient intake misclassified as inadequate when it is actually adequate.

fatty streak The initial step of atherosclerosis, usually beginning in childhood, in which lipids (primarily cholesterol and its esters) become deposited in macrophages and smooth muscle cells within the inner lining of large elastic and muscular arteries.

FDA Food and Drug Administration.

femtoliter (fL) A unit of volume in the metric system. One femtoliter equals 10^{-15} liter.

ferritin The combination of the protein apoferritin and iron that functions as the primary storage form for body iron. It is primarily found in the liver, spleen, and bone marrow.

ferritin model A model for assessing the prevalence of iron deficiency, requiring abnormal values for at least two of the following measurements: serum ferritin level, transferrin saturation, and erythrocyte protoporphyrin level.

fibrous plaque A collection of lipids within the arterial walls during adolescence and early adulthood, creating a projection into the channel, or lumen, of the artery, resulting in impaired blood flow and oxygen delivery to a tissue or an organ.

fL Femtoliter.

flag sign Alternating bands of depigmented and normal-colored hair produced by alternating periods of poor and relatively good nutritional status.

food balance sheet *See* balance sheet approach.

food exchange system A meal planning method, originally developed for the diabetic diet, that simplifies control of energy consumption, helps ensure adequate nutrient intake, and allows considerable variety in food selection.

food frequency questionnaire A questionnaire listing foods on which individuals indicate how often they consume each listed item during certain time intervals (daily, weekly, or monthly). Standard portion sizes are used and an estimate of nutrient intake is provided on the questionnaire. Sometimes referred to as the semi-quantitative food frequency or list-based diet history approach.

food inventory record An approach to household food consumption measurement in which total household food use is calculated by subtracting food on hand at the end of the survey period (ending inventory) from the sum of food on hand at the start of the survey period (beginning inventory) and food brought into the household during the survey.

food list-recall approach A method of measuring household food consumption in which an interviewer, using a detailed listing of foods, asks the respondent to recall the amount of food used by the household during the preceding week and the amount paid for purchased items. This approach has been used in the Nationwide Food Consumption Survey (NFCS).

food propensity questionnaire A questionnaire similar to a food frequency questionnaire that determines the probability that a person will consume a specific food or beverage on any given day over a designated time, usually the previous year.

fortification The addition of nutrients to food at a nutrient concentration greater than originally present and/or the addition of nutrients not initially existing in food.

four-compartment model A body composition model viewing the body as being composed of four chemical groups: water, protein, mineral, and fat.

Frankfort horizontal plane An imaginary plane intersecting the lowest point on the margin of the orbit (the bony socket of the eye) and the tragion (the notch above the tragus, the cartilaginous projection just anterior to the external opening of the ear). This plane should be horizontal with the head and in line with the spine.

Friedewald equation An equation that can be used to calculate the concentration of serum low-density lipoprotein cholesterol (LDL-C) when total cholesterol (TC), high-density lipoprotein cholesterol (HDL-C), and triglyceride (TG) are known. When solving for LDL-C the equation is: LDL-C = TC − HDL-C − (TG ÷ 5). It was named for William T. Friedewald, M.D. who developed it.

functional fiber Nondigestible carbohydrates that have beneficial physiological effects in humans but that have been isolated or extracted from foods and then added as an ingredient to food or taken as a dietary supplement.

g Abbreviation for gram.

generalized equations Regression equations for estimating body density or percent body fat from anthropometric measures that are applicable to population groups varying widely in adiposity and age.

globesity A term coined by the World Health Organization to describe the global epidemic of obesity.

glycated hemoglobin Hemoglobin that has glucose bound to it. Also referred to as hemoglobin A_{1C} or simply as an A1C test, it reflects average blood glucose levels during the past 8 to 12 weeks.

goiter Thyroid gland enlargement caused by dietary iodine deficiency.

gram A unit of mass in the metric system. One gram equals 10^{-3} kilogram, 1 pound equals 453.5924 grams, and 1 ounce equals 28.350 grams.

gynoid obesity Excess body fat that is predominantly within the hips and thighs, as opposed to within the abdomen and upper body. This is the usual pattern of female obesity.

HANES Health and Nutrition Examination Survey.

HDL High-density lipoprotein.

Healthy Eating Index An instrument developed by the U.S. Department of Agriculture to provide a single summary measure of overall dietary quality.

height-weight indices Various ratios or indices expressing body weight in terms of height. Among these are Quetelet's index and Benn's index.

hemoglobin The iron-containing protein pigment of red blood cells that carries oxygen to body cells. Blood hemoglobin levels can reflect iron status (e.g., abnormally low hemoglobin may mean anemia).

hemoglobin A$_{1C}$ *See* glycated hemoglobin.

HHANES Hispanic Health and Nutrition Examination Survey.

high-density lipoprotein (HDL) A serum lipoprotein synthesized by the liver and intestine that transports cholesterol within the bloodstream. As the serum level of HDL increases, risk of coronary artery disease decreases.

hydrostatic weighing Underwater weighing. The most widely used technique of determining whole-body density, based on Archimedes' principle.

hydroxyapatite Calcium and phosphate crystals providing rigidity to teeth and bones.

hyperlipidemia Excessively high levels of lipids in the blood.

hypermetabolism An increased rate of energy and protein metabolism accompanying trauma, infection, burns, or surgery.

hypertension Persistently elevated arterial blood pressure.

hypervitaminosis A An excessive consumption of vitamin A.

IDL Intermediate-density lipoproteins.

iliac crest The crest, or top, of the ilium (the largest of three bones making up the outer half of the pelvis). The crest is the bony spine located just below the waist. Used as an anatomic landmark in skinfold measurement sites.

impedance The opposition to an alternating current, composed of two elements: resistance and reactance.

imputed data Data used by compilers of food composition tables when certain nutrient data are unavailable. These data are obtained from similar foods or ingredients for which data are more complete.

incidence The number of new cases of a disease divided by the total number of persons at risk of the disease within a specific time period, usually one year. It indicates a person's risk or chances of developing the disease per year.

index of nutritional quality (INQ) A concept related to nutrient density that allows the quantity of a nutrient per 1000 kcal in a food, meal, or diet to be compared with a nutrient standard.

indirect colorimetry The determination of energy expenditure by measuring the body's oxygen consumption and carbon dioxide production.

infarction Death of tissue (necrosis) due to the upstream obstruction of the tissue's arterial blood supply. Infarction, which can occur in any organ, generally results from atherosclerosis. When it occurs in the heart, it is referred to as a myocardial infarction.

infectious disease Any disease caused by the invasion and multiplication of microorganisms, such as bacteria, fungi, or viruses.

infrared interactance When infrared light is projected through the skin, some of the energy is reflected from the skin and underlying tissues. Estimates of body composition are made by analyzing certain characteristics of this reflected energy.

INQ Index of nutritional quality.

intermediate-density lipoproteins (IDL) Lipoprotein particles created by the removal of triglycerides from VLDL. IDL is a midway product in the conversion of VLDL to LDL.

International Unit (IU) An amount defined by the International Conference for Unification of Formulae and used to express the quantity of certain substances.

International System of Units A system of measurement that is the most widely used internationally and that is almost universally used in science. It is abbreviated SI from the French term *Système International d'Unités*. It is derived and extended from the metric system; however, not all metric units of measurement are accepted as SI units.

intraindividual variability Change in an individual's nutrient intake from day to day.

in vivo neutron activation analysis *See* neutron activation analysis.

iron deficiency The depletion of body iron stores, corresponding to the second and third stages in the development of iron deficiency.

iron-deficiency anemia A low hemoglobin value found in association with iron deficiency. Theoretically, anemia corresponds to the third stage of iron deficiency.

iron overload An excessive accumulation of iron storage in tissues.

ischemia Impaired blood flow, causing oxygen-nutrition deprivation to associated tissues, resulting in pain (e.g., angina pectoris) or, if severe enough, tissue death, as in heart attack.

IU International Unit.

joule An SI unit of work or energy. The amount of work done by a force of 1 newton acting over the distance of 1 meter. One joule = 0.239 kcal. *See also* kilojoule.

kat/L The SI unit of enzyme activity. One katal per liter is the amount of enzyme necessary to catalyze a reaction at the rate of 1 mole of substrate per second per liter ($mol \cdot s-1 \cdot L-1$).

kcal Kilocalorie.

kg Kilogram.

kilocalorie (kcal) The amount of energy required to raise the temperature of 1 liter of water 1°C. A unit of heat equal to 1000 calories. Also known as a large calorie. One kcal equals 0.239 kilojoule.

kilogram (kg) A unit of mass in the metric system. One kilogram equals 1000 grams, or 2.2046 pounds.

kilojoule (kj) An SI unit of work or energy. A kilojoule equals 1000 joules. A kilojoule is equivalent to 4.18 kcal. *See also* joule.

kj Kilojoule.

kwashiorkor A protein deficiency, generally seen in children, characterized by edema, growth failure, and muscle wasting.

lapse A single or temporary recurrence of an unwanted habit or behavior that one has overcome or has turned from for a period of time.

LDL Low-density lipoprotein.

LDL receptors Molecules on the surface of plasma membranes of hepatic and peripheral cells that recognize and remove low-density lipoprotein from the blood.

leading question A question that contains an implicit or explicit suggestion about the expected desired answer.

life expectancy The average number of years of life remaining for a person of a given age and sex. In most countries, improvements in nutrition, public health, and medicine have resulted in more people, on average, living longer, thus increasing life expectancy.

lipoproteins Spherical macromolecular complexes of lipids (triglycerides, cholesterol, cholesterol esters, and phospholipids) and special proteins known as apoproteins that transport lipids from sites of absorption or synthesis to sites of storage or metabolism via the blood. They include chylomicrons, LDL, IDL, VLDL, and HDL.

list-based diet history *See* food frequency questionnaire.

longitudinal study Cohort study. A study design comparing future exposure to various factors in a group (cohort) of subjects in an attempt to determine how exposure with the factors relates to diseases that may develop.

low-density lipoprotein (LDL) A serum lipoprotein whose primary role is transporting cholesterol to the various cells of the body. LDL contains approximately 70% of the serum's total cholesterol, is considered the most atherogenic (atherosclerosis-producing) lipoprotein, and is the prime target of attempts to lower serum cholesterol. Low serum levels of LDL cholesterol are desirable.

μ The Greek letter mu, used as a prefix in such instances as μg (microgram) and μL (microliter), where it indicates 10^{-6}, or one-millionth.

m Meter.

magnetic resonance imaging (MRI) A technology allowing both imaging of the body and *in vivo* chemical analysis without radiation hazard to the subject.

malnutrition This can mean any nutrition disorder but usually refers to failing health caused by long-term nutritional inadequacies.

marasmic kwashiorkor A combination of chronic energy deficiency and chronic or acute protein deficiency.

marasmus Predominantly an energy (kilocalorie) deficiency presenting with significant loss of body weight, skeletal muscle, and adipose tissue mass, but with serum protein concentrations relatively intact.

MCV Mean corpuscular (red blood cell) volume.

MCV model A model for assessing the prevalence of iron deficiency that requires abnormal values for at least two of the following measurements: mean corpuscular volume, transferrin saturation, or erythrocyte protoporphyrin level.

mean A value calculated by summing all the observations in a sample and dividing the sum by the number of observations. Also referred to as the arithmetic mean or, simply, average. One of three measures of central tendency, along with median and mode.

median The observation that divides the distribution into equal halves, with 50% of the observations above and

50% of the observations below this point. Also known as the 50th percentile. One of the three measures of central tendency, along with mean and mode.

menopause The cessation of monthly menses.

meter (m) A unit of distance in the metric system. One meter equals 100 centimeters, 1000 millimeters, and 39.37 inches.

Metropolitan relative weight An individual's actual body weight divided by the midpoint value of weight range for a given height (obtained from a Metropolitan Life Insurance Company height-weight table) and then multiplied by 100. *See also* relative weight.

mg Milligram.

MI Myocardial infarction.

midaxillary line An imaginary line running vertically through the middle of the axilla, used as an anatomic landmark in skinfold measurements.

milligram (mg) A unit of mass in the metric system. 10^{-3} gram, or one-thousandth of a gram.

millimeter (mm) A unit of distance in the metric system. 10^{-3} meter, or 1/1000 of a meter.

millimole (mmol) 10^{-3} mole, or 1/1000 of a gram.

missing foods Foods eaten but not reported by participants of nutritional surveys.

mm Millimeter.

mmol Millimole.

mode The observation that occurs most frequently. One of the three measures of central tendency, along with mean and median.

modeling Observational learning, or imitation. A learning process in behavior modification in which observers learn new behaviors by watching the actions of a model.

morbidity Illness or sickness.

morphology The study of the shape and structure of organisms, organs, or parts.

mortality Death.

myocardial infarction (MI) Heart attack. The death of an area of heart tissue caused by blockage of the coronary artery feeding that area.

myocardium Heart muscle.

National Health and Nutrition Examination Survey (NHANES) A continuous, annual cross-sectional survey, conducted by the U.S. Department of Health and Human Services, that assesses food intake, height, weight, blood pressure, vitamin and mineral levels, and a number of other health parameters in a statistically selected group of Americans.

National Nutrition Monitoring System (NNMS) A congressionally mandated system in which the USDA and USDHHS are to work cooperatively in collecting data relating to health and nutritional status measurements, food composition measurements, dietary knowledge, attitude assessment, and surveillance of the food supply.

Nationwide Food Consumption Survey (NFCS) A periodic survey of food consumption at the household and individual levels, conducted by the USDA from 1977 to 1988.

NCEP National Cholesterol Education Program.

NCHS National Center for Health Statistics.

negative nitrogen balance A condition in which nitrogen loss from the body exceeds nitrogen intake. Negative nitrogen balance is often seen in the case of illness, trauma, burns, or recovery from major surgery.

negative reinforcer An unpleasant consequence of a behavior that maintains and strengthens the behavior by the negative reinforcer's being removed from the situation.

neutral questions Questions that allow a client to respond without pressure or direction from the interviewer.

neutron activation analysis A technology allowing in vivo measurement of the body's content of calcium, iodine, hydrogen, sodium, chloride, phosphorus, carbon, and other elements. A neutron beam is directed to the subject, and the response of various elements within the body allows estimation of the quantities of these elements.

NFCS Nationwide Food Consumption Survey.

NHANES National Health and Nutrition Examination Survey.

NHANES I The first National Health and Nutrition Examination Survey.

NHANES II The second National Health and Nutrition Examination Survey.

NHANES III The third National Health and Nutrition Examination Survey.

NHES National Health Examination Survey.

nitrogen balance A condition in which nitrogen losses from the body are equal to nitrogen intake. Nitrogen balance is the expected state of the healthy adult.

NLEA Nutrition Labeling and Education Act.

NMR Nuclear magnetic resonance.

nomogram A graphic device with several vertical scales allowing calculation of certain values when a straightedge is connected between two scales and the desired value is read from a third scale.

nonambulatory Unable to walk (ambulate).

nonquantitative food frequency questionnaire A food frequency questionnaire assessing frequency of food consumption but not the size of food servings.

nuclear magnetic resonance (NMR) Earlier name for magnetic resonance imaging (MRI).

nutrient database A compilation of data on the nutrient content of various foods. The database may exist in book form or as an electronic file accessible by computer.

nutrient density The nutritional composition of foods expressed in terms of nutrient quantity per 1000 kcal. If the quantity of nutrients per 1000 kcal is great enough, then the nutrient needs of a person will be met when his or her energy needs are met.

nutritional assessment The measurement of indicators of dietary status and nutrition-related health status of individuals or populations to identify the possible occurrence, nature, and extent of impaired nutritional status (ranging from deficiency to toxicity).

nutritional epidemiology The application of epidemiologic principles to the study of how diet and nutrition influence the occurrence of disease.

nutritional monitoring The assessment of dietary or nutritional status at intermittent times with the aim of detecting changes in the dietary or nutritional status of a population.

nutritional screening The process of identifying characteristics known to be associated with nutrition problems in order to pinpoint individuals who are malnourished or at risk for malnutrition.

nutritional surveillance Continuous assessment of nutritional status for the purpose of detecting changes in trend or distribution in order to initiate corrective measures.

Nutrition Labeling and Education Act (NLEA) A law passed by the U.S. Congress in 1990, mandating nutrition labeling for virtually all processed foods regulated by the U.S. Food and Drug Administration, authorizing appropriate health claims on food labels, and calling for activities to educate consumers about food labels.

obesity An excessive accumulation of body fat.

observational standards A dietary standard based on clinical observation, as opposed to scientific measurement of actual need.

olecranon process The bony projection of the distal ulna at the elbow. Used as an anatomic landmark in upper-arm anthropometric measurements.

open questions Questions providing individuals with considerable freedom in deciding the amount and type of information to give in answering an interviewer's questions.

osteopenia A condition in which bone mineral density is decreased but not to the point that a diagnosis of osteoporosis can be made. According to World Health Organization criteria, osteopenia occurs when the T-score is between −1.0 and −2.5.

osteoporosis A condition in which there is a marked decrease in bone mineral density and deterioration of bone microarchitecture, compromised bone strength, and an increased susceptibility to fracture and painful morbidity. According to World Health Organization criteria, osteoporosis occurs when the T-score is less than −2.5.

overnutrition The condition resulting from the excessive intake of foods in general or particular food components.

overweight Body weight in excess of a particular standard and sometimes used as an index of obesity.

parallax The apparent difference in the reading of a measurement scale (e.g., a skinfold caliper's needle) when viewed from various points not in a straight line with the eye.

parenteral nutrition The process of administering nutrients directly into veins to improve nutritional status.

pellagra A niacin deficiency syndrome characterized by inflamed mucous membranes, mental deterioration, diarrhea, and eruptions in skin areas exposed to light or injury.

PEM Protein-energy malnutrition.

percentiles Divisions of a distribution into equal, ordered subgroups of hundredths. The 50th percentile is the median. The 90th percentile, for example, is an observation whose value exceeds 90% of the set of observations and is exceeded by only 10%.

peripheral vascular disease Atherosclerotic changes within the aorta, iliac, and femoral arteries, affecting blood flow in the body's periphery.

pg Picograms.

phantom foods Foods not eaten but reported as having been eaten by participants of nutrition surveys.

picograms (pg) A unit of mass in the metric system. One picogram equals 10^{-12} gram, or one-trillionth of a gram.

plasma The liquid component of blood that has not clotted. An anticoagulant added to the glass tube used to draw blood from a subject's vein prevents clotting of the blood. This tube is then centrifuged, leaving the blood cells at the bottom of the tube and the plasma at the top. Unlike serum, plasma contains the clotting factors.

plethysmography *See* air displacement plethysmography.

population-specific equations Regression equations for estimating body density or percent body fat from anthropometric measures that can be applied only to population groups sharing certain features, such as sex, age, and adiposity.

positive nitrogen balance Nitrogen intake exceeds nitrogen loss from the body. This is commonly seen during growth, pregnancy, and recovery from trauma, surgery, or illness.

positive reinforcer Any consequence (reward) that maintains and strengthens behavior by its presence. (The positive reinforcer makes the behavior more likely to recur.)

postprandial After a meal.

power-type indices Indices such as Quetelet's index and Benn's index.

precision The difference in results when the same measurement is repeatedly performed on the same sample.

prediabetes A term used to represent impaired fasting glucose (IFG) or impaired glucose tolerance (IGT) based on the observation that most people have either IFG or IGT before they are diagnosed with type 2 diabetes.

prevalence The number of existing cases of a disease or condition divided by the total number of people in a given population at a designated time. It indicates the burden of a disease or how common it is.

propensity The probability that a person will consume a specific food or beverage on any given day over a designated time, usually the previous year.

protein-energy malnutrition (PEM) An inadequate consumption of protein and energy, resulting in a gradual body wasting and increased susceptibility to infection.

provisional tables Provisional data supplied by the United States Department of Agriculture for special nutrients or foods, such as dietary fiber, bakery foods, vitamin K, fatty acids, and sugar, that are often released years before more complete data are available.

proximal Toward the center of the body.

QCT Quantitative computed tomography.

quantitative computed tomography (QCT) An imaging technique consisting of an array of X-ray sources and radiation detectors aligned opposite each other. As the X-ray beams pass through the subject, they are weakened, or attenuated, by the body's tissues and eventually picked up by the detectors. Data from the detectors are then transmitted to a computer, which reconstructs the subject's cross-sectional anatomy, using mathematic equations adapted for computer processing.

quantitative food frequency questionnaire *See* semi-quantitative food frequency questionnaire.

quantitative ultrasound The transmission of high-frequency sound waves through bone to determine its fracture risk.

Quetelet's index Weight in kilograms divided by height in meters squared (kg/m^2). The most widely used weight-height or power-type index.

rational-emotive therapy (RET) A counseling approach based on the premise that emotional disturbances are a product of irrational thinking. RET holds that emotions are primarily the result of our beliefs, evaluations, interpretations, and reactions to life situations, which in turn determine our behavior. Behavior is altered by correcting the thought process using methods such as cognitive restructuring, language changing, cognitive rehearsal, and thought stopping.

RDA Recommended Dietary Allowance.

RDIs Reference Daily Intakes.

reality therapy A therapy based primarily on the work of psychiatrist William Glasser and his premise that every person's behavior is an attempt to fulfill his or her basic human needs (behavior driven completely from within). Emphasis is placed on individual responsibility for actions and client participation in decision making.

Recommended Dietary Allowance The average daily dietary intake level sufficient to meet the nutrient requirement of nearly all (97% to 98%) healthy individuals in a particular life stage or gender group. One of four nutrient reference intakes included in the Dietary Reference Intakes.

recumbent The position of lying down. Recumbent length, for example, is obtained with the subject lying down and is generally reserved for children younger than 24 months of age or for children between 24 and 36 months who cannot stand erect without assistance.

REE Resting energy expenditure.

reference amount The amount of a food typically consumed per eating occasion as determined by food consumption surveys and which is used when determining the serving size listed on that food's Nutrition Facts label. The serving size listed on the food's Nutrition Facts label is the amount in common household measures closest to the reference amount.

Reference Daily Intakes (RDIs) A set of dietary references that serves as the basis for the Daily Values and are based on the Recommended Dietary Allowances (RDAs) for essential vitamins and minerals and, in selected groups, protein. The RDIs replace the U.S. Recommended Daily Allowances (U.S. RDAs).

regression equations Equations developed by comparing a variety of anthropometric measures with measurements of body density (usually by hydrostatic weighing) to see which anthropometric measures are best at predicting body density. A statistical process called multiple-regression analysis is used to develop the equations.

relapse The resumption of an unwanted habit or behavior that one has, for a period of time, overcome or turned from.

relative weight A subject's actual body weight divided by the midpoint value of weight range for a given height and then multiplied by 100. *See also* Metropolitan relative weight.

reliability *See* reproducibility.

remodeling The dynamic process of skeletal change in which bones are constantly undergoing resorption and reformation.

reproducibility Also known as reliability. The ability of a method to yield the same measurement value on two or more different occasions, assuming that nothing has changed in the interim.

resting energy expenditure (REE) Also known as resting metabolic rate. This term is used for metabolic rate or energy expenditure in the awake, resting, and postabsorptive individual.

RET Rational-emotive therapy.

rickets A condition, especially found in infants and children, characterized by malformed bones, delayed fontanel closure, and muscle pain, due to a deficiency of vitamin D.

scurvy An ascorbic acid (vitamin C) deficiency disease characterized by anemia, spongy and bleeding gums, and capillary hemorrhages.

secular trend In epidemiology, changes in prevalence of a disease or condition over time.

self-contract An agreement an individual makes with himself or herself to help build commitment to behaviorial change.

semiquantitative food frequency questionnaire A food frequency questionnaire that assesses both frequency and portion size of food consumption. *See also* food frequency questionnaire.

sensitivity A test's ability to indicate an abnormality where there is one.

serum The liquid component of blood that has clotted. A plain glass tube is used to draw blood from a subject's vein, and after several minutes the blood clots. This tube is then centrifuged, leaving the blood cells at the bottom of the tube and the serum at the top. Unlike plasma, serum does not contain the clotting factors.

serum proteins Proteins present in serum (the liquid portion of clotted blood) that are often regarded as indicators of the body's visceral protein status (e.g., albumin).

shortfall nutrients Nutrients whose intakes are below recommended levels among a significant part of the population.

SI The abbreviation for the International System of Units, derived from the French term *Système International d'Unités*. *See* International System of Units.

signs Observations made by a qualified examiner during a physical examination.

single-photon absorptiometry (SPA) An approach for measuring bone mineral content using photons at a single energy level derived from a radioisotopic source (iodine-125).

skinfold thickness A double fold of skin that is measured with skinfold calipers at various body sites.

software program The entire set of programs, procedures, and related documentation associated with computer programs. The list of program commands that operate a particular program on the computer.

somatic protein Protein contained in the body's skeletal muscles.

SPA Single-photon absorptiometry.

specificity A test's ability to indicate normalcy where there is no abnormality.

stadiometer A device capable of measuring stature in children over 2 years of age and in adults. This measure is taken in a standing position.

standard deviation (SD) A measure of how much a frequency distribution varies from the mean.

stature Standing height.

stimulus control A behavior modification technique in which behavioral antecedents are recognized and modified or controlled to decrease the occurrence of negative behaviors and to increase the occurrence of positive behaviors.

stroke A blockage or rupture of a blood vessel supplying the brain, with resulting loss of consciousness, paralysis, or other symptoms.

stunting A decreased height-for-age. It is generally seen in long-term, mild to moderate protein-energy malnutrition.

Subjective Global Assessment A clinical approach to assessing the nutritional status of a patient using information gained from the patient's history and physical examination.

supine The position in which one is lying on his or her back.

surrogate source A source of information about a subject's behavior (e.g., dietary practices) from a source other than the subject. Typical surrogate sources include a spouse, child, close relative, and friend of the subject.

symptoms Disease manifestations that the patient is usually aware of and often complains of.

Système International d'Unités A French translation of International System of Units. *See* International System of Units.

TEF Thermal effect of food.

thermic effect of exercise Energy expenditure resulting from physical activity.

thermic effect of food (TEF) Also known as diet-induced thermogenesis or the specific dynamic action of food. TEF is the increased energy expenditure following food consumption or administration of parenteral or enteral nutrition caused by absorption and metabolism of food and nutrients.

TOBEC Total body electrical conductivity.

Tolerable Upper Intake Level The highest level of daily nutrient intake likely to pose no risk for adverse health effects for almost all apparently healthy individuals in the general population. As intake increases above this level, risk for adverse (toxic) effects increases. One of four nutrient reference intakes included in the Dietary Reference Intakes.

total body electrical conductivity (TOBEC) A method of assessing body composition in which a subject is placed in an electromagnetic field (EMF). Since electrolytes within the fat-free mass are capable of conducting electricity, the degree to which the EMF is disrupted is related to the amount of fat-free mass within the subject's body.

total fiber The sum of dietary fiber and functional fiber. *See* dietary fiber and functional fiber.

total water The total amount of water a person consumes which includes drinking water, water in other beverages, and water or moisture in food.

transferrin The form in which iron is transported within the blood.

tritium An isotope of hydrogen having three times the mass of ordinary hydrogen. It is commonly used as a tracer in the determination of total body water.

T-score A representation of the number of standard deviations above or below the mean value of a reference population. When used in evaluating bone mineral density (BMD), the T-score is the number of standard deviations above or below the mean BMD of the reference population, which is a large group of healthy young adults of the same sex. According to the World Health Organization, an adult can be diagnosed with osteoporosis if his or her bone mineral density corresponds to a T-score at or below −2.5.

24-hour recall A method of dietary recall in which a trained interviewer asks the subject to remember in detail all foods and beverages consumed during the past 24 hours. This information is recorded by the interviewer for later coding and analysis.

two-compartment model A body composition model that views the body as being composed of two compartments: fat mass and fat-free mass, or, according to an alternative approach, adipose tissue and lean body mass.

triglyceride A lipid composed of a glycerol molecule to which are attached three fatty acid molecules and the chemical form of most fat in food and in the body. Triglyceride is also found in the blood, primarily in very low-density lipoprotein particles and chylomicrons.

ulna The larger, inner bone of the forearm. Used as an anatomic landmark in arm anthropometry.

ultrasound A diagnostic method used for imaging internal organs and estimating the thickness of subcutaneous adipose tissue. High-frequency sound waves are transmitted into the body from a transducer (sound transmitter) applied to the skin surface. As ultrasound strikes the interface between two tissues differing in density (e.g., adipose tissue and muscle), some of it is reflected back and received by the transducer. Alterations between the signal as it is transmitted and received are used to image internal organs and to determine subcutaneous tissue thickness.

undernutrition A condition resulting from the inadequate intake of food in general or particular food components.

underwater weighing *See* hydrostatic weighing.

USDA United States Department of Agriculture.

USRDA U.S. Recommended Daily Allowances.

U.S. Recommended Daily Allowances (USRDA) A set of nutrition standards developed by the FDA for use in regulating the nutrition labeling of food. They were replaced by the Reference Daily Intakes.

validity The ability of an instrument to measure what it is intended to measure. Validating a method of measuring dietary intake, for example, involves comparing measurements of intake obtained by that method with intake measurements obtained by some other accepted approach.

very low-density lipoprotein (VLDL) A lipoprotein, present in blood, that is synthesized by the liver and primarily carries triglyceride to cells for storage and metabolism.

viscera Organs of the body (such as liver, kidneys, heart).

visceral protein Protein found in the body's organs or viscera, as well as that in the serum and in blood cells.

VLDL Very low-density lipoprotein.

waist circumference The distance around the horizontal plane through the abdomen at the level of the iliac crest of a standing subject. This measurement is used as an index of abdominal fat content.

wasting A decreased weight-for-age. It is generally seen in severe protein-energy malnutrition.

weighed food record A method of recording individual food intake in which the amounts and types of all food and beverages are recorded for a specific period of time, usually ranging from 1 to 7 days. Portion sizes are determined by accurate weighing.

weight-height indices *See* height-weight indices.

WIC Special Supplemental Nutrition Program for Women, Infants, and Children.

xerophthalmia An eye disease caused by vitamin A deficiency in which the conjunctiva and cornea dry and thicken, in part because of decreased mucus production. If not treated in earlier stages with vitamin A supplements, permanent damage may ensue, with softening of the cornea and subsequent blindness.

INDEX